NEUROBIOLOGY OF HEARING:
THE CENTRAL AUDITORY SYSTEM

Neurobiology of Hearing Series

Neurobiology of Hearing: The Cochlea, *edited by Richard A. Altschuler, Richard P. Bobbin, and Douglas W. Hoffman, 506 pp, 1986.*

Neurobiology of Hearing: The Central Auditory System, *edited by Richard A. Altschuler, Richard P. Bobbin, Ben M. Clopton, and Douglas W. Hoffman, 512 pp, 1991.*

Neurobiology of Hearing:
The Central Auditory System

Editors

Richard A. Altschuler, PH.D.
Associate Professor
Kresge Hearing Research Institute
Department of Otolaryngology and
Department of Anatomy and Cell Biology
University of Michigan
Ann Arbor, Michigan

Richard P. Bobbin, PH.D.
Professor
Department of Otorhinolaryngology and
Biocommunication
Kresge Hearing Research Laboratory of the South
Louisiana State University Medical Center
New Orleans, Louisiana

Ben M. Clopton, PH.D.
Associate Professor
Kresge Hearing Research Institute
Department of Otolaryngology
University of Michigan
Ann Arbor, Michigan

Douglas W. Hoffman, PH.D.
Associate Professor
Departments of Psychiatry and Pharmacology
Dartmouth Medical School
Hanover, New Hampshire

Raven Press 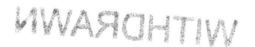 New York

Made in the United States of America

Library of Congress Cataloging-in-Publication Data

Neurobiology of hearing : the central auditory system / editors,
    Richard A. Altschuler . . . [et al.].
        p.   cm.
    Includes bibliographical references and index.
    ISBN 0-88167-806-6
    1. Auditory pathways. 2. Hearing. I. Altschuler, Richard A.
    [DNLM: 1. Auditory Pathways—physiology. 2. Brain Stem—
    physiology. 3. Hearing—physiology. 4. Neurobiology.
    WV 272 N4936]
    QP461.N42   1991
    612.8′5—dc20
    DNLM/DLC
    for Library of Congress   87-42836
                                                                    CIP

9 8 7 6 5 4 3 2 1

Contents

Contributing Authors

Richard A. Altschuler
Kresge Hearing Research Institute
Departments of Otolaryngology and Anatomy
*   and Cell Biology*
University of Michigan
1301 East Ann Street
Ann Arbor, Michigan 48109-0506

Jane A. Baran
Section of Otolaryngology and Audiology
Department of Surgery
Dartmouth-Hitchcock Medical Center
2 Maynard Street
Hanover, New Hampshire 03756
Department of Communication Disorders
University of Massachusetts
Amherst, Massachusetts

Carol C. Blackburn
The Center for Hearing Sciences
Department of Biomedical Engineering
The Johns Hopkins University
Traylor Building, Room 506
720 Rutland Avenue
Baltimore, Maryland 21205

John F. Brugge
Department of Neurophysiology
Waisman Center on Mental Retardation and
*   Human Development*
University of Wisconsin-Madison
Madison, Wisconsin 53706

David Caird
Zentrum der Physiologie
Theodor Stern Kai 7
6000 Frankfurt am Main
Federal Republic of Germany

Nell Beatty Cant
Department of Neurobiology
Duke University Medical School
Durham, North Carolina 27710

Donald M. Caspary
Department of Pharmacology
Southern Illinois University School of Medicine
P.O. Box 19230
Springfield, Illinois 62794-9230

Raymond H. Dye
The Parmly Hearing Institute
Loyola University of Chicago
6525 North Sheridan Road
Chicago, Illinois 60626

Carl L. Faingold
Department of Pharmacology
Southern Illinois University School of Medicine
P.O. Box 19230
Springfield, Illinois 62794-9230

Paul G. Finlayson
Department of Pharmacology
Southern Illinois University School of Medicine
P.O. Box 19230
Springfield, Illinois 62794-9230

Greta Gehlbach
Department of Pharmacology
Southern Illinois University School of Medicine
P.O. Box 19230
Springfield, Illinois 62794-9230

Robert H. Helfert
Kresge Hearing Research Institute
University of Michigan
1301 East Ann Street
Ann Arbor, Michigan 48109-0506

Don H. Johnson
Department of Electrical and Computer
*   Engineering*
Rice University
Houston, Texas 77001

J. M. Miller
Kresge Hearing Research Institute
University of Michigan
1301 East Ann Street
Ann Arbor, Michigan 48109-0506

David R. Moore
University Laboratory of Physiology
Parks Road
Oxford OX1 3PT, United Kingdom

Frank E. Musiek
Section of Otolaryngology and Audiology
Department of Surgery
Section of Neurology
Department of Medicine
Dartmouth-Hitchcock Medical Center
2 Maynard Street
Hanover, New Hampshire 03756

J. K. Niparko
Kresge Hearing Research Institute
University of Michigan
1301 East Ann Street
Ann Arbor, Michigan 48109-0506

Douglas L. Oliver
Department of Anatomy
The University of Connecticut Health Center
Farmington, Connecticut 06032

Dennis P. Phillips
Department of Psychology
Dalhousie University
Life Science Center
Halifax, Nova Scotia, Canada B3H 4J1

Richard A. Reale
Department of Neurophysiology
Waisman Center on Mental Retardation and
*   Human Development*
University of Wisconsin-Madison
Madison, Wisconsin 53706

William S. Rhode
Department of Neurophysiology
University of Wisconsin-Madison Medical
*   School*
273 Medical Sciences Building
1300 University Avenue
Madison, Wisconsin 53706

Murray B. Sachs
The Center for Hearing Sciences
Department of Biomedical Engineering
The Johns Hopkins University
Traylor Building, Room 506
720 Rutland Avenue
Baltimore, Maryland 21205

Amiram Shneiderman
Department of Anatomy
The University of Connecticut Health Center
Farmington, Connecticut 06032

Colleen R. Snead
Kresge Hearing Research Institute
University of Michigan
1301 East Ann Street
Ann Arbor, Michigan 48109-0506

Kevin M. Spangler
Department of Anatomy
Creighton University School of Medicine
Omaha, Nebraska 68178
(Currently at: Bowman Gray School of
*   Medicine*
Wake Forest University
Winston-Salem, North Carolina 27103)

Chiyeko Tsuchitani
Sensory Sciences Center
Graduate School of Biomedical Sciences
The University of Texas Health Sciences
*   Center*
6420 Lamar Fleming Avenue
Houston, Texas 77030

W. Bruce Warr
Center for Hearing Research
Boys Town National Research Hospital
555 North 30th Street
Omaha, Nebraska 68131

Robert J. Wenthold
Section on Neurochemistry
Laboratory of Molecular Otology
National Institute on Deafness and Other
*   Communication Disorders*
National Institutes of Health
Building 36, Room 5D08
Bethesda, Maryland 20892

Jeffery A. Winer
Division of Neurobiology, Room 289 LSA
Department of Molecular and Cell Biology
University of California
Berkeley, California 94720-2097

Donald Wong
Departments of Anatomy and Otolaryngology
*   and Head-Neck Surgery*
Indiana University School of Medicine
Medical Science Building, Room 204
635 Barnhill Drive
Indianapolis, Indiana 46202-5120

Xiaolin Xue
Kresge Hearing Research Institute
University of Michigan
1301 East Ann Street
Ann Arbor, Michigan 48109-0506

William A. Yost
The Parmly Hearing Institute
Loyola University of Chicago
6525 North Sheridan Road
Chicago, Illinois 60626

Preface

This second volume in the series, *Neurobiology of Hearing,* examines the central auditory system. As in the first volume on the cochlea, this book is designed to communicate recent advances at a level accessible to advanced students, researchers, physicians, and audiologists. It is intended for use as a current and comprehensive reference for background and review and as a text in courses in audiology, otolaryngology, neurobiology, and neurosciences programs. Each chapter incorporates background information necessary to understand the more advanced topics discussed in the chapter. The first two chapters provide an overview of the ascending and descending auditory pathways and subsequent chapters examine structure, physiology, pharmacology, and processing at the different levels of the central auditory system. Other chapters look more generally at neurotransmitters, sound localization, development, and plasticity as well as central auditory system audiological assessment and prosthetic stimulation. There have been significant increases in our understanding of the central auditory system, with parallel advances in our knowledge of neurotransmission, connections, processing, and assessment. This book gives the current concepts in the central auditory system function and, combined with the first volume, provides a thorough evaluation of the neurobiology of hearing.

The Editors

Acknowledgments

The editors would like to acknowledge support from the National Institute on Deafness and Other Communication Disorders, the National Science Foundation, and the Deafness Research Foundation.

NEUROBIOLOGY OF HEARING:
THE CENTRAL AUDITORY SYSTEM

Neurobiology of Hearing: The Central Auditory System, edited by R. A. Altschuler et al.
Raven Press, Ltd., New York © 1991.

1

The Ascending Auditory Pathways

Robert H. Helfert, Colleen R. Snead, and Richard A. Altschuler

Kresge Hearing Research Institute, University of Michigan, Ann Arbor, Michigan 48109

Considerable knowledge has been gained in recent years with regard to the structure and function of the nuclei composing the central auditory system, including their connectional and synaptic relationships. However, our understanding of the processing of auditory information beyond the organ of Corti remains in its infancy. This is due in part to our reliance on overly simplified circuit diagrams to describe the patterns of connections and relationships among the nuclei of the central auditory system and to attempt to accurately predict their function. We know now that the pathways from the cochlea to the auditory cortex are especially complex and that this elaborate organization must reflect the advanced level of auditory processing that occurs beneath the cerebral hemispheres. The ascending auditory system is comprised of several distinct parallel pathways, each involving multiple nuclei containing a variety of neuronal types and transmitters, the convergence and divergence of intrinsic and extrinsic circuits, monaural and/or binaural processing, and the crossing of a large percentage of the auditory information at several loci in the brainstem.

This chapter attempts to provide a current overview of the ascending auditory pathways, with emphasis placed on the neural connections along these pathways and, wherever possible, the putative neurotransmitters that might be associated with them. Details on the auditory midbrain and forebrain are given in the other chapters and are discussed only briefly here.

To date, the animal model most commonly used in auditory tract-tracing studies has been the cat, while much of the transmitter-related research used rodent models, such as the chinchilla, gerbil, guinea pig, and rat. Thus, if not mentioned otherwise, the neural connections and transmitter research described herein are based on cat and rodent studies, respectively.

SPIRAL GANGLION

The auditory nerve comprises first order neurons linking the sensory hair cells of the cochlea to the brainstem. It is the first major site of divergence in the auditory system, for every afferent fiber branches within the cochlear nucleus (CN) to form an obligatory synapse in each of its three major subdivisions (for reviews, see refs. 90,97). The auditory nerve contains axons from both type I and type II spiral ganglion cells, so named because their perikarya are located in the spiral ganglion of the cochlea. The type I cells compose the vast majority (90%–95%) of the spiral ganglion cell population. They are large, bipolar neurons. Their myelinated somata contain large, round nuclei, prominent nucleoli, and an abundance of rough endoplasmic reticulum. The remainder of the spiral ganglion neurons, type II cells, are smaller, pseudo-monopolar or bipolar (depending on the species), contain an abundance of neurofilaments, and possess a few loose layers of myelin around their somata. Several detailed reviews of the spiral ganglion cell types have been published (66,122,131, 143).

Type I spiral ganglion cells receive afferent input from inner hair cells (IHC) on the endings of their peripheral neurites, the so-called inner radial fibers. The output of the IHC is highly divergent, as each typically provides input to roughly 20 type I cells (84,153). In most species, the synapses between an IHC and type I cell are characterized by asymmetrical paramembranous densities, presynaptic bodies, and narrow synaptic clefts (14,84,122,140,149,154). All afferent contacts in the cat are below the level of the IHC nucleus, with twice as many located on the side of the IHC nearest the modiolus as on the opposite (pillar) side (84). The fibers that receive innervation from the pillar side of the IHC are usually larger than those on the modiolar side and contain more mitochondria (84). The differences in fiber size and number of mitochondria may be related to the spontaneous activity of the neuron. In the cat, high, medium, and low spontaneous rate (SR) fibers innervate a single IHC (85). The low SR fibers, which have the thinnest peripheral endings, are found on the modiolar side of the IHC, and the high SR fibers, which have the largest endings, are more frequently located on the pillar side. The characteristic frequency (CF) of a type I spiral ganglion cell correlates with the location along the organ of Corti of the IHC it contacts, i.e., spiral ganglion cells with the lowest CFs are found in the apical region of the cochlea, while those with the highest CFs are found in the base (72,86). The threshold of a single neuron at its CF corresponds to its spontaneous activity, with lower thresholds found for fibers with higher spontaneous rates, and vice versa (87).

Type II spiral ganglion cells receive convergent afferent input from outer hair cells. In the cat, the small type II peripheral fiber travels a small distance in the inner spiral bundle toward the base of the cochlea. After crossing the tunnel of Corti, it branches extensively to contact 5 to 28 outer hair cells (OHC) (17). Also in the cat, type II peripheral fiber lengths, diameters, and branching increase from the base of the cochlea to the apex (147). The type II peripheral endings are small and bouton-like, containing few mitochondria in a dense, granular matrix (148). Little is known about the physiological response properties and function of type II cells. One study produced a single recording from a labeled type II unit (128). This "silent" unit produced no spontaneous activity and was unresponsive to acoustic stimulation. However, many more recordings need to be made from documented type II spiral ganglion cells before any definitive hypothesis can be advanced regarding their function.

The axons of type I and type II spiral ganglion cells project centrally in the auditory nerve as a spiraling bundle. This bundle is organized tonotopically in that the center contains axons from spiral ganglion cells innervating the cochlear apex, while the periphery of the bundle possesses axons from spiral ganglion cells innervating the base (10,141). The nerve emerges from the internal acoustic meatus and enters the ipsilateral CN where each axon bifurcates to form ascending and descending branches (Fig. 1) (for reviews on the branching patterns of the auditory nerve, see refs. 90,97). The ascending branches curve laterally and dorsally as they pass toward the rostral end of the ventral CN (VCN). The descending branches course caudally through the VCN toward its posterior tip, where the fascicles of fibers then converge and continue into the dorsal CN (DCN). Along their courses through the VCN both branches give off regularly spaced axon collaterals. In the DCN, individual fascicles of axons turn toward the surface of the nucleus and terminate almost entirely in the central region of

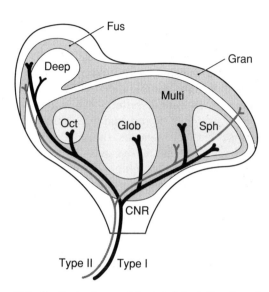

FIG. 1. Projections of type I (*black lines*) and type II (*gray lines*) spiral ganglion cell axons. CNR, cochlear nerve root; Deep, deep layer of the dorsal cochlear nucleus; Fus, fusiform cells; Glob, globular cells; Gran, granule cells; Multi, multipolar cells; Oct, octopus cells; Sph, spherical cells.

the DCN, with very few fibers reaching the fusiform cell or molecular layers (97). In the basal turns of rodent cochleae, the thin axons of type II neurons generally follow the pattern of type I fibers (17,18). However, unlike type I fibers, most type II fibers terminate in regions of the nuclei containing high densities of granule cells (Fig. 1).

As the auditory nerve bifurcates in the cochlear nerve root, the fibers maintain their topographic arrangement, projecting in a tonotopic manner to each subdivision of the nucleus. The fibers from the apical cochlea bifurcate ventrolaterally, near the point of entry of the nerve, while the most basal fibers bifurcate at the dorsomedial tip of the nerve root (38,83,109,143,166). Therefore, the ventral portion of each subdivision receives apical input and responds best to low-frequency stimulation, while the dorsal areas receive basal cochlear input and have high CFs (15,81). In the ante-

rior and posterior subdivisions of the VCN (AVCN and PVCN), the fibers from a specific frequency region of the cochlea spread to form oblique isofrequency planes across the nuclei. Although tonotopic representation is maintained in the DCN as well, the orientation of the isofrequency planes varies with species (97). Recent studies in the cat indicate that this tonotopic arrangement may be more complex. Spiral ganglion cells located closest to the scala tympani project to the lateral portion of the VCN isofrequency laminae and those nearest scala vestibuli to the medial portion, giving a vertical (scala tympani to scala vestibuli) dimension to the spiral ganglion representation in the organ of Corti (81).

There is considerable evidence that suggests that excitatory amino acids such as glutamate and/or aspartate may play an important role as neurotransmitter in type I spiral ganglion cells (for reviews, see refs. 28,46,171 and Chapter 11, *this volume*). However, no neurotransmitter has been identified conclusively in the auditory nerve. In the case of type II spiral ganglion cells, a transmitter candidate has yet to be assigned.

COCHLEAR NUCLEUS

The CN is the site of an obligatory synapse for all fibers of the auditory nerve. As such, it represents the first location in the central nervous system to process and relay acoustic information from the periphery. It is a site of divergence in that the auditory nerve branches to innervate the three subdivisions of the CN. Within each division, there is some convergence of several fibers innervating a single cell, and divergence as the collaterals innervate multiple cell types. The subdivisions of the CN contain a variety of cell types, most of which receive direct input from the auditory nerve. Thorough descriptions of these cell types can be found in several reviews (27,28,97).

Cell Types of the Cochlear Nuclei

Four major classes of projection neurons are found exclusively in the VCN: spherical bushy cells, globular bushy cells, octopus cells, and multipolar/stellate cells. Bushy cells, named for their appearance in Golgi preparations, are characterized by round cell bodies with tufted dendritic arbors. Spherical bushy cells are located in the AVCN. They lie between nerve fascicles and cluster in small groups with interlocking dendritic arbors. Spherical cell perikarya exhibit a ventral-to-dorsal gradation in size, with the largest located most ventrally in the cat (114) and several rodents (52,167,168). Large endbulb-type synaptic endings from one or more type I fibers contact each spherical cell perikaryon (16,52, 89). Spherical cells also receive noncochlear input via synaptic terminals that are thought to contain inhibitory neurotransmitters such as gamma-aminobutyric acid (GABA) and glycine, which is the case as well for the other principal cell types in the CN (111,172,173). Globular bushy cells are located within and adjacent to the nerve root and are basically similar to the spherical cells, with minor differences in somal shape and dendritic organization (97). They receive endbulb-type endings from the auditory nerve smaller than those contacting the spherical cells (38,39,89) and project to differ targets in the superior olivary complex (SOC). Because of the strong influence of their primary afferent input, the response patterns of both spherical and globular cells are "primary-like," which reflect their tight temporal coupling to the auditory nerve (73,125,180). This coupling may produce timing information essential for the encoding of cues for sound localization (30). Octopus cells are located in the posterior tip of the VCN and along the intermediate acoustic stria (97). These cells possess thick dendrites that arise from one side of the perikaryon, much like the arms of an octopus. The dendrites cross the descending branch of the CN axons. Most of the primary input to the octopus cells is from long, thin collaterals of the descending branch that run parallel to their dendrites and cover the soma and proximal dendrites with bouton-type endings (38,52,69,115). Their broad tuning reflects the wide frequency range of inputs, and the "onset" response pattern suggests that, along with the excitatory input, the octopus cells receive considerable inhibitory input (125, 135). Multipolar/stellate cells, found scattered throughout the VCN, vary in size and have long dendrites that extend across multiple isofrequency laminae. They receive input from long collaterals of the auditory nerve axons via scattered small bouton endings terminating mostly on their dendrites (38,39,89). The "chopper" response patterns of multipolar/stellate cells are, perhaps, manifested by a summation of input in time and space consistent with this morphology (125,135).

There are five major cell types unique to the DCN: fusiform, fan, radiate, cartwheel, and small stellate cells. Each is distributed in one or more of the three morphologically defined DCN layers. These layers are characteristic in the DCN of the nonprimate models studied and are commonly named molecular, fusiform cell, and deep layers. Fusiform cells, located in the middle (fusiform cell) layer, have two distinct dendritic arbors extending perpendicular to the surface of the DCN. The apical dendrites receive input from fibers in the outer (molecular) layer, while the soma and basal dendrites receive input from the auditory nerve in a restricted frequency lamina (11,126,175). Their complex "pauser" or "build-up" response patterns reflect an interaction between excitatory and inhibitory inputs (for review, see ref. 28). Fan cells (also known as corn cells) are medium-sized neurons scattered throughout the deep DCN, lying either orthogonal, parallel, or oblique to the surface and isofrequency planes of the nucleus. Their spiny dendrites ramify within the central region with few entering the granular layer and none beyond to the molecular layer. There is no evidence of direct auditory nerve input to the fan cells. Radiate neurons are also located in the deep DCN and are similar in appearance to the larger multipolar/ stellate cells in the VCN. Their long dendrites span wide areas of the nucleus and terminate before reaching the molecular layer. It is likely that these dendrites receive major input from the auditory nerve (97). Cartwheel neurons, with dendrites radiating from their somata in spoke-like patterns, are located in the molecular layer as well as in the fusiform cell layer near its boundary with the molecular layer. Cartwheel neurons receive major input from granule cells via axodendritic synapses (178,179). Small stellate cells possess thin dendrites and, like cartwheel neurons, are located in the fusiform cell and molecular layers and receive input from granule cells (described below). They appear to lack any direct input from the cochlear nerve (178,179). In some species, small stellate cells are also interconnected by dendrodendritic and dendrosomatic gap junctions (178).

Several cell types can be identified in both the VCN and DCN, such as giant cells and granule cells. In addition, depending on the species, there may be a heterogeneous population of small cell types in both divisions. These would include the Golgi cells (108) and a type in the guinea pig that is similar in appearance to small stellate cells (97). Giant neurons are present, in small numbers, in the deep DCN and are scattered throughout the VCN. Based on morphological criteria, they may actually comprise several subtypes (71). Giant cells are present in large numbers in the cat (114) and in smaller numbers in rodents and primates, including humans (52,53,99,168). Typically, their large dendrites penetrate even the granule cell layer of the VCN and the molecular layer of the DCN. Recordings from giant cells show unusually large frequency and dynamic ranges that reflect this enormous dendritic span (126). Gran-

ule cells consist of very small, spherical somata with short, thin dendrites. They form a layer covering the DCN and VCN, their long axons (often referred to as parallel fibers) compose most of the molecular layer in the DCN. There are scattered granule cells in the central region of the DCN as well. While most granule cells lie outside the main regions of auditory nerve input, recent evidence suggests that they may receive input from the type II spiral ganglion cells (18).

Projections of the Cochlear Nuclei

There are two principal, ascending pathways emanating from the CNs (Fig. 2). The first is a bilateral projection from the VCN to the nuclei of the SOC, and the second are projections from both the DCN and VCN to the contralateral inferior colliculus (IC) and nuclei of the lateral lemniscus (LL). In addition to the ascending pathways, there are several intrinsic projections that connect CN subdivisions as well as projections that cross over to the contralateral CN.

The binaural pathway consists of three projections (see review in ref. 164 and Chapter 5, *this volume*). The cell types from which these projections arise are similar in that they receive massive, direct input from the auditory nerve and, in turn, conduct excitatory output along large-caliber, fast-conducting axons. The spherical bushy cells provide ascending, tonotopic input to the lateral superior olive (LSO) ipsilaterally and to the medial superior olive (MSO) bilaterally. The globular bushy cells provide the same type of input to the contralateral medial nucleus of the trapezoid body (MNTB) via large calyceal endings on the principal cells, the contralateral dorsomedial periolivary nucleus (DMPO) and to the ipsilateral lateral nucleus of the trapezoid body (LNTB). The octopus cells project mostly via the intermediate acoustic stria to innervate the caudal and dorsal periolivary cell groups bilaterally (with

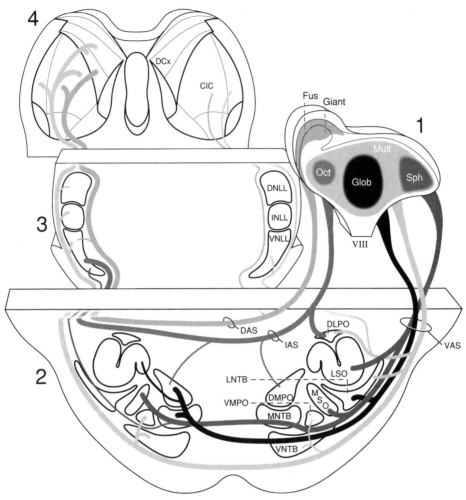

FIG. 2. Extrinsic projections from the cochlear nucleus. The lines originate from specific regions in the cochlear nucleus (**1**) and terminate in the superior olivary complex (**2**), the nuclei of the lateral lemniscus (**3**), and the inferior colliculus (**4**). *Thick, medium,* and *thin lines* indicate major, moderate, and minor projections, respectively. 1: Fus, fusiform cells; Giant, giant cells; Glob, globular cells; Mult, multipolar cells; Oct, octopus cells; Sph, spherical cells; VIII, cochlear nerve root. 2: DAS, dorsal acoustic stria; DLPO, dorsolateral periolivary nucleus; DMPO, dorsomedial periolivary nucleus; LSO, lateral superior olive; LNTB, lateral nucleus of the trapezoid body; MNTB, medial nucleus of the trapezoid body; MSO, medial superior olive; VMPO, ventromedial periolivary nucleus; VAS, ventral acoustic stria; VNTB, ventral nucleus of the trapezoid body. 3: DNLL, dorsal nucleus of the lateral lemniscus; INLL, intermediate nucleus of the lateral lemniscus; VNLL, ventral nucleus of the lateral lemniscus. 4: CIC, central nucleus of the inferior colliculus; DCx, dorsal cortex.

greater emphasis to the ipsilateral nuclei) and to the contralateral ventral nucleus of the lateral lemniscus (VNLL).

The heavy CN projections to both the contralateral IC and lemniscal nuclei arise from multipolar/stellate cells in the VCN, and giant cells and fusiform cells in the DCN. The multipolar/stellate cells are the only neurons in the VCN to project as far rostrally as the IC (24,164). These neurons, which are found in all divisions of the VCN, innervate periolivary nuclei (PON) bilaterally, particularly those surrounding the LSO. They then proceed via the contralateral LL, collateralize in the VNLL, and continue on to the central nucleus of the IC, where they terminate tonotopically (1,137, 164). There are also minor projections to the ipsilateral VNLL and IC, and the contralateral DNLL (43). The projections to the SOC may function as a component of a feedback loop, as virtually all of the periolivary groups they innervate project back to the CN (for a discussion of these loops, see Chapter 2, *this volume*). Most of the axons from the fusiform cells and giant cells of the DCN bypass the SOC, cross via the dorsal acoustic stria, and project tonotopically to the central nucleus and external cortex of the contralateral IC (136,137,161, 164). Fusiform and giant cells also send a minor projection to the ipsilateral IC (21, 110). As these fibers pass through the LL, they give off collaterals to the contralateral VNLL (43,176).

There are cells in both the VCN and DCN that are excited or inhibited by contralateral acoustic stimulation (91,92,120, 121). These responses are likely to be mediated, at least in part, by projections originating from the contralateral CN. Thus, the possibility exists that many cells in the CN receive binaural input. Large and medium-sized multipolar cells in the VCN and giant cells in the DCN project to the contralateral VCN and DCN (26,146,170). The cell types receiving this input appear to be the spherical bushy cells and octopus cells, as well as other cells in the PVCN and DCN (26). Immunocytochemical studies suggest that the pathway connecting the two CNs may in part be glycinergic (170), which concurs with the findings that inhibition in VCN occurs with contralateral acoustic stimulation (91,120). In the DCN, this input appears to contact fusiform cells and/or small cells in the fusiform cell layer as well as elements in the superficial layer, including apical dendrites of fusiform cells or cartwheel cells (26). While these direct and indirect pathways from the contralateral CN may play a role in enhancing intensity or timing differences at the level of the CN, their functional significance is only speculative at this time. In addition to the CN-to-CN projections, one must also consider the more substantial descending inputs to the CN from the SOC and IC (1,177), which are detailed in Chapter 2 of this volume.

Recently, several investigators have demonstrated the presence of intrinsic CN projections. Horseradish peroxidase (HRP) studies reveal that the DCN receives spatially restricted, tonotopic projections from large, multipolar/stellate cells and octopus cells in the PVCN, and more widely distributed, less tonotopic projections from multipolar cells, globular cells, and small spherical cells in the AVCN (2,146,151). The PVCN receives strong, tonotopic input from the DCN and substantial nontonotopic input from the caudal AVCN and within the PVCN itself (151). The AVCN receives substantial input from the ipsilateral DCN, limited input intrinsically, and none from the ipsilateral PVCN (90,151, 175). The cell types from which these internal projections arise have not been identified conclusively, with one possible exception being the fan cell. Fan cells appear to be the source of the tonotopically organized DCN projection to the AVCN (90,175). It is unlikely that cartwheel and fan cells project outside the CN complex, thus they are probably local circuit neurons. They possess short axons that project to restricted areas, and because cartwheel and fan cells are immunoreactive for inhibitory amino acid transmitters (4,68), they are likely to suppress the activity of their target neurons. The granule cells and small stellate cells, on the other hand, span the entire CN complex and may be involved in the longer intrinsic circuits. These internal circuits may be of minor importance in higher primates because granule cells, small stellate cells, and cartwheel cells are either very limited in number or vestigial in these animals (97).

SUPERIOR OLIVARY COMPLEX

The SOC is a major binaural processing center. A major function of the ascending component of the SOC is devoted to localizing sound along the azimuth. Its principal nuclei appear ideally suited to the task of processing cues for binaural sound localization, such as interaural time, phase, and intensity differences. The SOC typically contains three principal nuclei: the LSO, MSO, and MNTB. These nuclei are surrounded by several smaller, more diffuse nuclei, collectively termed PON. They are usually named according to their location in the SOC (e.g., Fig. 3). The PON comprise heterogeneous populations of neurons of great structural, physiological, and neurochemical diversity, possess complex patterns of neural connectivity, and contain elements of both the ascending and descending auditory pathways. The major projections of the SOC are illustrated in Fig. 4.

Medial Superior Olive

When viewed in transverse sections, the MSO consists of a central cell band in which the vast majority of neurons are stacked one atop the other with their dendrites extending laterally and medially. These neurons are either bipolar or multipolar (75,145). The central cell band is surrounded by smaller numbers of marginal neurons that lie beneath the myelinated axon envelope of the MSO orthogonal to the central cell band neurons. While the MSO responds to almost the entire range of frequencies detectable by a species, its tonotopic organization is biased toward low frequencies. Units responding to the lowest frequencies are located dorsally in the MSO and the highest frequency units are found ventrally (48,50,51).

The MSO plays an important role in sound localization by detecting interaural

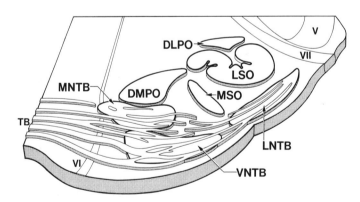

FIG. 3. Superior olivary complex (SOC). Illustration of the guinea pig SOC as it appears in transverse sections at the level of the lateral superior olive. DLPO, dorsolateral periolivary nucleus; DMPO, dorsomedial periolivary nucleus; LSO, lateral superior olive; LNTB, lateral nucleus of the trapezoid body; MNTB, medial nucleus of the trapezoid body; MSO, medial superior olive; TB, trapezoid body (ventral acoustic stria); VNTB, ventral nucleus of the trapezoid body; V, tract of the spinal trigeminal nucleus; VI, abducens nerve tract; VII, facial nerve tract. Not shown are the anterolateral periolivary nucleus (located rostral or rostrolateral to the LSO) and the posterior periolivary nucleus (located caudal to the LSO).

time, phase, and intensity differences (41, 48–51,107,181). Axons providing input to the MSO enter the nucleus from both the lateral and medial sides to produce paired rostrocaudally oriented sheets of terminal arborizations (145,155). The synaptic relation of these terminal sheets to most of the central cell band neurons is such that the lateral dendrites receive input primarily from spherical cells in the ipsilateral AVCN, while their medial dendrites are contacted by a similar number of terminals from the same cell type and region in the contralateral CN (155,163). Marginal neurons in the lateral pole of the MSO receive principal input from the ipsilateral AVCN and those located in the medial pole, from the contralateral AVCN (58). The presynaptic terminals from spherical cells contain round vesicles and multiple sites of synaptic membrane specialization (75,88,118,145), and probably employ an excitant amino acid as their neurotransmitter (see Chapter 9). Indeed, the bilateral AVCN input to the MSO is excitatory and evokes maximal facilitation from most central cell band units when the excitatory inputs arrive simultaneously (48–51).

Many MSO units are also inhibited if the inputs arrive out of phase (48–51). Under this circumstance, inhibition can be induced from either side, depending on the sequence in which the binaural stimuli are presented and/or their relative intensities (182). The neuronal circuitry responsible for both ipsilateral and contralateral inhibition of MSO neurons is proposed in Chapter 5. To summarize briefly, inhibition of MSO units may be mediated by neurons located in the ipsilateral LNTB and MNTB, which receive inputs from globular cells in the ipsilateral and contralateral VCNs, respectively. The LNTB and MNTB contain neurons that are immunoreactive for glycine (60). Thus, these neurons are likely sources of the flattened-pleomorphic vesicle synaptic terminals observed contacting MSO perikarya and proximal dendrites

(75,88,118,145) and probably contain glycine as an inhibitory neurotransmitter (59, 60).

Minor inhibitory input to the MSO may be provided by GABAergic neurons. Small numbers of GABA-immunoreactive synaptic terminals have been observed contacting the perikarya and dendrites of MSO neurons (60). They contain oval-pleomorphic synaptic vesicles and scattered dense core vesicles. Synaptic terminals matching this description and distribution had been previously described in the MSO (88,118, 145). Yet to be revealed are the origin(s) of the presumptive GABAergic input to the MSO and the role GABA plays in the processing of auditory information in this nucleus.

The vast majority of both central cell band and marginal neurons project to the ipsilateral central nucleus of the IC (1,21, 32,37,62,110,134,155) and to the nuclei of the LL, in particular the DNLL (43,62) (Fig. 4). However, the MSO also sends a minor projection to the contralateral IC (21,62,110). Preliminary studies indicate that most MSO neurons exhibit elevated immunoreactivity for aspartate and glutamate (55), while a very small number are intensely GABA immunoreactive, and none exhibits glycine immunoreactivity above background levels (60). In addition, biochemical studies indicate that glutamate and aspartate levels are elevated in the principal SOC nuclei, with glutamate concentrations greatest in the MSO (47). These findings suggest that an excitant amino acid transmitter is used by most MSO neurons and, therefore, that the major pathway originating from the MSO may be excitatory. The targets of the small number of GABA immunoreactive MSO neurons is unknown at this time. They might function within the nucleus as interneurons or they may project outside the MSO. It is conceivable that these neurons could correspond to the equally small number of MSO neurons whose axons cross over to the contralateral

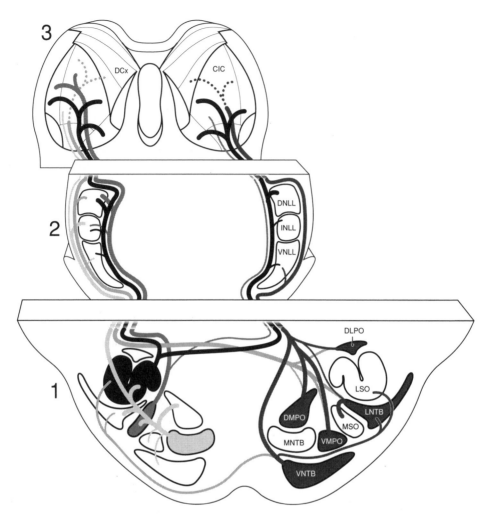

FIG. 4. Ascending projections from the nuclei of the superior olivary complex (SOC). The lines originate from the principal SOC nuclei (**1,** left) and from the periolivary nuclei (**1,** right) and terminate in the SOC, the nuclei of the lateral lemniscus (**2**), and the inferior colliculus (**3**). *Thick, medium,* and *thin lines* indicate major, moderate, and minor projections, respectively. *Solid lines* represent focused projections that terminate in a topographic or tonotopic manner; *broken lines* depict projections that terminate diffusely in their target. 1: DLPO, dorsolateral periolivary nucleus; DMPO, dorsomedial periolivary nucleus; LSO, lateral superior olive; LNTB, lateral nucleus of the trapezoid body; MNTB, medial nucleus of the trapezoid body; MSO, medial superior olive; VMPO, ventromedial periolivary nucleus; VNTB, ventral nucleus of the trapezoid body. 2: DNLL, dorsal nucleus of the lateral lemniscus; INLL, intermediate nucleus of the lateral lemniscus; VNLL, ventral nucleus of the lateral lemniscus. 3: CIC, central nucleus of the inferior colliculus; DCx, dorsal cortex. Not illustrated are projections from the anterolateral and posterior periolivary nuclei.

side, providing the contralateral IC with crossed inhibitory input. The functional significance of such a pathway, should it exist, is unknown.

Medial Nucleus of the Trapezoid Body

The MNTB is named for its position and location in the trapezoid body (ventral acoustic stria). Its neurons reside among the fascicles of trapezoid body axons passing through the nucleus. Of the three types of MNTB neurons described in the cat (106), principal neurons are, by far, the most prevalent type. This is likely to be the case as well for most, if not all, of the other mammalian species. Principal neurons are globular or oval shaped and possess two to four slender dendrites. They correspond to the equally large number of contralaterally driven, monaural units recorded in the MNTB (50,51). The remaining cell types, elongate neurons and stellate neurons, are encountered less frequently. The MNTB is tonotopically organized, with units responding to the highest frequencies located ventromedially and the lowest frequency units found dorsolaterally (12,50,51,152). Principal cells receive excitatory input from the globular cells of the contralateral VCN (54,160,161,163,164) via secure synaptic calyces (of Held) containing spherical vesicles and multiple synaptic contacts (67,82). In addition, collateral fibers arising either from the calyciferous axon, or from the calyx itself, ramify extensively within the cat MNTB (106,123). The collaterals probably terminate on somata and proximal dendrites of principal neurons other than the one contacted by the parent calyx (106). MNTB neurons also receive input from both flattened- and oval-pleomorphic vesicle terminals that immunolabel with glycine and GABA, respectively (59). The source of the glycine-immunoreactive terminals may be from within the MNTB itself, as several studies indicate that principal neurons are glycinergic (13,60,100,119,173) and

that these neurons produce axon collaterals that end on adjacent MNTB neurons (12, 106). The source of GABA input to the MNTB has not been identified.

The projection of the MNTB is almost entirely ipsilateral, and, as previously mentioned, most MNTB neurons are probably glycinergic, thus inhibitory, and receive input from the contralateral CN. In essence, these neurons compose an internuncial pool whose principal function is to reverse the sign of the contralateral globular cell output from excitatory to inhibitory. MNTB principal and elongate neurons send major projections around and through the MSO to the medial and intermediate limbs of the LSO (37,44,54,124,152). Axon collaterals branch off from this pathway to form substantial projections to the DMPO, MSO, and LNTB in the SOC, to the intermediate nucleus of the lateral lemniscus, and to the ventral nucleus of the lateral lemniscus (12,43,80,106,152). Small contributions are made to the ventromedial PON and ventral nucleus of the trapezoid body (12,79,152). Terminals from the MNTB are extremely sparse in the central nucleus of the IC (152). There is a topographic organization to the major MNTB projections that underlie their tonotopic organization (12,152). Neurons in the most ventromedial (high-frequency) portion of the MNTB project to the medial (high-frequency) limb of the LSO and to the medial regions of the DMPO and LNTB. The terminal fields of more dorsolaterally located (lower frequency) MNTB neurons are found further laterally along the tonotopic axis of the LSO and further laterally along the transverse axis of the DMPO and LNTB.

Lateral Superior Olive

In most species, the LSO can usually be distinguished from other SOC nuclei by its shape. It folds upon itself so that, when viewed transversely, the LSO forms a U, S, or W, depending on the number of folds.

The amount and degree of folding are species dependent. The gaps between the folds, the hila, are major sites through which afferent axons enter the LSO. In cats and several rodent species, for instance, the LSO is folded into a recumbent S-shape, and possesses two hila (Fig. 3). The cat and gerbil LSO contain at least five morphologically distinct cell types, of which one predominates (57,58). Principal neurons compose roughly three-quarters of the total neuronal population in the LSO. Also referred to as fusiform neurons because of their shape in transverse sections, principal neurons are indeed multipolar with a discoid dendritic organization. They are arranged in laminar sheets that are oriented perpendicular to the transverse axis of the LSO and appear to fan out from the hila of the LSO (57,58,142). The other cell types include the following: multiplanar neurons, with dendrites showing no preference for plane of orientation; marginal neurons, which lie immediately beneath the envelope of afferent axons surrounding the LSO, orthogonal in orientation to principal neurons; lateral olivocochlear neurons and neurons that are similar to principal neurons except that they possess fewer perisomatic synaptic contacts.

The ipsilateral afferents to the LSO are supplied by axons from the spherical cells of the AVCN (25,155,162,164). These axons form endbulb-type presynaptic terminals containing round vesicles and multiple, asymmetrical synaptic contacts. These synaptic terminals normally contact the dendrites of LSO neurons and are similar in appearance to round vesicle terminals found on the dendrites of MSO neurons (56). This should not be surprising considering that the LSO and MSO receive most of their excitatory input from the same cell type, spherical cells (see Chapter 5). The excitatory pathway to the LSO may use an excitant amino acid transmitter, because excitation of LSO neurons appears to be mediated by non-NMDA (*N*-methyl-*D*-aspartate) excitant amino acid receptors (29).

Further support for the role of excitant amino acids as transmitters in the LSO comes from immunocytochemical studies (56). High levels of glutamate immunoreactivity have been observed in round vesicle terminals in the LSO, indicating that these terminals may contain glutamate as a transmitter or as a precursor to one.

The principal source of contralateral input to the LSO is the population of globular cells in the opposite VCN, relayed via the inhibitory, putatively glycinergic principal neurons of the MNTB. Synaptic terminals from the MNTB contain flattened vesicles and contact mostly the somata and proximal dendrites of most LSO neurons. These terminals are immunoreactive for glycine (59). It is through this circuit that the LSO receives crossed inhibitory input representing the contralateral ear. In cats, however, the distribution of this input is not uniform across the entire tonotopic axis of the LSO as the lowest frequency region, located in the lateral limb of the LSO, receives less input from the MNTB (44,164). The cat MNTB contains few low-frequency units (50,51), which might explain the relative paucity of MNTB input to the LSO lateral limb in this animal. Studies in dogs and cats show that a second source of contralateral input is provided by a direct connection from the opposite globular cell region to the medial (high-frequency) limb of the LSO (44,49,164).

The physiological properties of LSO neurons are detailed in Chapter 6. The LSO responds tonotopically to tone presentations along discrete isofrequency planes, which are oriented perpendicular to its curvatures. That is, the isofrequency planes are aligned parallel to the orientation and dendritic organization of the principal neurons. The functional signs of the major afferent pathways to the LSO (ipsilaterally facilitatory, contralaterally inhibitory) are reflected in the response properties of most LSO neurons. These neurons, presumably principal cells, are sensitive to interaural intensity differences. They correspond to EI units, which are excited by ipsilateral tone presentations and are inhibited by the simultaneous presentation of a contralateral tone of similar frequency (50,51,159) and, in addition, probably possess inhibitory sidebands on either side of their best excitatory frequencies (19). Most of the EI units are also sensitive to time of arrival of the inputs such that they respond more intensely to an ipsilateral time lead (22). Multiplanar and marginal neurons possess several dendrites that run parallel to the tonotopic axis of the LSO (57,58). Thus, they probably respond to a greater range of frequencies than principal neurons, and one or both types may actually correspond to the LSO units with broad tuning curves recorded in other studies (50,51,158). The small olivocochlear neurons in or around the LSO comprise the lateral olivocochlear system, which is a component of the descending pathways discussed in Chapter 2.

The ascending fibers from the LSO project rostrally, bilaterally, and tonotopically, via the LL, to the central nucleus of the IC (1,21,32,37,45,110,134,155), dorsal nucleus of the lateral lemniscus (DNLL) and, to a much lesser extent, VNLL (37,43,45) (Fig. 4). In the cat, the LSO also gives rise to a connection to the MNTB (37). Both the crossed and uncrossed components of the ascending LSO projection produce banded terminal labeling patterns in the central nucleus of the IC, as described in Chapter 7.

A substantial proportion of the LSO projection neurons may be inhibitory. In the guinea pig, a majority of the LSO projection neurons exhibit intense immunoreactive labeling for GABA as well as moderate glycine immunoreactivity (60). Uptake and immunocytochemical studies in the cat suggest that many LSO neurons use glycine as a neurotransmitter (63,139). Further, these studies show that the projection of the same LSO neurons are restricted to the ipsilateral IC. The LSO may send a crossed excitatory projection to the contralateral IC and an uncrossed projection that contains both an excitatory and inhibitory component, with the

latter predominating (63,139). The net effect would be to facilitate unit activity in the contralateral IC and reduce activity in the ipsilateral side (139). Thus, the LSO may provide major input to the many units in the IC excited by contralateral sounds and inhibited by ipsilateral ones (for review, see ref. 65 and Chapter 8, *this volume*).

The Periolivary Nuclei

The PON are aggregates of neurons surrounding the principal nuclei of the SOC. As with the principal nuclei, the size and shape of each PON often vary among the mammalian species. The variance reflects interspecies differences in the geometry of the SOC. These differences are most likely related by the contribution of each PON toward specific tasks in central auditory processing, which in turn depends on the auditory requirements of a given species. Each PON possesses unique cytoarchitectonic and neurochemical attributes and distinctive patterns of input and output connections, and is often located in the same general SOC site across species.

The principal sources of ascending input to the PON are from the multipolar, octopus, and globular cells of the ipsilateral VCN (for review, see ref. 164). The multipolar cells, which project via the ventral acoustic stria to the contralateral IC, send collateral axons ipsilaterally to innervate the dorsal PON (DMPO excluded), LNTB, and, to a lesser extent, the ventral PON. After crossing the midline, collaterals from multipolar cell axons innervate the contralateral ventral PON groups. In cats, the octopus cell fibers project mostly by way of the intermediate acoustic stria, innervate the ipsilateral dorsal and posterior PON groups, cross to provide minor input to the contralateral DMPO, and then proceed rostrally to the VNLL. The globular cell axons send collaterals to the ipsilateral LNTB and posterior PON (150), and, via collaterals from branches that terminate as calyces of Held, the contralateral DMPO (106).

The PON, in addition to making major contributions to the descending auditory pathways (for a review, see Chapter 2), send bilateral ascending projections to the IC and, to a lesser extent, the nuclei of the LL (2,21,32,43,110) (Fig. 4). Studies in the cat suggest that the periolivary projections terminate diffusely in the IC (2). The ventral nucleus of the trapezoid body, ventromedial PON, and DMPO project primarily to the ipsilateral IC in rats and guinea pigs (32,55), while the LNTB projects mainly to the contralateral IC in guinea pigs (55). The remainder of the PON appear to have more evenly balanced bilateral projections to the IC. Some PON send projections that terminate within the SOC. The LNTB, for example, projects to the ipsilateral MSO (see Chapter 5) and LSO (80), while in the rat the ventral nucleus of the trapezoid body projects bilaterally to the LSO and LNTB (152,165).

Immunocytochemical evidence suggests that GABA and glycine might be used by many neurons in most of the PON (60). It is also conceivable that a significant portion of these neurons project to the IC as well as to the nuclei of the LL. If this is the case, and given the diffuse nature of their ascending projections, the PON may serve to regulate physiological setpoints of excitability in their target neurons.

NUCLEUS OF THE CENTRAL ACOUSTIC TRACT

The central acoustic tract is a pathway that runs medial to and parallel with the LL and brachium of the IC. It contains axons that bypass the IC and terminate directly in the medial geniculate nucleus (MGN) and superior colliculus (31,61,117,123). In bats, the source of most of these fibers, the nucleus of the central acoustic tract (NCAT), is located rostral to the MSO and ventromedial to the VNLL. Because of similari-

ties in location, cytoarchitecture, input, and projections (31), the NCAT most likely corresponds to the posteromedial division of the VNLL described in cats (6,36,61,162).

The NCAT consists mostly of large multipolar neurons (31,183). In bats, it receives bilateral ascending input from the AVCN, with greater emphasis from the contralateral side, and projects ipsilaterally to the deep and intermediate layers of the superior colliculus and to the suprageniculate nucleus, located adjacent to the medial geniculate body (31). There appear to be minor differences between the NCAT of the bat and cat. The latter differs from the former in that the cat NCAT receives ascending AVCN input only from the contralateral side (162) and projects bilaterally to the medial division of the MGN (61).

The NCAT of the mustache bat provides input to a circuit that connects the superior colliculus and MGN with the auditory and frontal cortices (31,76). This interplay between auditory, visual, and motor areas could be essential for the combined head, neck, pinna, and eye movements that enable the animal to track a source of sound.

NUCLEI OF THE LATERAL LEMNISCUS

The LL begins caudally where axons from the contralateral CN and ipsilateral SOC join rostral to the SOC to form a single tract. It passes rostrodorsally through the lateral pontine tegmentum and ends in the IC. The LL contains axons from both the ascending and descending auditory pathways, and intermingled among the lemniscal axons are the neurons that compose its nuclei. The ascending auditory fibers within the LL include those originating from the CN and SOC, as well as those from nuclei located within the LL. Most of these fibers terminate in the IC; however, a substantial number of axons originating from the nuclei of the LL pass through the IC to terminate in the superior colliculus and, to a much lesser extent, the MGN (62,78,156,174).

Three large, morphologically distinct lemniscal nuclei appose one another in such a way that they form a chain that, in essence, bridges the SOC and IC. They differ from each other cytoarchitectonically and connectionally and are named according to their location along the LL as VNLL, intermediate nucleus of the LL (INLL), and dorsal nucleus of the LL (DNLL). The nuclei of the LL and their input and output connections form multisynaptic pathways that parallel the other ascending pathways. The ascending connections of the nuclei of the LL are summarized in Fig. 5.

The differences in the connections between the lemniscal nuclei suggest that they are involved in completely different modes of auditory processing. The VNLL and INLL receive most of their ascending input from the contralateral CN and send their projections ipsilaterally, i.e., they are components of monaural circuits. The DNLL, on the other hand, is involved in binaural processing as it derives most of its input from the binaural nuclei in the SOC and in turn projects bilaterally.

Despite the potential importance of the nuclei of the LL in auditory processing, they have received little attention compared to the other nuclear complexes in the central auditory system. Our understanding of their synaptic organization in relation to their connections to brainstem nuclei is far from complete. Hence, their functional role in hearing is poorly understood at this time. Studies in the bat suggest that the VNLL is involved in encoding temporal features of biosonar signals, which are used by echolocating bats to detect the distance of objects in space (33,34). By virtue of its ability to detect variations in the temporal features of auditory input, the VNLL could be a

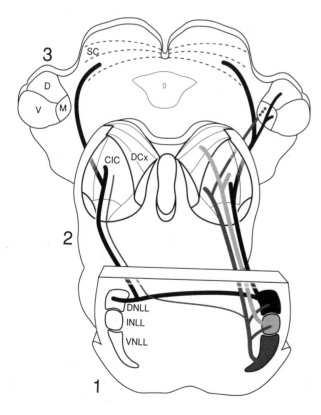

FIG. 5. Ascending projections from the nuclei of the lateral lemniscus (**1**). The projections terminate in the nuclei of the lateral lemniscus, the inferior colliculus (**2**), the medial geniculate nucleus (**3**; D, V, M), and the deep layers of the superior colliculus (**3, SC**). Line thickness indicates the relative magnitude of a given projection. 1: DNLL, dorsal nucleus of the lateral lemniscus; INLL, intermediate nucleus of the lateral lemniscus; VNLL, ventral nucleus of the lateral lemniscus. 2: CIC, central nucleus of the inferior colliculus; DCx, dorsal cortex. 3: D, dorsal; V, ventral; M, medial: divisions of the medial geniculate nucleus; SC, superior colliculus. Not shown are the nuclei of the central auditory tract and their projections.

fundamental component of the neural circuitry involved in language perception.

Ventral Nucleus of the Lateral Lemniscus

In many mammals, the VNLL can be divided into two areas based on cytoarchitectural differences. One area, the columnar division (33), contains multipolar neurons with round or oval somata, along with a few elongate and small neurons (1,33,183). These neurons are packed tightly into clusters or columns, which are demarcated by the fascicles of lemniscal fibers traversing the VNLL. The second area, the multipolar cell area, is less densely populated and is comprised of multipolar neurons with polygonal somata, along with some globular neurons and elongate neurons. The location of the two areas within the VNLL appears to vary among the species studied, even within a single mammalian order. In chiropterans, for example, the columnar division is found in the dorsal VNLL of the big brown bat (33) and in the ventral VNLL of the mustache bat (183).

The afferent innervation of the VNLL is dominated by projections from the contralateral CN (33,43). Octopus cells and multipolar cells of the VCN appear to be the major sources of this projection, with neurons from the DCN and spherical cell region of the AVCN also contributing (164). In the bat, the pathways from the AVCN diverge to tonotopically innervate both subdivisions of the VNLL so that, in the columnar division, low-frequency units are located dorsally and high-frequency ones are positioned ventrally (33,34). The remainder of the ascending afferents to the VNLL arise from the SOC on the ipsilateral side, particularly from the PON (43).

The heavy bias of the VNLL input toward the contralateral CN is reflected in the response properties of VNLL neurons, i.e., most if not all neurons in the VNLL are influenced only by contralateral stimulation (8,34,51,95). In the bat, most units in the

columnar area are broadly tuned and produce phasic responses of extremely short duration that are precisely locked to the stimulus onset (34). Neurons producing such responses would be ideally suited to convey stimulus onset information to the higher centers involved in the temporal analysis of auditory input (34).

VNLL neurons project to the ipsilateral central nucleus of the IC (CIC) (1,21,33, 78,110,133,174,184). Some fibers terminate in the ipsilateral DNLL (43,78), and a very minor projection crosses the brainstem to terminate in the contralateral CIC (1,21, 110). In many mammals, the VNLL contribution to the CIC is quite substantial. In the cat, for instance, the VNLL places a close second to the contralateral CN complex in the number of cells that send ascending fibers to the IC (1). While there is tonotopic organization to the projections of the VNLL, it is questionable whether this organization is as precise as that found in lower auditory centers such as the VCN and the principal nuclei of the SOC, and it may vary considerably among mammalian orders.

Immunocytochemical and uptake/transport studies suggest that a large number of VNLL neurons are glycinergic. In rats, gerbils, and cats the VNLL contains many immunoreactive perikarya (5,9), and their axons ascend to terminate in the IC (5). In guinea pigs and chinchillas, large numbers of VNLL neurons are labeled subsequent to the injection of tritiated glycine into the ipsilateral IC (138). Glycinergic VNLL neurons may function as interneurons that convey to their targets temporally coded, inhibitory input representing the contralateral ear.

Intermediate Nucleus of the
Lateral Lemniscus

To date, little information is available on the response properties of neurons in the INLL, and none regarding its function. The

INLL has been described as a transition zone between the VNLL and DNLL. The cells of the INLL resemble those in the DNLL (1) except that they are typically smaller. Yet, from the standpoint of input, the INLL is closely allied with the VNLL in that it receives monaural innervation from the contralateral ear. This monaural input arises directly from the contralateral VCN, and indirectly from this nucleus by way of the MNTB (43,152).

INLL neurons project to the dorsal cortex and adjacent central nucleus of the ipsilateral IC (174,184) and possibly to the medial division of the MGN (174). Whether or not the INLL cells are organized tonotopically may depend on the species. In the bat there is physiological (95) and connectional (184) evidence that tonotopy exists in the INLL, while in the cat the INLL does not appear to be tonotopically organized (8).

Dorsal Nucleus of the Lateral Lemniscus

The DNLL is a prominent cluster of neurons embedded in the fibers of the LL ventral to the IC. It contains several different cell types (1,70), most of which are preferentially oriented in horizontal planes (33, 70). At least nine cell types have been described in the cat DNLL based on differences in somal size and shape (70). The cell shapes have been classified as round, ovoid, or elongate, and each class has been further categorized based on whether the cell type possesses large, medium-sized, or small perikarya. Most of the medium-sized neurons and large, elongate cells are found in the caudal portion of the DNLL, while most of the large oval and large round neurons are located rostrally (70). This differential distribution of cell types may be related to the probability that the rostral DNLL projects to a different target than the caudal DNLL, as described later.

The capacity of the DNLL for binaural processing is reflected in its input. Major sources of ascending input to neurons of the DNLL are the MSO and LSO (43), nuclei in the SOC that are involved in sound localization. Substantial input to the DNLL also originates from the ipsilateral VNLL and contralateral DNLL (43,78), and minor sources include the contralateral VCN and PON (43).

The DNLL projects primarily to the IC and superior colliculus bilaterally, the contralateral DNLL, and, to a lesser extent, the medial and dorsal divisions of the ipsilateral medial geniculate body (1,35,78, 113,156,184). The axons projecting contralaterally cross in the dorsal midbrain tegmentum at the commissure of Probst. Neurons in the caudal portion of the DNLL project to the IC, while those of the rostral portion project to deep layers of the superior colliculus (78,156). The projections to the IC are tonotopic, with low-frequency neurons located dorsally and high-frequency neurons found ventrally (8,78,133). In the rat most neurons that project to the ipsilateral IC are located in the central region of the caudal DNLL, while those projecting contralaterally are typically found on either side of this central region (156).

Based on its principal sources of input (MSO and LSO) and a limited knowledge of the response characteristics of its neurons, it would be reasonable to assume that the DNLL plays a part in coding for sound localization. Its neurons are sensitive to interaural time and intensity differences (8, 20), and many of these units are excited by contralateral stimulation and inhibited by a similar stimulus applied ipsilaterally (20). Immunocytochemical evidence suggests that most of the DNLL neurons use GABA as a neurotransmitter and, therefore, provide inhibitory input to its targets (3,98,127, 157). Although the function of the DNLL in hearing is not clear, it most likely serves as a feed-forward inhibitory nucleus (3), regulating and modulating IC neurons, particularly those involved in the localization of sound in space (156).

The DNLL projects to the deep layers of

the superior colliculus, providing auditory input to this structure. Neurons in this region of the superior colliculus are known to respond not only to visual and somatosensory input, but to auditory stimuli as well. A map of auditory space has been described in the intermediate and deep layers of the superior colliculus of guinea pigs and cats (74,96,116). Neurons in these layers receiving binaural auditory input could be involved in the mediation of head, ear, and neck movements (156).

The next three complexes in the ascending auditory pathway are the IC, MGN, and auditory cortex. Each of these is considered in detail in later chapters and so are only briefly outlined here, with divisions and connections given but without consideration at the level of cell types. This additional information and more extensive references are found in Chapters 9, 12, and 14 of this volume.

INFERIOR COLLICULUS

The IC comprises the auditory midbrain, a site where the auditory pathways that have diverged from the CN into multiple ascending tracts now largely converge. While there are direct connections of second order fibers from both ipsilateral and contralateral CN, a large number of the fibers entering the IC represent pathways that synapsed once or twice in the SOC and/or lateral lemniscal nuclei interposed, and so are third, fourth, or possibly higher order fibers. While a few fibers from the lemniscal nuclei may bypass the IC and end directly in the MGN, the IC should be considered to house the terminal synapses for the vast majority of incoming fibers and, thus, provides a summation of lower auditory brainstem processing as well as an opportunity for additional processing.

The IC consists of a CIC, which is surrounded dorsally and caudally by the dorsal cortex (DCx) and on either side by the para-

central nuclei (PCN). The CIC is the largest and most extensively studied subdivision (40,42,93,112,129,130,134,169). It receives fibers from both ipsi- and contralateral CN, with much greater input from the latter. This second order input arises from multipolar/stellate cells of the VCN, fusiform cells of the DCN, and giant cells from both divisions. The CIC also receives input from lower binaural centers in the SOC and nuclei of the LL. This input arises bilaterally from the LSO, PON, and DNLL, and ipsilaterally from the MSO and VNLL. Many of these inputs terminate in discrete bands and clusters on the principal cell types, which together form the cytoarchitectonically distinct fibrodendritic laminae characteristic of the CIC. The CIC in turn gives rise to fibers that terminate tonotopically in the ventral division of the MGN (77,101, 102) (Fig. 6).

The DCx receives similar inputs from the CN and DNLL, but its input from the SOC is provided only by the PON (32). The DCx, as well as the PCN, gives rise to fibers that terminate in the dorsal and ventral divisions of the MGN (Fig. 6). There is a connection between left and right IC as well as connections to and from other modalities, e.g., to the visual system via the superior colliculus (see Chapter 9).

MEDIAL GENICULATE NUCLEUS

The MGN is the auditory thalamic relay to the cortex. It is conventionally divided into dorsal, ventral, and medial divisions (Chapter 12, *this volume;* 7,23,64,103–105). It is useful to think of the MGN as a component of the central pathway from the IC to the auditory cortex (see Chapter 9). This pathway originates in the CIC and terminates in the ventral division of the MGN, which in turn projects to the primary auditory cortex (AI) (Fig. 6). In cats, the anterior portions of the ventral division of the MGN connect anteriorly in AI, while more

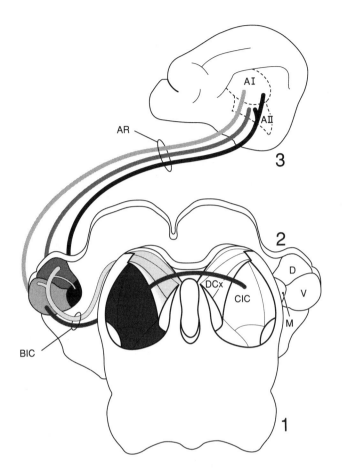

FIG. 6. Ascending projections from the inferior colliculus (**1**) to the medial geniculate nucleus (**2**), and from the latter to the auditory cortex (**3**). 1: CIC, central nucleus of the inferior colliculus; DCx, dorsal cortex. 2: D, dorsal; V, ventral; M, medial: divisions of the medial geniculate nucleus. 3: AR, auditory radiation; AI, primary auditory cortex; AII, secondary auditory cortex.

posterior portions project more posteriorly (132). This division is the largest, most tonotopic and organized part of the MGN. Thus, the tonotopic and topographic organization of the ascending auditory pathway is preserved to the level of AI. The ventral division possesses fibrodendritic laminae similar to those in the CIC, the nucleus from which it receives most of its input.

The dorsal and medial divisions are involved in more diffuse pathways. The dorsal division, which receives input predominantly from the DCx of the IC, projects to secondary auditory cortical fields (including AII). The medial division, which receives minor input from all IC divisions as well as nonauditory nuclei, projects to both primary and nonprimary auditory cortices.

AUDITORY CORTEX

The auditory cortex in humans is associated with the transverse temporal gyrus and is largely buried in the sylvian fissure. In the cat, much of the auditory cortex is exposed on the lateral surface of the brain, associated with the ectosylvian gyrus. The division of the cortex has been defined by evoked potentials as well as anatomical considerations into primary auditory cortex (AI) and secondary auditory cortex (AII), as well as several associational areas (auditory fields), which include the anterior, ventral, posterior, and ventroposterior auditory fields, and the posterior ectosylvian cortical field. Refer to Chapter 14 for a more detailed exposition of these associational areas. There are several tonotopic maps in the auditory cortex, the most complete one is located in AI. In the cat, low frequencies are represented posteriorly and high ones anteriorly (94). As previously mentioned, area AI receives its input from the ventral division of the MGN. All other nonprimary auditory cortex areas receive inputs from medial and dorsal divisions of the MGN.

REFERENCES

1. Adams JC. Ascending projections of the inferior colliculus. *J Comp Neurol* 1979;183:519–538.
2. Adams JC. Multipolar cells in the ventral cochlear nucleus project to the dorsal cochlear nucleus and the inferior colliculus. *Neurosci Lett* 1983;37:205–208.
3. Adams JC, Mugnaini E. Dorsal nucleus of the lateral lemniscus: a nucleus of GABAergic projection neurons. *Brain Res Bull* 1984;13:585–590.
4. Adams JC, Mugnaini E. Patterns of glutamate decarboxylase immunostaining in the feline cochlear nuclear complex studied with silver enhancement and electron microscopy. *J Comp Neurol* 1987;262:375–401.
5. Adams JC, Wenthold RJ. Immunostaining of ascending auditory pathways with glycine antiserum. *Absts Midwinter Mtg Assoc Res Otolaryngol* 1987;10:63.
6. Aitkin LM, Phillips C. Is the inferior colliculus an obligatory relay in the cat auditory system? *Neurosci Lett* 1984;44:259–264.
7. Aitkin LM, Webster WR. Medial geniculate body of the cat: organization and responses to tonal stimuli of neurons in ventral division. *J Neurophysiol* 1972;32:365–380.
8. Aitkin LM, Anderson DJ, Brugge JF. Tonotopic organization and discharge characteristics of single neurons in nuclei of the lateral lemniscus of the cat. *J Neurophysiol* 1970;122:421–440.
9. Aoki E, Semba R, Keino R, Kato H, Kashiwamata S. Glycine-like immunoreactivity in the rat auditory pathway. *Brain Res* 1988;442:63–71.
10. Arnesen AR, Osen KK. The cochlear nerve in the cat: topography, tonotopy, and fiber spectrum. *J Comp Neurol* 1978; 178:661–678.
11. Blackstad TW, Osen KK, Mugnaini E. Pyramidal neurons of the dorsal cochlear nucleus: a Golgi and computer reconstruction study in cat. *Neuroscience* 1984;13:827–854.
12. Bledsoe SC, Pandya P, Altschuler RA, Helfert RH. Axonal projections of PHA-L-labeled neurons in the medial nucleus of the trapezoid body. *Soc Neurosci Abstr* 1988;14:491.
13. Bledsoe SC, Snead CR, Helfert RH, Prasad V, Wenthold RJ, Altschuler RA. Immunocytochemical and lesion studies support the hypothesis that the projection from the medial nucleus of the trapezoid body to the lateral superior olive is glycinergic. *Brain Res* 1990;517:189–194.
14. Bodian D. Presynaptic bodies of auditory hair cells in Old World monkeys. *Anat Rec* 1980;197:379–386.
15. Bourk TR, Mielcarz JP, Norris BE. Tonotopic organization of the anteroventral cochlear nucleus of the cat. *Hear Res* 1981;4:215–241.
16. Brawer JR, Morest DK. Relation between auditory nerve endings and cell types in the cat's anteroventral cochlear nucleus seen with the Golgi method and Nomarski optics. *J Comp Neurol* 1975;160:491–506.
17. Brown MC. Morphology of labeled afferent fibers in the guinea pig cochlea. *J Comp Neurol* 1987;260:591–604.
18. Brown MC, Berglund AM, Kiang NY-S, Ryugo DK. Central trajectories of type II spiral ganglion neurons. *J Comp Neurol* 1988;278:581–590.
19. Brownell WE, Manis PB, Ritz LA. Ipsilateral inhibitory responses in the cat lateral superior olive S-segment. *Brain Res* 1979;177:189–193.
20. Brugge JF, Anderson DJ, Aitkin LM. Responses of neurons in the dorsal nucleus of the lateral lemniscus of cat to binaural tonal stimulation. *J Neurophysiol* 1970;33:441–458.
21. Brunso-Bechtold JK, Thompson GC, Masterton RB. HRP study of the organization of auditory afferents ascending to central nucleus of inferior colliculus in cat. *J Comp Neurol* 1981;197:705–722.
22. Caird D, Klinke R. Processing of binaural stimuli by cat superior olivary complex neurons. *Exp Brain Res* 1983;52:385–399.
23. Calford MB, Webster WR. Auditory representation within principal division of cat medial geniculate body: an electrophysiological study. *J Neurophysiol* 1981;45:1013–1028.
24. Cant NB. Identification of cell types in the anteroventral cochlear nucleus that project to the inferior colliculus. *Neurosci Lett* 1982;32:241–246.
25. Cant NB, Casseday JH. Projections from the anteroventral cochlear nucleus to the lateral and medial superior olivary nuclei. *J Comp Neurol* 1986;247:457–476.
26. Cant NB, Gaston KC. Pathways connecting the right and left cochlear nuclei. *J Comp Neurol* 1982;212:313–326.
27. Cant NB, Morest DK. The structural basis for stimulus coding in the cochlear nucleus of the cat. In: Berlin C, ed. *Hearing science*. San Diego: College-Hill Press. 1984;371–421.
28. Caspary DM. Cochlear nuclei: functional neuropharmacology of the principal cell types. In: Altschuler RA, Bobbin RP, Hoffman DW, eds. *Neurobiology of hearing: the cochlea*. New York: Raven Press, 1986;303–332.
29. Caspary DM, Faingold CL. Non-N-methyl-d-aspartate receptors may mediate ipsilateral ex-

citation at lateral superior olivary synapses. *Brain Res* 1989;503:83–90.

30. Casseday JH, Covey E. Central auditory pathways in directional hearing. In: Yost WA, Gourevitch G, eds. *Directional hearing.* New York: Springer-Verlag, 1987;109–145.

31. Casseday JH, Kobler JB, Isbey SF, Covey EC. Central acoustic tract in an echolocating bat: an extralemniscal auditory pathway to the thalamus. *J Comp Neurol* 1989;287:247–259.

32. Coleman JR, Clerici WJ. Sources of projections to subdivisions of the inferior colliculus in the rat. *J Comp Neurol* 1987;262:215–226.

33. Covey E, Casseday JH. Connectional basis for frequency representation in the nuclei of the lateral lemniscus of the bat *Eptesicus fuscus.* *J Neurosci* 1986;6:2926–2940.

34. Covey E, Casseday JH. Parallel monaural pathways to the midbrain in an echo-locating bat. *Soc Neurosci Abstr* 1989;15:746.

35. Covey E, Hall WC, Kobler JB. Subcortical connections of the superior colliculus in the mustache bat, *Pteronotus parnellii.* *J Comp Neurol* 1987;263:179–197.

36. Edwards SB, Ginsburgh CL, Henkel CK, Stein BE. Sources of subcortical projections to the superior colliculus in the cat. *J Comp Neurol* 1979;184:309–330.

37. Elverland HH. Ascending and intrinsic projections of the superior olivary complex in the cat. *Exp Brain Res* 1978;32:117–134.

38. Fekete DM, Rouiller EM, Liberman MC, Ryugo DK. The central projection of intracellularly labeled auditory nerve fibers in the cat. *J Comp Neurol* 1984;229:432–450.

39. Feldman M, Harrison JM. The acoustic nerve projection to the ventral cochlear nucleus in the rat. *J Comp Neurol* 1969;137:267–292.

40. FitzPatrick KA. Cellular architecture and topographic organization of the inferior colliculus of the squirrel monkey. *J Comp Neurol* 1975;164:185–208.

41. Galambos R, Schwartzkopff F, Rupert A. Microelectrode study of superior olivary nuclei. *Am J Physiol* 1959;197:527–536.

42. Geniec P, Morest DK. The neuronal architecture of the human posterior colliculus. A study with the Golgi method. *Acta Otolaryngol (Stockh) [Suppl]* 1971;295:1–33.

43. Glendenning KK, Brunso-Bechtold JK, Thompson GC, Masterton RB. Ascending auditory afferents to the nuclei of the lateral lemniscus. *J Comp Neurol* 1981;197:673–703.

44. Glendenning KK, Hutson KA, Nudo RJ, Masterton RB. Acoustic chiasm. II. Anatomical basis of binaurality in lateral superior olive of cat. *J Comp Neurol* 1985;232:261–285.

45. Glendenning KK, Masterton RB. Acoustic chiasm: efferent projections of the lateral superior olive. *J Neurosci* 1983;3:1521–1537.

46. Godfrey DA, Carter JA, Berger SJ, Lowry OH, Matschinsky FM. Quantitative histochemical mapping of candidate transmitter amino acids in cat cochlear nucleus. *J Histochem Cytochem* 1977;25:417–431.

47. Godfrey DA, Parli JD, Dunn JD, Ross CD. Neurotransmitter microchemistry of the cochlear nucleus and superior olivary complex. In: Syka J, Masterton RB, eds. *Auditory pathway.* New York: Plenum, 1988;107–121.

48. Goldberg JM, Brown PB. Functional organization of the dog superior olivary complex: an anatomical and electrophysiological study. *J Neurophysiol* 1968;31:639–656.

49. Goldberg JM, Brown PB. Response of binaural neurons of dog superior olivary complex to dichotic tonal stimuli: some physiological mechanisms of sound localization. *J Neurophysiol* 1969;32:613–636.

50. Guinan JJ, Guinan SS, Norris BE. Single auditory units in the superior olivary complex. I. Responses to sounds and classifications based on physiological properties. *Int J Neurosci* 1972;4:101–120.

51. Guinan JJ, Guinan SS, Norris BE. Single auditory units in the superior olivary complex. II. Locations of unit categories and tonotopic organization. *Int J Neurosci* 1972;4:147–166.

52. Harrison JM, Irving R. The anterior ventral cochlear nucleus. *J Comp Neurol* 1965;124:15–42.

53. Harrison JM, Irving R. The organization of the posterior ventral cochlear nucleus in the rat. *J Comp Neurol* 1966;126:391–403.

54. Harrison JM, Warr WB. The cochlear nucleus and ascending pathways of the medulla. *J Comp Neurol* 1962;119:341–380.

55. Helfert RH. Unpublished observations in guinea pig.

56. Helfert RH, Altschuler RA. Unpublished observations.

57. Helfert RH, Schwartz IR. Morphological evidence for the existence of multiple neuronal classes in the cat lateral superior olivary nucleus. *J Comp Neurol* 1986;244:533–549.

58. Helfert RH, Schwartz IR. Morphological features of five neuronal classes in the gerbil lateral superior olivary nucleus. *Am J Anat* 1987;179:55–69.

59. Helfert RH, Bonneau JM, Wenthold RJ, Altschuler RA. Distribution of GABA and glycine immunoreactive synapses in the guinea pig superior olivary complex. *Soc Neurosci Abstr* 1988;14:487.

60. Helfert RH, Juiz JM, Bledsoe SC, Bonneau JM, Wenthold RJ, Altschuler RA. Two classes of glutamate immunoreactive synapses in the guinea pig superior olivary complex. *Soc Neurosci Abstr* 1989;15:941.

61. Henkel CK. Evidence of subcollicular projections to the medial nucleus of the geniculate body in the cat: an autoradiographic and horseradish peroxidase study. *Brain Res* 1983;259:21–30.

62. Henkel CS, Spangler KM. Organization of the efferent projections of the medial superior olivary nucleus in the cat as revealed by HRP and autoradiographic tracing methods. *J Comp Neurol* 1983;221:416–428.

63. Hutson KA, Glendenning KK, Masterton RB.

Biochemical basis for the acoustic chiasm? *Soc Neurosci Abstr* 1987;13:548.

64. Imig TJ, Morel A. Organization of the thalamo-cortical auditory system in the cat. *Annu Rev Neurosci* 1983;6:95–120.

65. Irvine DRF. The auditory brainstem. In: Otto-son D, ed. *Progress in sensory physiology,* vol 7. Berlin: Springer-Verlag, 1986;79–121.

66. Javel E. Basic response properties of auditory nerve fibers. In: Altschuler RA, Bobbin RP, Hoffman DW, eds. *Neurobiology of hearing: the cochlea.* New York: Raven Press, 1986; 213–245.

67. Jean-Baptiste J, Morest DK. Transneuronal changes of synaptic endings and nuclear chro-matin in the trapezoid body following cochlear ablations in the cat. *J Comp Neurol* 1975;162: 111–134.

68. Juiz JM, Helfert RH, Wenthold RJ, De Blas AL, Altschuler RA. Immunocytochemical lo-calization of the GABAa/benzodiazepine re-ceptor in the guinea pig cochlear nucleus: evi-dence for receptor heterogeneity. *Brain Res* 1989;504:173–179.

69. Kane E. Octopus cells in the cochlear nucleus of the cat: heterotypic synapses upon homo-typic neurons. *Int J Neurosci* 1973;5:251–279.

70. Kane ES, Barone LM. The dorsal nucleus of the lateral lemniscus in the cat: neuronal types and their distribution. *J Comp Neurol* 1980; 192:797–826.

71. Kane ES, Puglisi SG, Gordon BS. Neuronal types in the deep dorsal cochlear nucleus of the cat. I. Giant neurons. *J Comp Neurol* 1981; 198:483–513.

72. Kiang NY-S, Watanabe T, Thomas EC, Clark LF. *Discharge patterns of single fibers in the cat's auditory nerve.* Cambridge, MA: MIT Press, 1965.

73. Kiang NY-S, Morest DK, Godfrey DA, Guinan JJ, Kane EC. Stimulus coding at caudal levels of the cat's auditory nervous system: I. Re-sponse characteristics of single units. In: Moller AR, ed. *Basic mechanisms in hearing.* New York: Academic Press, 1973;455–478.

74. King AJ, Palmer AR. Cells responsive to free-field auditory stimuli in guinea pig superior col-liculus: distribution and response properties. *J Physiol (Lond)* 1983;342:361–381.

75. Kiss A, Majorossy K. Neuron morphology and synaptic architecture in the medial superior oli-vary nucleus. *Exp Brain Res* 1983;52:315–327.

76. Kobler JM, Isbey SF, Casseday JH. Auditory pathways to the frontal cortex of the mustache bat, *Pteronotus parnellii. Science* 1987;236: 824–826.

77. Kudo M, Niimi K. Ascending projections of the inferior colliculus in the cat: an autoradio-graphic study. *J Comp Neurol* 1980;191:545–556.

78. Kudo M. Projections of the nuclei of the lateral lemniscus in the cat: an autoradiographic study. *Brain Res* 1981;221:57–69.

79. Kuwabara N, DiCaprio RA, Zook JM. Collat-eral axons of the medial nucleus of the trape-zoid body. *Soc Neurosci Abstr* 1989;15:745.

80. Kuwabara N, Zook JM. Medial and lateral su-perior olives receive projections from the me-dial and lateral nuclei of the trapezoid body. *Soc Neurosci Abstr* 1990;16:723.

81. Leake PA, Synder RL. Topographic organiza-tion of the central projections of the spiral gan-glion in cats. *J Comp Neurol* 1989;281:612–629.

82. Lenn NJ, Reese TS. The fine structure of nerve endings in the nucleus of the trapezoid body and the ventral cochlear nucleus. *Am J Anat* 1966;118:375–390.

83. Lewy FN, Kobrak H. The neural projection of the cochlear spirals on the primary acoustic centers. *Arch Neurol Psychiatr* 1936;35:839–852.

84. Liberman MC. Morphological differences among radial afferent fibers in the cat cochlea: an electron microscopic study of serial sec-tions. *Hear Res* 1980;3:45–63.

85. Liberman MC. Single-neuron labeling in the cat auditory nerve. *Science* 1982;216:1239–1241.

86. Liberman MC. The cochlear frequency map for the cat: labeling auditory-nerve fibers of known characteristic frequency. *J Acoust Soc Am* 1982;72:1441–1449.

87. Liberman MC, Simmons DD. Applications of neuronal labeling techniques to the study of the peripheral auditory system. *J Acoust Soc Am* 1985;78:312–319.

88. Lindsay BG. Fine structure and distribution of axon terminals from the cochlear nucleus on neurons in the medial superior olivary nucleus of the cat. *J Comp Neurol* 1975;160:81–105.

89. Lorente de Nó R. Anatomy of the eighth nerve. III. General plan of structure of the primary cochlear nuclei. *Laryngoscope* 1933;43:327–350.

90. Lorente de Nó R. *The primary acoustic nuclei.* New York: Raven Press, 1981.

91. Mast TE. Binaural interaction and contralateral inhibition in dorsal cochlear nucleus of the chinchilla. *J Neurophysiol* 1970;33:108–115.

92. Mast TE. Dorsal cochlear nucleus of the chin-chilla: excitation by contralateral sound. *Brain Res* 1973;62:61–70.

93. Merzenich MM, Reid MD. Representation of the cochlea within the inferior colliculus of the cat. *Brain Res* 1974;77:397–415.

94. Merzenich MM, Knight PL, Roth GL. Repre-sentation of cochlea within primary auditory cortex in the cat. *J Neurophysiol* 1975;38:231–249.

95. Metzner W, Radke-Schuller S. The nuclei of the lateral lemniscus in the horseshoe bat, *Rhinolophus rouxi:* a neurophysiological ap-proach. *J Comp Physiol* 1987;160:395–411.

96. Middlebrooks JC, Knudsen EI. A neural code for auditory space in the cat's superior colli-culus. *J Neurosci* 1984;4:2621–2634.

97. Moore JK. Cochlear nuclei: relationship to the auditory nerve. In: Altschuler RA, Hoffman DW, Bobbin RP, eds. *Neurobiology of hearing:*

the cochlea. New York: Raven Press, 1986; 283–301.

98. Moore JK, Moore RY. Glutamic acid decarboxylase-like immunoreactivity in brainstem auditory nuclei of the rat. *J Comp Neurol* 1987; 260:157–174.

99. Moore JK, Osen KK. The cochlear nuclei in man. *Am J Anat* 1979;154:393–418.

100. Moore MJ, Caspary DM. Strychnine blocks binaural inhibition in lateral superior olivary neurons. *J Neurosci* 1983;3:237–242.

101. Moore RY, Goldberg JM. Ascending projections of the inferior colliculus in the cat. *J Comp Neurol* 1963;121:109–136.

102. Moore RY, Goldberg JM. Projections of the inferior colliculus in the monkey. *Exp Neurol* 1966;14:429–438.

103. Morest DK. The neuronal architecture of the medial geniculate body of the cat. *J Anat* 1964;98:611–630.

104. Morest DK. The laminar structure of the medial geniculate body of the cat. *J Anat* 1965; 99:143–160.

105. Morest DK. The lateral tegmental system of the midbrain and the medial geniculate body: study with Golgi and Nauta methods in cat. *J Anat* 1965;99:611–634.

106. Morest DK. The collateral system of the medial nucleus of the trapezoid body of the cat, its neuronal architecture and relation to the olivo-cochlear bundle. *Brain Res* 1968;9:288–311.

107. Moushigian G, Rupert AL, Whitcomb MA. Brainstem neuronal response patterns to monaural and binaural tones. *J Neurophysiol* 1964; 27:1174–1191.

108. Mugnaini E, Warr WB, Osen KK. Distribution and light microscopic features of granule cells in the cochlear nucleus of cat, rat and mouse. *J Comp Neurol* 1980;191:581–606.

109. Noda Y, Pirsig W. Anatomical projection of the cochlea to the cochlear nuclei of the guinea pig. *Arch Oto-Rhino-Laryngol* 1974;208:107–120.

110. Nordeen KW, Killackey JP, Kitzes LM. Ascending auditory projections to the inferior colliculus in the adult gerbil. *Meriones unguiculatus. J Comp Neurol* 1983;214:131–143.

111. Oberdorfer MD, Parakkal MH, Altschuler RA, Wenthold RJ. Ultrastructural localization of GABA immunoreactive terminals in the anteroventral cochlear nucleus of the guinea pig. *Hear Res* 1988;33:229–238.

112. Oliver DL, Morest DK. The central nucleus of the inferior colliculus in the cat. *J Comp Neurol* 1984;222:237–264.

113. Oliver DL, Shneiderman A. An EM study of the dorsal nucleus of the lateral lemniscus: inhibitory, commissural, synaptic connections between ascending auditory pathways. *J Neurosci* 1989;9:967–982.

114. Osen KK. Cytoarchitecture of the cochlear nuclei in the cat. *J Comp Neurol* 1969;136:453–484.

115. Osen KK. Course and termination of the primary afferents in the cochlear nuclei of the cat.

116. Palmer AR, King AJ. The representation of auditory space in the mammalian superior colliculus. *Nature* 1982;299:248–249.

117. Papez JW. Central acoustic tract in cat and man. *Anat Rec* 1929;42:60.

118. Perkins RE. An electron microscopic study of synaptic organization in the medial superior olive of normal and experimental chinchillas. *J Comp Neurol* 1973;148:387–416.

119. Peyret D, Campistron G, Geffard M, Aran J-M. Glycine immunoreactivity in the brainstem auditory and vestibular nuclei of the guinea pig. *Acta Otolaryngol* 1987;104:71–76.

120. Pfalz RKJ. Centrifugal inhibition of afferent secondary neurons in the cochlear nucleus by sound. *J Acoust Soc Am* 1962;34:1472–1477.

121. Pirsig W, Pfalz R, Sadanaga M. Postsynaptic auditory crossed efferent inhibition in the ventral cochlear nucleus and its blocking by strychnine nitrate. *Kumamoto Med J* 1968;21: 75–82.

122. Pujol R, Lenoir M. The four types of synapses in the organ of Corti. In: Altschuler RA, Bobbin RP, Hoffman DW, eds. *Neurobiology of hearing: the cochlea.* New York: Raven Press, 1986;161–172.

123. Ramón y Cajal S. *Histologie du système nerveux de l'homme et des vertébrés,* vol I. Madrid: Inst. Ramon y Cajal (1952 reprint), 1909.

124. Rasmussen GL. The olivary peduncle and other fiber connections of the superior olivary complex. *J Comp Neurol* 1946;84:141–219.

125. Rhode WS, Oertel D, Smith PH. Physiological properties of cells labelled intracellularly with horseradish peroxidase in cat ventral cochlear nucleus. *J Comp Neurol* 1983;213:448–463.

126. Rhode WS, Smith PJ, Oertel D. Physiological response properties of cells labeled intracellularly with horseradish peroxidase in cat dorsal cochlear nucleus. *J Comp Neurol* 1983;213: 426–447.

127. Roberts RC, Ribak CE. GABAergic neurons and axon terminals in the brainstem auditory nuclei of the gerbil. *J Comp Neurol* 1987;258: 267–280.

128. Robertson D. Horseradish peroxidase injection of physiologically characterized afferent and efferent neurones in the guinea pig spiral ganglion. *Hear Res* 1984;15:113–121.

129. Rockel AJ, Jones EG. The neuronal organization of the inferior colliculus in the adult cat. I. The central nucleus. *J Comp Neurol* 1973;147: 11–60.

130. Rockel AJ, Jones EG. The neuronal organization of the inferior colliculus in the adult cat. II. The pericentral nucleus. *J Comp Neurol* 1973;149:301–334.

131. Romand R, Romand MR. The spiral ganglion. In: Friedmann I, Ballantyne J, eds. *Ultrastructural atlas of the inner ear.* London: Butterworths, 1984;165–183.

132. Rose JE, Woolsey CN. The relations of tha-

An experimental anatomical study. *Arch Ital Biol* 1970;108:21–51.

lamic connections, cellular structure and evocable electrical activity in the auditory region of the cat. *J Comp Neurol* 1949;91:441–466.

133. Ross LS, Pollack GD, Zook JM. Origin of ascending projections to an isofrequency region of the mustache bat's inferior colliculus. *J Comp Neurol* 1988;270:488–505.

134. Roth GL, Aitkin LM, Andersen RA, Merzenich MM. Some features of the spatial organization of the central nucleus of the inferior colliculus of the cat. *J Comp Neurol* 1978; 182:661–680.

135. Rouiller EM, Ryugo DK. Intracellular marking of physiologically characterized cells in the ventral cochlear nucleus of the cat. *J Comp Neurol* 1984;225:167–186.

136. Ryugo DK, Willard EH. The dorsal cochlear nucleus of the mouse: a light microscopic analysis of neurons that project to the inferior colliculus. *J Comp Neurol* 1985;242:381–396.

137. Ryugo D, Willard FH, Fekete DM. Differential afferent projections to the inferior colliculus from the cochlear nucleus in the albino mouse. *Brain Res* 1981;210:342–348.

138. Saint Marie RL, Baker RA. Neurotransmitter-specific uptake and retrograde transport of [³H]glycine from the inferior colliculus by ipsilateral projections of the superior olivary complex and nuclei of the lateral lemniscus. *Brain Res* 1990;524:244–253.

139. Saint Marie RL, Ostapoff E-M, Morest DK, Wenthold RJ. Glycine immunoreactive projection of the cat lateral superior olive: possible role in midbrain ear dominance. *J Comp Neurol* 1989;279:382–396.

140. Saito K. Fine structure of the sensory epithelium of guinea pig organ of Corti: subsurface cisternae and lamellar bodies in outer hair cells. *Cell Tissue Res* 1983;229:467–481.

141. Sando I. The anatomical relationships of the cochlear nerve fibers. *Acta Otolaryngol (Stock)* 1965;59:417–436.

142. Scheibel ME, Scheibel AB. Neuropil organization in the superior olive of the cat. *Exp Neurol* 1974;43:339–348.

143. Schwartz AM. Auditory nerve and spiral ganglion cells. In: Altschuler RA, Bobbin RP, Hoffman DW, eds. *Neurobiology of hearing: the cochlea.* New York: Raven Press, 1986; 271–282.

144. Schwartz IR. Dendritic arrangements in the cat medial superior olive. *Neuroscience* 1977;2: 81–101.

145. Schwartz IR. Axonal organization in the cat medial superior olive. *Contrib Sensory Physiol* 1984;8:99–129.

146. Shore SE, Godfrey DA, Helfert RH, Bledsoe SE Jr, Altschuler RA. Intrinsic and contralateral connections between cochlear nucleus subdivisions in the guinea pig. *Absts Midwinter Mtg Assoc Res Otolaryngol* 1990;13:335.

147. Simmons DD, Liberman MC. Afferent innervation of OHC's in adult cats: I. Light microscopic analysis of fibers labeled with horse-radish peroxidase. *J Comp Neurol* 1988;270: 132–144.

148. Simmons DD, Liberman MC. Afferent innervation of OHC's in adult cats: II. Electron microscopic analysis of fibers labeled with horseradish peroxidase. *J Comp Neurol* 1988;270: 145–154.

149. Smith CA, Sjöstrand FS. Structure of the nerve endings on the external hair cells of the guinea pig cochlea as studied by serial sections. *J Ultrastruct Res* 1961;5:523–556.

150. Smith PH, Carney LH, Yin TCT. Projections of globular bushy cells in the cat. *Soc Neurosci Abstr* 1987;13:547.

151. Snyder RL, Leake PA. Intrinsic connections within and between cochlear nucleus subdivisions in cat. *J Comp Neurol* 1988;278:209–225.

152. Spangler KM, Warr WB, Henkel CK. The projections of principal cells of the medial nucleus of the trapezoid body in the cat. *J Comp Neurol* 1985;238:249–262.

153. Spoendlin H. Innervation pattern of the organ of Corti of the cat. *Acta Otolaryngol (Stock)* 1969;67:239–254.

154. Spoendlin H. Primary neurons and synapses. In: Friedmann I, Ballantyne J, eds. *Ultrastructural atlas of the inner ear.* London: Butterworths, 1984;133–164.

155. Stotler WA. An experimental study of the cells and connections of the superior olivary complex of the cat. *J Comp Neurol* 1953;98:401–432.

156. Tanaka K, Otani K, Tokunaga A, Sugita S. The organization of neurons in the nucleus of the lateral lemniscus projecting to the superior and inferior colliculi in the rat. *Brain Res* 1985; 341:252–260.

157. Thompson GC, Cortez AM, Lam DM-K. Localization of GABA immunoreactivity in the auditory brainstem of guinea pigs. *Brain Res* 1985;339:119–122.

158. Tsuchitani C. Functional organization of lateral cell groups of the cat superior olivary complex. *J Neurophysiol* 1977;40:296–318.

159. Tsuchitani C, Boudreau JC. Single unit analysis of cat superior olive S-segment with tonal stimuli. *J Neurophysiol* 1966;29:684–697.

160. Tolbert LP, Morest DK, Yurgelun-Todd DK. The neuronal architecture of the anteroventral cochlear nucleus of the cat in the region of the cochlear nerve root: horseradish peroxidase labelling of identified cell types. *Neuroscience* 1982;7:3031–3052.

161. van Noort J. *The structure and connections of the inferior colliculus. An investigation of the lower auditory system.* Leiden: van Gorcum & Co., 1969.

162. Warr WB. Fiber degeneration following lesions in the anterior ventral cochlear nucleus of the cat. *Exp Neurol* 1966;14:453–474.

163. Warr WB. Fiber degeneration following lesions in the multipolar and globular cell areas in the ventral cochlear nucleus of the cat. *Brain Res* 1972;40:247–270.

164. Warr WB. Parallel ascending pathways from the cochlear nucleus: neuroanatomical evidence of functional specialization. *Contrib Sensory Physiol* 1982;7:1–38.

165. Warr WB, Spangler KM. A novel projection of the ventral nucleus of the trapezoid body in the rat. *Soc Neurosci Abstr* 1989;15:745.

166. Webster DB. Projection of the cochlea to cochlear nuclei in Merriam's kangaroo rat. *J Comp Neurol* 1971;143:323–340.

167. Webster DB, Ackerman RF, Longa GC. Central auditory system of the kangaroo rat, *Dipodomys merriami. J Comp Neurol* 1968;133:477–494.

168. Webster DB, Trune DR. Cochlear nuclear complex of mice. *Am J Anat* 1982;163:103–130.

169. Webster WR, Surviere J, Crewther J, Crewther D. Isofrequency-frequency 2-DG contours in the inferior colliculus of the awake monkey. *Exp Brain Res* 1984;56:425–437.

170. Wenthold RJ. Evidence for a glycinergic pathway connecting the two cochlear nuclei: an immunocytochemical and retrograde transport study. *Brain Res* 1987;415:183–187.

171. Wenthold RJ, Martin MR. Neurotransmitters of the auditory nerve and central auditory system. In: Berlin C, ed. *Hearing science.* San Diego: College-Hill Press, 1984;341–369.

172. Wenthold RJ, Zemple JM, Parakkal MH, Reeks KA, Altschuler RA. Immunocytochemical localization of GABA in the cochlear nucleus of the guinea pig. *Brain Res* 1986;380:7–18.

173. Wenthold RJ, Huie D, Altschuler RA, Reeks KA. Glycine immunoreactivity localized in the cochlear nucleus and superior olivary complex. *Neuroscience* 1987;2:897–912.

174. Whitley JM, Henkel CK. Topographical organization of the inferior collicular projection and other connections of the ventral nucleus of the lateral lemniscus in the cat. *J Comp Neurol* 1984;229:257–270.

175. Wickesberg RE, Oertel D. Tonotopic projection from the dorsal to the anteroventral cochlear nucleus of mice. *J Comp Neurol* 1988;268:389–399.

176. Willard TH, Ryugo DK. Anatomy of the central auditory system. In: Willett JT, ed. *The auditory psychobiology of the mouse.* Springfield, IL: Charles C. Thomas, 1983;201–303.

177. Winter IM, Robertson D, Cole KS. Descending projections from auditory brainstem nuclei to the cochlear nucleus of the guinea pig. *J Comp Neurol* 1989;280:143–157.

178. Wouterlood FG, Mugnaini E. Cartwheel neurons of the dorsal cochlear nucleus: a Golgielectron microscope study in rat. *J Comp Neurol* 1984;227:136–157.

179. Wouterlood F, Mugnaini E, Osen KK, Dahl AL. Stellate neurons in rat dorsal cochlear nucleus with combined Golgi impregnation and electron microscopy: synaptic junctions and mutual coupling by gap junctions. *J Neurocytol* 1984;131:639–664.

180. Wu SH, Oertel D. Intracellular injection with horseradish peroxidase of physiologically characterized stellate and bushy cells in slices of mouse anteroventral cochlear nucleus. *J Neurosci* 1984;4:1577–1588.

181. Yin TCT, Kuwada S. Neuronal mechanisms of binaural interaction. In: Edelman GM, Gall WE, Cowan WM, eds. *Dynamic aspects of neocortical function.* New York: Wiley, 1984;263–313.

182. Yin TCT, Chan JCK, Charney LH. Neural mechanisms of interaural time sensitivity in the cat's auditory brainstem nuclei. *International Union of Physiological Science Satellite Symposium on Hearing.* San Francisco: University of California, 1986;61.

183. Zook JM, Casseday JH. Cytoarchitecture of auditory system in lower brainstem of the mustache bat. *Pteronotus parnellii. J Comp Neurol* 1982;207:1–13.

184. Zook JM, Casseday JH. Origin of ascending projections to inferior colliculus in the mustache bat, *Pteronotus parnellii. J Comp Neurol* 1982;207:14–28.

Neurobiology of Hearing: The Central Auditory System, edited by R. A. Altschuler et al.
Raven Press, Ltd., New York © 1991.

2

The Descending Auditory System

*Kevin M. Spangler and †W. Bruce Warr

Department of Anatomy, Creighton University School of Medicine, Omaha, Nebraska 68178 (currently at Bowman Gray School of Medicine, Wake Forest University, Winston-Salem, North Carolina 27103); †Center for Hearing Research, Boys Town National Research Hospital, Omaha, Nebraska 68131

SCOPE OF THE CHAPTER

There are several levels at which the central nervous system can affect the process of audition. In most mammals, this includes efferent control of the pinna, the middle ear muscles, the organ of Corti, and the central auditory nuclei.

In this chapter, the descending auditory pathways are considered, particularly those allowing for centrifugal control of the auditory nuclei and the organ of Corti. Other reviews related in whole or in part to the descending auditory pathways include those by Pickles (84), Harrison and Howe (41), and Faye-Lund (27,28). More restricted accounts of certain aspects of the descending system can also be found in Warr et al. (119) on the olivocochlear (OC) system and by Winer (*this volume*) on the corticogeniculate system.

THE DESCENDING AUDITORY SYSTEM: REGIONAL FEEDBACK LOOPS OR A DESCENDING CHAIN?

Summary of the Descending Auditory System

The relationship between the main ascending and descending auditory pathways related to one ear are shown in schematic form in Fig. 1. The interconnections between the ascending and descending pathways at different levels are depicted as a series of triangular relationships or loops. Each arm of a loop may represent several separate pathways. For example, the lowest loop shows ascending projections from the cochlea, through the cochlear nucleus to the ipsilateral lateral and contralateral medial zones of the superior olivary complex. These areas in turn contain neurons that project back to the same cochlea and cochlear nucleus that are the source of their predominant afferent innervation.

Feedback Loop or Descending Chain?

The innervation of the cochlea by cells situated in the superior olivary complex was first described by Rasmussen (86), who called the pathway the olivocochlear bundle (OCB) (Fig. 1). Early studies employing electrical stimulation of the OCB found suppression of auditory nerve responses, suggesting that the OCB functions as the substrate for feedback control of the auditory receptor (31,32,127). This view of the OCB as a reflexive pathway has been extended to other parts of the descending auditory system, such that each stage of the descending pathway is considered to be part of a regional feedback loop (113).

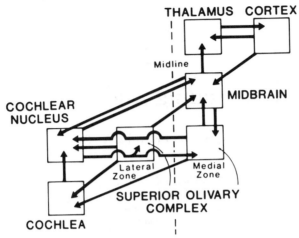

FIG. 1. Schematic representation of the major ascending and descending auditory pathways associated with the cochlea of one side. *Individual arrows* may represent several more than one pathway. Commissural pathways and lesser ipsilateral pathways have been omitted for the sake of clarity. The figure emphasizes the main contralateral flow of excitatory auditory information and the presence of parallel descending pathways. Note that the ascending and descending pathways are interconnected through a series of triangular relationships or loops.

In contrast to the foregoing "loop hypothesis," some studies have suggested that the descending pathways instead form a continuous chain of neurons extending from the auditory cortex to the organ of Corti. Evidence that one can evoke OCB-like effects by stimulating higher auditory centers (23) is especially important to this concept.

Of course, both of these arrangements may coexist. In this chapter we review, level by level, the interconnections of the descending and ascending auditory system. Additionally, we try to evaluate the strength of the descending chain hypothesis by examining the evidence for links between the loops at different levels of the auditory system.

PERIOLIVARY NEURONS OF THE SUPERIOR OLIVARY COMPLEX

The Superior Olivary Complex

The superior olivary complex of mammals consists of three principal nuclei: the medial and lateral superior olivary nuclei and the medial nucleus of the trapezoid body. These are surrounded by loosely arranged cell groups collectively called the periolivary nuclei or PON (Fig. 2). The PON in the cat have been named according to their location relative to either the medial superior olive or the trapezoid body (72). Cells groups homologous to the PON can be identified in other species, although the positions of cells and the nomenclature of the cell groups vary somewhat from species to species. For simplicity, periolivary neurons can be divided into lateral and medial periolivary groups, relative to a line drawn through the axis of the medial superior olive.

Feedback and Reflexive Connections of the Superior Olivary Complex

Based on the observations of the classical neuroanatomists, the principal olivary nuclei were thought to be involved in auditory reflexes (see ref. 85 for a review). However, studies employing anterograde

TABLE 1. *List of abbreviations*

AC	Auditory cortex
AAF	Anterior auditory field
AI	Primary auditory cortex
AII	Secondary auditory cortex
AES	Anterior ectosylvian gyrus
ALPO	Anterolateral periolivary nucleus
AVCN	Anteroventral cochlear nucleus
COCH. N.	Cochlear nucleus
CS	Corpus striatum
D	Dorsal division of the medial geniculate
DC	Caudal dorsal nucleus of the medial geniculate
DCN	Dorsal cochlear nucleus
DD	Deep dorsal nucleus of the medial geniculate
DL	Dorsal lateral nucleus of the pontine gray
DLPO	Dorsolateral periolivary nucleus
DMPO	Dorsomedial periolivary nucleus
DS	Superficial dorsal nucleus of the medial geniculate
EX PYR	Extrapyramidal motor system
G	Globular cells of the anteroventral cochlear nucleus
I	Insular cortex
IC	Inferior colliculus
ICC	Central nucleus of the inferior colliculus
ICCdm	Dorsomedial part of the central nucleus of the inferior colliculus
ICX	External nucleus of the inferior colliculus
ICP	Pericentral nucleus of the inferior colliculus
LNTB	Lateral nucleus of the trapezoid body
LSO	Lateral superior olivary nucleus
M1 & M2	Multipolar cells types in the anteroventral cochlear nucleus
MGB	Medial geniculate body
MGBd	Dorsal division of the medial geniculate
MGBsg	Suprageniculate nucleus of the medial geniculate
MGBv	Ventral division of the medial geniculate
MNTB	Medial nucleus of the trapezoid body
MSO	Medial superior olivary nucleus
NBIC	Nucleus of the brachium of the inferior colliculus
POl	Lateral part of the posterior thalamic group
PON	Periolivary nuclei
PPO	Posterior periolivary nucleus
PVCN	Posteroventral cochlear nucleus
S	Spherical cells of the anteroventral cochlear nucleus
SC	Superior colliculus
SNr	Substantia nigra, pars reticulata
T	Temporal cortex
TEG	Tegmentum of the midbrain
TRN	Thalamic reticular nucleus
VL	Lateral part of the ventral division of the medial geniculate body
Vo	Ovoid part of the ventral division of the medial geniculate body
VLPO	Ventrolateral periolivary nucleus
VMPO	Ventromedial periolivary nucleus
VNTB	Ventral nucleus of the trapezoid body

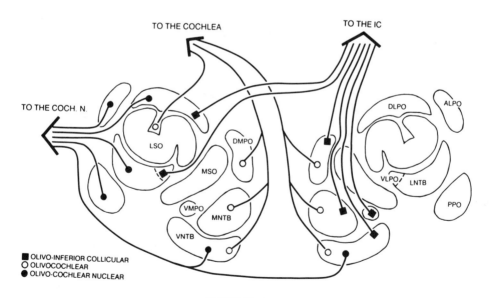

FIG. 2. A two-dimensional representation of the projections of periolivary nuclei. Periolivary nuclei lateral to the medial superior olive project ipsilaterally to the cochlea and cochlear nucleus but contralaterally to the inferior colliculus. Medial periolivary regions project bilaterally (mainly contralaterally) to the COCH. N. and cochlea, but ipsilaterally to the IC. (See Table 1 for abbreviations.)

and retrograde tracing methods in the cat have shown instead that they serve primarily as relays in ascending "lemniscal" pathways (e.g., 1,30,48,103,116). In contrast, the PON contain cells that project, among other places, to the cochlea, the cochlear nucleus, the superior and inferior colliculi, and the facial nucleus (2,22,25,26,86–89,98,115). The projections of the PON may therefore be responsible for reflexive and feedback functions of the superior olivary complex.

CONNECTIONS OF THE PERIOLIVARY NUCLEUS WITH THE COCHLEA

Definition of the Lateral and Medial Olivocochlear Systems

There is now substantial neuroanatomical justification for recognizing two systems of OC neurons, lateral and medial (for review, see ref. 119). The systems take their names from the respective locations of their parent neuronal cell bodies in the lateral and medial regions of the superior olivary complex (Figs. 1 and 2) (117).

Chief among the reasons for distinguishing between the two systems is that, within the organ of Corti, axon terminals of lateral OC neurons mainly contact radial afferent fibers in the inner hair cell region, whereas axon terminals of medial OC neurons form direct synaptic contacts with outer hair cells (Fig. 3). The functions of the lateral OC system are still unknown, but their connections suggest a direct axo-axonic effect on cochlear nerve fibers (60). The available evidence suggests that the medial OC system suppresses activity in cochlear nerve fibers indirectly through a mechanism involving outer hair cells, perhaps by modulating their motility (37). In the following

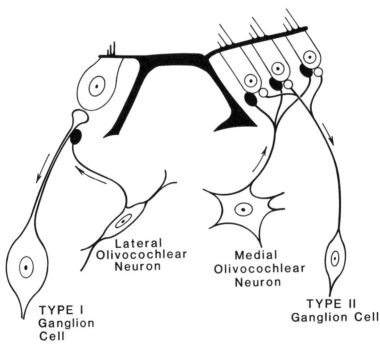

FIG. 3. Organization of the lateral and medial olivocochlear (OC) systems. Lateral OC neurons project to the region beneath the inner hair cells where they form axo-axonic contacts on the dendrites of Type I spiral ganglion cells. Medial OC neurons project to the region beneath the outer hair cells and synapse directly with them (38,61).

sections, the major neuroanatomical features of the lateral and medial OC systems are summarized.

The Lateral Olivocochlear System

Lateral OC neurons are small fusiform cells, approximately 1,000 of which project to each cochlea in the cat and guinea pig (91,115).

In all species studied to date, lateral OC neurons are characterized by having an intimate topographic relationship with the lateral superior olivary nucleus. This intimacy ranges from the extreme condition found in rodents, where they lie more or less entirely within the neuropil of the lateral superior olive, to the conditions found in primates (105) and bats (9), where these cells form a separate, but immediately adjacent, PON. In rodents, lateral OC neurons have an apparent tonotopic organization similar to that of the lateral superior olive (91, 109,110,124).

Because these lateral OC axons are un-myelinated, recordings of unit responses from these neurons have not yet been obtained. Projections of lateral OC neurons are primarily ipsilateral (Fig. 2) and form the bulk of the inner and tunnel spiral bundles of the organ of Corti (13,38,39,102). The principal postsynaptic targets of this projection are the radial afferent fibers, each of which is contacted by 5 to 30 synapses. The low spontaneous rate units are the most heavily innervated (60).

The sources of innervation of lateral OC neurons (Fig. 4) appear to reside in the ipsilateral ventral cochlear nucleus (106). Spherical and multipolar cells of the ipsilateral anteroventral cochlear nucleus have been found to project to the lateral superior olivary nucleus, which in the rat contains the lateral OC neurons (17,116,124). Synaptic terminals on the OC neurons are virtually lacking on the soma but are found sparsely on the proximal dendrites and contain mainly small round or pleomorphic vesicles (45,104,121). This type of axon terminal is identical to one of the three types of endings found on the principal neurons

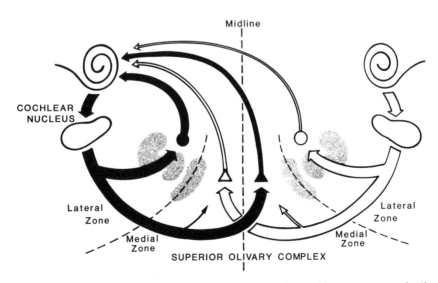

FIG. 4. The organization of ascending auditory inputs to the olivocochlear neurons projecting to one cochlea is schematically shown. *Solid arrows* show that major loops feedback to the side of stimulus origin. *Open arrows* depict lesser pathways underlying the influence of one cochlea on the other.

in the lateral superior olive of the rat and probably also the cat (16,121,123), meaning that the principal cells and the lateral OC neurons share a common source of synaptic input, probably arising from a class of multipolar cells in the ventral cochlear nucleus.

The Medial Olivocochlear System

Medial OC neurons are large to medium-sized stellate cells, some 500 of which project to each cochlea in the cat and guinea pig (15,91). In most species, medial OC neurons make up a somewhat scattered population within the medial periolivary zone, partially encircling the medial superior olivary nucleus. Most of these cells are found from middle to rostral levels of the superior olivary complex and some extend to the levels of the ventral nucleus of the lateral lemniscus (91,115,124). The dendrites of medial OC neurons form a meshwork through which most of the crossed and uncrossed axons of the trapezoid body pass (Fig. 2).

Inputs to medial OC neurons are derived from the ventral cochlear nucleus bilaterally, but mainly from the opposite side (106) and possibly also from the ipsilateral inferior colliculus (IC) (28). Several distinct types of synaptic terminals contact medial OC neurons. The most prevalent type contains round-to-oval vesicles, often accompanied by some dense-cored vesicles, depending on the species (45,104,122,123). In the rat, one type of ending has striking similarities to the calyces of Held found on neighboring principal cells of the medial nucleus of the trapezoid body, raising the possibility of an input arising from globular cells of the ventral cochlear nucleus (72, 123).

Most medial OC neurons project to the side from which they receive their excitatory afferent input. Since that input itself is crossed, some 60% to 70% of medial OC neurons have crossed projections (115) (Fig. 4). Paradoxically, therefore, the crossed OCB represents a feedback pathway to the side from which the medial OC neurons receive their acoustic input. As shown in Fig. 4, the projections of the remaining 30% to 40% of medial OC neurons, which are uncrossed, represent in reality an intercochlear pathway by which inputs from one ear can affect the functioning of the other ear (115,118).

Medial OC neurons give rise to myelinated fibers (10), which, like lateral OC axons, travel in the OCB to the cochlea (86,87). As they leave the brain via the vestibular nerve, they send collaterals to the ventral cochlear nucleus (80). After joining the cochlear nerve, the axons branch several times in their course through the intraganglionic spiral bundle, lose their myelin sheath upon entering the organ of Corti, cross the tunnel of Corti as upper tunnel radial fibers, and terminate at the bases of outer hair cells (13).

INTERCONNECTIONS OF THE COCHLEAR NUCLEUS, PERIOLIVARY NUCLEUS, AND INFERIOR COLLICULUS

The Periolivary Projection to the Cochlear Nucleus

Studies using both retrograde and anterograde transport have established that the PON have a massive projection to the cochlear nucleus. Terminals of this projection are found throughout the dorsal, anteroventral, and posteroventral subdivisions of the cochlear nuclear complex. The number of cells that project to the cochlear nucleus in the cat is estimated to be 6,800 (100). Although this number may include some OC neurons with collaterals to the cochlear nucleus, it is still several times greater than the number of neurons projecting to the cochlea in that species (10,115).

The majority of the neurons projecting to one cochlear nucleus (Fig. 2) are located ipsilaterally in the lateral nucleus of the trapezoid body or its extensions (the posterior periolivary nucleus and anterolateral periolivary nucleus) and contralaterally in the ventral nucleus of the trapezoid body (2,22,26,100). These neurons are the largest population of cells in the PON and are found in all periolivary regions except (a) the ventromedial PON, whose cells project only to the midbrain (2,99), (b) in the dorsal hilus of the lateral superior olive where lateral OC neurons are located (115), and (c) beneath the ventral hilus of the lateral superior olive (the ventrolateral PON, see Fig. 2), where, again, only midbrain projecting cells are found (2,99,109).

Many of the cells in the periolivary regions and many axon terminals within the cochlear nucleus are immunoreactive to antibodies specific for glycine (4), gamma-aminobutyric acid (GABA) (105), or its synthesizing enzyme glutamic acid decarboxylase (68,90). Many PON cells will also transport [3H]GABA in a retrograde fashion (81). These facts suggest that the descending PON projection is largely inhibitory.

In studies using anterograde transport of tritiated leucine, some evidence was found for a tonotopic organization of the projection from the PON to the cochlear nucleus. This indicates that although the individual PON project to all cochlear nuclear subdivisions, the projections are likely to be frequency specific (14,100).

Descending Projections from the Inferior Colliculus

Projections from the Inferior Colliculus and Related Structures to the Periolivary Nuclei

Several studies describe a colliculo-olivary projection with origins in the external and adjacent part of the central nucleus of the IC (8,69,88), while Hashikawa and Kawamura (44) found the cells of origin to be in the central, pericentral, dorsomedial, and commissural parts of the IC. Descending projections have also been described as arising from: (a) the ventral nucleus of the lateral lemniscus (56,125), (b) the superior colliculus (46), and (c) the nucleus of the brachium of the IC (47). The course and terminations of all of these projections are very similar in that axons descend in the lateral lemniscus and filter down through the medial periolivary region, giving some terminals to the dorsomedial PON and the ventral nucleus of the trapezoid body (or its homologue in rodents). Apparently the lateral periolivary region is altogether free of a direct projection from the midbrain in the cat and rat, although a midbrain influence could be mediated by way of a relay in the ventral nucleus of the trapezoid body since it projects to the lateral periolivary cell groups (Fig. 5) (100).

Although the specific postsynaptic targets for the colliculo-olivary axons have not been firmly established, the question of whether they contact OC neurons is crucial to the idea that the OC neurons are the last link in a descending chain. Anderson et al. (8) made combined injections of horseradish peroxidase (HRP) and tritiated leucine in the IC and found that the anterograde labeling of axon terminals was located only around HRP-filled cells in the ventral nucleus of the trapezoid body, suggesting that the descending inputs end on midbrain-projecting cells, making it a reciprocal projection. On the other hand, Faye-Lund (28) reported that in the rat the descending fibers end instead in the region containing the acetylcholinesterase- (AChE) positive OC neurons and neurons projecting to the cochlear nucleus. Clearly, this important issue needs further study.

Colliculocochlear Nuclear Projections

Numerous studies using anterograde transport (8,52) or anterograde degeneration (12,28,88,111) have demonstrated a bilateral projection of thin fibers from the IC

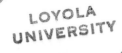

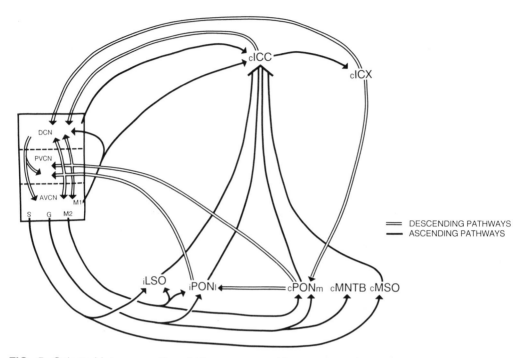

FIG. 5. Selected interconnections between one cochlear nucleus, the superior olivary nuclei bilaterally, and the contralateral inferior colliculus. Lower case "c" and "i" indicate contralateral and ipsilateral, and "m" and "l" medial and lateral, respectively. The cochlear nucleus, and its three subnuclei, the DCN, PVCN, and AVCN nuclei, are enclosed in the box at the left. In the AVCN, letters (S, G, M1, M2) represent individual cell types, whose projections are known. See text for description of projections. (See Table 1 for abbreviations.)

to the cochlear nuclei. Most fibers course through the caudal trapezoid body to terminate in the contralateral dorsal cochlear nucleus in a manner similar to the "centrifugal bundle" of Lorente de Nó (59). Kane and Conlee (52) reported that a few fibers also innervated the anteroventral cochlear nucleus. In these studies, the number of fibers projecting to the cochlear nucleus was thought to be rather small. In contrast, retrograde transport studies indicate that the number of neurons projecting to the cochlear nuclei is large (5,28,43,44). Faye-Lund (28) found four to five times the number of cells projecting to the cochlear nucleus as projecting to the superior olivary complex. A few fibers also apparently descend to the cochlear nuclei from the nuclei of the lateral lemniscus (21,56,125).

Cellular Aspects

The cells giving rise to the projection to the cochlear nuclear complex were reportedly found in the deep part of the external and throughout the central nucleus (28,43). They therefore have a slightly wider distribution than colliculo-olivary parent neurons. Conlee and Kane (21) reported that axons from cells in different parts of the colliculus had slightly different targets in the dorsal cochlear nucleus such that the pericentral and dorsal parts of the central nucleus projected to the outer fusiform and molecular layers, while ventral collicular regions projected to fusiform cell bodies and proximal dendrites as well as to giant cells in the deep layer of the dorsal cochlear nucleus.

Colliculopontine Projections

The IC also gives rise to a projection to the dorsolateral part of the pontine nucleus (43,53); this same region is the target of projections from the auditory cortex and the superior colliculus (6,7,53,67). Hashikawa (43) reported that most of the colliculopontine cells were found in the intercollicular zone, with a smaller number found in the central nucleus.

The Relationship of Ascending and Descending Pathways in the Lower Auditory System

1. *Loops in the lower auditory system.* In Fig. 5, selected interconnections of the cochlear nucleus, superior olivary complex, and the IC are illustrated, emphasizing the pathways that may be part of feedback loops.

2. *Projections of the cochlear nuclei to the PON.* There is substantial evidence that the cochlear nucleus of one side projects to the ipsilateral lateral and contralateral medial periolivary regions. These projections most probably originate from globular and multipolar cells in the cochlear nucleus (42, 85,107,116). Dorsal and caudal periolivary regions additionally receive input from the posteroventral cochlear nucleus via the intermediate acoustic stria (29,116). Globular and spherical cells (Fig. 5) provide input to the principal nuclei of the superior olivary complex (72,116).

3. *The connections of the PON and the cochlear nucleus.* The PON have descending projections to the cochlea and cochlear nucleus. At the cellular level the projections to the cochlear nucleus are probably only partially reciprocal (100). The periolivary projection to the cochlear nucleus terminates in virtually all regions of that structure, but the PON is only known to receive afferents from multipolar, globular cells and octopus cells of the ventral cochlear nucleus, as described above.

4. *Connections of the inferior colliculus with the PON and cochlear nucleus.* The IC receives input from, among other places, the contralateral lateral and ipsilateral medial periolivary regions (116), the multipolar cells of the anteroventral cochlear nucleus (3), and the dorsal cochlear nucleus (1,75,79) (see Fig. 5). For the most part, axons from lower auditory structures terminate in bands in the central nucleus of the IC and contact both the discoid and stellate cells found there (78). However, it is not known if ascending axons directly contact the collicular neurons that give rise to descending projections (see ref. 44), in addition to the colliculogeniculate and intrinsic neurons. In fact, none of the afferent inputs to IC neurons with descending projections has been specifically demonstrated.

Despite this, from Fig. 5, several possible loops involving the IC can be described. For example, the dorsal cochlear nucleus projects to the IC (75), which in turn projects back to the dorsal cochlear nucleus. The IC also is involved in a fairly simple loop with the medial PON. Several additional, more complex loops are possible if: (a) the central nucleus of the IC to the external nucleus of the IC projection is considered (57), (b) descending collicular axons contact the PON neurons that project to the cochlear nucleus, and (c) the collicular projection to the dorsal cochlear nucleus contacts the cells of origin of the intrinsic connections within the cochlear nucleus (18,59).

Functions of the Lower Auditory Feedback Loops

Few studies have devoted their attention to the function of the lower auditory feedback loops (see ref. 84 for review). Electrical stimulation of the lateral part of the superior olivary region produced inhibition of single units in the ipsilateral cochlear nucleus, while stimulation of more medial regions produced excitation. Some of these effects led to the release of acetylcholine or were influenced by the application of cholinergic blocking agents (19,20). Other studies demonstrated a modulatory effect of contralateral sound stimulation on the activity of neurons in the cochlear nucleus (83). Although these studies have provided us with some interesting clues to the function of the descending pathways, they are subject to several criticisms including a lack of specificity concerning which descending pathways were being stimulated and an overemphasis on the role of acetylcholine.

DESCENDING PROJECTIONS FROM THE AUDITORY CORTEX

Introduction

Studies in the cat and other mammals have amply documented the existence of projections from the auditory cortex to the medial geniculate body (MGB) and the IC. For reviews of the early literature, see papers by Morest (73), Whitlock and Nauta (126), and Faye-Lund (27). Within the past 30 years these corticofugal pathways in the cat have been re-examined with the methods of anterograde degeneration (24,51,58, 111,113); anterograde transport of radiolabeled protein (6,7) and retrograde transport of HRP (49,97). Additionally, because of the largely reciprocal nature of the corticogeniculate connections, papers on the ascending projections of the MGB also have import for consideration of the descending pathways (see elsewhere in this volume). The corticogeniculate projections have also been studied in other animal models (e.g., opossum [63,128], rat [11,27,112,130], monkey [34,126], tree shrew [76,77]).

General Considerations of the Corticofugal Pathways

Large numbers of efferent axons leave the auditory cortex and descend in the in-

ternal capsule. Some axons leave the internal capsule to terminate in the corpus striatum (24,111,120), the pulvinar, and the suprageniculate and thalamic reticular nuclei (24). The corticofugal fibers then continue ventrally and posteriorly and run through the lateral part of the posterior group and the ventral aspect of the MGB between the ventral and medial divisions. Terminals within the MGB are arranged in several continuous arrays, in the anterior-posterior axis (6,24). Some fibers continue through the MGB, entering the brachium of the IC, giving off terminals to its intrinsic nucleus and other neighboring structures, such as the superior colliculus (6,24,111). Eventually the corticofugal fibers enter the lateral aspect of the IC to spread out over its lateral and dorsal parts (excluding the central nucleus), with some also passing in the collicular commissure to the dorsomedial part of the contralateral IC. A few fibers descend in the cerebral peduncle, eventually terminating in tegmental structures or the dorsolateral pontine gray (6,7,24,111).

The auditory cortex, the MGB, and the IC each can be divided into several cytoarchitectonic and/or functional subdivisions. Several schemes have been used to divide the auditory cortex (6,7,95); for present purposes we will group cortical areas (after refs. 6,7) into tonotopic fields that include the primary auditory cortex (AI) and the anterior auditory field (AAF), and non-tonotopically organized fields ("diffuse system") represented by AII and the temporal area (T). The MGB has been divided into three divisions (71,129): dorsal, ventral, and medial, each of which can be subdivided (see Fig. 6). The ventral division is tonotopically organized and is the target of the main ascending "core" projection from the IC (57,70,111). The IC has been subdivided according to two main schemes (74,92,93); the simpler scheme recognizes a central nucleus with a central part and a dorsomedial part; a pericentral nucleus and an external nucleus (92,93). This nomencla-

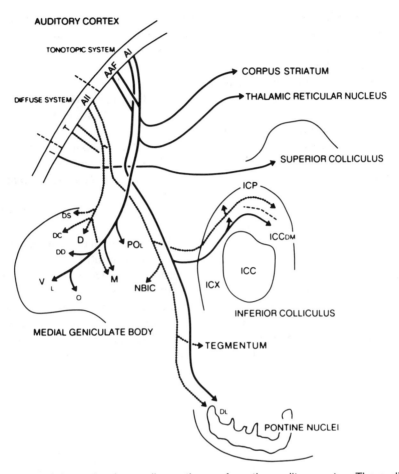

FIG. 6. Summary of the major descending pathways from the auditory cortex. The auditory cortex is subdivided here into a tonotopic system, represented by AI and the AAF, and a diffuse system, represented by AII and T. Insular cortex is also included. The projections of the tonotopic system and insula are illustrated by *solid lines*: those of the diffuse system by *dotted lines*. Both the tonotopic and diffuse systems have separate outflows, one to thalamic and/or forebrain structures and the other to midbrain and pontine structures. Refer to the text for further details. (See Table 1 for abbreviations.)

ture was adopted here because it is consistent with that used in several of the important connectional studies.

In the cat the results of numerous studies (6,7,24,111) suggest that (a) each subdivision of the auditory cortex projects mainly to one division of the MGB, (b) most cortical areas have subsidiary connections to other MGB divisions, (c) almost all subdivisions of the cortex project at least some fibers to the medial division, (d) the cortical subdivisions project not only to certain areas of the MGB but also to parts of the midbrain that in turn supply afferents to those same geniculate areas, and (e) tonotopically organized areas of the cortex and the MGB are reciprocally related, as is true for the nontonotopically organized regions of the two structures.

Cellular Aspects of the Corticofugal Projections

Overall, the descending projections are considered to be quite massive, involving many of the cells in layers V and VI of the auditory cortex (55,65,66,77,131). Indeed the number of cortical cells projecting to at least the ventral and dorsal divisions of the MGB are estimated to be roughly equal to the total number of cells contributing ascending inputs to those two same subdivisions (97). Cells from layers V that project to the IC are large pyramidal cells (65,131), while those projecting to the MGB are smaller cells in layers V and VI (65,131).

Descending corticogeniculate axons are relatively thin and, in the ventral division, end mainly on the dendrites of principal cells, outside of the synaptic nests (62,73), but they also contact Golgi type II cell bodies and proximal dendrites. The synaptic endings of presumed corticogeniculate axons are small (<0.5 μm), contain pleomorphic vesicles, and form asymmetric synapses (73). The terminals of corticofugal axons in dorsomedial part of the central nu-

cleus of the IC contain round synaptic vesicles and end in asymmetric synaptic contacts (94).

Loops Involving the Primary Auditory Cortex

The Main Connections of the Primary Auditory Cortex with the Medial Geniculate Body and the Inferior Colliculus

Corticogeniculate Limb

There seems to be general agreement that the primary auditory area (AI in cats) is reciprocally connected to the ventral division of the MGB (6,49) (see Fig. 7A). These connections are topographic and organized tonotopically (6,49,97). The cortical axons in the lateral part of the ventral division terminate in parallel sheets that correspond in

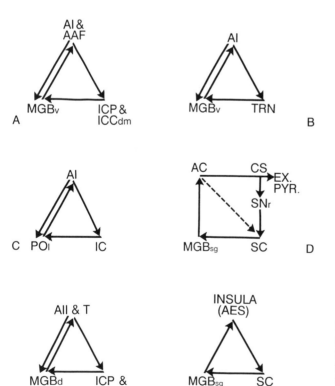

FIG. 7.A–F: The connections of the subdivisions of the auditory cortex with midbrain and thalamic structures can be illustrated as separate triangular relationships or loops. See text for details of specific loops.

a general way to the fibrodendritic laminae described in this subdivision (6,71). Terminal labeling found in pars ovidae is not obviously laminated. Likewise, in individual experiments, the topographic relationship between AI and the medial division is not apparent, although the position of labeling varies with different injection sites (6).

Injections of radiolabeled amino acids into one of the tonotopically organized parts of auditory cortex results in labeling that only partially fills an isofrequency region of the ventral division of the MGB (16,49). The remainder of the isofrequency region receives projections from the other tonotopically organized auditory cortical fields. So, by injecting several tonotopically related cortical areas in the same animal, Imig and Morel (49) were able to show that there are complex but continuous three-dimensional arrays connecting isofrequency regions of the medial and ventral subdivisions of the MGB. These arrays also extend rostrally into the lateral part of the posterior group, suggesting a functional continuity between the lateral part of the posterior thalamic group and the ventral division (6,49,50).

Corticocollicular Connections

In cats AI also projects to the IC in a topographic, tonotopic manner (7). The cortical projection ends in sheet-like arrays in the dorsomedial part of the central nucleus bilaterally and the lateral and deeper medial parts of the pericentral nucleus ipsilaterally (7,24). These regions correspond largely to the dorsal and caudal "cortices" of the IC (74). Axons from AI reach the IC through the brachium of the IC and course through the external nucleus, but give off few if any terminals in that region (7,24,111). It it also generally agreed that axons from AI do not enter the central nucleus (7,24,74,111). The anterior auditory field, also tonotopically organized, sends similar but lesser projections to the IC (7).

The same basic projections from the primary auditory cortex to the IC exist in other species (e.g., 27,63,77,128; but see Fitzpatrick and Imig [33] who show terminals in the central nucleus in the monkey).

Colliculogeniculate Projections

The areas that receive input from AI (pericentral and dorsomedial part of central nucleus) receive a portion of their auditory input from the central nucleus (57) or from lower auditory structures in the main ascending pathway (1,79). They also project to basically the same areas of the MGB that are the targets of the central nucleus (ventral and medial divisions). These projections close the loop described in Fig. 7A and suggest that the cortex can affect not only a specific area of the MGB but also the nuclei providing ascending input to that area of the MGB.

Corticoreticulogeniculate Loop

At least in the cat, a loop connecting AI, the thalamic reticular nucleus, and the MGB can be defined (Fig. 7B). AI is known to project to a specific part of the thalamic reticular nucleus (6,24,111). The thalamic reticular nucleus, which contains neurons with glutamic acid decarboxylase-like and somatostatin-like immunoreactivities (36, 101) projects to parts of ventral and dorsal divisions of the MGB (96). These areas are also reciprocally connected to the auditory cortex. This loop provides a means for another, probably inhibitory, influence of the cortex on the MGB.

Cortical Loop with the Inferior Colliculus and the Lateral Posterior Thalamic Group

The connectional loop of the auditory cortex with the lateral part of the posterior thalamic group is shown in Fig. 7C. Jones and Powell (51) have suggested that the posterior thalamic group acts as an extension of the intralaminar nuclei, since they are reciprocally connected with the lateral cortical regions between area 4 and the visual cortex (in the cat) and they receive ascending sensory input (69,70). Others have suggested instead that the POL is simply an extension of the ventral division (50) or the deep dorsal nucleus (6).

Corticostriatal Pathways

Auditory cortex, especially AI, projects, somewhat topographically, onto the caudate and putamen (corpus striatum, ref. 120). As suggested by Fig. 7D, this leads to several effector pathways. The striatum has numerous extrapyramidal connections and could in this way mediate auditory cortical influence on the motor systems. Among these pathways is the striatonigral projection that terminates in the substantia nigra (SN), pars reticulata. It is this portion of the SN that gives rise to the nigrotectal projection (25,40). By this route, the striatonigral projection may convey certain auditory cortical information (pertinent to motor events) to the superior colliculus, in much the same way that May and Hall (64) have suggested is the case for some saccade-related visual cortical information.

Projections of Nonprimary Cortex

Connections of Nontonotopically Organized Fields and the Temporal Area

A loop involving AII and T is illustrated in Fig. 7E. AII and T are grouped together because of, and can be distinguished from other auditory cortical areas by, their lack of tonotopic organization and distinct binaural interaction columns, the broad tuning curves of their neurons, and their lack of and strong connections with the dorsal division of the MGB (6). As shown in Figs. 6 and 7E, they are reciprocally connected to portions of the dorsal (especially caudal

dorsal and ventral lateral nuclei) and medial divisions of the MGB. They also project to the medial and lateral parts of the pericentral nucleus of the IC, as well as to certain tegmental structures, including NBIC, and the regions near the dorsal nucleus of the lateral lemniscus (e.g., 6,24,111). Except for the medial division of MGB and parts of the IC, these connections are largely separate from those of AI. In the IC, the projections to the dorsal cortex reportedly end in more superficial portions than those from AI (7). AII also apparently lacks projections to the thalamic reticular nucleus and the posterior group, although it does project to the same pontine nuclei as AI (7). The tectal and tegmental targets of AII have ascending projections to the MGB, particularly the dorsal subdivision, thereby closing the loop.

A Loop Involving Insular Cortex

Parts of the anterior and posterior sylvian gyri, including what has been called the "insular" cortex in the cat, are among the cortical areas that project to the superior colliculus (54,108; but see ref. 82). Auditory cortical projections to the superior colliculus are thought to terminate mainly in the deep layers (e.g., 111), although some reports suggest terminations in superficial layers as well (82). The intermediate and deep layers of the superior colliculus in turn project to the suprageniculate nucleus of the dorsal division of MGB and many other targets (35). As indicated in Fig. 7F, the suprageniculate nucleus projects to the insular cortex. Unlike most thalamocortical connections, the projection of the suprageniculate to the insular cortex is apparently not reciprocal (see Winer, *this volume*). It may be that this loop has an homology in the connections of area D in the tree shrew auditory cortex, where (a) area D projects to the suprageniculate and to the superior colliculus, (b) the superior colliculus projects to the suprageniculate, and (c) the suprageniculate projects back to area D (76,77).

Functional Considerations

The functions of the descending pathways from the cortex to MGB and the IC are not known. Stimulation of AI has generally been found to have an inhibitory effect on cells in the ventral nucleus of the MGB, although facilitation has also been reported (98,114). Wantanabe et al. (114) reported a large number of MGB cells that were not responsive to cortical stimulation, a finding that is difficult to reconcile with other studies and with the reported density of innervation. The functions in the MGB that are most or least affected by cortical inputs are not known, but it is thought that some of the discontinuities and slight nonreciprocities in the projections may be related to some aspect of processing such as binaural interactions or frequency selectivity (see Winer, *this volume*).

Neurons of the IC can either be inhibited or facilitated by cortical stimulation (67). A portion of both the cortically inhibited and facilitated cells in turn project to the MGB (67). If the cortex is modulating the MGB indirectly through pathways described by the loop, the functions of these connections are not known. The cells that receive cortical input but do not project to the MGB may be Golgi type II neurons or cells participating in the descending pathways (44). Direct electrophysiological evidence is lacking for cortical excitatory (or inhibitory) effects on IC neurons with descending projections.

SUMMARY AND COMMENT

1. The descending auditory system can be described most conservatively as a series of loosely interconnected regional feedback loops. In general, a population of descending neurons will project back to the side (ipsilateral or contralateral), to the nucleus or subnucleus, and often to the very cells that, directly or indirectly, provide their ascending excitatory input. Most of the descending projections have been found to be more or less tonotopic.

2. Few links between loops at different levels of the auditory system have been established, although several are possible. Indeed, some populations of descending neurons appear to be free of input from higher auditory centers. If a descending chain of neurons exists, much work remains before its component neurons can be defined from the auditory cortex to the inner ear.

3. The activity in almost any auditory neuron in the central nervous system could be affected, directly or indirectly, because of the extensive nature of the descending projections. Especially extensive are the projections to the cochlea, cochlear nucleus, and the medial geniculate. However, several individual nuclei such as the central nucleus of the IC, and the medial and lateral superior olives do not receive direct descending input.

REFERENCES

1. Adams JC. Ascending projections to the inferior colliculus. *J Comp Neurol* 1979;183:519–538.
2. Adams JC. Cytology of periolivary cells and the organization of their projections in cat. *J Comp Neurol* 1983;215:275–289.
3. Adams JC. Multipolar cells in the ventral cochlear nucleus project to the dorsal cochlear nucleus and the inferior colliculus. *Neurosci Lett* 1983;37:205–208.
4. Adams JC, Wenthold RJ. Immunostaining of GABA-ergic and glycinergic inputs to the anteroventral cochlear nucleus. *Neurosci Abstr* 1987;13:1259.
5. Adams JC, Warr WB. Origins of axons in the cat's acoustic striae determined by injection of horseradish peroxidase into severed tracts. *J Comp Neurol* 1976;170:107–122.
6. Anderson RA, Knight PL, Merzenich MM. The thalamocortical and corticothalamic connections of AI, AII, and the anterior auditory field (AAF): in the cat: evidence for two largely segregated systems of connections. *J Comp Neurol* 1980;194:663–701.
7. Anderson RA, Snyder RL, Merzenich MM. The topographic organization of corticocollicular projections from physiologically identified loci in the AI, AII, and anterior auditory

fields of the cat. *J Comp Neurol* 1980;191:479–494.

8. Andersen RA, Roth GL, Aitkin LM, Merzenich MM. The efferent projections of the central nucleus and the pericentral nucleus of the inferior colliculus in the cat. *J Comp Neurol* 1980;194:649–662.

9. Aschoff A, Ostwald J. Different origins of cochlear efferents in some bat species, rats and guinea pigs. *J Comp Neurol* 1987;264:56–72.

10. Arnesen AR, Osen KK. Fibre population of the vestibulocochlear anatomosis in the cat. *Acta Otolaryngol* 1984;98:25–269.

11. Beyerl BD. Afferent projections to the central nucleus of the inferior colliculus in the rat. *Brain Res* 1978;145:209–223.

12. Borg E. A neuroanatomical study of the brainstem auditory system of the rabbit. Part II: Descending connections. *Acta Morphol Neerl Scand* 1983;11:49–62.

13. Brown MC. Morphology of labeled efferent fibers in the guinea pig cochlea. *J Comp Neurol* 1987;260:605–618.

14. Bourk TR, Mielcarz JP, Norris BE. Tonotopic organization of the anteroventral cochlear nucleus of the cat. *Hear Res* 1981;4:215–241.

15. Buno W Jr. Auditory nerve fibre activity influenced by contralateral ear sound stimulation. *Exp Neurol* 1978;59:67–74.

16. Cant NB. The fine structure of the lateral superior olivary nucleus of the cat. *J Comp Neurol* 1984;227:63–77.

17. Cant NB, Casseday JH. Projections from the anteroventral cochlear nucleus to the lateral and medial superior olivary nuclei. *J Comp Neurol* 1986;247:457–477.

18. Cant NB, Gaston KC. Pathways connecting the right and left cochlear nuclei. *J Comp Neurol* 1982;212:313–326.

19. Comis SD. Centrifugal inhibitory processes affecting neurons in the cat cochlear nuclei. *J Physiol (Lond)* 1970;210:751–760.

20. Comis SD, Whitfield IC. Influence of centrifugal pathways on unit activity in the cochlear nucleus. *J Neurophysiol* 1968;31:62–68.

21. Conlee JW, Kane ES. Descending projections from the inferior colliculus to the dorsal cochlear nucleus in the cat: an autoradiographic study. *Neuroscience* 1982;7:161–178.

22. Covey E, Jones DR, Casseday JH. Projections from the superior olivary complex to the cochlear nucleus in the tree shrew. *J Comp Neurol* 1984;226:289–305.

23. Desmedt JE. Physiological studies of the efferent recurrent auditory system. In: Keidel WD, Neff WD, eds. *Handbook of sensory physiology*, vol V/II. Berlin: Springer-Verlag, 1975;219–246.

24. Diamond IT, Jones EG, Powell TPS. The projection of the auditory cortex upon the diencephalon and brainstem in the cat. *Brain Res* 1969;15:305–340.

25. Edwards SB, Ginsburg CL, Henkel CK, Stein BE. Sources of subcortical projections to the superior colliculus in the cat. *J Comp Neurol* 1979;184:309–330.

26. Elverland HH. Descending connections between superior olivary and cochlear nuclear complexes in the cat studied by autoradiographic and horseradish peroxidase methods. *Exp Brain Res* 1977;27:397–412.

27. Faye-Lund H. The neocortical projection to the inferior colliculus in the albino rat. *Anat Embryol* 1985;173:53–70.

28. Faye-Lund H. Projection from the inferior colliculus to the superior olivary complex in the albino rat. *Anat Embryol* 1986;175:35–52.

29. Fernandez C, Karapas F. Course and termination of the striae of Monakow and Held in the cat. *J Comp Neurol* 1967;131:371–386.

30. Glendenning KK, Masterton RB. Acoustic chiasm: efferent projections of the lateral superior olive. *J Neurosci* 1983;3:1521–1537.

31. Fex J. Auditory activity in centrifugal and centripetal fibres in cat. A study of the feedback system. *Acta Physiol Scand* 1962;55(suppl 189):1–68.

32. Fex J. Auditory activity in uncrossed centrifugal cochlear fibres in cat. *Acta Physiol Scand* 1965;64:43–57.

33. Fitzpatrick KA, Imig TA. Projections of auditory cortex upon the thalamus and midbrain in the owl monkey. *J Comp Neurol* 1978;177:537–556.

34. Forbes BF, Moskowitz N. Projections of auditory responsive cortex in the squirrel monkey. *Brain Res* 1974;64:239–254.

35. Graham J. An autoradiographic study of the efferent connections of the superior colliculus in the cat. *J Comp Neurol* 1977;173:629–654.

36. Graybiel AM, Elde RP. Somatostatin-like immunoreactivity characterizes neurons of the nucleus reticularis thalami in the cat and monkey. *J Neurosci* 1983;3:1308–1321.

37. Guinan JJ. Effect of efferent neural activity on cochlear mechanics. *Scand Audiol Suppl* 1986;25:53–62.

38. Guinan JJ Jr, Warr WB, Norris BE. Differential olivocochlear projections from lateral versus medial zones of the superior olivary complex. *J Comp Neurol* 1983;221:358–370.

39. Guinan JJ Jr, Warr WB, Norris BE. Topographic organization of the olivocochlear projections from the lateral and medial zones of the superior olivary complex. *J Comp Neurol* 1984;226:21–27.

40. Hall WC, May PJ. The anatomic basis for sensorimotor transformations in the superior colliculus. In: Neff WD, ed. *Contributions to sensory physiology*, vol 8. New York: Academic Press, 1984;1–40.

41. Harrison JM, Howe ME. Anatomy of the descending auditory system (mammalian). In: Keidel WD, Neff WD, eds. *Handbook of sensory physiology*, vol V/I. Berlin: Springer-Verlag, 1974;363–388.

42. Harrison JM, Warr WB. A study of the cochlear nuclei and the ascending auditory path-

ways of the medulla. *J Comp Neurol* 1962; 119:341–380.

43. Hashikawa T. The inferior colliculopontine neurons of the cat in relation to other collicular descending neurons. *J Comp Neurol* 1983; 219:241–249.

44. Hashikawa T, Kawamura K. Retrograde labeling of ascending and descending neurons in the inferior colliculus. A fluorescent double labeling study in the cat. *Exp Brain Res* 1983; 49:457–461.

45. Helfert RH, Schwartz IR, Ryan AF. Ultrastructural characterization of gerbil olivocochlear neurons based on differential uptake of 3H-D-aspartic acid and a wheatgerm agglutinin-horseradish peroxidase conjugate of the cochlea. *J Neurosci* 1988;8:3111–3123.

46. Henkel CK, Edwards SB. The superior colliculus control of pinna movements in the cat: possible anatomical connections. *J Comp Neurol* 1978;182:763–776.

47. Henkel CK, Whitley JW. Descending projections of the nucleus of the brachium of the inferior colliculus. *Anat Rec* 1981;199:110.

48. Henkel CK, Spangler KM. Organization of the efferent projections of the medial superior olivary nucleus in the cat as revealed by HRP and autoradiographic tracing methods. *J Comp Neurol* 1983;221:415–428.

49. Imig TJ, Morel A. Topographic and cytoarchitectonic organization of thalamic neurons related to their targets in low-, middle- and high-frequency representations in cat auditory cortex. *J Comp Neurol* 1984;227:511–539.

50. Imig TJ, Morel A. Tonotopic organization in lateral part of posterior group of thalamic nuclei in the cat. *J Neurophysiol* 1985;53:836–851.

51. Jones EG, Powell TPS. An analysis of the posterior group of thalamic nuclei on the basis of its afferent connections. *J Comp Neurol* 1971; 143:185–216.

52. Kane ES, Conlee JW. Descending inputs to the caudal cochlear nucleus of the cat: degeneration and autoradiographic studies. *J Comp Neurol* 1979;187:759–784.

53. Kawamura K. The pontine projection from the inferior colliculus in the cat. An experimental anatomical study. *Brain Res* 1975;95:309–322.

54. Kawamura K, Konno T. Various types of corticotectal neurons of cats as demonstrated by means of retrograde axonal transport of horseradish peroxidase. *Exp Brain Res* 1979;35:161–175.

55. Kelly JP, Wong D. Laminar connections of the cat's auditory cortex. *Brain Res* 1981;212: 1–15.

56. Kudo M. Projections of the nuclei of the lateral lemniscus in the cat: an autoradiographic study. *Brain Res* 1981;221:57–69.

57. Kudo M, Niimi K. Ascending projections of the inferior colliculus in the cat: an autoradiographic study. *J Comp Neurol* 1980;191:545–556.

58. Kusama T, Otani K, Kawana E. Projections of

the motor, somatic sensory, auditory and visual cortices in cats. *Prog Brain Res* 1966;21A:292–322.

59. Lorente de Nó R. Anatomy of the eighth nerve. III. General plan of structure of the primary cochlear nuclei. *J Comp Neurol* 1933;43:327–350.

60. Liberman MC. Efferent synapses in the inner hair cell area of the cat cochlea: an electron-microscopic study of serial sections. *Hear Res* 1980;3:189–204.

61. Liberman MC, Brown MC. Physiology and anatomy of single olivocochlear neurons in the cat. *Hear Res* 1986;24:17–36.

62. Majorossy K, Rethelyi M. Synaptic architecture in the medial geniculate body (ventral division). *Exp Brain Res* 1968;6:306–323.

63. Martin GF. The pattern of neocortical projections to the mesencephalon of the opossum *Didelphis virginiana*. *Brain Res* 1968;11:593–610.

64. May PJ, Hall WC. The sources of the nigrotectal pathway. *Neuroscience* 1986;19:159–181.

65. Mitani A, Shimokouchi M, Itoh K, Nomura S, Kudo M, Mizuno M. Morphology and laminar organization of electrophysiologically identified neurons in the primary auditory cortex in the cat. *J Comp Neurol* 1985;235:430–447.

66. Mitani A, Shimokouchi M. Neuronal connections in the primary auditory cortex: an electrophysiological study in the cat. *J Comp Neurol* 1986;235:417–429.

67. Mitani A, Shimokouchi M, Nomura S. Effects of stimulation of the primary auditory cortex upon colliculogeniculate neurons in the inferior colliculus of the cat. *Neurosci Lett* 1983;42: 185–189.

68. Moore JK, Moore RY. Glutamic acid decarboxylase-like immunoreactivity in brainstem auditory nuclei of the rat. *J Comp Neurol* 1987; 260:157–174.

69. Moore RY, Goldberg JM. Projections of the inferior colliculus in the monkey. *Exp Neurol* 1966;14:429–438.

70. Moore RY, Goldberg JM. Ascending projections of the inferior colliculus in the cat. *J Comp Neurol* 1963;121:109–135.

71. Morest DK. The neuronal architecture of the medial geniculate body of the cat. *J Anat* 1964; 98:611–630.

72. Morest DK. The collateral system of the medial nucleus of the trapezoid body of cat, its neuronal architecture, and relation to the olivocochlear bundle. *Brain Res* 1968;9:288–311.

73. Morest DK. Synaptic relationship of Golgi type II cells in the medial geniculate body of the cat. *J Comp Neurol* 1975;162:157–194.

74. Morest DK, Oliver DL. The neuronal architecture of the inferior colliculus in the cat: defining the functional anatomy of the auditory midbrain. *J Comp Neurol* 1984;222:209–236.

75. Oliver DL. Dorsal cochlear nucleus projections to the inferior colliculus in the cat: a light and electron microscopic study. *J Comp Neurol* 1984;224:155–172.

76. Oliver DL, Hall WC. The medial geniculate

body of the tree shrew *Tupaia glis*. I. Cytoarchitecture and midbrain connections. *J Comp Neurol* 1978;182:423–458.

77. Oliver DL, Hall WC. The medial geniculate body of the tree shrew *Tupaia Glis*. II. Connections with the neocortex. *J Comp Neurol* 1978; 182:459–494.

78. Oliver DL, Morest DK. The central nucleus of the inferior colliculus in the cat. *J Comp Neurol* 1984;222:237–264.

79. Osen KK. Projection of the cochlear nuclei on the inferior colliculus in the cat. *J Comp Neurol* 1972;144:355–372.

80. Osen KK, Mugnaini E, Dahl AL, Christiansen AH. Histochemical localization of acetylcholinesterase in the cochlear and superior olivary nuclei. A reappraisal with emphasis on the cochlear granule cell system. *Arch Ital Biol* 1984; 122:169–212.

81. Ostapoff EM, Morest DK, Potashner SJ. Retrograde transport of 3H-GABA from the cochlear nucleus to the superior olive in guinea pig. *Soc Neurosci Abstr* 1985;11:1051.

82. Paula-Barbosa MM, Sousa-Pinto A. Auditory cortical projections to the superior colliculus in the cat. *Brain Res* 1973;50:47–51.

83. Pfalz RKJ. Centrifugal inhibition of afferent secondary neurons in the cochlear nucleus by sound. *J Acoust Soc Am* 1962;34:1472–1477.

84. Pickles JO. *Introduction to the physiology of hearing*. New York: Academic Press, 1982.

85. Ramon Y Cajal S. *Histologie du Système Nerveux de l'homme et des Vertébrés,* vol I. Instituto Ramon y Cajal, Madrid, pp. 774–838.

86. Rasmussen GL. The olivary peduncle and other fiber projections of the superior olivary complex. *J Comp Neurol* 1946;84:141–219.

87. Rasmussen GL. Further observations of the efferent cochlear bundle. *J Comp Neurol* 1953; 99:61–74.

88. Rasmussen GL. Anatomic relationships of the ascending and descending auditory systems. In: Field WS, Alford BR, eds. *Neurological aspects of auditory and vestibular disorders*. Springfield, IL: Charles C. Thomas, 1964;5–19.

89. Rasmussen GL. Efferent connections of the cochlear nucleus. In: Graham AB, ed. *Sensorineural hearing processes and disorders*. Boston: Little, Brown, 1967;61–75.

90. Roberts RC, Ribak CE. GABAergic neurons and axon terminals in the brainstem auditory nuclei of the gerbil. *J Comp Neurol* 1987; 258:267–280.

91. Robertson D. Brainstem location of efferent neurons projecting to the guinea pig cochlea. *Hear Res* 1985;20:79–84.

92. Rockel AJ, Jones EG. The neuronal organization of the inferior colliculus of the adult cat. I. The central nucleus. *J Comp Neurol* 1973;147: 11–60.

93. Rockel AJ, Jones EG. The neuronal organization of the inferior colliculus of the adult cat. II. The pericentral nucleus. *J Comp Neurol* 1973;149:301–334.

94. Rockel AJ, Jones EG. Observations on the fine structure of the central nucleus of the inferior colliculus of the cat. *J Comp Neurol* 1973;147: 61–92.

95. Rose JE, Woolsey CN. Cortical connections and functional organization of the thalamic auditory system of the cat. In: Harlow HF, Woolsey CN, eds. *Biological and biochemical bases for behavior*. Madison: University of Wisconsin Press, 1958;127–150.

96. Rouiller EM, Colomb E, Capt M, de Ribaupierre F. Projections of the reticular complex of the thalamus onto physiologically characterized regions of the medial geniculate body. *Neurosci Lett* 1985;53:227–232.

97. Rouiller EM, de Ribaupierre F. Origin of afferents to physiologically defined regions of the medial geniculate body of the cat: ventral and dorsal divisions. *Hear Res* 1985;19:97–114.

98. Ryugo DK, Weinberger NM. Corticofugal modulation of the medial geniculate body. *Exp Neurol* 1976;51:377–391.

99. Spangler KM. The organization and efferent projections of the periolivary nuclei in the cat. Unpublished doctoral thesis, Wake Forest University, Winston-Salem, NC.

100. Spangler KM, Cant NB, Henkel CK, Farley GR, Warr WB. Descending projections from the superior olivary complex to the cochlear nucleus of the cat. *J Comp Neurol* 1987;259: 452–465.

101. Spangler KM, Morley BJ. Somatostatin-like immunoreactivity in the midbrain of the cat. *J Comp Neurol* 1987;260:87–97.

102. Spangler KM, Warr WB. Transneuronal changes in cochlear radial afferent fibers following destruction of lateral olivocochlear neurons. *Soc Neurosci Abstr* 1987;13:1258.

103. Spangler KM, Warr WB, Henkel CK. The projections of principal cells of the medial nucleus of the trapezoid body in the cat. *J Comp Neurol* 1985;238:249–261.

104. Spangler KM, White JS, Warr WB. Electron microscopic features of axon terminals on olivocochlear neurons in the cat. *Absts 9th Midwinter Mtg Assoc Res Otolaryngol.* 1986;37.

105. Thompson GC, Cortez AM, Lam DM. Localization of GABA immunoreactivity in the auditory brainstem of guinea pigs. *Brain Res* 1985;339:119–122.

106. Thompson AM, Thompson GC. Posteroventral cochlear nucleus projections to olivocochlear neurons. *J Comp Neurol* 1991;303:267–285.

107. Tolbert LP, Morest DK, Yurgelun-Todd DA. Neuronal architecture of the anteroventral cochlear nucleus of the cat. Horseradish peroxidase labeling of identified cell types. *Neuroscience* 1983;7:3031–3052.

108. Tortelly A, Reinoso-Suarez F, Llamas A. Projections from nonvisual cortical areas to the superior colliculus demonstrated by retrograde transport of HRP in the cat. *Brain Res* 1980; 188:543–549.

109. Tsuchitani C. Functional organization of lateral cell groups of cat superior olivary complex. *J Neurophysiol* 1977;40:296–318.

110. Tsuchitani C, Boudreau JC. Single unit analysis of cat superior olive S-segment with tonal stimuli. *J Neurophysiol* 1966;29:684–697.

111. van Noort J. *The structure and connections of the inferior colliculus*. Netherlands: Van Gorcum & Co., 1969.

112. Vaughn DW. Thalamic and callosal connections of the rat auditory cortex. *Brain Res* 1983; 260:181–189.

113. Walther JB, Rasmussen GL. Descending connections of auditory cortex and thalamus of the cat. *Fed Proc* 1960;19:291.

114. Wantanabe T, Yanagisawe K, Kanzaki J, Katsuki Y. Cortical efferent flow influencing unit responses of medial geniculate body to sound stimulation. *Exp Brain Res* 1966;2:302–317.

115. Warr WB. Olivocochlear and vestibular efferent neurons of the feline brainstem: their location, morphology, and number determined by retrograde axonal transport and acetylcholinesterase histochemistry. *J Comp Neurol* 1975; 161:159–182.

116. Warr WB. Parallel ascending pathways from the cochlear nucleus: neuroanatomical evidence of functional specialization. In: Neff WD, ed. *Contributions to sensory physiology*, vol 7. New York: Academic Press, 1982;1–38.

117. Warr WB, Guinan JJ Jr. Efferent innervation of the organ of Corti: two separate systems. *Brain Res* 1979;173:152–155.

118. Warr WB, White JS, Nyffeler MJ. Olivocochlear neurons: quantitative comparison of the lateral and medial efferent systems in adult and newborn cats. *Soc Neurosci Abstr* 1982;8:346.

119. Warr WB, Guinan JJ, White JS. Organization of the efferent fibers: the lateral and medial systems. In: Altschuler RA, Bobbin RP, Hoffman DW, eds. *Neurobiology of hearing: the cochlea*. New York: Raven Press, 1986;333–348.

120. Webster KE. The cortico-striatal projection in the cat. *J Anat* 1965;99:329–337.

121. White JS. Fine structure of the lateral superior olivary nucleus. *Soc Neurosci Abstr* 1983;9: 765.

122. White JS. Fine structural features of medial olivocochlear neurons in the rat. *Neurosci Abstr* 1984;10:393.

123. White JS. Differences in the ultrastructure of labyrinthine efferent neurons in the albino rat. *Absts 9th Midwinter Mtg Assoc Res Otolaryngol.* 1986;34.

124. White JS, Warr WB. The dual origins of the olivocochlear bundle in the albino rat. *J Comp Neurol* 1983;219:203–214.

125. Whitley JM, Henkel CK. Topographical organization of the inferior collicular and other connections of the ventral nucleus of the lateral lemniscus in the cat. *J Comp Neurol* 1984;229: 257–270.

126. Whitlock DG, Nauta WJH. Subcortical projections from the temporal neocortex in *Macacca mulatta*. *J Comp Neurol* 1956;106:182–212.

127. Wiederhold ML, Kiang NY-S. Effects of electric stimulation of the crossed olivocochlear bundle on single auditory-nerve fibers in the cat. *J Acoust Soc Am* 1970;48:950–965.

128. Willard FH, Martin GF. Collateral innervation of the inferior colliculus in the North American opossum: a study using fluorescent markers in a double labeling paradigm. *Brain Res* 1984; 303:171–182.

129. Winer JA. The medial geniculate body of the cat. *Adv Anat Embryol Cell Biol* 1985;86.

130. Winer JA, Larue DT. Patterns of reciprocity in auditory thalamocortical and corticothalamic connections: study with horseradish peroxidase and autoradiographic methods in the rat medial geniculate body. *J Comp Neurol* 1987; 257:282–315.

131. Wong D, Kelly JP. Differentially projecting cells in individual layers of the auditory cortex. *Brain Res* 1981;230:362–366.

Neurobiology of Hearing: The
Central Auditory System, edited by
R. A. Altschuler et al.
Raven Press, Ltd., New York © 1991.

3

Physiological-Morphological Properties of the Cochlear Nucleus

William S. Rhode

*Department of Neurophysiology, University of Wisconsin-Madison Medical School,
Madison, Wisconsin 53706*

The cochlear nucleus (CN) occupies a key location in the auditory central nervous system, being the first in a chain of nuclei that operates on auditory information in both a parallel and hierarchical fashion. Parallelism is apparent in that the auditory nerve (AN) has two branches that innervate three major cytoarchitectural divisions (1, 2). Lorente de Nó (2) described the CN as a brain with its own cerebellum and suggested that a hierarchical organization is present in the CN resulting from the substantial intrinsic connections.

The anatomy is covered only briefly here as several reviews are available (2–4). The AN enters the CN and bifurcates into an ascending branch that innervates the anteroventral CN (AVCN) and a descending branch that innervates both the posteroventral CN (PVCN) and the dorsal CN (DCN). AN terminals have regional specializations in the CN, the most salient feature being the large end-bulbs of Held in the anterior AVCN that constitute the AN synaptic connection with the large spherical/bushy cells. This specialization is thought to be important in preserving temporal information present in AN fiber discharges. Although the temporal response properties of AN fibers are fairly stereotypical, there are differences that have been tied to the rate of spontaneous activity (5) (see Fig. 1, PL

and PL_S). Similarly, recent morphological studies of AN fibers, which were first characterized physiologically, then labeled with horseradish peroxidase (HRP), suggest that high and low spontaneous rate fibers differ in their terminal distribution within the CN (6).

A variety of cell types are present in each major subdivision of the CN. While Lorente de Nó (2) described more than 50 cell types, more tractable classification schemes are based on nine major cell types described by Osen (7) or the 22 cell types described by Brawer et al. (8). The major neuronal types of the CN are called bushy, stellate, octopus, multipolar, fusiform, and granule cells, each having a distinctive dendritic and axonal morphology. Because each type also has distinctive patterns of synaptic input, both excitatory and inhibitory, separate computations are presumably being carried out in parallel in the CN. Information leaves the CN via three pathways: the ventral acoustic stria (VAS), projecting from the AVCN and PVCN; the intermediate acoustic stria (IAS), serving the PVCN; and the dorsal acoustic stria (DAS), carrying axons of the DCN fusiform and giant cells.

The early microelectrode studies of Rose et al. (1) demonstrated three tonotopically organized regions of the CN corresponding

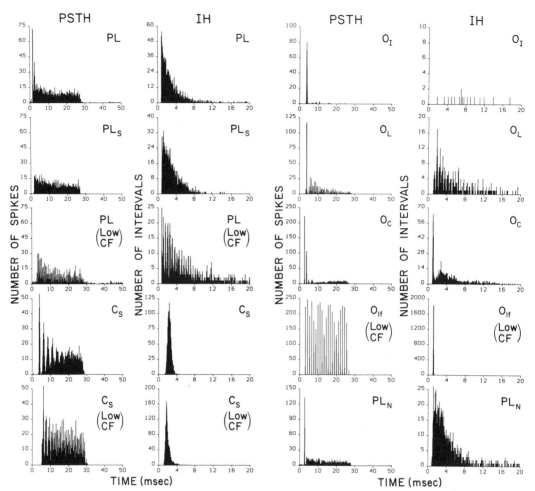

FIG. 1. Representative sample of response patterns (peristimulus time histograms [PSTH]) and interspike interval histogram (IH) configurations seen in the cochlear nucleus. PL, primary-like pattern; PL$_S$, primary-like pattern seen in auditory nerve fibers with low spontaneous firing rates (SR near zero); PL (low CF), primary-like response showing phase locking, PSTH modes are separated by times corresponding to the tone period (T), modes in the corresponding IH are also separated by T; C$_S$, a sustained chopper pattern, corresponding IH is narrow and symmetric; C$_S$ (low CF), a sustained chopper that shows phase locking, yet is easily distinguished from PL$_S$ by its IH, which is narrow, symmetric, and unimodal; O$_I$, onset pattern with little late activity; O$_L$, onset unit with sustained activity that is also phase locked, the modes of the IH are separated by the stimulus period; O$_C$, onset unit with an initial chopper response (sometimes called C$_T$ [transient] units when the late activity is particularly vigorous), IH reflects both the chopping behavior and the later activity in its two modes; O$_{lf}$, an onset unit with low CF, IH at saturation is unimodal and very narrow; PL$_N$, primary-like with notch has a prominent onset component, its IH is similar to that of PL units. (From ref. 22, with permission.)

to the three anatomical divisions. Other physiological studies have described response properties of individual cells in the CN (9–13). These studies have made it possible to infer how morphological cell types

respond to sound (14) in regions of the CN with a dominant cell type. However, we still have a rudimentary knowledge of the role that many cell types play in this complex structure.

In addition to the principal cells of each region, there are many small neurons in the CN. These are mostly interneurons such as the granule cells in the DCN that send their axons parallel to the surface of the DCN and contact cartwheel and fusiform cells (15). Additional complexity is introduced by a flow of information between regions via a number of internuclear tracts (2).

The principal concern of the present review is the relationship of structure and function in the CN. Intracellular labeling of neurons that have been physiologically characterized allows a definitive correlation of physiological response properties with neuronal morphology, with the added benefit of the visualization of adult neuronal morphology in its entirety (16). It is a technique that can be combined with immunocytochemical labeling and can be used at both the light and electron microscopic levels (17–19).

PHYSIOLOGICAL RESPONSE DIVERSITY

Temporal Response Pattern

Two classification schemes for the physiological response properties of CN neurons are used frequently: (a) the first, proposed by Pfeiffer (9), is a description of the temporal patterns in poststimulus time histograms in response to short tones (25 msec) at the characteristic frequency of neurons; (b) the other scheme was introduced by Evans and Nelson (20) and extended by Young and Voigt (21) and describes the "receptive field" or regions of excitation and inhibition on a frequency-intensity plane. In addition, the unit response to a wideband noise (WBN) stimulus is often used to help distinguish types. Each scheme has strengths and weaknesses. In some instances in which the classification of a unit is difficult, both have to be employed to identify cells. In the DCN, the response pattern of some neurons change as

a function of signal frequency, intensity, stimulus on/off times, and anesthetic state, making the scheme of Evans and Nelson more useful than that of Pfeiffer (22, 23).

The principal temporal response patterns recorded in the AN and CN in response to short tones at the unit's characteristic frequency (CF) are illustrated in Figs. 1 and 2, along with the interspike interval histograms (IH). The primary-like (PL) pattern is recorded from the majority of AN fibers and from many cells in AVCN bushy cells (18,24). It consists of an initial transient that rapidly adapts to a steady level. There is a second pattern, PL_S, found in AN fibers with low spontaneous rates (<0.5 spikes/sec) that exhibits only the sustained portion of the PL pattern (25). Additionally, at low stimulus frequencies (<5 kHz), AN fiber and CN unit discharges may synchronize to a particular phase of the stimulating sinusoid, producing peaks in the poststimulus time histogram (PSTH) at the same frequency as the sound stimulus. It is also observed in the interspike IH in which peaks occur at integral multiples of the stimulus period. The PL with notch pattern (PL_N) exhibits a short pause (<2 msec) after the initial spike; the pause is thought to be related to the refractory period of the cell. This pattern is found in the area of the entrance of the AN to the CN and is associated with globular/bushy cells found in this region. Globular cells are slightly elongated and have an eccentrically positioned nucleus that makes it relatively easy to distinguish these cells in Nissl-stained material.

A temporal response pattern that is pervasive throughout the CN is termed chopper (C) because of the temporal regularity of its response. Intervals between PSTH modes depend on stimulus intensity, rather than on stimulus frequency. Choppers generally behave as free-running, driven oscillators. However, choppers do phaselock to low-frequency signals, although more poorly than other ventral CN (VCN) cell types. Interspike IH of choppers are distinctive: sustained choppers (C_S) have a

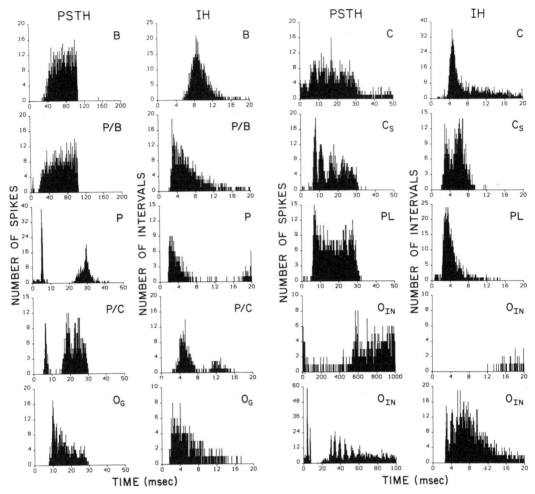

FIG. 2. Examples of peristimulus time histograms (PSTH) and interspike interval histograms (IH) found in the dorsal cochlear nucleus (DCN). Buildup (B) units occur most often in the fusiform cell layer with relatively symmetric IHs. Short latency spikes may be followed by the buildup pattern (P/B); existence of the first spike is dependent on a sufficiently long recovery time. Pausers (P) are characterized by the cessation of discharges following the initial spike that lasts from 5 to more than 20 msec. Pauser pattern can have a chopper pattern superimposed (P/C). Chopper pattern can also be superimposed on a buildup pattern. This category of onset units with the graded decrease in discharge rate was designated O_G by Bourk (12) and C_S by Godfrey et al. (11). These units usually have pronounced nonmonotonic spike rate vs. intensity curves. Chopper (C) patterns are seen frequently in the DCN. Here the C pattern is often seen at low intensities and high intensities in units that display pauser patterns at mid-intensities. Sustained chopper patterns (C_S) are also frequently seen. A pattern that is similar to primary-like patterns (PL) is occasionally seen. These units also have nonmonotonic rate-intensity curves. Type IV units show suppression to tonal stimuli. They may show an onset response (O_{IN}) with suppression of activity throughout the tone. Second O_{IN} (Type IV) unit illustrated also shows a C at stimulus offset. Stimulus tone onset is at *time zero* and stimulus tone duration is equal to half the duration of the time scale shown on the *abscissa* for PSTHs in this and all the following figures, unless otherwise noted. The second O_{IN} in this figure has a stimulus duration equal only to one-fourth the duration of the time scale (25 msec). Normally 25-msec tones are presented every 105 msec. Buildup units can have very long latencies, up to 200 msec, requiring longer duration tones. (From ref. 58, with permission.)

narrow, symmetric IH and a small coefficient of variation (CV = standard deviation/mean) of the IH; transient choppers (C_T) usually show a similar IH (narrow and symmetric) only during the onset portion of their response, their discharges becoming less regular after several milliseconds. Plots of the CV versus time (12,26) help to distinguish these subtypes. The increase in CV with time after stimulus onset prominent in C_Ts may be related to inhibitory inputs arriving and disrupting the "pacemaker-like" behavior of the choppers (27). These cells chop in response to swept tones (22) and amplitude-modulated (AM) tones (low modulating frequencies) (28), respond primarily to the envelope of speech stimuli (29), and chop when depolarized by a current applied intracellularly (30). It appears that the chopper behavior is a basic property of their neuronal membrane.

Another frequently occurring response pattern is termed onset. It is seen throughout the VCN, although it is most often associated with the PVCN. There are several distinct onset patterns: O_I, O_L, and O_C. The O_I pattern is so called because there is little activity after the initial onset spike. The O_L pattern is similar to PL_N but occurs largely in the PVCN. O_L units, in contrast to O_I units, can exhibit sustained rates comparable to those of AN fibers. The third onset pattern is O_C or onset-chopper and is characterized by one to four modes occurring early in the PSTH. The discharges of onset units often "entrain" (fire once per stimulus cycle) to low-frequency sinusoids ($f < 1$ kHz). This is evident when the IH consists of a single, very narrow mode with a mean equal to the stimulus period. This behavior could be of special significance for encoding low pitch and amplitude modulation.

In the DCN, a number of distinct response patterns can be seen (Fig. 2). The buildup pattern (B) is one in which the firing rate gradually increases over 10 to 100 msec. Another pattern is the pauser (P), in which, after an initial spike, a delay between 3 and 25 msec occurs, after which a buildup response occurs. Frequently a chopper pattern is superimposed on the pauser and buildup pattern and may be an inherent property of many DCN cells. The chopper pattern occurs frequently in the DCN, but the discharge rate is lower than that seen in the VCN. Occasionally, there is an initial narrow mode followed by widening of the modes, as is seen for the sustained chopper in Fig. 2 (C_S). There are also PL and onset patterns in the DCN. The onset pattern varies considerably from an O_G (graded decrease in response) to one that is marked by inhibition of spontaneous activity labeled O_{IN} (onset-inhibitory) (Fig. 2), both of which indicate that strong inhibitory influences are present.

Response Field Classification

Evans and Nelson (20) developed a classification scheme based on the presence or absence of inhibitory sidebands and the response to noise that has been further developed by Young and colleagues (26). Five types of response maps are illustrated in Fig. 3. Type I is characteristic of PL units of the AVCN and AN fibers. It has no inhibitory sidebands and the rate-intensity curve is monotonic. Type II has inhibitory sidebands, but because they have little or no spontaneous activity the sidebands are not readily apparent. However, their nonmonotonic rate curves and poor responses to wideband noise are indicative of inhibitory inputs. Type III is similar to Type I except that it has inhibitory sidebands around the excitatory tip of the response map. Type IV has a low-threshold, excitatory tip and prominent inhibition over a wide range. Several islands of excitation may exist at higher intensities. Type V differs from Type IV in that it does not have a low-level excitatory region. Types IV and V are found in the DCN. Young and Voigt (21) report seeing relatively few Type V maps. Types IV and V are seen more frequently in the decerebrate preparation than in anesthe-

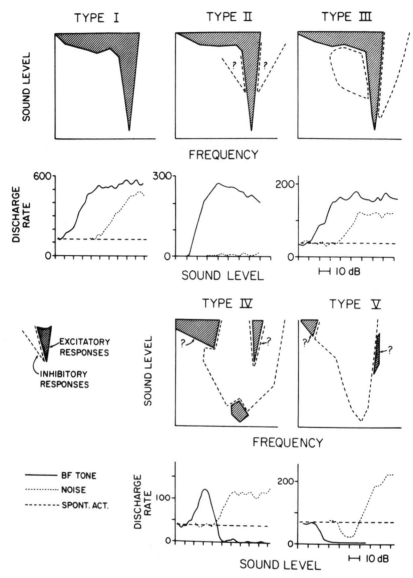

FIG. 3. Examples of response maps (**top**) and rate versus sound level functions (**bottom**) for the five response map types. Types are labeled above each response map. Response maps are schematic, showing the general layout of response maps for each type. Question marks indicate variable or unknown features. Excitatory response (increase in discharge rate) regions are shaded; inhibitory response (decrease in discharge rate) regions are unshaded, enclosed in dashed lines. Rate versus level functions are actual examples of average discharge rate during 200-msec BF tone bursts (*solid lines*) or noise bursts (*dotted lines*), plotted as a function of the sound pressure level of the stimulus. *Horizontal dashed lines* show spontaneous rate. (From ref. 67, with permission.)

tized animals, indicating that barbiturate anesthetics reduce the inhibitory inputs (20). Young and Brownell (13) demonstrated that administering a barbiturate to a decerebrate cat while recording from a Type IV unit reduced the inhibitory zone and expanded the excitatory part of the response map with the result that the unit was then better classified as Type III.

Spectral Selectivity

One of the attributes of interest in any part of the auditory system is the ability to separate spectral components of a complex stimulus. There are three ways of preserving the exquisite frequency selectivity seen in the AN. First, strong excitatory connections between AN fibers and postsynaptic CN cells, as occurs in the rostral AVCN

(bushy cells), preserve most of the information contained in AN inputs. Second, convergence of several AN fibers on CN cells can correct or even sharpen timing information. Third, inhibitory sidebands can also sharpen spectral selectivity. Inhibitory sidebands are observed throughout the CN but are most prominent in the DCN where inhibitory mechanisms can totally suppress unit activity. The frequency selectivity is usually given as the quality factor Q_{10} ($= CF/BW$, where BW is the bandwidth at 10 dB above threshold). Figure 4 illustrates the Q_{10}s for some of the major cell types in the VCN (AVCN + PVCN). All cell types have Q_{10}s similar to those of AN fibers. However, there are two exceptions O_Is (not shown) and O_Cs have much lower Q_{10}s (larger bandwidths), indicating innervation by multiple AN fibers spanning a range of CFs.

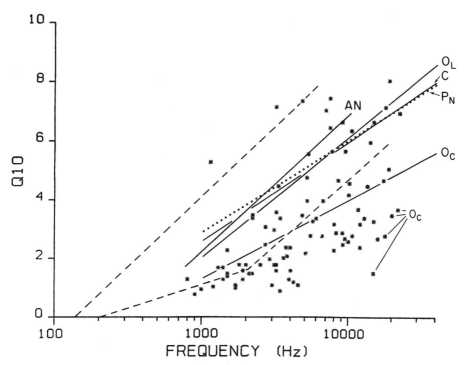

FIG. 4. Scatter diagram of Q_{10} (characteristic frequency/bandwidth [CF/BW]) vs. CF for O_C units. *Dashed lines* indicate the limits of Q_{10} for auditory nerve (AN) fibers found. The regression line fits to Q_{10} data for AN, O_L, C, and P_N are also shown. The regression lines are shown only between 1 and 20 kHz since the data have breaks in the curves below and above these values.

There is some difficulty in determining Q_{10}s for DCN cells especially if they are Type IV or V units with nonmonotonic rate curves. The tuning curves for seven DCN cells are shown in Fig. 5 and clearly indicate that the spectral selectivity can be exquisite with high-frequency slopes of up to 2,000 dB/octave—far better than typically seen in AN fibers (150–500 dB/octave). The difference in slopes, along with the suppression of spontaneous neural activity by a tone, indicates that a sharpening mechanism is present. Because the reduction in activity occurs around a central excitatory region, the mechanism has often been described as lateral inhibition, by analogy with that seen in the visual system.

The variety of gain functions (rate curves) found in the CN require that response areas be collected to adequately describe a unit's behavior throughout the frequency-intensity plane. A response area is a series of isointensity firing rate versus stimulus-frequency curves that allow Q_{10}s, threshold tuning curves, monotonicity, and the existence of inhibitory sidebands (if spontaneous rate is nonzero) to be determined. If the spontaneous rate is zero, then a "bias signal," WBN is applied and the response area collected in the same manner to determine whether there are inhibitory sidebands. The WBN also serves the role of a masker and allows one to determine how this part of the auditory system deals with background noise.

There are different levels of inhibition (the term "suppression" is sometimes used instead of "inhibition" because the latter assumes the operation of a specifically neural mechanism and suppression is present in the AN) illustrated in Figs. 6 through 9 where both response areas and "masked" response areas are shown for three types of VCN units: O_L, O_C, and C_S, and one DCN unit, an O_G/Type II. The O_L unit (Fig. 6) shows marked suppression, both above and below CF, with nearly complete suppression in some regions. Onset units show a range of sideband suppression from nonexistent (Fig. 7B) to large (as in Fig. 6B). The O_C unit masked response area in Fig. 7B has no (or very weak) sidebands. This is common for O_Cs, but the low CF is also a factor because sidebands are generally smaller for low CF units in all categories. Typically, chopper units have prominent inhibitory sidebands whether they are C_Ts or C_Ss (nearly 100% inhibition of WBN activ-

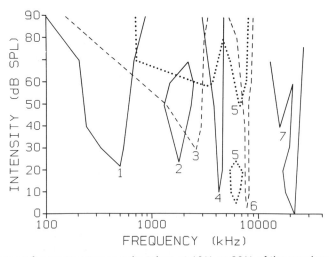

FIG. 5. Isorate curves for seven pauser units taken at 10% or 20% of the maximum discharge rate. (From ref. 58, with permission.)

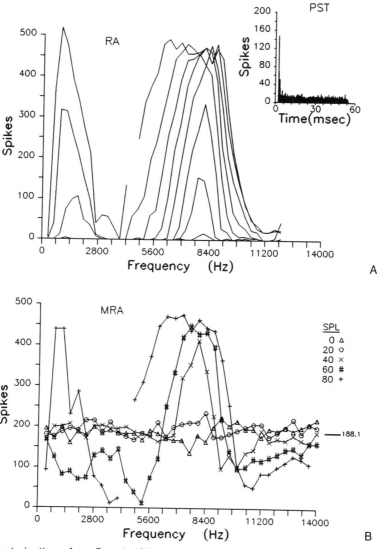

FIG. 6. Characterization of an O_L unit (CF=8,100 Hz; TH=10 dB SPL). **A:** Response area (RA) plot for an intensity range of 10 to 80 dB, in 10-dB steps. Inset shows PSTH at CF, 60 dB SPL. **B:** Response area with a noise masker (MRA) that produces 188 spikes/sec alone. Tones: 0 to 80 dB, 10-dB steps. Only data for 20-dB steps are shown for purposes of clarity. Same in Figs. 7–9.

ity, e.g., Fig. 8). When there is spontaneous activity present in choppers, it is common to see inhibitory sidebands (Fig. 15). In the DCN, some O_G units have nonmonotonic rate curves and show no response to WBN and therefore are similar to Type II (e.g., Fig. 9). The effect of applying WBN is to decrease the overall responsiveness of this

unit (Fig. 9B) and to reduce the frequency range that excites the unit.

These sidebands indicate that it is possible to inhibit nearly 100% of the noise-induced activity in many cells. This is different from two-tone suppression found in AN fibers, where the reduction is usually between 10% and 75% (31). Supporting

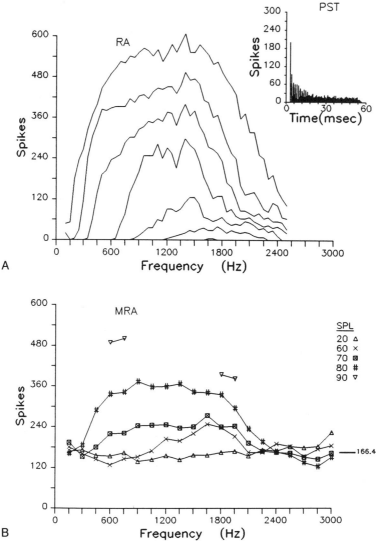

FIG. 7. Characterization of an O_C unit (CF = 1,700 Hz; TH = 28 dB SPL). **A:** Response area plot for a 20- to 80-dB range. Inset shows PSTH at CF and 60 dB SPL. **B:** Response area with a wideband noise masker that produces 166 spikes/sec alone. Tones: 20 to 90 dB, 10-dB steps.

evidence for inhibitory processes originates from intracellular recording in DCN neurons where hyperpolarizing potentials (32) and inhibitory postsynaptic potentials (IPSPs) (33) are observed. IPSPs are also recorded in the VCN (34,35). Further, AN fibers never exhibit suppression of spontaneous activity (except after stimulus offset), whereas the chopper unit in Fig. 15 shows prominent suppression of spontaneous activity over a wide frequency range. Occasionally, the upper cutoff frequency for an inhibitory effect is over an octave higher than the unit's CF, much wider than the suppression regions of AN fibers. DCN units have the widest sidebands, while O_C neurons show small, if any, inhibitory sidebands (Fig. 7). Many PL units in the AVCN

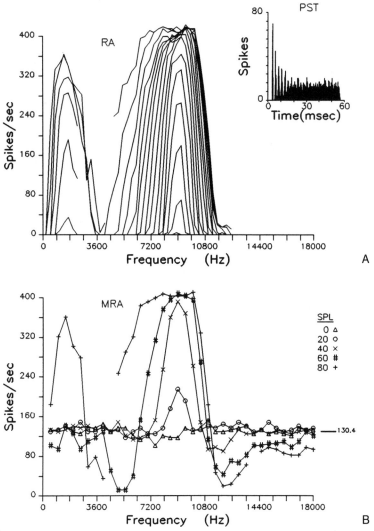

FIG. 8. Characterization of a C_S unit (CF = 9,000 Hz; TH = 1 dB SPL). **A:** Response area plot for an intensity range 10 to 80 dB SPL, 5-dB steps. Inset shows PSTH at CF and 60 dB SPL. **B:** Response area with a wideband noise masker that produces 130 spikes/sec alone. Tones: 0 to 80 dB, 20-dB steps.

show weak suppression of noise-driven responses.

Together these latter observations indicate the suppression seen in AN fibers is not the underlying explanation for most of the suppression in the CN. Excitatory-inhibitory interactions in the CN are common. Inhibitory sidebands maintain and at times improve the exquisite frequency selectivity of AN fibers.

Temporal Response Properties

Phase Locking

There are several measures of the ability of the auditory system to encode temporal signal features. The most commonly used one involves the use of the synchronization coefficient (SC), a measure of phase locking that varies from 0 (random behavior) to

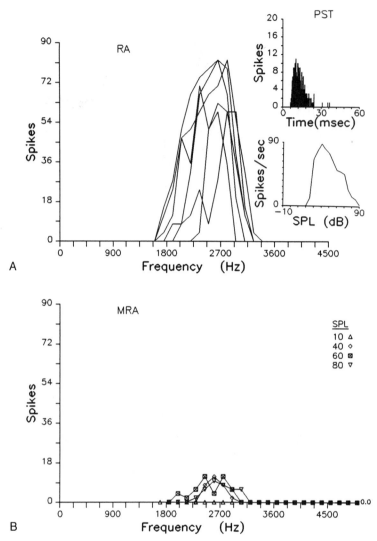

FIG. 9. Characterization of a O_G unit in dorsal cochlear nucleus (CF = 2,050 Hz; TH = 22 dB SPL). **A:** Response area plot for an intensity range 20 to 80 dB, 10-dB steps. Inset shows PSTH at 2,700 Hz and 70 dB SPL. **B:** Response area with a wideband noise masker that produces no driven spikes.

1 (perfect locking). A benchmark number to remember is 0.785, the SC for perfectly encoding a half-rectified sine wave. The frequency dependence of SCs for AN fibers and for C, $P_N (= PL_N)$, O_L, and O_C neurons in the VCN is illustrated in Fig. 10.

SCs for AN discharges can be larger than 0.785 for CFs <1,000 Hz. Further, AN fibers with low spontaneous rates can phase lock better at high intensities than high spontaneous rate fibers. This feature may be especially important for encoding the temporal information in complex signals such as speech. VCN cells are able to phase lock to nearly as high a frequency as AN fibers. O_Ls, O_Cs, and PL_Ns all phase lock poorly beyond 3 kHz, but below 2 kHz they synchronize as well as, or better than, AN

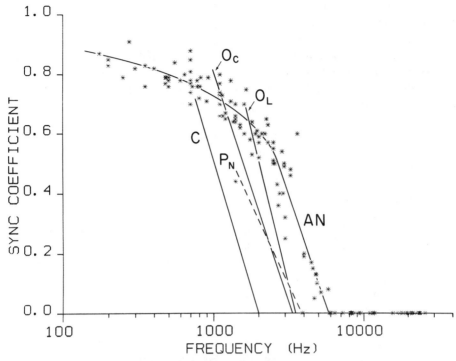

FIG. 10. Scatter diagram of the synchronization coefficients for auditory nerve fibers along with the regression line fit. The regression line fits to the synchronization coefficients for O_L, O_C, P_N, and C units are also shown. Maximum synchronization coefficient at characteristic frequency (CF) is plotted. Line fits were performed only over the frequency range in which the synchronization coefficient vs. log frequency relation appeared linear (roughly 0.05<sync< 0.6). (From ref. 22, with permission.)

fibers. The onset units may entrain to frequencies below 1 kHz, achieving SCs as high as 0.99.

Chopper units cease to phase lock to frequencies higher than 2 kHz, the lowest frequency limit of any unit type in the VCN. They also display the smallest SCs of any VCN population, rarely exceeding 0.6 at any frequency. In the DCN, phase locking is very weak, weaker than VCN choppers, with little synchronization beyond 1 kHz. Often there is no significant phase-locked activity even at CF in units with CFs <1 kHz. Temporal encoding of the stimulus frequency or fine structure cannot be the function of DCN units.

The phase-locking behavior of CN cells relates to their ability to encode more complex signals such as speech. Onset cells have been shown to encode voice pitch very well, while choppers encode the envelope of complex signals and PL neurons are able to preserve fine temporal structure (29).

Amplitude Modulation

The appeal of pure tones and clicks as auditory stimuli lies in their spectral and temporal simplicity. However, they occur infrequently in nature. Animal vocalizations, including human speech, contain AM and frequency-modulated components. Encoding of AM sounds has been investigated at many stages in the auditory pathway from the AN to the auditory cortex (36–38).

Various methods of presentation of the data in the form of a modulation function (MF) have been employed. Basically, an MF shows the degree to which the neural response encodes the modulation (envelope).

AM responses up to several kHz at the auditory periphery decrease progressively as the auditory system is ascended until at the level of the auditory cortex; the best modulating frequency for AM coding is 10 to 100 Hz. At the level of the CN, the maximum frequency for AM encoding varies from a few hundred hertz to several kilohertz depending on the type of unit and its CF. Møller (39) has made extensive studies of AM responses in the CN of rats but made no correlation with temporal response pattern or receptive field type. Frisina et al. (28) did make such a correlation in the gerbil and found that all unit types (in the VCN) exhibit an improvement in AM coding over that seen in the AN, and that the preferential order of unit types for AM encoding was $O_N > C > PL_N > PL$ units.

AM transfer characteristics in the CN are mostly low pass or bandpass when the SC for phase locking to the modulating frequency is graphed (Fig. 11). There are several features that are important in an AM-MF: the shape, maximum value, best modulating frequency (BMF), and the cutoff frequency (operationally defined as that modulating frequency for which the SC falls below 0.1). Few neurons phase lock to the modulating frequency at a 0.785 level for any combination of frequency and intensity when the modulation coefficient is 1.0 (in which case the spectral sidebands are 6 dB below the sound pressure level (SPL) of the carrier).

The ability to encode AM seems to be present in all CN cells. However, the manner in which they respond to changes in intensity and modulating frequency varies. In each instance it is of interest to compare the unit's MF to that of an AN fiber (Fig. 11A).

Most AN-MFs extend out to around 2 kHz, are low pass in shape, show a pronounced decrease in their ability to encode the modulating signal as stimulus intensity is increased, and the largest SCs for the fiber are usually between 0.6 and 0.7. The modulation transfer function (MTFs) for five CN units, shown in Fig. 11, make it clear that significant temporal processing is occurring: (a) The SCs for some units are significantly larger (up to 0.95) than those in AN fibers. This is especially true in onset units (e.g., Fig. 11D). (b) Often AM coding is relatively independent of intensity (e.g., Fig. 11B, D, and E). (c) Both low-pass and bandpass filter characteristics can be seen even in the same unit at different intensities.

There are marked variations of AM coding within each CN unit category. Most chopper units have a low-pass MF before they reach rate saturation (low SPLs) and become bandpass as intensity is increased. Some chopper units will follow AM to levels 60 dB beyond their threshold, while some behave more like AN fibers in that by 70 dB SPL there is no significant AM encoding. Frisina et al. (28) reported similar findings for chopper units. Examination of the response of choppers to AM with low modulating frequencies indicates that they chop during each half cycle of AM. As intensity increases, the chopping becomes continuous, thus accounting for the observed drop in synchronization. As the modulation frequency increases, the sidebands of the AM no longer fall within the unit's passband. Hence, the unit responds only to the carrier frequency.

Of the onset subtypes, O_Cs appear to be best adapted for AM encoding, having a wide dynamic range and often little reduction in AM encoding as the intensity is increased (Fig. 11D and E). However, O_Ls can display similar properties (Fig. 11B). Some O_Ls demonstrate a marked reduction in AM encoding as intensity is increased similar to that seen in AN fibers.

A factor that affects AM coding is the CF

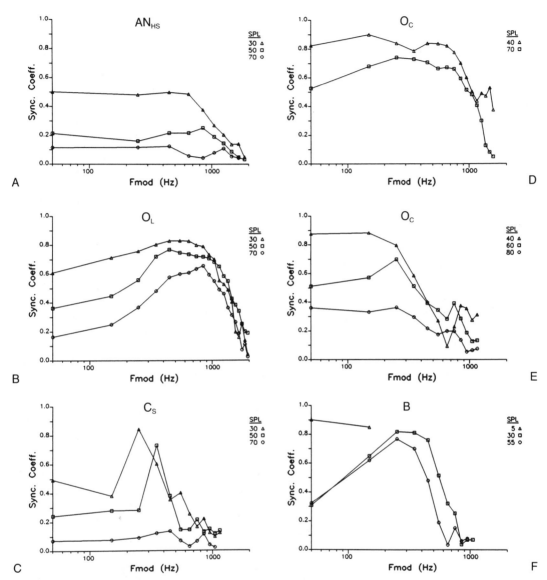

FIG. 11. The sinusoidal amplitude modulation transfer functions for six auditory units plotted as the synchronization coefficient vs. the modulation frequency. The unit type, CF, threshold (in dB SPL) and spontaneous rate are specified for each panel. **A:** AN_{HS}, 10,300 Hz, 8 dB, 76 spikes/sec. **B:** O_L, 7,900 Hz, 8 dB, 1 spike/sec. **C:** C_S, 9,000 Hz, 8 dB, 0 spikes/sec. **D:** O_C, 5,500 Hz, 22 dB, 0 spikes/sec. **E:** O_C, 1,750 Hz, 23 dB, 0 spikes/sec. **F:** B, 7,300 Hz, −4 dB, 0 spikes/sec.

of the unit. When the CF is low enough that the unit phase locks to the carrier frequency (=CF), then the SC for the modulating frequency is lower. As the modulating frequency is increased, the SC drops off rapidly so that the highest modulating frequency coded is lower than that for high CF units.

In the DCN, pausers and buildup units are similar to choppers and onsets (O_Ls) in their MFs. Some are relatively insensitive to intensity increases, while others completely lose the ability to encode AM as the SPL is increased beyond 60 dB. The relatively robust AM encoding in the cat DCN stands in contrast to that of the gerbil, where there appears to be no AM encoding (28).

The cutoff frequency (modulation frequency for which SC<0.1) varies with unit type in the following order: $PL > O_C = O_L > PL_N > C > P/B$; PLs (AN fibers) attain values between 1,500 and 2,500 Hz, whereas most chopper units are limited to less than 1 kHz. The magnitude of the SCs for AM is largest for O_Cs with the following order: $O_C > O_L > PL_N > C > P/B > PL$. But exceptions are frequent: each parameter has a distribution of values and the tails of the distribution overlap.

Møller (39) did not find any consistent relation between BMF and the maximum discharge rate, but we note a tendency in some chopper units (mostly sustained choppers) to achieve the maximum SC when f_{mod} equals the discharge rate to tone at the carrier frequency and the same intensity. Whether there is any systematic spatial mapping of BMF in the CN is unclear and may be difficult to resolve due to the variety of unit types and responses.

Extended Dynamic Range

A perennial problem in auditory research has been to explain our ability to hear over a range in excess of 100 dB when most AN fibers have only a 20 to 30-dB dynamic range. This has been termed the dynamic range problem by Palmer and Evans (40). They demonstrated that a background of notched noise biases the rate response of the majority of neurons in the CN toward higher SPLs, effectively extending the system's dynamic range. They argued that this extended dynamic range occurred beyond the AN. However, Gibson et al. (41) provide evidence that, under the condition of a continuous noise background, the dynamic range adjustment occurs primarily in the cochlea. We find that in the DCN there is a wide range of variability with some units remarkably better at dynamic range adjust-

ment in the presence of simultaneous noise than others.

Furthermore, the O_C cells have largely solved the dynamic range problem. It is our hypothesis that there are unique membrane properties in O_C multipolar neurons that underlie the integration of the synaptic activity originating from inputs of the AN. While we have not been able to study these cells intracellularly long enough to uncover the underlying biophysical principles, we have sufficient data to suggest a simple model. First, O_C neurons have the smallest Q_{10}s (widest bandwidths) of any neuron in the CN. This suggests that several AN fibers with different CFs converge on O_C neurons. Second, the large dynamic range (up to 80 dB) suggests that these additional inputs are "recruited" at different levels as SPL increases. This could occur in a number of ways involving nerve fibers with different thresholds, different dynamic ranges, and/or different types of saturation.

While there could be many (even hundreds) of AN fibers converging on an O_C unit, a simple model, employing three AN fibers (A, B, C), is shown in Fib. 12A as originating from three inner hair cells in the cochlear partition. The O_C neuron is contacted at three sites by these fibers and sums the incoming postsynaptic potentials via the dendrites and soma. Model threshold tuning curves for the AN fibers are shown in Fig. 12B. At an arbitrary stimulus frequency such as indicated by the dotted vertical line, these threshold curves are contacted at different levels (points of their curves), which are indicated on the ordinate of Fig. 12B. Assuming the same rate curve for each fiber but with the thresholds indicated and that synaptic activity is summed, the output caused by the three fibers would produce the rate curve indicated in Fig. 12C where the rate curve of the O_C cell has a much greater dynamic range than any one AN fiber.

There are a variety of O_C rate curves and dynamic ranges. The particular input com-

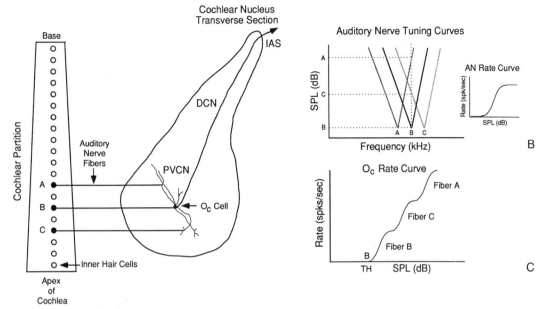

FIG. 12. A: Schematic of an uncoiled cochlea with three inner hair cells (A, B, C) from which three nerve fibers arise and innervate an O_C cell shown in a transverse section of the cochlear nucleus. The O_C axon exits via the intermediate acoustic stria (IAS). **B:** Tuning curves for the three auditory nerve (AN) fibers in part A. The *dashed vertical line* intersects the tuning curves at points brought out on the ordinate indicating the SPL at which each fiber begins to respond at that frequency. **C:** The resultant rate curve when the output of the three AN fibers is summed by the O_C cell.

bination could account for a large measure of the variability since there is no reason why the range of CFs and the uniformity of CFs would not vary in some random manner.

MORPHOLOGICAL-PHYSIOLOGICAL CORRELATIONS

The introduction of intracellular labeling with HRP after cells have been characterized physiologically has proven to be extremely useful (16). It has also contributed to the study of adult neuronal morphology since it can include axonal morphology. In addition, the combination of extracellular and intracellular physiological studies with the morphology makes a start toward understanding the circuitry of the CN. Furthermore, another feature of HRP studies is

that electron microscopy can be applied to the tissue, providing valuable information about synaptic distributions on the labeled cell along with vesicle shape and the synaptic terminations of the labeled cell (17–19). Much of this work corroborated the earlier population studies in the CN (1, 9–12).

Anteroventral Cochlear Nucleus—Bushy Cells

The AVCN contains a number of cell types including bushy, stellate, and granule cells (42–44). Bushy cells can be divided into large spherical cells in the very anterior region of AVCN, small spherical cells in the more dorsal AVCN, and globular cells in the medial region of the AN entrance to the CN, all of which exhibit a PL temporal response pattern. The globular/ bushy cells provide the input to the medial nucleus of the trapezoid body (MNTB). Their axons are among the largest in the CN. Their synapses on the principal cells in the MNTB, called the calyces of Held, are probably the largest synaptic structures in the nervous system, providing a secure path for information transmission to the contralateral lateral superior olivary nucleus (14). Smith and Rhode (17) studied and labeled 14 globular/bushy cells with

HRP and found that they exhibited a PL or PL_N pattern in response to tone pips at CF. Five cells labeled by Rouiller and Ryugo (45) exhibited a variety of response patterns including PL_N, onset, and one chopper.

Three globular/bushy cells are shown in Fig. 13, illustrating a variety of dendritic shapes and extents, from a fairly compact dendritic tree to one that extends over 300 μm. These cells are characterized by beaded dendrites arranged in a compact, dense bush, along with their elliptically

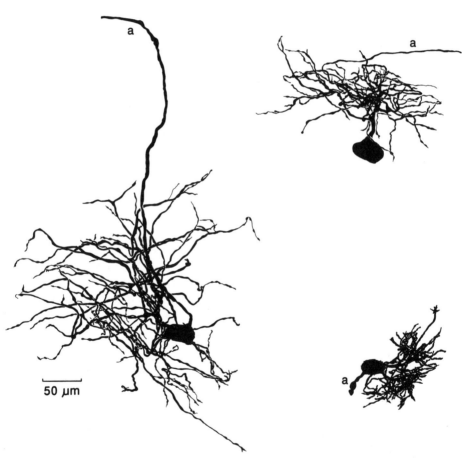

FIG. 13. Camera lucida drawings of three typical bushy cells that were physiologically characterized and labeled with HRP. Recording and injection site for the bushy cell on the left (82118, U44, CF = 16 kHz) was in the axon just past the point where the camera lucida drawing ends. Records from cell in upper right (81154, U31, CF = 500 Hz) taken from soma region. Swelling in axon of cell at lower right (82067, U33, CF = 13.5 kHz) is recording and injection site. Note terminal specialization on uppermost dendrite. a, axon. Scale bar applies to all three drawings. (Adapted from ref. 18.)

shaped soma and eccentrically positioned nucleus (apparent in Nissl-stained material). The AN synapses, containing large, round vesicles in electron micrographs, are primarily on the somas and proximal dendrites. Synapses on the dendrites often contain pleomorphic or flat vesicles, which are probably inhibitory inputs (by analogy with other systems).

The response pattern of globular-bushy cells to CF tones can vary from a PL pattern at 10 dB above threshold (Fig. 14A) to the PL_N pattern observed at high intensities (Fig. 14B). The prominent onset peak is probably a result of convergence of at least two fibers. Each of these can discharge the cell at onset but may not be as effective afterward due to the activity of inhibitory circuits (35). The relatively low discharge rates observed in some PL_N units (Fig. 14C) could be due to inhibitory inputs. At low frequencies the discharges are phase locked substantially better than those of individual AN fibers, with SCs reaching 0.99 (Fig.

14D). A threshold-crossing detector could account for this superior phase-locking behavior if several AN fibers provide synchronous input to the cell.

The number of AN fibers converging on each globular/bushy cell is thought to be one to four based on the Golgi studies of Lorente de Nó (2). Other indirect evidence is the correlation between spontaneous rate and maximum discharge rate shown earlier (Fig. 13) (22). The data clustered in groups, suggesting one to four inputs to each PL_N cell and allowing both high and low spontaneous active fibers to synapse on these cells. Also, the height of excitatory postsynaptic potentials (EPSPs) recorded intracellularly/intraaxonally clustered into several amplitude groups. None of these observations is conclusive, but they lend support to the idea that relatively small numbers of AN fibers converge onto globular/bushy cells. In the low-frequency region of the anterior AVCN, it has been known for some time that the bushy cells

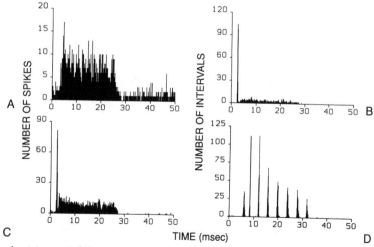

FIG. 14. PL_N short tone at CF responses (250 × 25 msec). **A** and **B:** Response at TH + 10 and TH + 40 dB; CF = 26 kHz. Only the onset rate has changed as the stimulus level is increased. **C:** Response at TH + 60 in a unit with CF = 9.8 kHz that has the same onset rate as the unit in A and B but a much lower sustained rate. **D:** Response at TH + 35 in a unit with low CF (= 250 Hz). (Adapted from ref. 18.)

behave similarly to AN fibers. In this region some spherical bushy cells receive only one large end-bulb (2).

The most extensive intracellular studies of these cells come from a mouse tissue-slice preparation (35,46). They demon-strated that bushy cells had a nonlinear current-voltage relationship such that in a slightly depolarized state the membrane impedance is low, resulting in a small time constant, exactly what would be required to preserve fine temporal encoding of com-

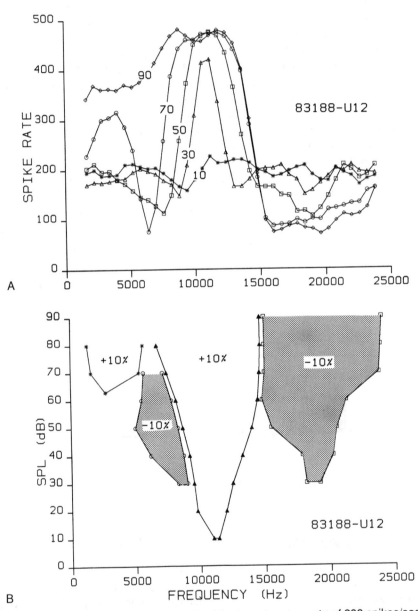

FIG. 15. A: Response area for a chopper unit with a spontaneous rate of 200 spikes/sec illustrating prominent inhibitory sidebands. **B:** Isorate curves taken at SR ± 10%. Inhibitory region is in shaded area. (Adapted from ref. 22.)

plex signals. A second population of cells in AVCN that had a linear I-V (current-voltage) curve discharged regularly when depolarized and summed EPSPs. These were shown to be stellate cells by labeling with HRP and are the same cell types we earlier demonstrated to be chopper units in the PVCN and DCN.

Ventral Cochlear Nucleus—Stellate Cells

There are a variety of chopper response patterns that undoubtedly reflect the balance between excitatory and inhibitory inputs. Some cells that display chopper behavior have prominent inhibitory sidebands that are obvious when they are spontaneously active (e.g., Fig. 15). A couple of

C_Ss proved to be stellate cells that had relatively long, unbranched and smooth dendrites (e.g., Fig. 16B). The C_T pattern was recorded from stellate cells with somewhat shorter, more branched dendrites (e.g., Fig. 16A). Other variations of chopper patterns have not been tied to any morphological features.

The electron microscopic studies of Smith and Rhode (19) showed that the C_S cells had very sparse synaptic coverage of the somas and a lot of small AN terminals on the proximal dendrites of these cells. Oertel (47) illustrated that the time course of the EPSPs on stellate cells was sufficiently slow to allow spatial and temporal summation, thereby providing a substrate for the sustained depolarization recorded in choppers.

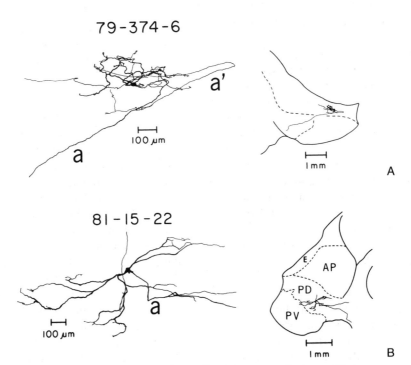

FIG. 16. A: Camera lucida reconstruction of a stellate/chopper unit along with transverse section of the cochlear nucleus of a stellate/chopper located in the PVCN. **B:** Camera lucida reconstruction of a stellate/chopper unit located in the posterodorsal division of the AVCN along with an inset illustrating the dendritic extent in a transverse section of the cochlear nucleus. E, granule cells; AP, anteroposteral region; PD, posterodorsal region of AVCN; PV, posteroventral region of AVCN. a, axon. (Adapted from ref. 24.)

Posteroventral Cochlear Nucleus

Multipolar Cells

The part of the VCN just posterior to the AN and innervated by the descending branch of the AN has been known to display two principal response patterns: chopper and onset (10). The chopper response pattern was associated with stellate cells and the onset pattern was associated with octopus cells (48). Each of these patterns can be further subdivided and each is likely associated with a distinct cellular morphology.

A large class of cells in the PVCN are the multipolar cells that appear to have an onset response pattern and are primarily located in the anterior PVCN. Traditionally, onset cells were divided into two populations: O_I and O_L. O_I units respond almost exclusively with a single onset spike and are characterized by an asymmetric response to an FM swept tone. No O_I units have been labeled, due probably to the infrequency of encountering them. The traditional O_L population has been shown to consist of two subgroups, both of which have a well-timed initial spike followed by a sustained response that ranges from 30 to 700 spikes/second. One group of these onset cells has the added feature of having two to four modes of "chopping" at the onset of the response (although occasionally a single onset peak is seen) and displaying a wide dynamic range. We called this pattern O_C and found it in roughly 50% of the onset cells in the PVCN.

To date, our most extensive labeling data are for O_C cells in the PVCN. Five labeled cells (more than 100 studied physiologically) provide a good picture of these multipolar cells. The distinguishing feature of these cells is their low Q_{10} and wide dynamic ranges, often in excess of 80 dB. An identified O_C cell is illustrated in Fig. 17. It has large dendrites, extending over nearly the entire dorsolateral to ventromedial extent of the PVCN in a transverse plane, al-

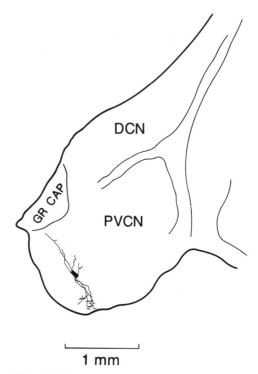

FIG. 17. Camera lucida drawing of an O_C cell in a transverse section of the cochlear nucleus. CF = 2.7 kHz. GR CAP, granule cap region. (Adapted from ref. 19.)

lowing access to inputs from AN fibers with different CFs. The membrane properties of O_C cells integrate (summate) the input EPSPs over a wide dynamic range. The intracellular response for an O_C is illustrated in Fig. 18C and D, along with its PSTH (Fig. 18D). A striking feature is the lack of saturation in the sound-evoked depolarization, even at 90 dB SPL. This relatively linear growth is a logical correlate of the large dynamic rate response of the sort shown in Fig. 18A. A simple model that could account for this behavior is shown in Fig. 12. For illustrative purposes, three fibers are shown to provide the necessary dynamic range of input by virtue of their different thresholds at a particular frequency due to having different CFs. Probably many fibers converge because the timing of O_C initial spikes is the least variable of any unit type in the CN, while the low Q_{10} (large band-

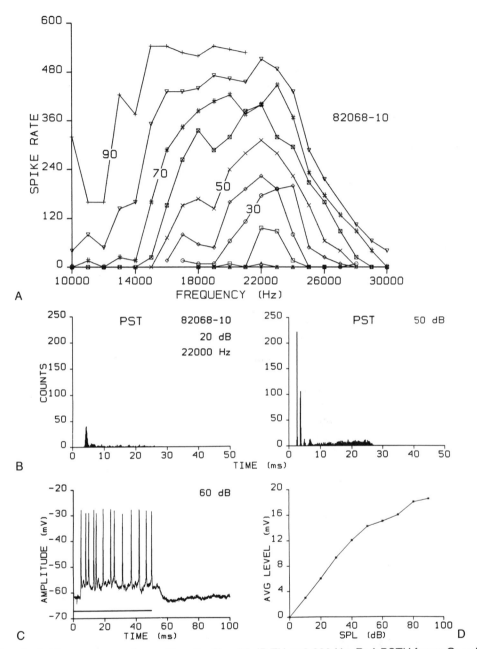

FIG. 18. A: Response area for an O_C cell with a 12 dB TH at 2,200 Hz. **B:** A PSTH for an O_C cell at 50 dB SPL. **C:** A single intracellular trace for the same cell whose PSTH is illustrated in B. **D:** The average membrane potential versus SPL for the same cell as in B and C. (Adapted from ref. 22.)

width) implies the convergence of AN fibers spanning a range of CFs. The standard deviation of the first spike latency is as low as 20 μsec in some units, suggesting that either these units can respond to individual EPSPs or that there are a substantial number of AN fiber inputs, or both.

Many synapses, containing large, round vesicles and thus probably arising from AN fibers, cover the cell soma and proximal dendrites of O_Cs. Further away from the soma such synapses are less common (19). Unfortunately, there is no practical way of counting the number of afferents. We have observed little indication of inhibitory behavior. However, in one cell (1 of 100) spontaneous firing was slightly suppressed below CF. Little sign of lateral inhibition has been seen in the masked response areas for O_C units (e.g., Fig. 7B). Some other O_Cs exhibited a reduction on the high-frequency side of CF. It was not unusual to see a slight reduction in driven rate after the onset spikes, followed by a return to higher rates within a few milliseconds (1–15 msec), again suggesting a "weak" inhibitory input.

In conjunction with the presence of both flat and pleomorphic vesicles in synapses on O_Cs, a tentative hypothesis is that inhibitory inputs depress the average discharge rate. While the average rate can attain 600 to 700 spikes/sec, some O_Cs also have low sustained rates (100 spikes/sec). Some of these cells can discharge at high rates (up to 1,000 spikes/sec) at low frequencies where their SCs may reach 0.99. These large SCs could be explained in a number of ways: (a) the input from the AN at low frequencies is synchronous, hence generating larger EPSPs that pass through a zero or threshold detector; (b) the inhibitory input is more effective at higher frequencies, reducing the efficacy of any synchronous input; (c) there is a relatively greater convergence of EPSPs as a consequence of the extensive low-frequency input at higher intensities due to the tails of AN fiber filter characteristics, which override the inhibitory input.

The role of O_Cs is unknown, but the fact that they possess pleomorphic vesicles in their boutons and have extensive collaterals in the CN (19) suggests that they may provide inhibitory input to other cells in the CN. Their axons have been shown to enter the IAS, but the targets of their projections have not yet been identified.

O_Cs encode the fundamental frequency of vowels very well (36) and could play a role in periodicity coding (49). For AM signals they often possess a low-pass filter characteristic and have better phase locking to the modulating frequency than other unit types. They also encode the modulating frequency to higher frequencies than other cells in the PVCN or DCN.

O_L neurons represent a substantial proportion (nearly 50%) of the PVCN population. It is likely that the octopus cells in this region are responsible for this pattern. These cells have been shown to have a large percentage of their somas covered by synapses with large, round vesicles (AN input) by Kane (48) in her electron microscopic studies. We labeled an octopus cell that we characterized as O_L (24). O_L cells exhibit average sustained rates of firing of 102 spikes/sec for those with no spontaneous activity and 215 spikes/sec for those with spontaneous activity (mean spontaneous rate = 43 spikes/sec).

The third type of onset cell, O_I, seen in the PVCN, is distinguished by a number of features. O_Is have an asymmetric response to a swept tone, low Q_{10}s, and the smallest dynamic range of any cell in the VCN (as low as 10 dB). Broad tuning curves imply that AN fibers with substantially different CFs provide converging input. Kane (48) suggested that octopus cells exhibit an onset pattern. These cells are located on the caudal aspect of the PVCN and have their dendrites oriented toward the center of the neuropil. A possible explanation for the asymmetric response to swept tones was offered by Gerstein in Szentagothai and Arbib (50): for a sweep in one direction, the excitatory effects of each EPSP could be enhanced if later-arriving EPSPs occur closer to the soma, resulting in a cascade of EPSPs. For a sweep in the other direction, later-arriving EPSPs, occurring farther from the soma, will have to travel through already depolarized dendrites and their arrival times at the soma will not be optimum for summation. However, O_Is do not appear to occur very often (6% of onset cells in PVCN in our sample), while Ritz and Brownell (51) virtually never saw them in the decerebrate cat. This latter study also indicates anesthesia could affect the proportions of cell types. One other feature common to O_Is and O_Ls is that at low frequencies their output can entrain to the stimulus at rates ranging between 400 and 1,000 spikes/sec. This implies that if the in-put is sufficiently synchronous, then these cells are capable of firing at high rates.

Dorsal Cochlear Nucleus—Fusiform Cells

The DCN is layered, with a molecular layer, a fusiform cell layer, and a deep layer. The principal cells are the fusiform cells and the giant cells in the deep layer that project to higher centers via the DAS (52–54). In anesthetized cats these cells display a variety of temporal response patterns, including pauser/buildup/chopper patterns (Fig. 2), which can all occur in a single fusiform cell depending on the stimulus parameters.

The response areas in Fig. 19 illustrate

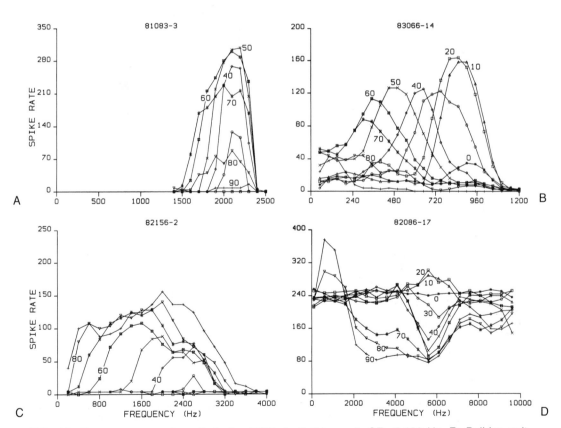

FIG. 19. Response areas for cells in the DCN. **A:** Buildup unit, CF = 2,100 Hz. **B:** Buildup unit, CF = 650 Hz. **C:** Pauser, CF = 2,600 Hz. **D:** Type 4, CF = 5,800 Hz. (Adapted from ref. 58.)

some of the variety of response areas for DCN cells. These responses are often non-monotonic as a function of intensity (Fig. 19A) and may exhibit a shift in CF as intensity increases (Fig. 19B). They can also have well-behaved response areas (monotonic rate curve), as in Fig. 19C. The response area in Fig. 19D would be classified as Type IV based on its receptive field. In decerebrate cats, Type IV is the predominant receptive field, characterized by a small, excitatory region at CF and low in-

tensities and one (some) region(s) of excitation at higher intensities (13).

The physiological variety is equaled by the morphological diversity. The four fusiform cells in Fig. 20 covers a range of locations from very lateral (Fig. 20D) to caudal (Fig. 20C) to rostral (Fig. 20A) and a placement in the center of the fusiform cell layer (Fig. 20B). The laterally located fusiform cell (Fig. 20D) had nearly no basal dendrites.

Fusiform and giant cells of the DCN pro-

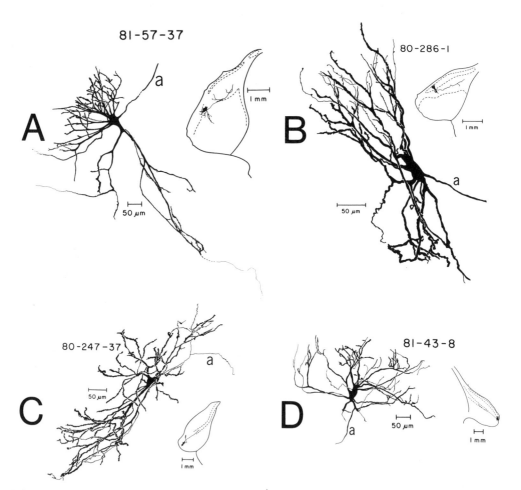

FIG. 20. Four fusiform cells and their locations within the transverse sections of the CN. **A:** Pauser unit, CF = 11,000 Hz, TH = 18 dB SPL, SR = 70 spikes/sec. **B:** Buildup unit, CF = 1,500 Hz, TH = −2 dB SPL, SR = 0 spikes/sec. **C:** Buildup unit, CF = 1,500 Hz, TH = 0 dB SPL, SR = 10 spikes/sec. **D:** Type IV receptive field, CF = 1,500, TH = 10 dB SPL, SR = 50 spikes/sec.

ject to the contralateral inferior colliculus (52,54,55). The fusiform cells are characterized by spinous, apical dendritic tufts that can extend to the ependymal layer (and even run a short distance parallel to it). We estimate that some of these cells may have as many as 10,000 spines. The somas are typically large (up to 50 μm) and elongate. The basal dendrites ramify little and are relatively free of spines. It has been demonstrated, using an electron microscope, that the predominant location of terminals with large, round synaptic vesicles is on the basal dendrites, with few on the soma, and virtually none on the apical dendrites. All of the fusiform cells we have labeled had axonal collaterals within the deep DCN. In mice, fusiform cells have no collaterals within the CN (56).

It is clear, in these cells, that inhibition plays a prominent role in their behavior (32,57,58). Intracellular records indicate that spike output can be suppressed even when the cell is depolarized to levels that normally elicit spikes. This suggests that the inhibitory input at the axon initial segment can possibly override the excitation.

Voigt and Young (59) cross-correlated spike trains from pairs of cells recorded with a single metal microelectrode and demonstrated that type II cells inhibit type IV. Type IV cells are almost certainly fusiform cells. Type II cells are possibly small stellate cells. This conjecture is supported by a current view of DCN circuitry (56,60).

The fusiform circuit could be implemented in a number of ways based on current data. In a minimal circuit, in addition to the AN input, there could be a single interneuron with a CF near the CF of the fusiform cell but with a higher threshold than the excitatory threshold. The gain function for the inhibitory input would have to be greater than the gain for the excitatory input to effect a nonmonotonic rate curve. Alternately, there could be two inhibitory interneurons with CFs above and below the CF of the fusiform cell. The relative gains (inhibitory vs. excitatory) could easily

account for a variety of response areas. Response areas with shifting CFs versus intensity could require a large number of neurons in the circuit.

Several studies have contributed to our present understanding of circuits involving fusiform cells (e.g., 15,61). Computer reconstruction of a number of fusiform cells by Blackstad et al. (62) demonstrated a high degree of flatness and parallel organization in their basal arbor. This could be a way of preserving frequency selectivity. Mugnaini and colleagues (15,61) suggest several circuits involving the cartwheel, Golgi, granule, and stellate cells. The granule cells have long axons traveling parallel to the stria and synapsing primarily on the spines of the apical dendrites of the fusiform cells. Golgi cells participate with granule cells in glomerular complexes, along with mossy fibers very similar to those complexes observed in the cerebellum. Cartwheel cells have been shown to label positively for glutamic acid decarboxylase, the precursor for gamma-aminobutyric acid, and are likely to be inhibitory interneurons, based on their synaptic contacts (symmetric synapse and pleomorphic vesicles). However, one should exhibit some caution in generalizing findings in one species to the cat.

Type II Response Type

One of the response types found in the DCN is called Type II (see Fig. 3). While Young and colleagues (59,67) have found it to be located near Type IV cells and likely to provide one of the inhibitory inputs to the Type IV, one variety is also found in the deep DCN and displays an O_G temporal pattern. These cells have nonmonotonic rate curves and usually respond poorly to WBN. The presence of WBN acts to suppress any tonal response. It appears that an inhibitory input to Type IIs has a greater influence than the excitatory portion of the input. Unlike many other cells where a tone at CF can cause a cell to discharge at the same rate with or without a noise present, WBN reduces the maximum discharge rate that an O_G/Type II cell can attain. An inhibitory input may be from stellate cells in the PVCN (63,64).

While Kane et al. (55) subdivided the giant cell population into four categories on the basis of dendritic morphology, their physiology is largely unknown. If we speculate that recordings are most likely to be made from the largest cells, then our data suggest that giant cells respond with O_G (PM) patterns, those observed most often in the deep layer. These are cells that exhibit type II noise response properties and are nonmonotonic in their rate curves.

SUMMARY

The diagram in Fig. 21 summarizes much of what we have learned about both the physiology and anatomy of the CN. It is obvious that only the principal (large) cell types are represented. This is likely due to a sampling bias introduced by the electrode and the difficulty of performing intracellular recording and labeling on all but large cells, especially *in vivo*. However, the past 10 years have been very productive in providing details of the anatomy and physiological responses to a wide battery of acoustic signals in a variety of species.

Figure 21 indicates that there are projec-

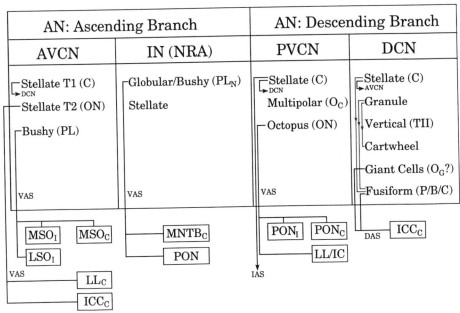

FIG. 21. A summary of known connectivity of the principal cell types in the cochlear nucleus along with their temporal response types or receptive field types listed alongside the morphological type. Anatomical abbreviations: AN, auditory nerve; AVCN, anteroventral cochlear nucleus; DAS, dorsal acoustic stria; DCN, dorsal cochlear nucleus; IAS, intermediate acoustic stria; IC, inferior colliculus; ICC_C, contralateral central nucleus of the inferior colliculus; IN, interstitial nucleus; LL, lateral lemniscus; MSO, medial superior olive; LSO, lateral superior olive; NRA, nerve root area; PON, periolivary nuclei; PVCN, posteroventral cochlear nucleus; VAS, ventral acoustic stria. Subscripts: I, ipsilateral; C, contralateral. Physiological abbreviations: B, buildup response pattern; C, chopper pattern; O_C, onset, chopper pattern; O_G, graded onset pattern; ON, onset pattern; P, pauser pattern; PL, primary-like; PL_N, primary-like with notch pattern; TII, type II receptive field; T1, type 1 stellate cell has relatively few synapses on soma; T2, type 2 stellate cell has dense synaptic coverage of the soma.

tions from each division of the CN that have fairly specific targets in the auditory brainstem. Each of these may provide higher auditory structures with the encoded features of the acoustic input necessary to perform their special task. What is equally clear is that this is a much simplified diagram, ignoring much of the internuclear pathways (2,65–67) and likely unaware of the full complexity of the projections from each major cell type.

The detailed interconnections of intrinsic cells along with multiple efferent projections need to be worked out. The application of techniques from disciplines such as immunocytochemistry and neural systems analysis will be required to take the next major steps in understanding this complex, parallel processing structure.

ACKNOWLEDGMENTS

This work was supported by NIH grant 5 PO1 NS12732. We appreciate the efforts of D. Geisler, S. Greenberg, D. Oertel, and R. Wickesberg in reviewing this chapter. The efforts of B. Sorensen for typing and T. Stewart for photography are appreciated.

REFERENCES

1. Rose JE, Galambos R, Hughes JR. Microelectrode studies of the cochlear nuclei of the cat. *Bull Johns Hopkins Hosp* 1959;104:211–251.
2. Lorente de Nó R. *The primary acoustic nuclei.* New York: Raven Press, 1981.
3. Cant NB, Morest DK. The structural basis for stimulus coding in the cochlear nucleus of the cat. In: Berlin C, ed. *Hearing sciences.* San Diego: College-Hill Press, 1984;371–421.
4. Moore JK. Cochlear nuclei: relationship to the auditory nerve. In: Altschuler RA, Hoffman DW, Bobbin RP, eds. *Neurobiology of hearing: the cochlea.* New York: Raven Press, 1986; 303–332.
5. Liberman MC. Auditory nerve responses from cats raised ina low noise chamber. *J Acoust Soc Am* 1978;63:442–455.
6. Fekete DM, Rouiller EM, Liberman MC, Ryugo DK. The central projections of intracellularly labeled auditory nerve fibers in cats. *J Comp Neurol* 1984;229:432–450.
7. Osen KK. Cytoarchitecture of the cochlear nuclei in the cat. *J Comp Neurol* 1969;136:453–484.
8. Brawer JR, Morest DK, Kane EC. The neuronal architecture of the cochlear nucleus of the cat. *J Comp Neurol* 1974;155:251–300.
9. Pfeiffer RR. Classification of response patterns of spike discharges for units in the cochlear nucleus: tone burst stimulation. *Exp Brain Res* 1966;1:220–235.
10. Godfrey DA, Kiang NYS, Norris BE. Single unit activity in the posteroventral cochlear nucleus of the cat. *J Comp Neurol* 1975;162: 247–268.
11. Godfrey DA, Kiang NYS, Norris BE. Single unit activity in the dorsal cochlear nucleus. *J Comp Neurol* 1975;162:269–284.
12. Bourk TR. Electrical responses of neural units in the anteroventral cochlear nucleus of the cat. Ph.D. thesis, MIT, 1976.
13. Young ED, Brownell WE. Responses to tones and noise of single cells in dorsal cochlear nucleus of unanesthetized cats. *J Neurophysiol* 1976;39:282–300.
14. Morest DK, Kiang NYS, Kane EC, Guinan JJ, Godfrey DA. Stimulus coding at the caudal levels of the cat auditory nervous system. II. Patterns of synaptic organization. In: Møller AR, ed. *Basic mechanisms of hearing.* New York: Academic, 1973;479–504.
15. Wouterlood FG, Mugnaini E. Cartwheel neurons of the dorsal cochlear nucleus: a Golgi-electron microscopic study in rat. *J Comp Neurol* 1984;277:136–157.
16. Muller KJ, McMahan UJ. The shapes of sensory and motor neurons and their distribution of their synapses in ganglia of the leech: a study using intracellular injection of horseradish-peroxidase. *Proc R Soc Lond [Biol]* 1976;194:481–499.
17. Smith PH, Rhode WS. Electron microscopic features of physiologically characterized, HRP-labeled fusiform cells in the cat dorsal cochlear nucleus. *J Comp Neurol* 1985;237:127–143.
18. Smith PH, Rhode WS. Characterization of HRP-labeled globular bushy cells in the cat anteroventral cochlear nucleus. *J Comp Neurol* 1987;266:360–375.
19. Smith PH, Rhode WS. Structural and functional properties distinguish two types of multipolar cells in the cat ventral cochlear nucleus. *J Comp Neurol* 1989;282:595–616.
20. Evans EF, Nelson PG. The responses of single neurons in the cochlear nucleus of the cat as a function of their location and anesthetic state. *Exp Brain Res* 1973;117:402–427.
21. Young ED, Voigt HF. The internal organization of the dorsal cochlear nucleus. In: Syka J, Aitkin L, eds. *Neuronal mechanisms of hearing.* New York: Plenum Press, 1981;127–133.
22. Rhode WS, Smith PH. Encoding timing and intensity in the ventral nucleus of the cat. *J Neurophysiol* 1986;56:261–286.
23. Rhode WS, Kettner RE. Physiological study of

neurons in the dorsal and posteroventral cochlear nucleus of the unanesthetized cat. *J Neurophysiol* 1987;57:414–442.

24. Rhode WS, Oertel D, Smith PH. Physiological
response properties of cells labeled intracellularly with horseradish peroxidase in the cat
ventral cochlear nucleus. *J Comp Neurol* 1983;
213:448–463.

25. Rhode WS, Smith PH. Characteristics of tone-
pip response patterns in relationship to spontaneous rate in auditory nerve fibers. *Hear Res*
1985;18:159–168.

26. Young ED, Robert JM, Shofner WP. Regularity
and latency of units in ventral cochlear nucleus:
implications for unit classification and generation of response properties. *J Neurophysiol*
1988;60:1–29.

27. Banks M, Sachs MB, Blackburn CC, Rice JJ.
Compartmental model for chopper units in the
ventral cochlear nucleus (VCN): preliminary
analysis of interspike interval regularity. *ARO
Abstr, Twelfth Midwinter Research Meeting*
1989;59.

28. Frisina RD, Smith RL, Chamberlain SC. Differential encoding of rapid changes in sound amplitude by second-order auditory neurons. *Exp
Brain Res* 1985;60:417–422.

29. Kim DO, Rhode WS, Greenberg S. Responses
of cochlear nucleus neurons to speech signals:
neural encoding of pitch, intensity and other
parameters. In: Moore BCJ, Patterson RD,
eds. *Auditory frequency selectivity.* New York:
Plenum, 1986;281–288.

30. Oertel D, Wu SH, Hirsch JA. Electrical characteristics of cells and neuronal circuitry in the
cochlear nuclei studied with intracellular recordings from brain slices. In: Edelman GM, Einar
Gall W, Cowan WM, eds. *Auditory function.*
New York: John Wiley, 1988;313–336.

31. Rhode WS, Geisler CD, Kennedy DK. Auditory
nerve fiber responses to wide-band noise and
tone combinations. *J Neurophysiol* 1978;41:
692–704.

32. Rhode WS, Smith PH, Oertel D. Physiological
response properties of cells labeled intracellularly with horseradish peroxidase in cat dorsal
cochlear nucleus. *J Comp Neurol* 1983;213:
426–447.

33. Hirsch JA, Oertel D. Synaptic connections in
the dorsal cochlear nucleus of mice, *in vitro. J
Physiol (Lond)* 1988;396:549–562.

34. Wu SH, Oertel D. Intracellular injection with
horseradish peroxidase of physiologically characterized stellate and bushy cells in slices of
mouse anteroventral cochlear nuclei. *J Neurosci*
1984;4:1577–1588.

35. Wu SH, Oertel D. Inhibitory circuitry in the
ventral cochlear nucleus is probably mediated
by glycine. *J Neurosci* 1986;6:2691–2706.

36. Capranica RR, Rose G, Brenowitz EA. Time
resolution in the auditory system of anurans.
In: Michelsen A, ed. *Time resolution in auditory
systems.* New York: Springer-Verlag, 1983;
58–73.

37. Kay RH. Hearing of modulation in sounds.
Physiol Rev 1982;62:894–975.

38. Plomp R. On the role of modulation in hearing.
In: Klinke R, Hartman R, eds. *Hearing—phys-
iological bases and psychophysics.* Heidelberg:
Springer-Verlag, 1983.

39. Møller AR. Coding of time-varying sounds in the
cochlear nucleus. *Audiology* 1977;17:446–468.

40. Palmer AR, Evans EF. Intensity coding in the
auditory periphery of the cat: responses of cochlear nerve and cochlear nucleus neurons to
signals in the presence of bandstop masking
noise. *Hear Res* 1982;7:305–323.

41. Gibson DJ, Young ED, Costalupes JA. Similarity of dynamic range adjustment in auditory
nerve and cochlear nuclei. *J Neurophysiol* 1985;
53:940–958.

42. Cant NB, Morest DK. Organization of the neurons in the anterior division of the anteroventral
cochlear nucleus of the cat, light-microscopic
observations. *Neuroscience* 1979;4:1904–
1923.

43. Mugnaini E, Warr WB, Osen KK. Distribution
and light microscopic features of granule cells in
the cochlear nuclei of cat, rat, and mouse. *J
Comp Neurol* 1980;191:581–606.

44. Tolbert LP, Morest DK, Yurgelum-Todd DA.
The neuronal architecture of the anteroventral
cochlear nucleus of the cat in the region of the
cochlear nerve root: horseradish peroxidase labelling of identified cell types. *Neuroscience*
1982;7:3031–3052.

45. Rouiller EM, Ryugo DK. Intracellular marking
of physiologically characterized cells in the ventral cochlear nucleus of the cat. *J Comp Neurol*
1984;225:167–186.

46. Oertel D. Synaptic response and electrical properties of cells in brain slices of the mouse anteroventral cochlear nucleus. *J Neurosci* 1983;
3:2043–2053.

47. Oertel D. Use of brain slices in the study of the
auditory system: spatial and temporal summation of synaptic inputs in cells in the anteroventral cochlear nucleus of the mouse. *J Acoust Soc
Am* 1985;78:328–333.

48. Kane EC. Octopus cells in the cochlear nucleus
of the cat: heterotypic synapses upon homotypic
neurons. *Int J Neurosci* 1973;5:251–279.

49. Greenberg S, Rhode WS. Periodicity coding in
cochlear nerve and ventral cochlear nucleus. In:
Yost WA, Watson CS, eds. *Auditory processing
of complex sounds.* Hillsdale, NJ: Lawrence
Erlbaum, 1987;225–236.

50. Szentagothai J, Arbib MA. *Conceptual models
of neural organization.* Cambridge, MA: MIT
Press, 1975.

51. Ritz LA, Brownell WE. Single unit analysis of
the posteroventral cochlear nucleus of the decerebrate cat. *Neuroscience* 1982;7:1995–2010.

52. Adams JC. Single unit studies on the dorsal and
intermediate acoustic striae. *J Comp Neurol*
1976;170:97–106.

53. Kane EC. Synaptic organization in the dorsal
cochlear nucleus of the cat: a light and electron

microscopic study. *J Comp Neurol* 1974;155: 301–329.

54. Roth GL, Aitkin LM, Anderson RA, Merzenich MM. Some features of the spatial organization of the central nucleus of the inferior colliculus of the cat. *J Comp Neurol* 1978;182:661–680.

55. Kane EC, Puglisi SG, Gordon BS. Neuronal types in the deep dorsal cochlear nucleus of the cat: I. Giant neurons. *J Comp Neurol* 1981;198: 483–513.

56. Oertel D, Wu SH. Morphology and physiology of cells in slice preparations of the dorsal cochlear nucleus of mice. *J Comp Neurol (in press)*.

57. Hirsch JA, Oertel D. Intrinsic properties of neurons in the dorsal cochlear nucleus of mice, *in vitro*. *J Physiol (Lond)* 1988;396:535–548.

58. Rhode WS, Smith PH. Physiological studies on neurons in the dorsal cochlear nucleus of cat. *J Neurophysiol* 1986;56:287–307.

59. Voigt HF, Young ED. Evidence of inhibitory interactions between neurons in the dorsal cochlear nucleus. *J Neurophysiol* 1980;44:76–96.

60. Mugnaini E. GABA neurons in the superficial layers of the rat dorsal cochlear nucleus: light and electron microscopic immunocytochemistry. *J Comp Neurol* 1985;235:61–81.

61. Wouterlood FG, Mugnaini E, Osen KK, Dahl A-L. Stellate neurons in rat dorsal cochlear nucleus studied with combined Golgi impregnation and electron microscopy: synaptic connections and mutual coupling by gap junctions. *J Neurocytol* 1984;13:639–664.

62. Blackstad TU, Osen KK, Mugnaini E. Pyramidal neurons of the dorsal cochlear nucleus: a Golgi and computer reconstruction in cat. *Neuroscience* 1984;13:827–854.

63. Snyder RL, Leake PA. Intrinsic connections within and between cochlear nucleus subdivisions in cat. *J Comp Neurol* 1988;278:209–225.

64. Oertel D, Wickesberg RE, Wu SH, Hirsch JA. The cochlear nuclear complex in brain slice preparations. *Assoc Res Otolaryngol Abstr* 1989;12:4.

65. Evans EF, Nelson PG. On the functional relationship between the dorsal and ventral divisions of the cochlear nucleus of the cat. *Exp Brain Res* 1973;17:428–442.

66. Shofner WP, Young ED. Inhibitory connections between AVCN and DCN: evidence from lidocaine injection in AVCN. *Hear Res* 1987;29: 45–53.

67. Young ED. Response characteristics of neurons of the cochlear nuclei. In: Berlin C, ed. *Hearing sciences*. San Diego: College-Hill Press, 1984; 423–460.

Neurobiology of Hearing: The Central Auditory System, edited by R. A. Altschuler et al. Raven Press, Ltd., New York © 1991.

4

Processing of Complex Sounds in the Cochlear Nucleus

Murray B. Sachs and Carol C. Blackburn

Center for Hearing Sciences, Department of Biomedical Engineering, The Johns Hopkins University, Baltimore, Maryland 21205

The function of the peripheral auditory system is to convert sound into patterns of spike discharges in the population of auditory-nerve fibers. The role of the central auditory system is to interpret those discharge patterns in order to produce the perception of sound and other appropriate behavior. During the past decade considerable progress has been made toward the goal of specifying the auditory-nerve representation of sounds as complex as human speech (39). The focus of research into the neural processing of complex stimuli has now shifted to the cochlear nucleus, the first brainstem auditory center. In this chapter we briefly review the fundamental properties of the representation of complex stimuli in the auditory nerve and then explore our current understanding of the processing of that representation in the cochlear nucleus.

FUNDAMENTALS OF THE REPRESENTATION OF COMPLEX STIMULI IN THE AUDITORY NERVE

The concept of representation of sensory stimuli has a long history in both the neurosciences and cognitive sciences (8,24). We use the term representation to mean a display of neural responses across a tonotopi-cally organized array of single auditory neurons. By neural signal processing we mean the transformation between the stimulus representation on the array of neurons that serve as inputs to a cell group and the representation across the tonotopically organized axons that are the output of the cell group.

Figure 1 illustrates this concept of representation at the level of the auditory nerve. The spectrum of the synthesized steady-state vowel /ɛ/ (as in *bet*) is shown in Fig. 1A; we use this vowel to illustrate most of the important aspects of representation not because it is specifically a speech sound but because it is a good example of a spectrally complex sound. There are, however, several aspects of this sound that limit the generality of results obtained with it. First, it is perfectly periodic, clearly an unnatural constraint. However, studies with aperiodic sounds (consonants [9,22,42]; whispered vowels [49]), have produced similar representations. Second, whereas this vowel is a steady-state sound, naturally occurring sounds are generally time-varying. Studies of the representation of transient speech-like sounds are just beginning at the level of the cochlear nucleus.

Because the vowel is periodic, its spectrum contains energy only at the fundamental frequency (128 Hz) and its harmonics.

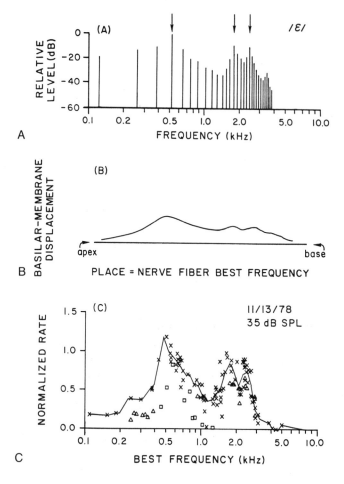

FIG. 1. A: Amplitude spectrum of vowel /ɛ/. This spectrum has been modified to compensate for the effects of the external ear resonance. **B:** Hypothetical plot of basilar membrane displacement versus place in response to the /ɛ/. **C:** Plot of normalized rate versus best frequency (BF) for ANF units studied on 11/13/78, with the /ɛ/ as the stimulus. Each point is the rate of one unit plotted at the unit's BF. Low spontaneous rate fibers (less than 1/sec) plotted with squares, medium spontaneous rate fibers (between 1 and 20/sec) with triangles, and high spontaneous rate fibers (greater than 20/sec) with Xs. *Solid line* is moving window average of high spontaneous rate fibers.

The most prominent feature of the spectrum are the peaks at 512, 1,792, and 2,432 Hz; these are the formant frequencies of the vowel. The perceptual identity of such vowels is directly related to these formant frequencies (30,31). In this chapter, we concentrate on the issue of how these energy peaks are represented in the auditory nerve and cochlear nucleus.

The general idea of spectral representation in the peripheral auditory system is illustrated in Fig. 1B. The idea is that peaks in the spectrum produce peaks in basilar membrane displacement at corresponding best frequency (BF) places. These peaks in basilar membrane displacement in turn produce peaks of response in the auditory-nerve population at the same BF places as

are shown in Fig. 1C. In considering representation across the auditory-nerve population, we must be careful to define just what we mean by a "response." The response measure used in Fig. 1C is normalized average discharge rate; the normalization is such that a value of one corresponds to the saturation rate of the fiber, while zero corresponds to spontaneous rate. We refer to plots of normalized rate versus BF as rate-place profiles.

Such an average rate measure neglects important information contained in the temporal details of the auditory-nerve fiber spike trains as illustrated in Fig. 2. The temporal waveform of the /ɛ/ is shown in Fig. 2A. Its fundamental period is 7.8 msec (its fundamental frequency is 128 Hz). The first

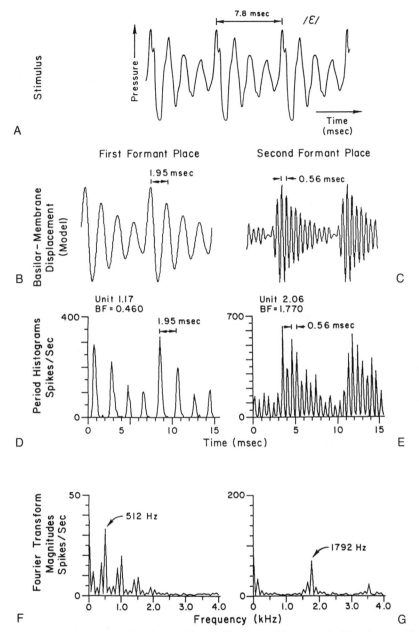

FIG. 2. A: Pressure versus time for the /ε/. **B** and **C:** Plots of hypothetical basilar membrane displacement at the first (512 Hz) and second (1,792 Hz) formant places, respectively. **D** and **E:** Period histograms for responses of ANF units with BFs near the first and second formant places. **F, G:** Magnitudes of the Fourier transforms of the corresponding period histograms.

formant frequency, which is the fourth harmonic of the fundamental, contains more energy than other spectral components, and it therefore dominates the temporal waveform. Hence there are four prominent peaks per fundamental period in the waveform. Figure 2B and C shows a crude representation of the temporal waveform seen by auditory-nerve fibers with BFs at the first and second formants of the vowel. Because of the mechanical properties of the basilar membrane (and perhaps because of interaction between basilar membrane motion and mechanical/electrical responses of hair cells [5]), the stimulus to the auditory-nerve fiber is a bandpass version of the acoustic signal. Thus, at the first formant place the waveform of basilar membrane displacement is dominated by the first formant, whereas at the second formant place it is dominated by the second formant. As shown by the period histograms in Fig. 2D and E, auditory-nerve fibers tuned to these formants are phase-locked to the corresponding formant. A quantitative measure of the phase-locked response of a single auditory-nerve fiber to any stimulus spectral component can be obtained from the Fourier transform of the period histogram, as shown in Fig. 2F and G. We use the magnitude of the Fourier transform at any frequency as a measure of a single fiber's phase-locking at that frequency.

We define the temporal (phase-locked) response of the population of auditory-nerve fibers at any stimulus frequency to be the average of the magnitudes of Fourier transform components at that frequency, taken over all fibers whose BFs are near (usually plus/minus one-quarter octave) the frequency of interest. We call this measure the ALSR for average localized (the average is taken only over fibers with BFs near the frequency) synchronized (reflecting the phase-locked response) rate (magnitude of the Fourier transform is given as absolute spikes per second). We refer to plots of ALSR versus stimulus frequency as temporal-place profiles. Figure 3 shows temporal-place profiles for the /ɛ/ presented at three sound levels. The data come from the same experiment as those presented in Fig. 1C. These temporal-place profiles provide a very precise representation of the stimulus spectrum up to the highest sound level tested (75 dB SPL). In fact, the prominence of spectral peaks in the profiles (e.g., peak to trough differences) increases as stimulus

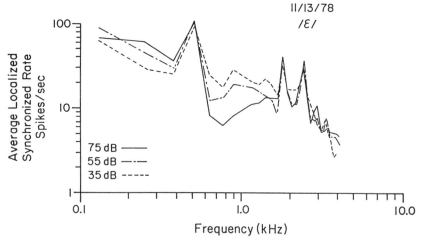

FIG. 3. Average localized synchronized rate (ALSR) for the /ɛ/ at 35, 55, and 75 dB SPL. See text for an explanation of the ALSR measure.

level increases. Thus, a temporal-place representation of stimulus spectrum is robust over stimulus level. We have also shown that such a representation is robust in the presence of background noise (38).

By contrast, rate-place profiles depend strongly on stimulus level and on signal to noise ratio. Figure 4A shows rate-place profiles for /ɛ/ presented over a range of stim-

ulus levels. Data points for individual fibers have been omitted and only plots of data averaged across fibers are shown; averages include only fibers with spontaneous rates greater than 20 spikes/sec (the "high spontaneous rate" fibers of Liberman (19); see Fig. 1 caption for details). At 25 and 35 dB SPL (same data as Fig. 1C) the rate-place profile provides an accurate representation

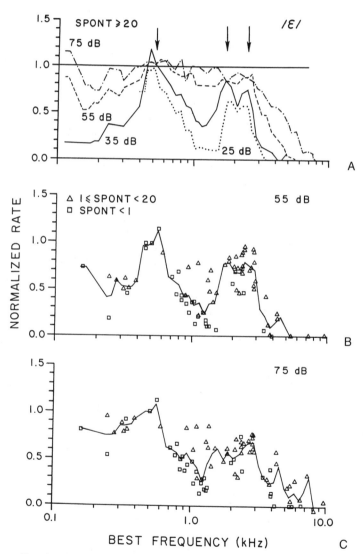

FIG. 4. A: Rate profiles (average data only) for /ɛ/ at 25, 35, 55, and 75 dB SPL for high spontaneous rate ANF units. **B** and **C:** Rate profiles for low and medium spontaneous rate units at 55 and 75 dB SPL, respectively.

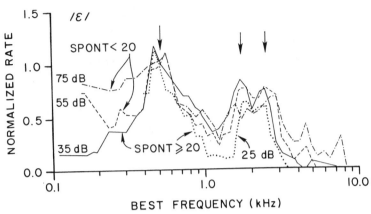

FIG. 5. Rate profiles for /ɛ/ for high spontaneous rate fibers at 25 and 35 dB SPL; low and medium spontaneous rate fibers at 55 and 75 dB SPL, respectively.

of stimulus spectrum. However, the prominence of formant peaks in the profile is very much reduced at 55 dB SPL, and at 75 dB SPL there is no sign of formant peaks at all. This loss of spectral features is a result of rate saturation and two-tone suppression (37). As shown in Fig. 4B and C, on the other hand, rate profiles computed from the low and medium spontaneous rate fibers maintain a representation of formant peaks even at the highest level tested (75 dB SPL). These fibers have higher thresholds (19) and broader dynamic ranges than high spontaneous rate fibers (29,40). Comparing parts A, B, and C of Fig. 4, we can see that the rate-place profiles for the low and medium spontaneous fibers are similar to one another at 55 and 75 dB and are similar to the profile for high spontaneous rate fibers for 25 and 35 dB SPL. This similarity is emphasized in Fig. 5 where these four profiles have been superimposed. This result suggests that a rate-place representation that is robust over stimulus level could be provided by a weighted sum of the rates of the low, medium, and high spontaneous rate fibers; the rates of high spontaneous (low threshold) fibers must be given greatest weight at low sound levels and the low spontaneous (high threshold) fibers weighted most heavily at high sound levels.

REPRESENTATION OF COMPLEX SPECTRA IN THE ANTEROVENTRAL COCHLEAR NUCLEUS

We thus arrive at two complementary auditory-nerve representations for the spectra of complex stimuli. It is important to note, however, that both of these representations place certain demands on central processing. In order that a rate-place representation be stable over even a moderate range of stimulus levels, the weighted sum of rates of high, medium, and low spontaneous fibers must be computed. In order that a temporal-place representation be viable the central nervous system must be able to deal with phase-locked spike trains up to frequencies at least in the range of the third formant frequencies (about 3.0 kHz). In this section we consider the processing of both of these representations by two populations of cells in the anteroventral cochlear nucleus (AVCN): bushy cells and stellate cells.

Two morphologically defined principal cell types, called bushy and stellate cells, have been described in the AVCN (Fig. 6A) (7). These differ from one another in terms of their cellular morphology, patterns of synaptic organization, sources of descending efferent input, and the patterns of their

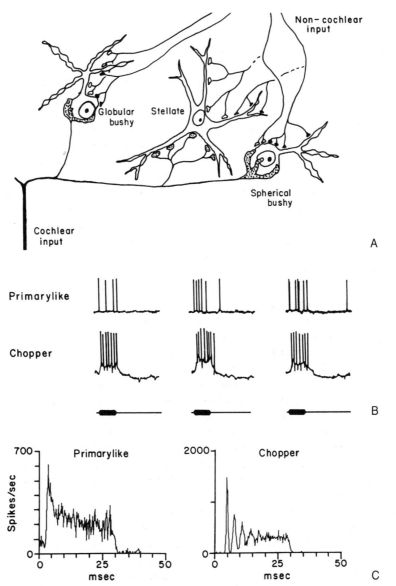

FIG. 6. A: Schematic illustration of afferent connections and synaptic organization of spherical bushy cells, globular bushy cells, and stellate cells in the anteroventral cochlear nucleus (From ref. 7, with permission.) **B:** Examples of spike trains recorded intracellularly from a primarylike unit (top) and chopper unit (middle). The bottom row shows the timing of the stimulus bursts, which were 25 msec BF tone bursts. (Redrawn from ref. 34.) **C:** Poststimulus time (PST) histograms for a primarylike unit and a chopper unit for 25 msec BF tone bursts.

axonal projections onto more central auditory nuclei. Corresponding differences in the complexity of their physiological responses have also been demonstrated. The bushy cells receive relatively few large synaptic terminals (the endbulbs of Held) from the auditory nerve directly on their somas (7,36). They have small dendritic trees that receive few synaptic terminals. Bushy cells differ in the number and size of their end-bulbs; spherical bushy cells have a few, larger endbulbs and globular bushy cells have more, smaller endbulbs (3). Intracellular labeling studies have allowed at least a preliminary identification of some response characteristics of bushy cells (32, 35). As a result of this synaptic input pattern, responses of bushy cells appear to be very similar to those of auditory-nerve fibers. Figure 6B and C illustrates those response properties that are relevant to this discussion and that we take as the physiologically distinguishing features of bushy cells. At the onset of a tone burst, they give a high rate of discharge followed by a gradual decline to a more or less steady level (Fig. 6C). This tone burst response is called primarylike and is associated with spherical bushy cells (32,35). The tone burst response of globular bushy cells is similar to the primarylike pattern except that there is a brief pause ("notch," about 1 msec) in firing after the initial rapid increase in rate; this pattern is called primarylike with notch (44). The responses of the great majority of spherical and globular bushy cells to the complex stimuli of interest here are thus far indistinguishable and so we consider them to be one class that we call *primarylike*. An important distinguishing feature of the primarylike units is the extent to which their firing patterns are irregular. As shown in Fig. 6B, the responses of these units to successively presented, identical stimuli are not the same; even the number of spikes during the stimulus interval varies from presentation to presentation. Furthermore the intervals between spikes are highly variable.

Stellate cells, on the other hand, receive a large number of small bouton inputs on their dendritic trees and, in some cases, on their cell bodies (Fig. 6A) (7). Stellate cells appear to produce chopper response patterns to BF tones (Fig. 6C) (32). This pattern is characterized by fluctuations in response rate synchronized to the stimulus onset. The spike trains of these units are very regular. The number of spikes is quite constant from one stimulus presentation to the next and the interval between spikes shows little variability (Fig. 6B). The chopping pattern in their tone burst responses is related to this regularity of firing. These units have a very precise onset time to the tone bursts and the following rate fluctuations simply reflect the regularity of the spike trains following the onset spike.

AVCN primarylike (bushy) cells and choppers (stellate) can be compared in their response maps (Fig. 7). A response map is a plot of a unit's receptive field, on coordinates of frequency (abscissa) and sound level (ordinate). Shaded regions show frequency-sound level combinations that give excitatory responses, i.e., increases in discharge rate above the spontaneous rate. Unshaded areas enclosed in dashed lines are areas of inhibitory responses, i.e., decreases in discharge rate from spontaneous rate. Almost all primarylike units recorded from spherical bushy in AVCN have Type I response maps (4,13). These maps have only a V-shaped excitatory area centered on the unit's BF. There are no inhibitory response areas. Auditory-nerve fibers have Type I response maps. Most chopper units that have spontaneous activity have Type III response maps. Some primarylike with notch units show Type III response maps (2,4,47). These maps have excitatory areas like those of Type I maps but are flanked on one or both sides by inhibitory areas (59).

An important functional difference between primarylike and chopper units is found in their ability to phase-lock to tones. As shown in Fig. 8, the ability of choppers to phase-lock is limited to lower frequencies than is that of primarylike units. The dependence of phase-locking on stimulus frequency in primarylike units is indistinguishable from that found for auditory-nerve fibers (14). In both cases, phase-locking decreases at tone frequencies above about 1 kHz and is unmeasurable above about 6.0 kHz. Thus, very little temporal information is lost across the auditory nerve to bushy cell synapse. This efficiency

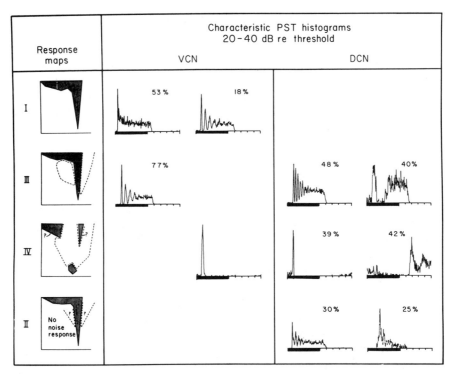

FIG. 7. The left column shows four types of response maps observed in cochlear nucleus units. The abscissae show stimulus frequency, the ordinates show stimulus level. The *shaded regions* are excitatory areas, the *unshaded regions* enclosed by *dashed lines* are inhibitory areas. Each row shows PST histogram types most commonly observed in units of each response map type in decerebrate preparations in the VCN (middle column) and DCN (right column). Percentages are fractions of each response map type displaying a particular PST type in each cochlear nucleus division. (From ref. 60, with permission.)

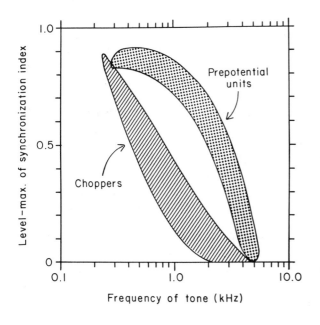

FIG. 8. Maximum phase-locking to tones as a function of frequency for prepotential units (bushy cells) and chopper units in the ventral cochlear nucleus of anesthetized cats. (From ref. 60 [redrawn from ref. 2], with permission.)

in transmitting temporal information is related both to the large, secure synaptic endings on the bushy cell soma and to specializations of the postsynaptic cell membrane, which allow it to follow rapid changes in synaptic potentials (27).

Phase-locking in chopper cells, on the other hand, declines at frequencies above 200 Hz and is very much smaller than that of primarylike units at higher frequencies (Fig. 8). This loss of phase-locking in choppers is consistent with the dendritic configuration of the stellate cells. The effect of large dendritic trees on synaptic inputs far from the soma can be viewed as a low pass filter effect (17,60). For example, under assumptions consistent with what is known about stellate cell membrane properties, Young et al. (60) computed the voltage response at the soma of a current source located on a dendritic tree 1½ space constants from the soma. At a frequency of 1.0 kHz, the soma voltage is attenuated more than 40 dB relative to the voltage generated by a 1.0 kHz current applied directly to the soma.

On the basis of these structural and physiological differences between bushy cells and stellate cells, we might expect that the signal processing carried out by populations of these cells would be very different. For example, we would expect that primarylike units with their strong phase-locking ability would preserve the temporal-place representation of complex spectra in the auditory nerve. Choppers clearly should not maintain this representation, but their more complex dendritic structure and related receptive fields could produce significant processing of rate-place representations.

Figure 9 compares the temporal representation of /ɛ/ in a primarylike unit with that in a chopper unit recorded in the same experiment. Figure 9C and D shows period histograms of the responses of the two units with /ɛ/ as the stimulus. The primarylike unit shows strong phase-locking to the second formant, as indicated by the closely spaced peaks (0.56 msec, equals the period

of the second formant, 1.792 kHz). The envelope of second formant response is strongly modulated by the fundamental frequency (112 Hz) of the vowel. The Fourier transform of the period histogram (Fig. 9E) shows a large component at the second formant with smaller components at frequencies just above and below the second formant. There is another component at the fundamental, and small peaks at the second harmonic of the second formant and its neighbors. We have previously referred to these latter harmonic components as "rectifier distortion products," because in the auditory nerve they appear to be the result of a transducer rectifying nonlinearity (56).

The period histogram for the chopper unit in Fig. 9D, on the other hand, shows no obvious phase-locking at the second formant frequency and its Fourier transform (Fig. 9F) shows a second formant peak barely above the noise level. Instead, the period histogram for this unit shows a strong modulation at the fundamental frequency. There is a corresponding large Fourier transform component at the fundamental frequency and a cluster of small peaks around the first formant frequency, specifically at 448 and 560 Hz, the two harmonics of the fundamental (112 Hz), which surround the first formant. There are two peaks in the period histogram separated by roughly the period of the first formant frequency (1.95 msec), which reflect these two harmonic components. This chopper response is consistent with the hypothesis that the auditory-nerve input signal to the chopper is low pass filtered by the dendritic tree of the stellate cell. Regardless of the mechanism, however, temporal response to the second formant is much weaker for the chopper than for the primarylike unit.

This difference between chopper and primarylike temporal representation is illustrated further in Fig. 10, which compares ALSRs for the two unit types. Recall that the ALSR gives the average synchronized rate at each frequency of all the units with BFs within one-quarter octave of the fre-

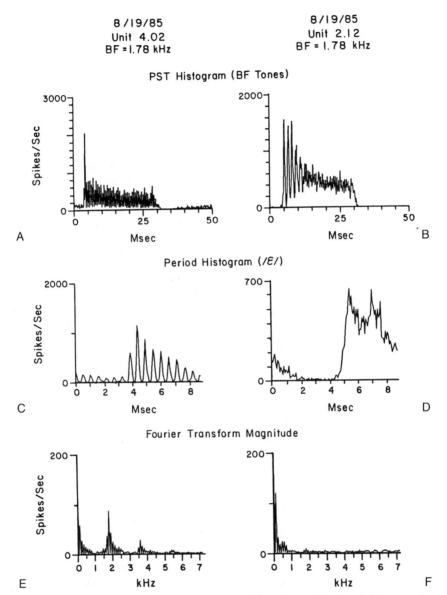

FIG. 9. Histograms and Fourier transform magnitudes for a primarylike unit (left) and a chopper unit (right) with same BFs (1.78 kHz). **A, B:** PST histograms for responses to BF tones. **C** and **D:** Period histograms for responses to /ε/ at 45 dB SPL. **E** and **F:** Fourier transform magnitudes computed from the period histograms. (From ref. 1, with permission.)

quency. The ALSR for the primarylike population is similar to those for auditory-nerve fibers, with clear peaks at each of the formant frequencies. The ALSR for the chopper population shows no such formant related peaks and decreases roughly monotonically with increasing frequency above about 500 Hz. This failure of the chopper ALSR to represent the vowel spectrum presumably reflects the loss of phase-locking in the chopper population as illustrated in Fig. 8.

As we pointed out above, although the complex dendritic structure of the stellate

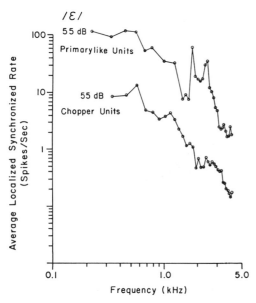

FIG. 10. ALSR plots for a population of primarylike units and a population of chopper units. Stimulus was /ε/ at 35 dB SPL. (From ref. 1, with permission.)

cell is the likely cause of this failure of phase-locking in the chopper population, this structure could be the basis for processing that could preserve or even sharpen rate-place profiles over a wide range of stimulus levels. Figure 11 shows rate-place profiles for a population of chopper units (ChT units) for the /ε/ at four stimulus levels. (The chopper population can be subdivided according to regularity of spike trains into ChS and ChT, for "sustained" and "transient" chopper [59].) The ChT profiles are compared with those for auditory-nerve fibers in Fig. 11. At 25 dB SPL the ChT rate profile is similar to that for the high spontaneous rate auditory nerve population. At higher levels, the ChT profiles are similar to those for the low and medium spontaneous rate population and very different from the high spontaneous rate population. Specifically, at 55 and 75 dB SPL the ChT profiles show peaks at the first formant and in the region of the second and third formants. In the high spontaneous auditory-nerve population these peaks are scarcely noticeable at 55 dB and are gone at 75 dB.

These data are consistent with the hypothesis that the ChT units weight high spontaneous rate inputs heavily at low sound levels and low spontaneous rate inputs at high levels. Interestingly, virtually all the ChT units in this population had little or no spontaneous activity, so that one might question whether these units receive any high spontaneous rate auditory-nerve inputs. There is some preliminary evidence on this point. Young and Sachs (57) recorded simultaneously from auditory-nerve and cochlear nucleus units, using a micropipette electrode in the auditory nerve and a platinum-plated platinum iridium electrode in the AVCN. They used cross-correlation analysis to search for functional interactions between auditory-nerve fibers and cochlear nucleus cells. They have found evidence of excitatory interactions between auditory-nerve fibers and both chopper and primarylike cochlear nucleus units. Such interactions were observed between chopper units and auditory-nerve fibers from low, medium, and high spontaneous rate groups, suggesting, within the limitations of cross-correlation analysis, that choppers do receive high spontaneous rate inputs.

If the chopper units do receive high spontaneous rate auditory-nerve inputs, then we must invoke some mechanism for their ignoring these inputs at high sound levels. As shown in Fig. 7, chopper units are inhibited by off-BF tones and such inhibition could certainly play a role in turning off the effect of high spontaneous inputs. Winslow et al. (50) hypothesized a simple neural circuit capable of turning off the effect of high spontaneous inputs at high stimulus levels. This circuit is based on the principle of direct path inhibition (18). High spontaneous rate, low threshold fibers with BFs equal to the chopper BF are assumed to form excitatory synapses distal in the dendritic tree and low spontaneous rate, high threshold fibers with similar BFs are assumed to form

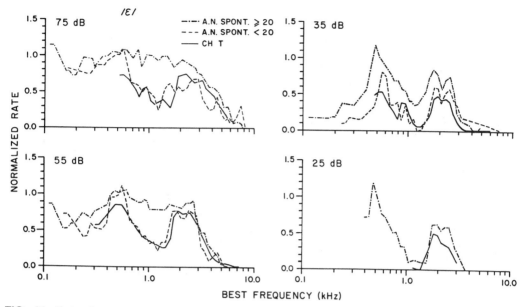

FIG. 11. Rate-place profiles for a population of ChT units and populations of high and low/medium spontaneous rate auditory-nerve fibers. Stimulus was /ɛ/ at four sound levels. (From ref. 1, with permission.)

excitatory synapses closer to the soma. Finally high spontaneous rate, off-BF fibers are assumed to project to interneurons, which in turn form inhibitory synapses on the direct path that current must take when flowing from the distal synapses to the soma. Consider the response of this circuit to the BF tones. Winslow et al. speculate that at stimulus levels low enough that there is little spread of excitation along the cochlear partition, the rate responses of this circuit will be similar to those of its on-BF high spontaneous rate inputs. The low spontaneous rate fibers will not be excited because their thresholds are too high; the off-BF fibers will not be stimulated if there is little spread. However, as stimulus level increases, spread of excitation activates the high spontaneous rate off-BF fibers, which indirectly inhibit the chopper unit. Direct path shunting inhibition is very effective in preventing current from more distal synapses from reaching the soma, but has little effect on synaptic current from more proximal locations. Thus, at stimulus levels high

enough to activate off-BF, high spontaneous fibers, synaptic currents from the distal synapses of high spontaneous fibers will short across the cell membrane at the site of inhibition, allowing currents due to the more proximal synapses of the low spontaneous, BF fibers to drive the cell.

REPRESENTATION OF BROADBAND STIMULI IN THE DORSAL COCHLEAR NUCLEUS

The existence of inhibitory sidebands in the ventral cochlear nucleus (VCN) chopper response maps strongly suggests the existence of inhibitory interneurons in the neural networks responsible for shaping the responses of these units. Both bushy cells and stellate cells receive axons from noncochlear sources (6,41), and some VCN cells have local axon collaterals (20,32,33, 52). Nonetheless, the VCN does not seem to contain large or complex internal neural networks. The dorsal cochlear nucleus

(DCN), on the other hand, contains a number of different types of interneurons that form a very complex internal structure (15, 20,25,26,28,51). The DCN principal cells, the fusiform cells in particular, receive a variety of inputs. The somas and both the apical and basal dendritic trees of these neurons are covered with synaptic contacts (15,43). Auditory-nerve fibers and possibly other inputs form terminals directly on fusiform cells; granule cells relay inputs from mossy fibers of undetermined origin; and axons of several types of interneurons distribute within the DCN.

Presumably because of this complex neuronal circuitry, there is a very increased prominence of inhibitory responses in the

DCN relative to the VCN (10,54). Evidence suggests that Type IV responses are recorded from DCN principal cells in decerebrate cats (fusiform and giant cells [53]). Type IV response maps (Fig. 7) have an excitatory region around the BF and at near threshold sound levels. At higher levels they have inhibitory response areas, which include BF. Excitatory areas at higher levels and away from BF (marked "?" in Fig. 7) are sometimes observed. Type IV responses are seen commonly in decerebrate animals but only infrequently in anesthetized animals (10,55). As can be seen from the response map in Fig. 12, tones at BF are excitatory near threshold and inhibitory at higher levels for these Type IV units; that

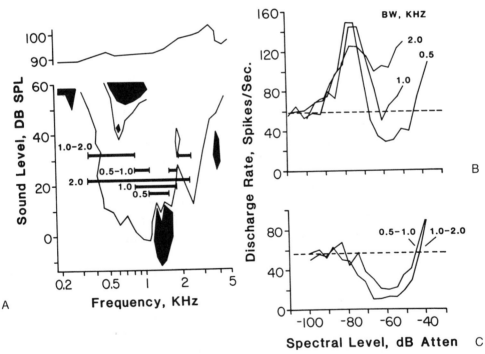

FIG. 12. **A:** Response map of a type IV unit recorded in dorsal cochlear nucleus of a decerebrate cat. Bars indicate the width of noise bands used to get the data in parts **B** and **C**. The line plot at the top shows the acoustic calibration that determines the detailed spectral shape of the noise bands. **B:** Rate versus level functions for three bandwidths of noise. *Dashed line* shows spontaneous rate. **C:** Rate versus level functions for two pairs of residual noise bands, which contain the frequencies added to the 0.5 kHz band to make the 1.0 kHz band and the frequencies added to the 1.0 kHz band to make the 2.0 kHz band. *Dashed line* shows spontaneous rate. (From ref. 60, with permission.)

is, BF tone rate level functions for Type IV units are nonmonotonic. (Narrow bands of noise centered at BF produce similar results.) A surprising result is that broadband noise produces excitatory responses from these units, even though the energy in the band may lie completely in the unit's inhibitory areas. Figure 12 analyzes this situation. Figure 12B shows rate versus level functions for responses of this Type IV unit to noise bands of different widths. The three bands are shown on the response map as single bars labeled 0.5, 1.0, and 2.0. As bandwidth is widened the unit's rate at moderate and high spectral levels increases. This rate increase implies that the frequency components added to the noise as bandwidth is widened should have an excitatory effect when presented alone. Figure 12C shows that this conclusion is not correct. When pairs of noise bands formed by excluding the 0.5 kHz band from the 1.0 kHz band or excluding the 1.0 kHz band from the 2.0 kHz band are presented alone their effect is inhibitory over a wide range of sound levels. Over this same range of levels, energy in these marginal bands has an excitatory effect when added to the 0.5 or 1.0 kHz bands (Fig. 12B). The frequency components in the marginal bands have an inhibitory effect when presented alone, but an excitatory effect when presented with frequency components near BF. Clearly Type IV units do not respond linearly in the sense of summation of inputs over their response maps.

Young and colleagues (54,60) presented a model that explains these features of the Type IV responses. The model is based on the idea that the major inhibitory input to the Type IV unit comes from Type II DCN units (48). Type II units (Fig. 7) have excitatory response areas like those of Type I and Type III, but they have little or no spontaneous activity and give little or no response to broadband noise stimuli (58). Because Type II units are not spontaneously active it is not possible to determine directly if they have inhibitory sidebands.

However, their weak responses to noise are most easily explained by powerful inhibitory inputs (marked "?" in Fig. 7) (58). Evidence that Type II units are inhibitory interneurons comes from a variety of studies (21,48,55).

Figure 13 shows the model of the DCN Type II-Type IV circuit. Axons a and b represent excitatory auditory nerve input to Type II and Type IV units. Axon e represents the strong inhibitory Type II-Type IV connection. Axons c and d represent inhibitory sidebands on Type II units (strong) and on Type IV units (weak). The axons coming from the bottom line are auditory-nerve fibers arrayed from left to right according to their BFs. The Type II unit in this model would respond to BF tones through the effects of axon a but would not respond to broadband noise because of the strong inhibitory actions of axons c and d.

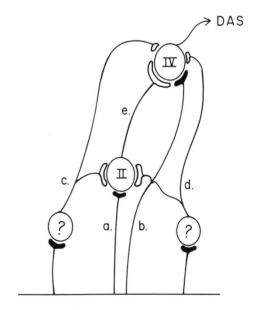

Best frequency

FIG. 13. Schematic model of the dorsal cochlear nucleus Type II-Type IV circuit. Excitatory terminals are shown as *solid* and inhibitory terminals are *unfilled*. Terminal size indicates strength of effect. Auditory-nerve input (bottom) shown arranged along basilar membrane. Letters identify axons for discussion in the text. (From ref. 60, with permission.)

The noise data in Fig. 12 can be explained in terms of the model in Fig. 13. As the noise bands are widened from 0.5 to 2.0 kHz, the response of the Type II cell to its excitatory input on axon a is progressively weakened by its inhibitory inputs on axons c and d. Thus the inhibition on the Type IV cell via axon e is reduced, allowing the Type IV unit to respond to its monotonically increasing excitatory input from the auditory nerve (axon b [40]). In this case, the weak inhibitory inputs to the Type IV (axons c and d) are assumed to be overpowered by the strong excitatory drive. When the residual noise bands (0.5–1.0 kHz or 1.0–2.0 kHz) are presented alone, the Type II unit is strongly inhibited by axons c and d, and there is no activity on axon e. The net effect is that the Type IV unit is inhibited through axons c and d. Excitatory activity does not reach the Type IV through axon b because there is no energy in the center of the marginal noise bands.

Thus, the rather surprising observation that adding stimulus energy in the inhibitory area of a Type IV response map leads to an increased excitatory response is explained by the neural circuit in Fig. 13, which could be realized in terms of known DCN circuitry. Even more complex stimulus transformations have been observed and can be similarly explained (60), although some observations may require modification of the model (46). The functional significance of these DCN transformations is not yet clear.

REPRESENTATION OF TEMPORAL FEATURES OF STIMULI

Thus far we have considered the encoding and processing of spectral features of complex sounds. Even though we have looked in detail at the temporal (phase-locked) information in spike trains, this information was used to represent spectral features of the stimuli, rather than what are commonly referred to as temporal features of the stimuli. Examples of such temporal features include envelope modulation by tones, and onset transients and formant transitions in consonant-vowel syllables. Representation of formant transitions have been studied extensively in the auditory nerve (9,22,42) but not in the cochlear nucleus. As was to be expected from the work of Smith and colleagues on adaptation in the auditory nerve (45), rate profiles for consonant-vowel syllables preserve formant structure during the onset formant transition but not during the steady-state vowel segment (22). The temporal-place representation also follows the formant frequency changes with great precision (22).

One feature of the representation of steady-state vowels that we have not discussed is the pitch or fundamental frequency. There are two ways in which this pitch could be represented: as peaks at harmonics of the fundamental frequency in a representation of the vowel spectrum or as a fundamental frequency modulation of period histograms of individual units. Miller and Sachs (23) showed that a very precise measure of pitch could be extracted from the harmonic structure of the temporal-place representation (ALSR). Modulation of the period histograms of some individual units also provided a good pitch measure, but this representation deteriorated with stimulus level for some units (primarily those dominated by a formant frequency) and for all but very low BF units in the presence of background noise. Such pitch modulation is clearly evident in both primarylike and chopper units in the AVCN (Fig. 9). Kim and colleagues (16) have shown similar histogram modulation for various unit types in the posteroventral cochlear nucleus (PVCN) and DCN. They show an example of an onset cell that follows the pitch period on an almost one spike per cycle basis and with very little jitter in the phase of firing; Blackburn and Sachs (1) observed similar behavior in onset units and choppers with BFs between the first two formants.

Frisina et al. (11) studied the ability of various VCN units to represent the envelope modulation of an amplitude modulated tone. The specific issue addressed was how such envelope modulation is coded at high sound levels where most auditory-nerve fibers are saturated. They computed histograms locked to the modulating tone, and defined percent modulation as the ratio of the Fourier transform component at the modulating frequency to the mean discharge rate of the unit. They reported a unit's modulation-locked response as "response gain" defined to be the ratio (in dB) of percent modulation in the response to percent modulation in the stimulus. Figure 14 shows an example of their results, plotted as three-dimensional surfaces displaying response gain versus amplitude modulation frequency and carrier level re each unit's threshold. The carrier frequency was the unit's BF. The unit depicted was identified as an Onset type-L in the classification of Godfrey et al. (12). Comparison of the modulation profile for this onset unit (solid line) with that for an auditory-nerve fiber (dotted line) indicates that the modulation gain is greater for the Onset unit, the difference being greatest at high carrier levels. Enhancement of amplitude modulation is seen for chopper, primarylike with notch, and primarylike units. The enhancement is greatest for onset units followed in order by chopper, primarylike with notch, and primarylike. These results, as well as those related to speech pitch, suggest the hypothe-

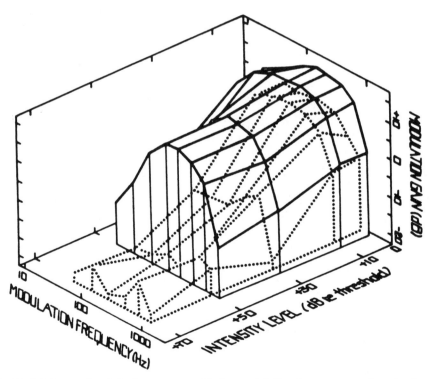

FIG. 14. Modulation gain plotted versus amplitude modulation frequency and carrier level for a cochlear nucleus. Onset type-L unit (*solid line*) and an auditory-nerve fiber (*dotted line*). Carrier frequency was at unit's BF and modulation depth was 35%. The BF of the Onset unit was 12.0 kHz; its threshold was 35 dB SPL. The BF of the auditory-nerve fiber was 6.5 kHz and its threshold was 2 dB SPL. (From ref. 11, with permission.)

sis that some cochlear nucleus cell types may be involved in sharpening the representation of stimulus temporal features.

SUMMARY: FUTURE DIRECTIONS

Let us briefly summarize this discussion by suggesting some future research directions. The study of the neural processing of complex sounds has led to some specific hypothesis regarding the function of two groups of cells in the AVCN, bushy cells, and stellate cells. On the one hand, we need to focus down on the mechanisms of signal processing in these cell groups. The goal here is to make precise enough measurements of the structure of these cells, of their interconnections with other cells, and of their electrical properties that we will be able to construct detailed mathematical models of their signal processing function. This aspect of the work is attempting to analyze the *components* of the neural machinery responsible for auditory signal processing.

While part of our effort should now focus on such mechanistic issues, there is also reason to look more globally at stimulus representation. We have arrived at the following concept of representation in the auditory system. Sound spectra are represented across the tonotopically arrayed population of auditory-nerve fibers. This "place" representation contains two components: rate and temporal. In the cochlear nucleus, the auditory-nerve representation generates multiple representations. For example, the temporal and rate components seem to be separately represented in the bushy cell and stellate cell populations. Success in describing these representations should encourage us now to shift part of our focus to higher level processing of complex stimuli, moving in the direction of what has been called "higher auditory function." One of the most intriguing questions will be how spectral features are extracted from the representations developed and sharpened in the periphery.

REFERENCES

1. Blackburn CC, Sachs MB. Speech encoding in the anteroventral cochlear nucleus. IBRO Satellite Symposium, Prague, Czechoslovakia, 1987.
2. Bourk TR. Electrical responses of neural units in the anteroventral cochlear nucleus of the cat. Ph.D. thesis, Massachusetts Institute of Technology, Cambridge, MA, 1976.
3. Brawer JR, Morest DK. Relations between auditory nerve endings and cell types in the cat's anteroventral cochlear nucleus seen with the Golgi method and Nomarski optics. *J Comp Neurol* 1975;160:491–506.
4. Brownell WE. Organization of the cat trapezoid body and the discharge characteristics of its fibers. *Brain Res* 1975;94:413–433.
5. Brownell WE, Bader CR, Bertrand D, de Ribaupierre Y. Evoked mechanical responses of isolated cochlear outer hair cells. *Science* 1985; 227:194–196.
6. Cant NB, Morest DK. Axons from non-cochlear sources in the anteroventral cochlear nucleus of the cat. A study with the rapid Golgi method. *Neuroscience* 1978;3:1003–1029.
7. Cant NB, Morest DK. The structural basis for stimulus coding in the cochlear nucleus of the cat. In: Berlin CI, ed. *Hearing science.* San Diego: College-Hill Press, 1984;374–422.
8. Churchland PS. *Neurophilosophy: toward a unified science of the mind-brain.* Cambridge, MA. MIT Press, 1986.
9. Delgutte B, Kiang NYS. Speech coding in the auditory nerve: IV. Sounds with consonant-like dynamic characteristics. *J Acoust Soc Am* 1984;75:897–907.
10. Evans EF, Nelson PG. The responses of single neurones in the cochlear nucleus of the cat as a function of their location and the anaesthetic state. *Exp Brain Res* 1973;17:402–427.
11. Frisina RO, Smith RL, Chamberlain SC. Differential encoding of rapid changes in sound amplitude by second-order auditory neurons. *Exp Brain Res* 1985;60:417–427.
12. Godfrey DA, Kiang NYS, Norris BE. Single unit activity in the posteroventral cochlear nucleus of the cat. *J Comp Neurol* 1975;162:247–268.
13. Goldberg JM, Brownell WE. Discharge characteristic of neurons in anteroventral and dorsal cochlear nuclei of cat. *Brain Res* 1973;64:35–54.
14. Johnson DH. The relationship between spike rate and synchrony in responses of auditory-nerve fibers to single tones. *J Acoust Soc Am* 1980;68:1115–1122.
15. Kane EC. Synaptic organization in the dorsal cochlear nucleus of the cat: a light and electron

microscopic study. *J Comp Neurol* 1974;155: 301–330.

16. Kim DO, Leonard G. Pitch-period following response of cat cochlear nucleus neurons to speech sounds. 8th International Symposium on Hearing, 1988.

17. Koch C. Cable theory of neurons with active, linearized membranes. *Biol Cybern* 1984;50: 15–33.

18. Koch C, Poggio T, Torre V. Retinal ganglion cells: a functional interpretation of dendritic morphology. *Philos Trans R Soc Lond [B]* 1982;298:227–264.

19. Liberman MC. Auditory-nerve response from cats raised in a low-noise chamber. *J Acoust Soc Am* 1978;63:442–455.

20. Lorente de Nó R. *The primary acoustic nuclei.* New York: Raven Press, 1981.

21. Manis PB, Brownell WE. Synaptic organization of eighth nerve afferents to the cat dorsal cochlear nucleus. *J Neurophysiol* 1983;50:1156–1181.

22. Miller MI, Sachs MB. Representation of stop consonants in the discharge patterns of auditory-nerve fibers. *J Acoust Soc Am* 1983;74: 502–517.

23. Miller MI, Sachs MB. Representation of voice pitch in discharge patterns of auditory-nerve fibers. *Hear Res* 1984;14:257–279.

24. Mountcastle VB. The neural mechanisms of cognitive functions can now be studied directly. *Trends Neuorsci* 1986;9:505–508.

25. Mugnaini E. GABA neurons in the superficial layers of the rat dorsal cochlear nucleus: light and electron microscopic immunocytochemistry. *J Comp Neurol* 1985;235:61–81.

26. Mugnaini E, Warr WB, Osen KK. Distribution and light microscopic features of granule cells in the cochlear nuclei of cat, rat and mouse. *J Comp Neurol* 1980;19:581–606.

27. Oertel D. Synaptic responses and electrical properties of cells in brain slices of the mouse anteroventral cochlear nucleus. *J Neurosci* 1983;3:2043–2053.

28. Osen KK, Mugnaini E. Neuronal circuits in the dorsal cochlear nucleus. In: Syka J, Aitkins L, eds. *Neuronal mechanisms of hearing.* New York: Plenum Press, 1981;119–125.

29. Palmer AR, Evans EF. Cochlear fiber rate-intensity functions: no evidence for basilar membrane nonlinearities. *Hear Res* 1980;2:319–326.

30. Peterson GE, Barney HL. Control methods used in the study of vowels. *J Acoust Soc Am* 1952;24:175–184.

31. Pols LCW, Tromp HRC, Plomp R. Frequency analysis of Dutch vowels from 50 male speakers. *J Acoust Soc Am* 1973;53:1093–1101.

32. Rhode WS, Oertel D, Smith PH. Physiological response properties of cells labeled intracellularly with horseradish peroxidase in the cat ventral cochlear nucleus. *J Comp Neurol* 1983;213: 448–463.

33. Rhode WS, Smith PH, Oertel D. Physiological response properties of cells labeled intracellu-

larly with horseradish peroxidase in cat dorsal cochlear nucleus. *J Comp Neurol* 1983;213:426–447.

34. Romand R. Survey of intracellular recording in the cochlear nucleus of the cat. *Brain Res* 1978;148:43–65.

35. Roullier EM, Ryugo DK. Intracellular marking of physiologically characterized cells in the ventral cochlear nucleus of the cat. *J Comp Neurol* 1984;229:432–450.

36. Roullier EM, Cronin-Schreiber R, Fekete DM, Ryugo DK. The central projections of intracellularly labelled auditory nerve fibers: an analysis of terminal morphology. *J Comp Neurol* 1986;249:261–273.

37. Sachs MB, Young ED. Encoding of steady-state vowels in the auditory nerve: representation in terms of discharge rate. *J Acoust Soc Am* 1979;66:470–479.

38. Sachs MB, Voigt HF, Young ED. Auditory nerve representation of vowels in background noise. *J Neurophysiol* 1983;50:27–45.

39. Sachs MB, Blackburn CC, Young ED. Rate-place and temporal-place representations of vowels in the auditory nerve and anteroventral cochlear nucleus. *J Phonet* 1988;16:37–53.

40. Schalk TB, Sachs MB. Nonlinearities in auditory-nerve fiber responses to bandlimited noise. *J Acoust Soc Am* 1980;67:903–913.

41. Schwartz AM, Gulley RL. Non-primary afferents to the principal cells of the rostral anteroventral cochlear nucleus of the guinea pig. *Am J Anat* 1978;153:489–508.

42. Sinex DG, Geisler CD. Responses of auditory-nerve fibers to consonant-vowel syllables. *J Acoust Soc Am* 1983;73:602–615.

43. Smith PH, Rhode WS. Electromicroscopic features of physiologically characterized, HRP-labelled fusiform cells in the cat dorsal cochlear nucleus. *J Comp Neurol* 1985;237:127–143.

44. Smith PH, Rhode WS. Characterization of HRP labelled globular bushy cells in the cat anteroventral cochlear nucleus. *J Comp Neurol* 1987; 266:360–376.

45. Smith RL, Brachman ML. Dynamic responses of single auditory-nerve fibres: some effects of intensity and time. In: van den Brink G, Bilsen FA, eds. *Psychophysical, physiological and behavioral studies in hearing.* Delft: Delft University Press, 1980.

46. Spirou GA, Young ED. Receptive field organization of DCN neurons: interpreting responses to bandlimited noise. Abstract, Eleventh Midwinter Meeting, Association for Research in Otolaryngology, 1988.

47. Spirou GA, Brownell WE, Zidanic M. Recordings from cat trapezoid body and HRP labeling of globular bushy cell axons. *J Neurophysiol* 1990;63:1169–1190.

48. Voigt HF, Young ED. Evidence of inhibitory interactions between neurons in dorsal cochlear nucleus. *J Neurophysiol* 1980;44:76–96.

49. Voigt HF, Sachs MB, Young ED. Representation of whispered vowels in discharge patterns of au-

ditory-nerve fibers. *Hear Res* 1982;8:49–58.

50. Winslow RL, Barta PE, Sachs MB. Rate coding in the auditory nerve. In: Yost WA, Watson CS, eds. *Auditory processing of complex sounds.* Hillsdale, NJ: Lawrence Erlbaum, 1987;212–224.

51. Wouterlood FG, Mugnaini E. Cartwheel neurons of the dorsal cochlear nucleus: a Golgi-electron microscopic study in rat. *J Comp Neurol* 1984;227:136–157.

52. Wu SH, Oertel D. Intracellular injection with horseradish peroxidase of physiologically characterized stellate and bushy cells in slices of mouse anteroventral cochlear nucleus. *J Neurosci* 1984;4:1577–1588.

53. Young ED. Identification of response properties of ascending axons from dorsal cochlear nucleus. *Brain Res* 1980;200:23–37.

54. Young ED. Response characteristics of neurons of the cochlear nuclei. In: Berlin CI, ed. *Hearing science.* San Diego: College-Hill Press, 1984;423–460.

55. Young ED, Brownell WE. Responses to tones and noise of single cells in dorsal nucleus of unanesthetized cats. *J Neurophysiol* 1976;39:282–300.

56. Young ED, Sachs MB. Representation of steady-state vowels in the temporal aspects of the discharge patterns of populations of auditory-nerve fibers. *J Acoust Soc Am* 1979;66:1381–1403.

57. Young ED, Sachs MB. Interactions of auditory nerve fibers and ventral cochlear nucleus cells studied with crosscorrelation. Abstract, 18th annual meeting, Society for Neuroscience, Toronto, Ontario, Canada, 1988.

58. Young ED, Voigt HF. Response properties of type II and type III units in the dorsal cochlear nucleus. *Hear Res* 1982;6:153–159.

59. Young ED, Robert J-M, Shofner WP. Regularity and latency of units in ventral cochlear nucleus: implications for unit classification and generation of response properties. *J Neurophysiol* 1988;60:1–29.

60. Young ED, Shofner WP, White JA, Robert J-M, Voigt HF. Response properties of cochlear nucleus neurons in relationship to physiological mechanisms. In: Edelman GM, Gall WE, Cowan WM, eds. *Auditory function: neurophysiological bases of hearing.* New York: John Wiley, 1988;277–312.

Neurobiology of Hearing: The
Central Auditory System, edited by
R. A. Altschuler et al.
Raven Press, Ltd., New York © 1991.

5

Projections to the Lateral and Medial Superior Olivary Nuclei from the Spherical and Globular Bushy Cells of the Anteroventral Cochlear Nucleus

Nell Beatty Cant

Department of Neurobiology, Duke University Medical School, Durham, North Carolina 27710

The lateral and medial superior olivary nuclei (LSO and MSO, respectively) appear to play central roles in the processing of binaural auditory stimuli. Evidence from anatomical, physiological, pharmacological, and behavioral studies indicates that neurons in these two nuclei receive binaural inputs and encode interaural differences in the intensity and in the time of arrival of acoustic stimuli (reviewed in refs. 1,2). The differential response patterns of neurons in the LSO and MSO depend on the integration of excitatory and inhibitory synaptic inputs carrying information about activity in the two cochleas. Before the mechanisms through which binaural inputs to the olivary nuclei are integrated can be understood, the synaptic organization of the excitatory and inhibitory inputs must be established. The purpose of this chapter is to describe current knowledge of the organization of both the direct and indirect projections to the LSO and MSO from the cochlear nucleus, which receives the primary auditory input. The physiology of the nuclei is discussed in other chapters in this volume.

The central thesis of this chapter is that the cochlear nucleus gives rise to a *spherical cell pathway* that provides direct excitatory input to the MSO and LSO and a *globular cell pathway* that provides these same nuclei with indirect inhibitory inputs that are relayed via interneurons in the periolivary nuclei, specifically, in the lateral and medial nuclei of the trapezoid body. In the first part of the chapter, the two types of bushy cells and their inputs from the cochlea and other sources are described. The second part focuses on their projections to the LSO and MSO and to the relevant periolivary nuclei.

THE SPHERICAL AND GLOBULAR BUSHY CELLS OF THE VENTRAL COCHLEAR NUCLEUS

Study of the anatomy and physiology of neuronal pathways in the brain is complicated by the fact that multiple neuronal types, defined on the basis of differences in their morphology, physiology, or connections and, presumably, also their function, are often intermingled within a single nucleus. Many published wiring diagrams of brainstem pathways, especially those in textbooks, are misleading because they illustrate projections from one nucleus to another rather than from one specific neuronal type to another. Fortunately, in the brainstem auditory system, many different cell types can be easily distinguished from one another based on criteria recognizable in ordinary cell stains (e.g., 3,4). Osen recognized that the cochlear nucleus, unlike many sensory nuclei in the brain, contains numerous neuronal types that can be distinguished easily and unambiguously in Nissl-stained material. The ease of identification enables us to describe the spatial organization of each cell type in the nucleus. Since each type has a unique distribution, this information is extremely useful in the interpretation of the results of many kinds of experimental procedures (5,6). For example, it has been possible to show that the very complex lower auditory pathways are made up of a number of parallel pathways involving different cell types (e.g., 7). Detailed knowledge of the distribution and connections of the different cell types has made possible correlations between neurons with documented morphology and physiological response properties and components of the particular pathways (8–11). Most information about the synaptic organization and connections of the cells of the lower auditory brainstem has derived from studies of the auditory pathways of the cat and the discussion that follows pertains to that species unless otherwise noted.

Two of the most easily distinguished cell types in the cochlear nucleus are the spherical and globular bushy cells (3). As will be discussed, these cells appear to provide the major direct and indirect cochlear nucleus inputs to the lateral and medial superior olivary nuclei. Although spherical and globular cells are quite distinct in Nissl stains, the appearance of the two types is very similar in Golgi preparations, where both can be classified as bushy cells as defined by Brawer et al. (12). The bushy cell is an odd cell type morphologically; a similar cell type is found in few other places in the brain. The distinguishing feature is a tuft of stringy appendages that arise from a short primary dendrite or dendrites and branch extensively in the vicinity of the cell body (Fig. 1). As discussed below, there appear to be variations in the extent of branching of the dendritic appendages and of the size of the dendritic fields that might, if studied quantitatively, lead to subdivision of the bushy cells into more than one group.

The spherical and globular cells are almost completely segregated from one another in the cochlear nucleus. In Fig. 2, the distribution of these two cell types is shown on a drawing of a Nissl-stained section. The spherical cells are distinguished from other neurons by a distinct "cap" of Nissl substance apposed to their nuclear membrane and large Nissl bodies distributed evenly throughout the perikaryon (3,13,14). They are located in the anterior division of the anteroventral cochlear nucleus (AVCN). The globular cells, unlike the other cells with which they are interspersed, contain abundant free ribosomes distributed throughout the perikaryon but lack complex arrays of Nissl bodies (3,15).

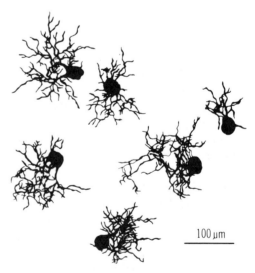

FIG. 1. Bushy cells in the anterior division of the anteroventral cochlear nucleus of an adult cat. Golgi-Kopsch impregnation.

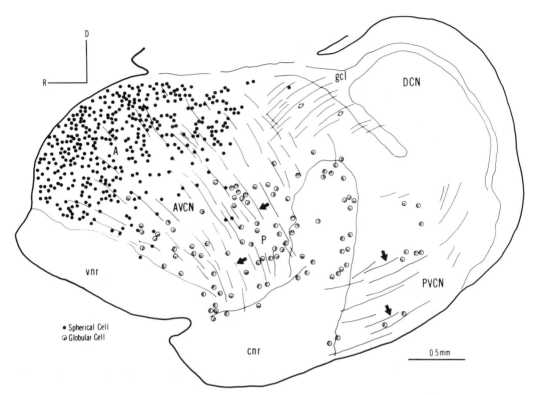

FIG. 2. Drawing of a sagittal section through the cochlear nucleus of an adult cat. Nissl-stained preparation. AVCN, anteroventral cochlear nucleus; A, anterior division of the AVCN; P, posterior division of the AVCN; PVCN, posteroventral cochlear nucleus; DCN, dorsal cochlear nucleus; gcl, granule cell layer; cnr, cochlear nerve root; vnr, vestibular nerve root; D, dorsal; R, rostral. The position of every spherical cell with an intact nucleus is indicated by a *filled circle*; that of every globular cell, by a *large circle enclosing a smaller one. Filled arrows* indicate ascending (in AVCN) and descending (in PVCN) branches of the auditory nerve (visualized in an adjacent section stained for myelin). *Open arrows* indicate axons that interconnect the AVCN and dorsal cochlear nuclei.

They are located in the posterior division of the AVCN, including the region of the nerve root. Similar cells are also found in the anterior parts of the posteroventral cochlear nucleus. In Golgi preparations (Fig. 3), both regions of the AVCN contain neurons classified as bushy cells (12,15,16). It has been shown that the bushy cells correspond to the spherical cells in the anterior part of the AVCN (16) and to globular cells in the posterior part (15,17). This difference in cell type is one basis for the subdivision of the AVCN into anterior and posterior divisions (12). To indicate the equivalence of the types defined in the two staining meth-

ods, the cells may be referred to as spherical bushy cells and globular bushy cells (14).

The Spherical Bushy Cells

Light Microscopic Observations

The spherical bushy cells can themselves be subdivided into two groups, large and small spherical cells, that have a different distribution in the nucleus (3). The distinction may have functional significance since the projection patterns of the large and

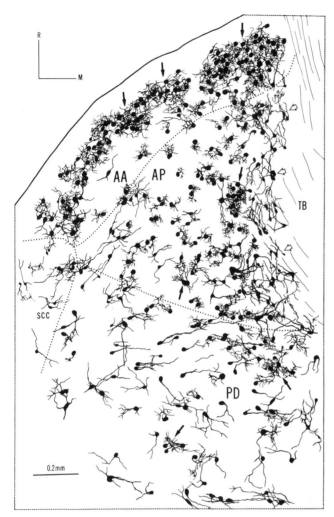

FIG. 3. Composite drawing of several horizontal sections through the anteroventral cochlear nucleus of an adult cat. Golgi-Kopsch impregnation. AA, anterior part of the anterior division; AP, posterior part of the anterior division; PD, dorsal part of the posterior division; TB, trapezoid body; scc, small cell cap; R, rostral; M, medial. *Filled arrows* indicate clusters of bushy cells in AA, AP, and PD. Multipolar or stellate cells with longer, less highly branched dendrites are intermingled with the bushy cells in AP and PD. *Open arrows* indicate multipolar cells that form the internal marginal layer of Lorente de Nó (22).

small cells differ (18, discussed below). Quantitative data illustrating the differences in size of the spherical cells in the different subdivisions of the anterior division of the AVCN are presented in Figs. 4 and 5. Figure 4 illustrates that the spherical bushy cells in the anterior part of the anterior division (subdivision AA of Brawer et al. [12]) are, on the average, larger than those in the other two subdivisions (APD and AP). The average size of the cells appears to vary systematically *within* the subdivisions as well (Fig. 5). The largest cells in all three subdivisions are concentrated in their more ventral parts (where lower frequen-

cies are represented) and the smaller cells are found more dorsally. In Golgi preparations, similar size differences are seen (16), but otherwise there appears to be little morphological diversity among the spherical bushy cells.

Fine Structure of the Spherical Bushy Cells

The spherical bushy cells appear to receive their major synaptic input onto their cell bodies and proximal dendrites. The synaptic terminals that contact the cells are

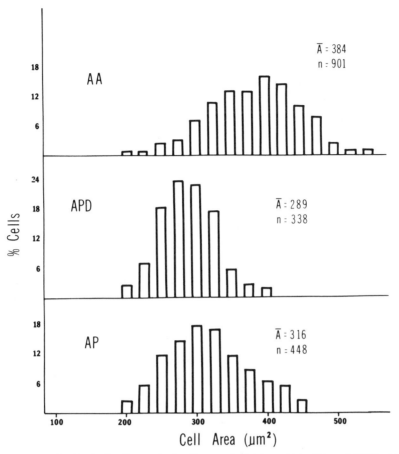

FIG. 4. Histograms of spherical cell area in the three subdivisions (AA, AP, and APD) of the anterior division of the anteroventral cochlear nucleus. The cross-sectional area of all spherical cells with an intact nucleus and nucleolus was measured in five evenly spaced sagittal sections through the cochlear nucleus. The figure shows the percentage of the total number of cells in each subdivision (n) with a given area in μm^2. The average area ($\bar{A}$) for each subdivision is given to the right of the histogram.

most conveniently subdivided on the basis of the size and shape of their synaptic vesicles in aldehyde-fixed material. Correlation between the types defined on this basis and (a) terminals arising from specific sources or (b) the presence of specific transmitter-related molecules lends substantial support to the use of these criteria for classification of synaptic terminals in electron micrographs (discussed in later paragraphs). Four basic types of synaptic terminals contact the spherical bushy cells. These are terminals with (a) large, round

synaptic vesicles; (b) small, round vesicles; (c) small, oval or pleomorphic vesicles; and (d) small, distinctly flattened vesicles. The pre- and postsynaptic densities associated with each type are characteristic for that type. The types of synaptic endings apposed to the neurons in the other nuclei to be considered are very similar, although their mode of distribution on the receptive surfaces varies and is characteristic for each cell type.

At least 70% (usually more) of the somatic surface of the spherical bushy cells is

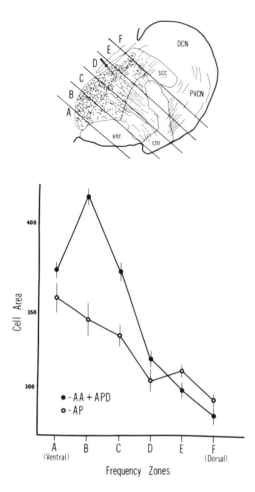

FIG. 5. The data shown in Fig. 4 replotted to illustrate the spatial distribution of the cells of various sizes (in terms of their cross-sectional area). **Top:** Illustration of one of five sagittal sections through the cochlear nucleus from which the measurements were made (abbreviations as in Fig. 2). The diagonal lines drawn through the anteroventral cochlear nucleus were placed based on the isofrequency lines calculated by Bourk et al. (87); comparable zones were matched on the five sections through the nucleus by matching our sections to theirs. The *arrow* in zone D shows the boundary between AA (ventral) and APD (dorsal). **Bottom:** The mean cell areas (in μm^2) in each "frequency zone" of the three subdivisions are plotted (bars indicate the standard errors of the means). Zone A, the most ventral, was present in the more lateral sections and would contain cells responsive to low frequencies. Zone F, the most dorsal, was present in the more medial sections and would contain cells responsive to the highest frequencies. (Unlike the section illustrated, which cuts through approximately the middle of the nucleus, the other four sections in which cells were measured did not contain all six zones.)

contacted by synaptic terminals (13). The most prominent terminals are the end-bulbs of Held, which attain their largest size in the most anterior part of the AVCN. Each end-bulb forms multiple synaptic contacts with the somatic surface. The fine structure of the cochlear endings is similar throughout the cochlear nuclear complex (17,19–21), although, as is obvious from Golgi and intra-axonal marking studies, the size of the terminals varies greatly (22–24). Synaptic terminals arising from cochlear axons contain large, round synaptic vesicles. These cochlear inputs to the spherical bushy cells are excitatory (25). In the anterior division of AVCN, at least, it appears that all terminals of this type disappear after cochlear ablation (19). The dendrites of the spherical bushy cells are also contacted by inputs from the cochlea, either processes of the end-bulb or boutons arising from collateral branches.

Recent investigations demonstrating diversity in the physiology and morphology of auditory nerve fibers lead to a number of unresolved questions. The cochlear input to the cochlear nucleus is of at least two types, known as type I and type II (26). The end-bulbs arise from the type I auditory axons (24). Whether the much less common type II axons form synapses with spherical bushy cells is not known. In the gerbil and mouse, the central course followed by type II spiral ganglion neurons is very similar to that of the type I neurons (27) so the possibility exists that some of the cochlear input to the spherical bushy cells is via the type II axon. A further unresolved question is whether there are differences in the morphology or distribution of the inputs from the several types of type I axons that have been described recently (24,28,29).

Much of the surfaces of the soma and proximal dendrites of the spherical bushy cells also form synapses with terminals that survive cochlear ablation. These noncochlear terminals can be distinguished from the cochlear inputs by the distinctly smaller size of their synaptic vesicles (19,21,30) and include the terminals with flattened or pleomorphic vesicles and, rarely, those with small, round vesicles. The development of immunocytochemical techniques for detecting the presence of transmitter molecules or of transmitter-related enzymes has led to the hypothesis that all or most of the noncochlear inputs are inhibitory (e.g., 31). In the guinea pig, neurons throughout the ventral cochlear nucleus are labeled with an antibody to the glycine receptor (32,33) and the terminals opposite these receptors contain oval or pleomorphic vesicles (33). Terminals containing round vesicles are not found opposite the receptors. The terminals with oval or pleomorphic vesicles may also exhibit immunoreactivity for GABA (34) or for the enzyme glutamic acid decarboxylase (GAD) (35,36), either alone or co-localized with glycine (33). The terminals containing glycine or gamma-aminobutyric acid (GABA) are abundant on spherical cells in the ventral cochlear nucleus of the guinea pig. Possible sources of these presumably inhibitory inputs are discussed in later sections.

The bushy dendritic appendages characteristic of spherical bushy cells appear to be contacted by relatively few terminals (19) so that the physiological responses of this cell type probably reflect primarily the or-

ganization of inputs on the somatic surface and the proximal dendrite(s).

The Globular Bushy Cells

Light Microscopic Observations

The globular bushy cells in Golgi material (15) or those filled intracellularly with horseradish peroxidase (37,38) appear more diverse morphologically than do the spherical bushy cells. While some globular bushy cells resemble the more anteriorly located spherical bushy cells, others exhibit considerably larger or sparser dendritic trees. Also in the posterior division of the AVCN, some of the cell bodies of globular bushy cells are covered with long somatic appendages giving them a shaggy appearance. No functional or connectional correlates of the morphological diversity have yet been described.

The Fine Structure of the Globular Bushy Cells

An average of 83% of the somatic and proximal dendritic surface of the globular bushy cells is apposed by synaptic terminals, which appear to be of the same basic types identified in the more anterior spherical cell areas (17). The small end-bulbs described in this region in Golgi material (22,23) appear in the electron microscope as large endings with large, round vesicles. Like the larger end-bulbs, they form multiple synaptic contacts, presumably excitatory, and degenerate after cochlear ablation (17). The input to the distinctive somatic appendages seen on some of the globular bushy cells is predominantly of this type (17).

About 40% of the terminals contacting the soma and proximal dendrites of the globular bushy cells have smaller vesicles and, since they remain unchanged after cochlear ablation, appear to be of noncochlear origin. Like the noncochlear terminals more anteriorly, these terminals contain either a pleomorphic mix of vesicles or distinctly flattened vesicles. Some of the terminals with pleomorphic vesicles are immunoreactive to antibodies to GAD (35,36). Since, in the guinea pig, most cell bodies in the ventral cochlear nucleus of the guinea pig are surrounded by puncta immunoreactive for glycine (39), it is likely that there is a glycinergic input to the globular bushy cells as well, although they have not been studied in the same detail as the spherical bushy cells. The distal dendritic appendages of the globular bushy cells, like those of the spherical bushy cells, are contacted by relatively few synaptic terminals, most of which contain flattened or pleomorphic synaptic vesicles (38,40).

Sources of Noncochlear Inputs to the Spherical and Globular Bushy Cells

Identified sources of noncochlear inputs to neurons of the ventral cochlear nucleus are the superior olivary complex, the contralateral cochlear nucleus, and other parts of the same cochlear nucleus (22,41–50). A few neurons in the ventral nucleus of the lateral lemniscus project to the cochlear nucleus (45,51), and the inferior colliculus projects to the caudal parts of the cochlear nucleus (22,52), but in neither case has a projection to the AVCN been described. The details of some of the noncochlear projections are better known than others, but it is not known with certainty whether any specific input contacts spherical or globular bushy cells. As discussed in the following paragraphs, all of the known sources of noncochlear inputs to the ventral cochlear nucleus could give rise to the terminals that contain glycine or GABA and would be, therefore, presumably inhibitory.

Projections to the ventral cochlear nucleus from the superior olivary complex arise in all of the periolivary areas but not from the MSO or LSO (46,50). The heaviest projections arise in the ipsilateral lateral nucleus of the trapezoid body (LNTB) and in both the ipsilateral and contralateral ventral nuclei of the trapezoid body (VNTB). These nuclei send dense projections into the anterior division of the AVCN, where the spherical bushy cells are located and sparse projections into the posterior AVCN, where the globular bushy cells are located (50). The LNTB and VNTB are possible sources of the GABAergic inputs to the bushy cells since neurons in both nuclei are immunoreactive for GABA (31). The LNTB may also be a source of the glycinergic terminals that contact the bushy cells (31).

Projections to the ventral cochlear nucleus from the contralateral cochlear nucleus arise from a group of large cells scattered widely but sparsely throughout both the dorsal and ventral nuclei (45,48). The main site of termination in the AVCN appears to be the anterior division or spherical cell area, but sparse input is also found in the area that contains the globular bushy cells (48). In the guinea pig, it appears that this pathway connecting the two cochlear nuclei is a source of the glycine-immunoreactive terminals that contact cells in the ventral cochlear nucleus (53).

A likely source of at least some of the glycinergic and GABAergic inputs to the bushy cells is the ipsilateral dorsal cochlear nucleus. Many small cells in the dorsal cochlear nucleus contain glycine, GABA, or GAD (31,36,54). In some but not all cases, labeled cells contain both GABA and glycine (31). Small cells in the dorsal cochlear nucleus are a source of input to the posterior division of the AVCN where the globular cells are located (47,55,56). Although it has been questioned whether the dorsal cochlear nucleus projects to the rostral part of the AVCN, where the spherical bushy cells are located (56), several investigators have noted such a projection (31; *unpublished observations*).

Projections from the Cochlear Nucleus to Other Parts of the Auditory System

Studies by Warr (7,57–59) and by van Noort (43) established the general patterns of efferent projections from the subdivisions of the cochlear nucleus of the cat. A detailed review of more recent findings is available (1). The AVCN has projections to the superior olivary nuclei on both sides of the brainstem, to the dorsal and ventral nuclei of the lateral lemniscus, and to the central nucleus of the inferior colliculus. The different neuronal types in the cochlear nucleus have very different patterns of projection, although in no case are all of the projections of a single cell type known with certainty. Much work remains to determine exactly which cell types are responsible for the known projections of the cochlear nucleus.

The major projections of both the spherical and globular bushy cells appear to be into the olivary nuclei and are discussed below. These cells probably project to additional auditory areas such as the nuclei of the lateral lemniscus, but those projections will not be examined here in detail.

NUCLEI OF THE SUPERIOR OLIVARY COMPLEX

The superior olivary complex comprises a number of cell groups, the most prominent of which are the LSO and MSO and the MNTB. Around these nuclei are a number of periolivary cell groups, many of which are almost nondescript in Nissl-stained sections but which are often clearly distinguishable in Golgi-impregnated sections (Fig. 6). The rest of this discussion is restricted to a consideration of four nuclei that appear to play major roles as recipients of the projections from globular and spherical bushy cells, namely the MSO, the LSO, the MNTB, and the LNTB. First, the cellular constituents of these nuclei and their

synaptic organization are described briefly. The rest of the section is devoted to a consideration of the sources of the synaptic inputs that contact each cell type and to the interconnections between the nuclei.

The Neurons and Their Fine Structure in Four Superior Olivary Nuclei That Receive Inputs from Bushy Cells

The Lateral Superior Olivary Nucleus

The LSO of the cat is made up of several neuronal types, the most common of which is the fusiform cell or principal cell (60–62) (Fig. 6). These cells give rise to dendrites that extend away from each pole of the cell body toward the margins of the nucleus (60,63). There the dendrites give rise to several spine studded branches. The long axis of the neurons appears to lie within the isofrequency planes defined physiologically (64). The neurons of the LSO respond with an increased firing rate to acoustic stimulation of the ipsilateral ear, an increase that can be inhibited by simultaneous stimulation of the contralateral ear (see elsewhere in this volume).

The synaptic organization of the LSO is relatively simple (63). The somas of the fusiform cells are contacted by many synaptic terminals, almost all of which contain flattened synaptic vesicles. These terminals appear to be glycinergic (39,65,66) and presumably provide inhibitory input to the neurons (67). The dendrites of the fusiform cells are also contacted by numerous terminals with flattened vesicles, but in addition, they are contacted by terminals that contain large, round synaptic vesicles. The distal dendrites appear to be contacted by such terminals almost exclusively. These terminals are presumably the source of excitatory inputs to the fusiform cells (discussed in ref. 63). The excitatory transmitter is not known. A very few terminals with

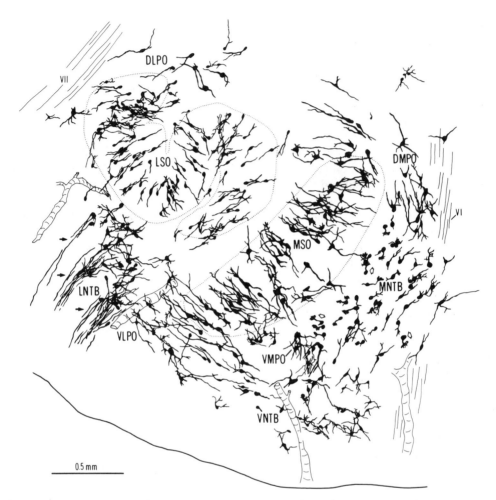

FIG. 6. Composite drawing of several transverse sections through the superior olivary complex of an adult cat. Golgi-Kopsch impregnation. Dorsal is to the top; lateral is to the left. The *solid line* at the bottom indicates the ventral brainstem surface. DLPO, dorsolateral periolivary nucleus; LSO (*outlined in dots*), lateral superior olivary nucleus; LNTB, lateral nucleus of the trapezoid body; VLPO, ventrolateral periolivary nucleus; MSO (*outlined in dots*), medial superior olivary nucleus; DMPO, dorsomedial periolivary nucleus; MNTB, medial nucleus of the trapezoid body; VMPO, ventromedial periolivary nucleus; VNTB, ventral nucleus of the trapezoid body; VII, seventh nerve root; VI, sixth nerve root. The *open arrows* in the MNTB indicate some of the principal cells with their bushy dendritic trees. The *arrows* in LNTB indicate the long dendrites of some of the neurons of that nucleus.

small, round vesicles also contact the fusiform cells.

The Medial Superior Olivary Nucleus

Most of the principal cells of the MSO, like those of the LSO, have oriented dendritic fields (60) (Fig. 6). Dendrites arise from each pole of the fusiform cell bodies and extend medially and laterally away from the cell body toward the margins of the nucleus (60,68). The neurons appear to lie within the isofrequency planes of the nucleus as defined in physiological experiments (69,70). The neurons in the MSO respond to acoustic stimulation of either ear with an increased firing rate but respond most vigorously when binaural inputs arrive at the ears with a time delay characteristic for each cell. Nonoptimal delays may result in firing rates below that caused by stimulation of either ear, suggesting that inhibition also plays a role in the function of the MSO (2,69). The physiology of this nucleus is discussed elsewhere in this volume.

In the electron microscope, the dendrites and cell bodies of the principal cells are contacted by many large terminals that contain large, round synaptic vesicles (71–73). These terminals are similar, if not identical, in their fine structure to the terminals with large, round vesicles in the LSO. As discussed below, some or all of these terminals in the two nuclei arise from the same source and they are most likely excitatory in effect. The cell bodies are also contacted by several types of terminals with small, pleomorphic or flattened vesicles (71–74), a morphology that is often characteristic of inhibitory synapses. It is likely that many of these terminals use glycine as a transmitter. Strychnine uptake, a marker for glycine receptor sites, is very high in the nucleus (65), and some terminals take up glycine from the medium with high affinity (68).

The Medial Nucleus of the Trapezoid Body

The MNTB is a complex nucleus, containing at least three cell types (75). The principal cells, the most common cell type, are bushy cells, similar to the globular and spherical bushy cells of the cochlear nucleus (Fig. 6). Their short, highly branched dendrites lie close to the cell body. In the guinea pig, these bushy cells are intensely immunoreactive for glycine (39). The principal cells are organized tonotopically and respond to acoustic stimuli of the contralateral ear with an increased firing rate (70,76,77).

In the electron microscope, the cell body of the principal cell is dominated by input from the calyces of Held. The calycine terminals contain large, round synaptic vesicles and contact the cell bodies at multiple synaptic sites (21,78). Except for their larger size, these terminals are very similar in their fine structure to the terminals with large, round synaptic vesicles that are common in both the MSO and LSO. The cell bodies of the principal cells are also contacted by a heterogeneous population of smaller terminals with smaller pleomorphic or flattened synaptic vesicles (78). The synaptic organization of the bushy dendrites of the principal cells has not been described.

The Lateral Nucleus of the Trapezoid Body

Ramón y Cajal (60) is still the source of the most complete description of the LNTB, which he called the semilunar nucleus. The LNTB contains large, multipolar neurons, many of which send long dendrites deep into the fibers of the trapezoid body as they pass ventral to the nucleus (60) (Fig. 6). In the guinea pig, many of the neurons in the LNTB contain high levels of glycine (31; Fig. 6A in ref. 39) or GABA 31,79). The LNTB appears to be tonotopically organized and its neurons respond with an increased firing rate to ipsilateral acoustic stimulation; most of the neurons do not appear to be affected by contralateral stimulation (80).

A description of the fine structure of the LNTB is not available in the literature. Neurons in the nucleus are contacted by several types of synaptic terminals including some with large, round vesicles and others with smaller pleomorphic or flattened vesicles (*unpublished observations*), but the relative proportion and distribution of the different synaptic types are not known. Some of the inputs to the LNTB are presumably glycinergic since labeling for glycine receptor sites is substantial in the nucleus (65).

Projections to the Lateral and Medial Superior Olivary Nuclei: Excitatory Inputs Arise from the Spherical Bushy Cells of the Cochlear Nucleus; Inhibitory Inputs Arise from the Medial and Lateral Nuclei of the Trapezoid Body

Projections to the Lateral Superior Olivary Nucleus

The projection from the AVCN to the LSO arises in at least four subdivisions of the nucleus (18) (Fig. 7). Spherical bushy cells in subdivisions AA and APD project to the LSO; it is most likely that these are the same cells that project to the MSO (18; see below), although this has not been demonstrated directly. Projections to LSO also arise from spherical bushy cells in subdivision AP, cells that do not project to the MSO. Because spherical bushy cells are not present in PD, which also contributes to the projection, another cell type must be involved as well. PD contains globular bushy cells and large multipolar or stellate cells. Which of these types provides the inputs to LSO is not known. Thus, while it is possible that globular cells project to the LSO, it is not known that they do so.

The different subdivisions of the AVCN could have different targets in the LSO. The several types of neurons in the LSO (61,62) would be included in any injection into the nucleus so that the finding of multiple sources of inputs to the LSO does not necessarily imply multiple sources of inputs to individual cell types. The terminals with large, round vesicles that terminate on the dendrites of fusiform cells probably arise primarily, if not entirely, from the spherical bushy cells (18), but it could be that the large, spherical cells of AA and the small, spherical cells of AP project differentially.

The MNTB is a major source of inhibitory terminals in the LSO. The projection arises in the principal cells and is organized so that tonotopicity is preserved (81,82). The terminals from the MNTB appear to be distributed mainly on the soma and proximal dendrites of the principal cells (82) and so coincide in location with the terminals with flattened vesicles that use glycine as a transmitter. No other source of these terminals has been described. According to Glendenning and colleagues (81), more than 95% of the neurons providing input to the LSO are located either in the cochlear nucleus or in the MNTB. A few inputs may arise in other periolivary nuclei (81), but details of these inputs, if they exist, are lacking.

Projections to the Medial Superior Olivary Nucleus

The MSO receives input from both cochlear nuclei (42,57,83,84). The lateral dendrites of the bipolar neurons of the MSO receive the ipsilateral inputs and the medial dendrites receive the contralateral inputs. These cochlear nuclear inputs appear to arise exclusively from the spherical bushy cells in subdivisions AA and APD of the AVCN (18) (Fig. 8). The spherical bushy cells give rise to the terminals in the MSO with large, round synaptic vesicles (72,73), which provide most of the inputs to the dendrites. The spherical bushy cells in subdivision AP (i.e., the small, spherical cells [Figs. 4 and 5]) do *not* project to MSO (Fig. 8).

The terminals with flattened or pleomorphic vesicles that contact the cell soma of cells in the MSO do not arise in the cochlear nucleus (72,73). The possible sources of these terminals are limited and some may be intrinsic to the MSO. However, there appear to be at least two intraolivary sources of inputs to MSO, and it can be reasonably argued that both of these are inhibitory. The first of these is the MNTB. It has been suggested that axons from the MNTB give off collaterals to the MSO as they pass through that nucleus on their way to the LSO (82). Since the axons from the

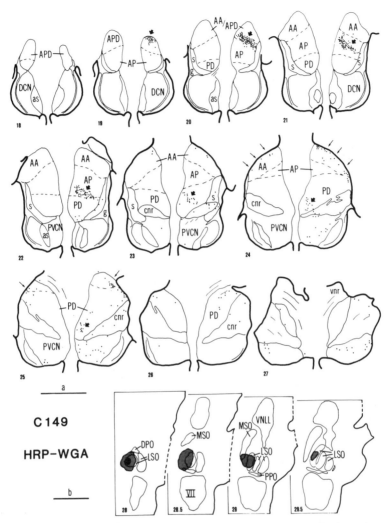

FIG. 7. Projections from the anteroventral cochlear nucleus (AVCN) to the lateral superior olivary nucleus (LSO) revealed by injections of horseradish peroxidase-labeled wheat germ agglutinin into the LSO. Horizontal sections through the left and right cochlear nuclei (section pairs 18–27) and through the right superior olivary complex (sections 28–29.5). The injection site in the superior olivary complex is indicated by *hatching*; the center of the injection site, where the concentration of horseradish peroxidase was the highest, is indicated by the *solid black fill.* In each pair of sections, the left nucleus is on the left; section pair 18 is the most dorsal, and progressively higher section numbers indicate progressively more ventral sections. Anterior is to the top of the figure; lateral is to the left of the left nuclei and to the right of the right nuclei. Sections were 70 μm thick; every fourth section through the cochlear nucleus and every other section through the superior olivary complex are illustrated. Labeled neurons in the cochlear nuclei are indicated by *dots,* each dot representing at least one cell. Subdivision boundaries in the AVCN are indicated by *dashed lines. Solid arrows* on sections 19–25 indicate "rows" of densely labeled neurons extending from anteromedial to posterolateral across the AVCN. *Thin arrows* on sections 24 and 25 indicate "rows" of lightly labeled neurons extending from anteromedial to posterolateral across subdivision AA. a, scale bar for sections through the cochlear nuclei = 2.0 mm; b, scale bar for sections through the superior olivary complex = 2.0 mm. as, acoustic stria; s, small cell cap; g, granule cell layer; VNLL, ventral nucleus of the lateral lemniscus; PPO, posterior periolivary nucleus; other abbreviations as in previous figures. (From ref. 18, with permission.)

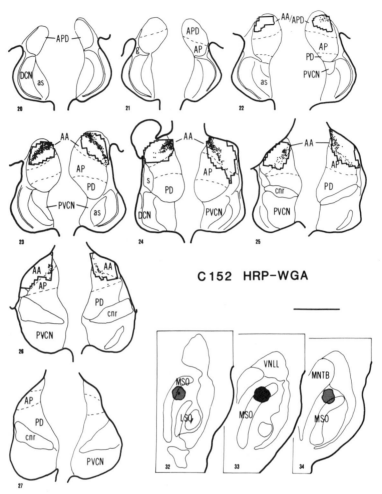

FIG. 8. Projections from the anteroventral cochlear nucleus (AVCN) to the medial superior olivary nucleus (MSO) as revealed by injections of horseradish peroxidase-labeled wheat germ agglutinin into the MSO. Horizontal sections through the left and right cochlear nuclei (section pairs 20–27) and through the right superior olivary complex. Details as in legend for Fig. 7. Only the most heavily labeled neurons are indicated by *dots*. In addition, the *heavy lines* traced around the area containing these cells enclose an area in which many more lightly labeled cells were located. Outside these lines, no neurons were labeled unless otherwise indicated by a *dot*. Within these lines, almost every neuron was labeled. Scale bar = 2.0 mm for all sections. Abbreviations as in previous figures. (From ref. 18, with permission.)

MNTB to the LSO are glycinergic and inhibitory, it is reasonable to suggest that this is also true of the terminal branches in the MSO.

The other potential source of inhibitory input to the MSO, the LNTB, has not been described previously. Cells in the LNTB

are intensely labeled when tracer injections are confined to the MSO (*unpublished observations*)`(Fig. 9). In the case illustrated in Fig. 9, the only labeled cells observed were in the two AVCN (shown in Fig. 8) and in the ipsilateral LNTB and MNTB. The question whether the labeling of cells

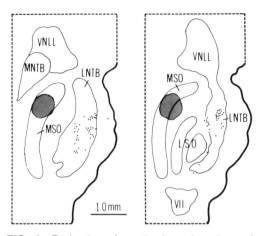

FIG. 9. Projections from the lateral nucleus of the trapezoid body (LNTB) to the medial superior olivary nucleus (MSO) revealed by injections of horseradish peroxidase-labeled wheat germ agglutinin into the MSO. This is the same cat as illustrated in Fig. 8. Horizontal sections through the right superior olivary complex. The section on the right is more dorsal. The *hatched area* represents the injection site; each *dot* represents one labeled neuron. VNLL, ventral nucleus of the lateral lemniscus; MNTB, medial nucleus of the trapezoid body; LSO, lateral superior olivary nucleus; VII, motor nucleus of the seventh nerve.

The Medial and Lateral Nuclei of the Trapezoid Body Receive Inputs from the Globular Bushy Cells of the Cochlear Nucleus

Projections to the Medial Nucleus of the Trapezoid Body

It has long been suspected that the globular cells of the posterior AVCN are the source of the calyces of Held that project into the MNTB (e.g., 85). Tolbert et al. (37) demonstrated this projection by injecting horseradish peroxidase into the MNTB and observing the subsequent labeling of globular bushy cells. The calyces (Fig. 10) form synapses with the principal cells (75). Like the globular and spherical bushy cells, the principal cells of the MNTB receive numerous other inputs, many presumably inhibitory since they contain flattened or pleomorphic synaptic vesicles. The sources of these inputs are not known, but subdivisions of the cochlear nucleus other than the globular cell areas do not appear to project to the MNTB (7). The function and physiological effects of the excitatory synapses on the principal cells of the MNTB seem clear, but the source(s) and function of the presumably inhibitory inputs are not known.

Projections to the Lateral Nucleus of the Trapezoid Body

The only known source of input to the LNTB is the cochlear nucleus (7,57,59). Most of the input is from the area of the nerve root (7,59), although there is a projection to the anterior part of the LNTB from the anterior AVCN (57). At least some of this input arises from the large axons of the globular cells as they pass through the trapezoid body on their way to the opposite side of the brain (37,85,86) (Fig. 10). The terminals with large, round vesicles that contact the neurons in the LNTB are simi-

is due to labeling of axons of passage is an important one in an area containing as many fiber bundles as the superior olivary complex. It does not seem likely in the case illustrated that the axons of cells in the LNTB were nicked on their way to another target, since injections only slightly lateral to the one illustrated in Fig. 10 would presumably pass through the same axon bundles but then enter LSO rather than MSO. In such cases numerous cells in the MNTB are labeled but cells in the LNTB are not labeled. The glycinergic cells of the LNTB (31,79) could be a source of the glycinergic terminals described in the MSO. The only other known projection of the LNTB is to the ipsilateral cochlear nucleus (46,50). Adams and Wenthold (31) have demonstrated that at least some of this input is probably glycinergic.

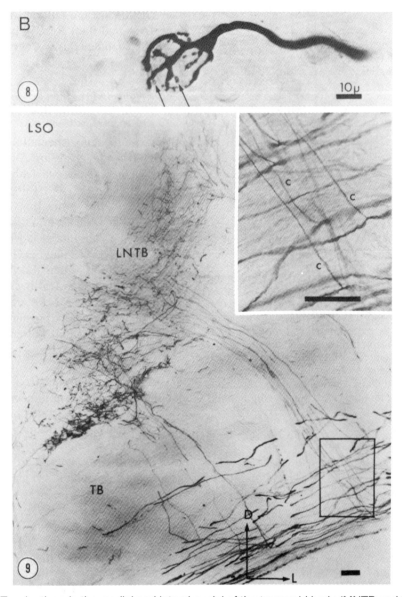

FIG. 10. Terminations in the medial and lateral nuclei of the trapezoid body (MNTB and LNTB) that arise from globular cells. **Upper panel:** Horseradish peroxidase-filled calyx in the MNTB of an adult cat. *Arrows* indicate grape-like calycine appendages. **Lower panel:** Thick horizontal fibers of the trapezoid body (TB) forming vertical collaterals that arborize in the lateral nucleus of the trapezoid body (LNTB) of an adult cat. Thinner, unfilled fibers are visible in the trapezoid body. Scale = 50 μm. Inset: Enlargement of the area within the rectangle showing origin of the vertical collaterals (c) from thick trapezoid fibers. Scale 50 μm. LSO, lateral superior olivary nucleus. (From ref. 37, with permission.)

lar in their fine structure to the calycine terminals in the MNTB *(unpublished observations)*. Smith et al. (86) injected single, physiologically characterized globular cells with horseradish peroxidase and showed that almost all axons that give rise to a calyx in the contralateral MNTB also give rise to terminals in the ipsilateral LNTB. Thus, it may be that the cells that provide inhibitory inputs to the LSO and MSO get their input from the same cells in the cochlear nucleus.

SUMMARY

The pathways discussed above are summarized in simplified form in Fig. 11. The principal neurons in the LSO and MSO receive direct excitatory inputs from the spherical bushy cells of the AVCN. These neurons also receive inhibitory inputs. Those to the LSO arise in the MNTB and

those to the MSO appear to arise in the LNTB and perhaps also in the MNTB. Both the MNTB and LNTB, in turn, receive excitatory inputs from the globular bushy cells of the AVCN. Both the spherical and globular bushy cells receive their major, if not only, excitatory input from the cochlea. Both types of bushy cells also receive inhibitory inputs that appear to be from multiple sources and include both GABAergic and glycinergic synapses. Work remains to determine the details of the connectivity of all the cell types discussed here.

A concept central to our current understanding of neuronal function is that information transfer in the central nervous system depends on the ability of individual neurons to integrate activity at multiple excitatory and inhibitory synapses. A major effort in neuroscience has been devoted to understanding the mechanisms by which neurons effect this integration. Neurons in

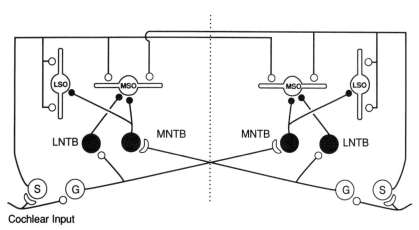

FIG. 11. Diagram of some of the connections discussed in this chapter. Both sides of the brain are represented; the *dotted line* indicates the midline. The connections illustrated are discussed in detail in the text. Briefly, cochlear input forms the major excitatory input to both spherical (S) and globular (G) bushy cells. The spherical cells provide excitatory inputs to the ipsilateral lateral superior olivary nucleus (LSO) and to both the ipsilateral and contralateral medial superior olivary nucleus (MSO). The globular cells provide excitatory inputs to the ipsilateral lateral nucleus of the trapezoid body (LNTB) and to the contralateral medial nucleus of the trapezoid body (MNTB). The MNTB projects ipsilaterally to the LSO where the effect is inhibitory. Both the MNTB and LNTB appear to send projections into the ipsilateral MSO where the effect may be inhibitory. Presumably excitatory inputs are indicated by the *open* terminal symbols, the larger of these representing calycine endings. Presumably inhibitory inputs are indicated by the *filled* terminal symbols.

the LSO and MSO offer an advantage for analysis of neuronal integration in that, compared to most of the nuclei of the mammalian central nervous system, they are relatively simple. Each contains only a few cell types and receives only a few well-defined inputs (e.g., 18,62,63,68,74,81). Schwartz and colleagues correctly point out that the earlier view that the MSO and LSO contain only one cell type is too simple (62,68). Nevertheless, compared to structures such as the cochlear nucleus, the lateral geniculate, the cerebral cortex, and the retina, the superior olivary cell groups do appear to be much less complex. In the superior olive, different types of neurons are, to a great extent, segregated into separate nuclei. Thus, the "interneurons" of the MNTB and LNTB are physically separated from their "principal" neurons in the LSO and MSO. This should make it easier than it has been in other parts of the brain to address the question of the synaptic organization of both the principal neurons and the local circuit neurons and to then relate the neuronal circuitry to the neuronal response properties.

ACKNOWLEDGMENTS

Research by the author is supported by a grant from the National Institutes of Health (R01 DC00135).

REFERENCES

1. Irvine DRG. *The auditory brainstem.* In: Ottoson D, ed. *Progress in sensory physiology,* vol 7. Berlin: Springer-Verlag, 1986;1–279.
2. Yin TCT, Chan JCK. Neural mechanisms underlying interaural time sensitivity to tones and noise. In: Edelman GM, Gall WE, Cowan WM, eds. *Auditory function. Neurobiological bases of hearing.* New York: John Wiley and Sons, 1988;385–430.
3. Osen KK. Cytoarchitecture of the cochlear nuclei in the cat. *J Comp Neurol* 1969;136:453–484.
4. Adams JC. Cytology of periolivary cells and the organization of their projections in the cat. *J Comp Neurol* 1983;215:275–289.
5. Kiang NYS, Morest DK, Godfrey DA, Guinan JJ, Kane EC. Stimulus coding at caudal levels of the cat's auditory nervous system. I. Response characteristics of single units. In: Møller AR, ed. *Basic mechanisms in hearing.* New York: Academic Press, 1973;455–478.
6. Morest DK, Kiang NYS, Kane EC, Guinan JJ, Godfrey DA. Stimulus coding at caudal levels of the cat's auditory nervous system. II. Patterns of synaptic organization. In: Møller AR, ed. *Basic mechanisms in hearing.* New York: Academic Press, 1973;479–504.
7. Warr WB. Parallel ascending pathways from the cochlear nucleus: neuroanatomical evidence of functional specialization. *Contrib Sens Physiol* 1982;7:1–38.
8. Rhode WS, Smith PH, Oertel D. Physiological response properties of cells labeled intracellularly with horseradish peroxidase in cat dorsal cochlear nucleus. *J Comp Neurol* 1983;213:426–447.
9. Rhode WS, Oertel D, Smith PH. Physiological response properties of cells labeled intracellularly with horseradish peroxidase in cat ventral cochlear nucleus. *J Comp Neurol* 1983;213:448–463.
10. Rouiller EM, Ryugo DK. Intracellular marking of physiologically characterized cells in the ventral cochlear nucleus of the cat. *J Comp Neurol* 1984;225:167–186.
11. Smith PH, Rhode WS. Electron microscopic features of physiologically characterized, HRP-labeled fusiform cells in the cat dorsal cochlear nucleus. *J Comp Neurol* 1985;237:127–143.
12. Brawer JR, Morest DK, Kane E. The neuronal architecture of the cochlear nucleus of the cat. *J Comp Neurol* 1974;155:251–300.
13. Cant NB. The fine structure of two types of stellate cells in the anterior division of the anteroventral cochlear nucleus of the cat. *Neuroscience* 1981;6:2643–2655.
14. Cant NB, Morest DK. The structural basis for stimulus coding in the cochlear nucleus. In: Berlin C, ed. *Hearing sciences: recent advances.* San Diego: College-Hill Press, 1984;371–421.
15. Tolbert LP, Morest DK. The neuronal architecture of the anteroventral cochlear nucleus of the cat in the region of the cochlear nerve root: Golgi and Nissl methods. *Neuroscience* 1982;7:3013–3131.
16. Cant NB, Morest DK. Organization of the neurons in the anterior division of the anteroventral cochlear nucleus of the cat. Light-microscopic observations. *Neuroscience* 1979;4:1909–1923.
17. Tolbert LP, Morest DK. The neuronal architecture of the anteroventral cochlear nucleus of the cat in the region of the cochlear nerve root: electron microscopy. *Neuroscience* 1982;7:3053–3067.
18. Cant NB, Casseday JH. Projections from the anteroventral cochlear nucleus to the lateral and medial superior olivary nuclei. *J Comp Neurol* 1986;247:457–476.
19. Cant NB, Morest DK. The bushy cells in the anteroventral cochlear nucleus of the cat. A study

with the electron microscope. *Neuroscience* 1979;4:1925–1945.

20. Kane ESC. Synaptic organization in the dorsal cochlear nucleus of the cat: a light- and electron-microscopic study. *J Comp Neurol* 1974;155: 301–330.

21. Lenn NJ, Reese TS. The fine structure of nerve endings in the nucleus of the trapezoid body and the ventral cochlear nucleus. *Am J Anat* 1966; 118:375–390.

22. Lorente de Nó R. *The primary acoustic nuclei.* New York: Raven Press, 1981.

23. Brawer JR, Morest DK. Relations between auditory nerve endings and cell types in the cat's anteroventral cochlear nucleus seen with the Golgi method and Nomarski optics. *J Comp Neurol* 1975;160:491–506.

24. Rouiller EM, Cronin-Schreiber R, Fekete DM, Ryugo DK. The central projections of intracellularly labeled auditory nerve fibers in cats: an analysis of terminal morphology. *J Comp Neurol* 1986;249:261–278.

25. Pfeiffer RR. Anteroventral cochlear nucleus: waveforms of extracellularly recorded spike potentials. *Science* 1966;154:667–668.

26. Spoendlin H. Degeneration behavior of the cochlear nerve. *Arch Klin Exp Ohr Nas Kehlk Heilk* 1971;200:275–291.

27. Brown MC, Berglund AM, Kiang NYS, Ryugo DK. Central trajectories of type II spiral ganglion neurons. *J Comp Neurol* 1988;278:581–590.

28. Liberman MC. Auditory-nerve response from cats raised in a low-noise chamber. *J Acoust Soc Am* 1978;63:442–455.

29. Fekete DM, Rouiller EM, Liberman MC, Ryugo DK. The central projections of intracellularly labeled auditory nerve fibers in cats. *J Comp Neurol* 1984;229:432–450.

30. Schwartz AM, Gulley RL. Non-primary afferents to the principal cells of the rostral anteroventral cochlear nucleus of the guinea-pig. *Am J Anat* 1978;153:489–508.

31. Adams JC, Wenthold RJ. Immunostaining of GABA-ergic and glycinergic inputs to the anteroventral cochlear nucleus. *Neurosci Abstr* 1987;13:1259.

32. Altschuler RA, Betz H, Parakkal MH, Reeks KA, Wenthold RJ. Identification of glycinergic synapses in the cochlear nucleus through immunocytochemical localization of the postsynaptic receptor. *Brain Res* 1986;369:316–320.

33. Wenthold RJ, Parakkal MH, Oberdorfer MD, Altschuler RA. Glycine receptor immunoreactivity in the ventral cochlear nucleus of the guinea pig. *J Comp Neurol* 1988;276:423–435.

34. Oberdorfer MD, Parakkal MH, Altschuler RA, Wenthold RJ. Ultrastructural localization of GABA-immunoreactive terminals in the anteroventral cochlear nucleus of the guinea pig. *Hear Res* 1988;33:229–238.

35. Saint Marie RL, Morest DK, Brandon C. The pattern of GAD-like immunoreactivity on identified cell types in the cat ventral cochlear nucleus. *Neurosci Abstr* 1985;11:1049.

36. Adams JC, Mugnaini E. Patterns of glutamate decarboxylase immunostaining in the feline cochlear nuclear complex studied with silver enhancement and electron microscopy. *J Comp Neurol* 1987;262:375–401.

37. Tolbert LP, Morest DK, Yurgelun-Todd DA. The neuronal architecture of the anteroventral cochlear nucleus of the cat in the region of the cochlear nerve root: horseradish peroxidase labelling of identified cell types. *Neuroscience* 1982;7:3031–3052.

38. Smith PH, Rhode WS. Characterization of HRP-labeled globular bushy cells in the cat anteroventral cochlear nucleus. *J Comp Neurol* 1987; 266:360–375.

39. Wenthold RJ, Huie D, Altschuler RA, Reeks KA. Glycine immunoreactivity localized in the cochlear nucleus and superior olivary complex. *Neuroscience* 1987;22:897–912.

40. Ostapoff EM, Morest DK. Analysis of synapses to bushy cells in the posterior anteroventral cochlear nucleus (AVCN-P) of the cat. *Neurosci Abstr* 1984;10:842.

41. Rasmussen GL. Efferent fibers of the cochlear nerve and cochlear nucleus. In: Rasmussen GL, Windle W, eds. *Neural mechanisms of the auditory and vestibular system.* Springfield, IL: Charles C. Thomas, 1960; 105–115.

42. Rasmussen GL. Efferent connections of the cochlear nucleus. In: Graham AB, ed. *Sensorineural hearing processes and disorders.* Boston: Little, Brown, 1967;61–75.

43. van Noort J. *The structure and connections of the inferior colliculus.* Assen: Van Gorcum, 1969.

44. Osen KK, Roth K. Histochemical localization of cholinesterase in the cochlear nuclei of the cat, with notes on the origin of acetylcholinesterase-positive afferents and the superior olive. *Brain Res* 1969;16:165–185.

45. Adams JC, Warr WB. Origins of axons in the cat's acoustic striae determined by injection of horseradish peroxidase into severed tracts. *J Comp Neurol* 1976;170:107–122.

46. Elverland HH. Descending connections between the superior olivary and cochlear nucleus complexes in the cat studied by autoradiographic and horseradish peroxidase methods. *Exp Brain Res* 1977;27:397–421.

47. Cant NB, Morest DK. Axons from non-cochlear sources in the anteroventral cochlear nucleus of the cat. A study with the rapid Golgi method. *Neuroscience* 1978;3:1003–1029.

48. Cant NB, Gaston KC. Pathways connecting the right and left cochlear nuclei. *J Comp Neurol* 1982;212:313–326.

49. Oliver DL. Dorsal cochlear nucleus projections to the inferior colliculus in the cat. *J Comp Neurol* 1984:224:155–172.

50. Spangler KM, Cant NB, Henkel CK, Farley GC, Warr WB. Descending projections from the superior olivary complex to the cochlear nucleus of the cat. *J Comp Neurol* 1987;259:452–465.

51. Whitley JM, Henkel CK. Topographical organization of the inferior colliculus projection and

other connections of the ventral nucleus of the lateral lemniscus in the cat. *J Comp Neurol* 1984;229:257–270.

52. Kane ES, Conlee JW. Descending inputs to the caudal cochlear nucleus of the cat: degeneration and autoradiographic studies. *J Comp Neurol* 1979;187:759–784.

53. Wenthold RJ. Evidence for a glycinergic pathway connecting the two cochlear nuclei: an immunocytochemical and retrograde transport study. *Brain Res* 1987;415:183–187.

54. Mugnaini E. GABA neurons in the superficial layers of the rat dorsal cochlear nucleus: light and electron microscopic immunocytochemistry. *J Comp Neurol* 1985;235:61–81.

55. Wickesberg RE, Oertel D. Tonotopic projection from the dorsal to the anteroventral cochlear nucleus of mice. *J Comp Neurol* 1988;268:389–399.

56. Synder RL, Leake PA. Intrinsic connections within and between cochlear nucleus subdivisions in cat. *J Comp Neurol* 1988;278:209–225.

57. Warr WB. Fiber degeneration following lesions in the anterior ventral cochlear nucleus of the cat. *Exp Neurol* 1966;14:453–474.

58. Warr WB. Fiber degeneration following lesions in the posteroventral cochlear nucleus of the cat. *Exp Neurol* 1969;23:140–155.

59. Warr WB. Fiber degeneration following lesions in the multipolar and globular cell areas in the ventral cochlear nucleus of the cat. *Brain Res* 1972;40:247–270.

60. Ramón y Cajal S. *Histologie du système nerveux de l'homme et des vertébrés,* vol I (1972 reprint). Madrid: Instituto Rámon y Cajal, 1909.

61. Warr WB. Olivocochlear and vestibular efferent neurons of the feline brain stem. Their location, morphology, and number determined by retrograde axonal transport and acetylcholinesterase histochemistry. *J Comp Neurol* 1975;161:159–182.

62. Helfert RH, Schwartz IR. Morphological evidence for the existence of multiple neuronal classes in the cat lateral superior olivary nucleus. *J Comp Neurol* 1986;244:533–549.

63. Cant NB. The fine structure of the lateral superior olivary nucleus of the cat. *J Comp Neurol* 1984;227:63–77.

64. Tsuchitani C, Boudreau JC. Single unit analysis of cat superior olive S-segment with tonal stimuli. *J Neurophysiol* 1966;29:684–697.

65. Glendenning KK, Baker BN. Neuroanatomical distribution of receptors for three potential inhibitory neurotransmitters in the brainstem auditory nuclei of the cat. *J Comp Neurol* 1988;275:288–308.

66. Sanes DH, Geary WA, Wooten GF, Rubel EW. Quantitative distribution of the glycine receptor in the auditory brain stem of the gerbil. *J Neurosci* 1987;7:3793–3802.

67. Moore MJ, Caspary DM. Strychnine blocks binaural inhibition in lateral superior olivary neurons. *J Neurosci* 1983;3:237–242.

68. Schwartz IR. Axonal organization in the cat me-

dial superior olivary nucleus. *Contrib Sens Physiol* 1984;8:99–129.

69. Goldberg JM, Brown PB. Functional organization of the dog superior olivary complex: an anatomical and electrophysiological study. *J Neurophysiol* 1968;31:639–656.

70. Guinan JJ, Guinan SS, Norris BE. Single auditory units in the superior olivary complex. II. Locations of unit categories and tonotopic organization. *Int J Neurosci* 1972;4:147–166.

71. Clark GM. The ultrastructure of nerve endings in the medial superior olive of the cat. *Brain Res* 1969;14:293–305.

72. Perkins RE. An electron microscopic study of synaptic organization in the medial superior olive of normal and experimental chinchillas. *J Comp Neurol* 1973;148:387–416.

73. Lindsey BC. Fine structure and distribution of axon terminals from the cochlear nucleus on neurons in the medial superior olivary nucleus of the cat. *J Comp Neurol* 1975;160:81–103.

74. Schwartz IR. The differential distributions of synaptic terminals on marginal and central cells in the cat medial superior olivary nucleus. *Am J Anat* 1980;159:25–31.

75. Morest DK. The collateral system of the medial nucleus of the trapezoid body of the cat, its neuronal architecture and relation to the olivo-cochlear bundle. *Brain Res* 1968;9:288–311.

76. Guinan JJ, Guinan SS, Norris BE. Single auditory units in the superior olivary complex. I. Responses to sounds and classifications based on physiological properties. *Int J Neurosci* 1972;4:101–120.

77. Li RYS, Guinan JJ. Antidromic and orthodromic stimulation of neurons receiving calyces of Held. Quarterly Progress Report No. 100, Research Laboratory of Electronics, Massachusetts Institute of Technology, 1971; 227–234.

78. Jean Baptiste M, Morest DK. Transneuronal changes of synaptic endings and nuclear chromatin in the trapezoid body following cochlear ablations in cats. *J Comp Neurol* 1975;162:111–134.

79. Helfert RH, Altschuler RA, Wenthold RJ. GABA and glycine immunoreactivity in the guinea pig superior olivary complex. *Neurosci Abstr* 1987;13:544.

80. Tsuchitani C. Functional organization of lateral cell groups of cat superior olivary complex. *J Neurophysiol* 1977;40:296–318.

81. Glendenning KK, Hutson KA, Nudo RJ, Masterton RB. Acoustic chiasm. II: Anatomical basis of binaurality in lateral superior olive of cat. *J Comp Neurol* 1985;232:261–285.

82. Spangler KM, Warr WB, Henkel CK. The projections of principal cells of the medial nucleus of the trapezoid body in the cat. *J Comp Neurol* 1985;238:249–262.

83. Stotler WA. An experimental study of the cells and connections of the superior olivary complex of the cat. *J Comp Neurol* 1953;98:401–431.

84. Osen KK. Afferent and efferent connections of three well-defined cell types of the cat cochlear

nuclei. In: Andersen P, Jansen JKS, eds. *Excitatory synaptic mechanisms*. Oslo: Universitetforlaget, 1970;295–300.

85. Harrison JM, Warr WB. A study of the cochlear nuclei and ascending auditory pathways of the medulla. *J Comp Neurol* 1962;119:341–379.

86. Smith PH, Carney LH, Yin TCT. Projections of globular bushy cells in the cat. *Neurosci Abstr* 1987;13:547.

87. Bourk TR, Mielcarz JM, Norris BE. Tonotopic organization of the anteroventral cochlear nucleus of the cat. *Hear Res* 1981;4:215–241.

Neurobiology of Hearing: The Central Auditory System, edited by R. A. Altschuler et al. Raven Press, Ltd., New York 1991.

6

Neurotransmitters of Brainstem Auditory Nuclei

Robert J. Wenthold

Section on Neurochemistry, Laboratory of Molecular Otology, National Institute on Deafness and Other Communication Disorders, National Institutes of Health, Bethesda, MD 20892

Our knowledge of neurotransmitters in the auditory system has increased significantly over the past 10 years. Much of the early neurotransmitter research was directed at determining which neurotransmitters were present in the auditory system, with the cochlear nucleus being the only structure receiving a systematic approach to this question. This effort has continued over recent years, but the more specific question, concerning which neurons contain these neurotransmitters and where receptors for them are found, is also being addressed, especially in the cochlear nucleus. Several experimental techniques can be applied to such studies, but immunocytochemistry using specific antibodies against neurotransmitters, neurotransmitter-related enzymes, and neurotransmitter receptors has been very productive. For several neurotransmitters, including the catecholamines, acetylcholine, and gamma-aminobutyric acid (GABA), antibodies are available against the neurotransmitter itself, biosynthetic and degradative enzymes, and their postsynaptic receptors (Table 1). Glycine (gly), as well as the gly receptor, has been localized with antibodies. The neuroactive peptides can also be localized directly with antibodies. Therefore, with a few exceptions as discussed below, most known neurotransmitters can be identified with immu-nocytochemistry, thereby providing a convenient and reliable approach to characterizing auditory system neurotransmitters.

In the auditory nuclei of the brainstem, there is evidence from several lines of research that amino acids play major roles in neurotransmission, while many more traditional transmitters, such as catecholamines or serotonin, are present at low concentrations. For example, in the cochlear nucleus of the guinea pig, choline acetyltransferase (ChAT) and tyrosine hydroxylase are present at 40% and 8%, respectively, of the concentrations found in the cerebrum (26). On the other hand, glutamate decarboxylase (GAD) is about 50% higher in the cochlear nucleus and gly levels in the cochlear nucleus are among the highest found in the central nervous system (32). Recently, antibodies have become available for studying amino acid neurotransmitters, particularly the inhibitory amino acids GABA and gly. Antibodies are now available against GABA, gly, GAD, the gly postsynaptic receptor, and the GABA postsynaptic receptor, the $GABA_A$ receptor. These antibodies have been used to obtain detailed data concerning the distribution of neurons believed to use GABA and gly as neurotransmitters. There has also been recent progress on the identification of neurons using excitatory

TABLE 1. *Immunocytochemical approaches to neurotransmitter identification*

	Antibodies		
Neurotransmitter	Neurotransmitter-conjugate	Related enzyme	Receptor
GABA	GABA (105)	GAD (14), GABA-T (14)	GABA (82)
Acetylcholine	Acetylcholine (30), epinephrine (44,102)	ChAT (50)	Nicotinic (97), muscarinic (54)
Catecholamines	Norepinephrine (44,102), dopamine (22)	PNMT (44) DBH (44,88), TH (44,79)	β-Adrenergic (11)
Serotonin	Serotonin (94,102)	TrH (79)	
Gly	Gly (81,107)		Gly (100,112)
Excitatory amino acids	Glutamate (42,55,74,95), asp (12,74)	Glutaminase (105) AAT (105) GDH (105)	Kainate (106), glutamate (109)

GAD, glutamic acid decarboxylase; GABA-T, GABA-transaminase; ChAT, choline acetyltransferase; PNMT, phenylethanolamine *N*-methyl transferase; DBH, dopamine-β-hydroxylase; TH, tyrosine hydroxylase; TrH, tryptophan hydroxylase; Gly, glycine; asp, aspartate; AAT, aspartate aminotransferase; GDH, glutamate dehydrogenase.
References are indicated by number in parentheses.

amino acid (EAA) neurotransmitters. Antibodies against glutamate (glu) and aspartate (asp), as well as against enzymes involved in the metabolism of these amino acids, are available and have demonstrated the wide distribution of these amino acids in the nervous system. However, such antibodies do not differentiate between the neurotransmitter pools and the metabolic pools of the amino acids. With the recent cloning of postsynaptic EAA receptors, antibodies will now be available for localizing these receptors.

This review focuses on recent immunocytochemical work on inhibitory neurotransmitters in the auditory nuclei of the brainstem and briefly discusses other neurotransmitters found in these areas. The literature has been reviewed through 1988, and the chapter includes critical references published after that date. Information on earlier studies can be found in a previous review (110).

IMMUNOCYTOCHEMISTRY AND NEUROTRANSMITTER LOCALIZATION

The immunocytochemical characterization of a neurotransmitter is usually directed at three areas: the localization of the neurotransmitter itself, localization of an enzyme that is reasonably specific for the neurotransmitter, and localization of a postsynaptic receptor for the neurotransmitter. Any other characteristic that is specific for the particular neurotransmitter, such as proteins that are part of an uptake or release mechanism, could also be used to map the distribution of a neurotransmitter, but thus far, this has not been routinely done with immunocytochemistry. The transmitter degrading enzymes acetylcholinesterase and GABA transaminase (GABA-T) have also been used for transmitter characterization, but in some cases, the selective association with their respective neurotransmitter has been questioned.

Successful localization of the transmitter depends primarily on whether or not that substance is found predominantly in neurons where it functions as a neurotransmitter, or if it is generally found throughout the nervous system and involved in roles unrelated to neurotransmission. In this regard the relative concentration of the neurotransmitter appears to be critical, as seen in the case of gly. Gly, for example, is present in every cell in the nervous system, but the high concentrations found in neurons that release gly as a neurotransmitter serve as a useful marker for the immunocytochemical localization of these neurons with anti-gly antibodies. Unfortunately, there is a tendency to generalize and disregard the possibility that in some cases a high concentration of a substance such as gly in a neuron could be unrelated to a neurotransmitter function. Several substances, such as acetylcholine (ACh), GABA, and many neuroactive peptides, are used primarily as neurotransmitters and can be reliably localized with immunocytochemistry.

Immunocytochemical localization of enzymes related to neurotransmitter synthesis or degradation has been widely applied. A major limitation is that highly purified enzymes are needed to make the antibodies, and these enzymes are usually present in small amounts in tissue and difficult to purify. Furthermore, many neurotransmitters are not produced locally through the action of a specific enzyme.

Immunocytochemical localization of neurotransmitter receptors has received relatively little attention primarily because of the lack of available antibodies against receptors. Receptors are difficult to purify because they are present in small amounts and closely associated with the membrane, and only recently have specific antibodies against a limited number of receptors been available. However, receptor localization is certain to receive increased attention because of their importance in neurotransmission and the fact that soon we can expect most receptors to be purified and cloned. The cloning studies have shown that most receptor families are made up of multiple subtypes, often with different distributions and pharmacological subtypes. The postsynaptic receptor is potentially the most selective marker for transmitter identification. While some neurotransmitters can be involved in functions in addition to neurotransmission, it has not been shown that postsynaptic receptors subserve other roles. However, there are reports based on autoradiographic receptor localization indicating that distributions of the neuro-

transmitter and the receptor often do not match (43). This may be due to the technical limitations of autoradiography but requires further investigation. Immunocytochemical studies have already revealed unexpected findings on the distribution of receptors such as suggesting that neurotransmitter receptors are not always found on the postsynaptic membrane. For example, it has been reported that the $GABA_A$ receptor is present on both the pre- and postsynaptic membranes (82). Adrenergic receptors have been found on astrocytes (11).

Antibodies against several small molecule neurotransmitters are now available (Table 1). These antibodies are made against the neurotransmitter, which is coupled to a larger molecule, usually a protein, with a chemical that is also used as a fixative in perfusing the animal. For example, we have made antibodies against the amino acids GABA, gly, glu, and asp, by coupling them to bovine serum albumin (BSA) with glutaraldehyde. These conjugates are extensively dialyzed to remove free glutaraldehyde and amino acid and injected into rabbits. While the antiserum has a high concentration of antibody that recognizes the neurotransmitter conjugate, it is usually necessary to purify the antibodies to reduce nonspecific staining as well as cross-reactivity with other molecules. This can be done using affinity chromatography, taking advantage of the antibody molecule's high affinity for the antigen. The antigen is attached to a support resin, and the antiserum is passed through. Antibodies recognizing the antigen are bound and others pass through. Either the antigen of interest or substances expected to be recognized by contaminating antibodies can be attached to the resin. It is impossible to anticipate every possible molecule with which the antibody may crossreact; in our study using antibodies against amino acids, we used conjugates of other amino acids that are known to be abundant in the brain and attached these conjugates to the resin. Antibodies recognizing these compounds bind and remain on the resin, while those that are not bound presumably will be more specific for the original antigen. While this works well for GABA (113), we have found that using two affinity columns is required for gly (107). Antiserum is first passed through a column containing gly conjugated to ovalbumin (the original antigen was gly-glutaraldehyde-BSA). Only antibodies that recognize gly-glutaraldehyde should bind and these are then eluted with weak acid, which is known to disrupt the antigen-antibody interaction. These antibodies are then passed through a column of GABA-glutaraldehyde-BSA, and the antibodies that do not recognize GABA pass through. This latter procedure assures that any antibodies that recognize GABA are removed. We now prepare our antibodies against GABA in an analogous way to give staining with lower background.

Antibodies made in this way have a low affinity for the free amino acid since even high concentrations of amino acid do not block staining. Rather, the antibodies recognize the amino acid-glutaraldehyde complex. In determining the specificity of the antibody, we have used immunoblots in which the conjugate is immobilized on strips of nitrocellulose. Other techniques can also be used to give quantitative data on specificity. In these studies, conjugates of other amino acids and structurally related compounds are tested. The possibility of a protein contributing to the staining can be studied using a western blot. In this procedure, total proteins from a tissue are separated on an acrylamide gel and then electrophoretically transferred to a sheet of nitrocellulose paper on which they tightly bind. Using methods similar to those used in immunocytochemistry, proteins that bind particular antibodies can now be identified.

In considering the options for immunocytochemical characterization of neurotransmitters, it is apparent that this approach could lead to incorrect results due to lack of specificity of the antibody or lack of appropriateness of the marker. This necessitates the use of more than one immunocytochemical marker when possible. Therefore, the combined localization of a neurotransmitter, its biosynthetic enzyme, and its postsynaptic receptor is far stronger evidence in determining the neurotransmitter of a particular neuron than the localization of any one of these alone.

COCHLEAR NUCLEUS

GABA

Because it is relatively straightforward to assay and localize immunocytochemically, GABA is now the best characterized putative neurotransmitter in the cochlear nucleus. Biochemical studies were first to show moderate levels of GABA, GAD, and GABA-T in the cochlear nucleus compared to other brain nuclei. The distribution of GABA in the cochlear nucleus is not uniform as Godfrey et al. (32) found a 40-fold range in concentrations with highest levels in the dorsal cochlear nucleus (DCN). Release of both endogenous and exogenous GABA from cochlear nucleus slices has been demonstrated (80,103). Pharmacological studies have shown that GABA exerts an inhibitory action on neurons of the cochlear nucleus (21), while autoradiographic (28,31) and immunocytochemical (49) analyses have demonstrated that GABA receptors are present in the cochlear nucleus. Together, these data provide convincing evidence that GABA is acting as a neurotransmitter in the cochlear nucleus, but give little information concerning the identification of GABAergic neurons and synapses. Certain pathways may be amenable to surgical lesion followed by analysis for changes in any of these parameters, but these are generally difficult studies, can often give ambiguous results, and can be applied only rarely.

Using antibodies against GABA and GAD, the distribution of putative GABAergic cells and terminals has been reported at the light and ultrastructural levels in the cochlear nucleus in a number of species including the cat (4,6,84), guinea pig (108, 113), rat (60,62,90), mouse (73), gerbil (83,88), and human (2). Immunoreactive terminals appear as labeled puncta at the light microscopic level. In some cases, especially in the ventral cochlear nucleus (VCN), such puncta can be seen outlining unlabeled cell bodies (Fig. 1A). While generally similar results are obtained for different species, as well as with the two different antibodies, some important differences emerge. Antibodies against GABA stain cell bodies more intensely than do antibodies against GAD. Most investigators have used colchicine pretreatment to obtain satisfactory cell body staining with GAD, while such treatment seems to have little effect when using the GABA antibody. The reason for the high GABA levels in the cell soma is not apparent; it does not appear that GABA in the cell body is a major source of neurotransmitter for the presynaptic terminals since GAD is concentrated in the presynaptic terminal. More likely, cell body GABA could arise from an unregulated GAD, which is synthesized in the

cell body for transport to the terminal. It may also suggest functions unrelated to neurotransmission. Satisfactory terminal labeling can be obtained with either antibody.

In comparing results among different species, a major limitation is that neuronal cell types in auditory nuclei have not been rigorously identified in most species. In general, immunoreactivity is found in all areas of the nucleus, cell body labeling is found mostly in the superficial layers of the DCN, large projection neurons and granule cells are not immunoreactive, and immunoreactive terminals are found on cell bodies throughout the magnocellular region of the VCN. In the cat, where neuronal cell types have been described, Adams and Mugnaini (4) and Saint Marie et al. (84) have recently described GAD immunoreactivity in the VCN. Immunoreactive terminals were identified on bushy cells, globular cells, and octopus cells. Although GAD immunoreactivity is not present in auditory nerve terminals, Adams and Mugnaini report that the size and distribution of pericellular staining with anti-GAD antibodies are positively correlated with those of au-

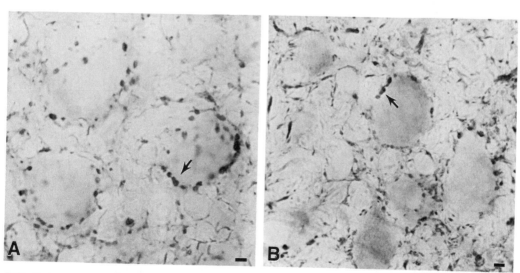

FIG. 1. Immunoreactive puncta (*arrows*) around unlabeled cells in the guinea AVCN using antibodies against GABA (**A**) and gly (**B**). Bars = 3.5 μm (A) and 3.2 μm (B). (From refs. 107, 113, with permission.)

ditory nerve terminals. Bushy cells in the rostral VCN were densely innervated by large GAD-positive terminals, while octopus cells were moderately innervated by small GABA-positive terminals. The true significance of this finding awaits the quantitative determination of size and number of terminals associated with these cell types. Such a pattern is not apparent in the guinea pig.

Studies in the cochlear nucleus at the ultrastructural level show that GAD or GABA immunoreactivity is found in presynaptic terminals with oval/pleomorphic synaptic vesicles (Fig. 2A). In the guinea pig VCN, not all such terminals contain GABA immunoreactivity, suggesting that this class of synaptic terminal is heterogeneous with respect to the neurotransmitter released (67,68).

GAD-immunoreactive cells in the superficial DCN have been identified in the rat as Golgi, stellate, and cartwheel neurons (62,65). Similar cell types have been reported in the superficial DCN of the cat, guinea pig, mouse, and gerbil, although identification of the cells was not thoroughly carried out. In the guinea pig, three classes of immunoreactive neurons can be identified based on size and shape. The distribution of these cells is illustrated in Fig. 3. GABA-immunoreactive neurons in the deeper regions of the DCN have been reported, but not described in detail. However, some of these may also contain gly immunoreactivity, as discussed below.

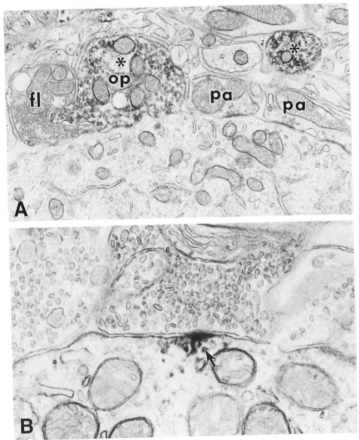

FIG. 2. Ultrastructural localization of GABA (**A**) and gly receptor (**B**) immunoreactivities in the guinea pig AVCN. GABA immunoreactivity (*asterisks*) is found in terminals with oval/pleomorphic (op) synaptic vesicles, while primary afferent terminals (pa) and terminals with flattened synaptic vesicles (fl) are unlabeled. Gly receptor immunoreactivity is found postsynaptic of terminals with flattened synaptic vesicles (*arrow*) as well as terminals with oval/pleomorphic vesicles. (From ref. 8, with permission.)

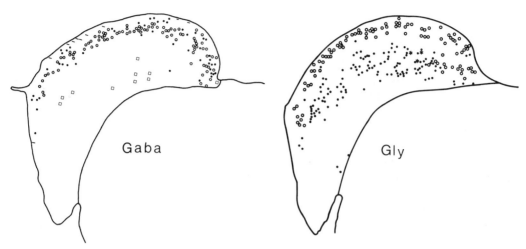

FIG. 3. Distribution of GABA and gly-immunoreactive cell bodies in the guinea pig DCN. *Open circles* indicate cell bodies with average diameters of 16 μm and *solid circles* indicate cells of 9–10 μm. Such labeled cells are found with both antibodies. *Bars* show small flattened GABA-immunoreactive cell bodies, while *squares* and *asterisks* show other GABA- or gly-immunoreactive cells, respectively, which do not fit into the above categories. (From refs. 107, 113, with permission.)

We still know very little about the origins of the GABA-immunoreactive terminals found throughout the cochlear nucleus. Studies cutting the auditory nerve show that GABA (80) and GAD (111) levels in the cochlear nucleus do not change, nor does release of endogenous GABA (103), suggesting that the auditory nerve is not a major source of GABA in the cochlear nucleus. Descending inputs to the cochlear nucleus account for some of the GABA, but it is not clear how much. Lesions of the trapezoid body do not change GAD levels in the cochlear nucleus (27), while lesions of the dorsal acoustic stria lead to small changes in GAD in the cochlear nucleus (23). Uptake and release of GABA do not change in the anteroventral cochlear nucleus (AVCN), and only about 30% changes in the DCN and posteroventral cochlear nucleus (PVCN) after lesioning all descending inputs to the cochlear nucleus (80). However, Godfrey et al. (36) report that GABA levels are reduced to about half in the rostral AVCN following cutting all descending inputs to the cochlear nucleus in the cat. Adams and Mugnaini (4) suggest that some

periolivary neurons may send GABA-containing inputs to the AVCN. A study by Ostapoff (72) using retrograde transport of ^{3}H-GABA to measure uptake and retrograde transport in GABAergic neurons suggests that cells in the superior olivary complex (SOC) are a source of GABAergic terminals in the cochlear nucleus. Destruction of the inferior colliculus (IC) does not significantly reduce the release of GABA from cochlear nucleus slices (15). Since GABA- and GAD-immunoreactive cell bodies are sparse in the VCN, the DCN is the other major source of GABA input to the VCN. Mugnaini (62) indicates that the GAD-immunoreactive cells in the superficial DCN send projections only locally and not to the VCN. GABA cells in the deep DCN probably project to the VCN, but their small number, at least in some species, suggests that these could not be major contributors to the GABA in the VCN. The available data do not appear to fully account for GABA in the VCN. Therefore, it remains possible that not all descending inputs were severed in some of the lesion studies and that some of the GABA-containing cells in the superficial DCN project to the VCN. These are questions that can be studied using combined immunocytochemistry and retrograde transport. It cannot be ruled out that additional neurons within the cochlear nucleus give rise to GABA-containing processes but do not contain detectable GABA or GAD in their cell bodies.

The distribution of the $GABA_A$ receptor was studied in the cochlear nucleus of the guinea pig using monoclonal antibodies (49). Labeling was sparse in VCN, but intense in the DCN, especially in the superficial layer. Intense cell body labeling was seen, and, at the ultrastructural level, pre- and postsynaptic labeling was present.

Glycine

Studies on the analysis of gly distribution, gly uptake and release, and the effects of iontophoretically applied gly agonists and antagonists suggested that gly is a major inhibitory neurotransmitter in the cochlear nucleus (21,92,93,110,115). Two immunocytochemical approaches are now available to address questions concerning the specific localization of gly and glycinergic synapses in the cochlear nucleus. The first is the direct localization of gly using antibodies against conjugates of gly. The second is the localization of the gly postsynaptic receptor. This receptor complex was purified in 1985 and several monoclonal antibodies that recognize the various subunits are available (77,78).

Using antibodies against gly conjugated to BSA with glutaraldehyde, gly-containing neuronal cell bodies and other structures have been localized immunocytochemically in the cochlear nucleus of the guinea pig (76,107) and the rat (13). Punctate labeling is present throughout the cochlear nucleus. In the VCN such labeling is often found outlining unlabeled cell bodies (Fig. 1B). Gly-immunoreactive cell bodies are most abundant in the DCN where two classes of cells are present (Fig. 3) (107). The larger

neurons, with cell soma diameters of 16 μm, are abundant in the superficial layers, while the smaller neurons, with cell soma diameters of 10 μm, are found in the deeper layers (107). As discussed below, gly-immunoreactive cells in the superficial layer are similar to a population of GABA-immunoreactive cells. Based on size and distribution, these appear to be cartwheel cells. In the VCN numerous gly-immunoreactive cell bodies are present, in contrast to patterns seen with anti-GABA antibodies where few immunoreactive cells are seen. Large gly-immunoreactive neurons are found throughout the VCN but are most abundant near the eighth nerve root. A second class of gly-immunoreactive cells, consisting of small spherical cells, is most abundant in the granule cell cap of the AVCN.

Gly receptor immunoreactivity has been studied in the cochlear nucleus at the light and electron microscopic levels (8,112). With fluorescence microscopy immunoreactivity appeared as puncta, and, like that seen with anti-gly antibodies, this labeling was seen around cell bodies in the VCN. A similar pattern of labeling is obtained using horseradish peroxidase (HRP)-conjugated secondary antibody (Fig. 4). Gly receptor-immunoreactive cell bodies were not present. At the ultrastructural level, immunoreactivity is concentrated at postsynaptic sites on dendrites and cell bodies (Fig. 2B). All large cell types in the VCN contain gly receptor immunoreactivity on their cell bodies or proximal dendrites (112). Analysis of presynaptic terminal types in the VCN shows gly receptor immunoreactivity is postsynaptic to terminals containing flattened synaptic vesicles as well as those containing oval/pleomorphic synaptic vesicles.

The origins of gly-immunoreactive terminals in the cochlear nucleus are not completely known. Many may arise from immunoreactive cell bodies within the cochlear nucleus; the greatest concentration of gly-immunoreactive cell bodies is in the

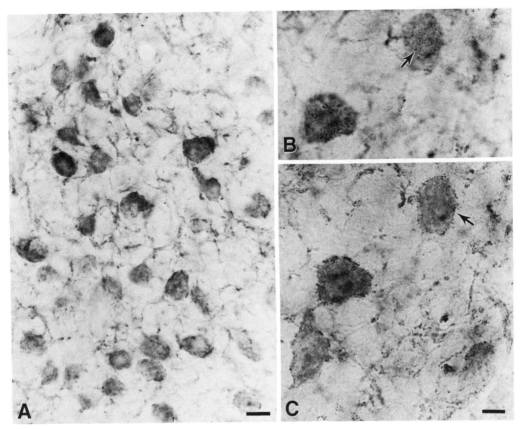

FIG. 4. A: Gly receptor immunoreactivity in the guinea pig VCN localized with a horseradish peroxidase labeled second antibody. Punctate labeling (*arrows*) associated with dendrites and cell bodies is apparent using different levels of focus (**B** and **C**). Bars = 14 μm (A) and 8 μm (B,C).

DCN, and it appears that at least some of the small gly-immunoreactive cells in the deep DCN project to the AVCN (6). Other small cells in the superficial DCN and the VCN are also characteristic of intrinsic neurons. Lesioning descending inputs to the cochlear nucleus in the guinea pig leads to a significant decrease in the release of accumulated ^{14}C-gly from slices of the DCN and PVCN, while auditory nerve lesioning does not change the release of gly from cochlear nucleus slices (92,93). Gly levels in the cochlear nucleus of the cat do not change significantly when descending pathways are cut (36). One glycinergic input to the cochlear nucleus appears to originate in the contralateral cochlear nucleus. Com-

bined retrograde HRP analysis and immunocytochemistry indicate that the large gly-immunoreactive neurons in the VCN, which are most abundant in the auditory nerve root, project to the contralateral cochlear nucleus (104). These cells, which were studied in the guinea pig, may be similar to the giant cells described in the cat, which have been shown to project to the contralateral cochlear nucleus (19). Gly-immunoreactive neurons are present in the ventral nucleus of the trapezoid body (VNTB) (104), and neurons in this nucleus are reported to project to the cochlear nuclei in the cat (91). In the guinea pig, after injection of HRP into the cochlear nuclei, gly-immunoreactive cells in the VNTB are also labeled with HRP (Fig. 5), suggesting that these cells may also be a source of glycinergic input to the cochlear nucleus.

Relationship Between Glycine and GABA in the Cochlear Nucleus

As noted above, a population of neurons in the superficial DCN of the guinea pig, tentatively identified as cartwheel cells, appeared to be immunoreactive for both GABA and gly. These immunoreactive cells also have a similar distribution in the DCN (Fig. 3). Double-labeling studies using primary antibodies made in different species and fluorescent second antibodies were done to confirm that both immunoreactivities are present within the same neuron (Fig. 6) (113). These studies also show punctate colabeling, suggesting these neurotransmitters are colocalized in presynaptic terminals. However, not all neuronal cell bodies or puncta in the DCN contain both immunoreactivities; some neurons contain GABA immunoreactivity only or gly immunoreactivity only, which suggests that these results are not simply due to antibody cross-reactivity. It remains possible that these results are due to a cross-reaction of the gly antibody with a molecule

that is present in only a subpopulation of GABAergic neurons. The colocalization of GABA and gly has also been reported for subpopulations of neurons in the cerebellum and spinal cord (75) and has recently been described in the cochlear nucleus of the cat (71).

The unexpected finding of the colocalization of GABA and gly immunoreactivities raises questions about the functions of these two putative neurotransmitters. The most basic question, whether or not both GABA and gly are released from the same terminal in the cochlear nucleus, is technically very difficult to address. The localization of receptors for these amino acids on or postsynaptic to these terminals can provide insight into their functions. Postsynaptically, there may be both receptors, one receptor with which both neurotransmitters interact or one receptor with which only one neurotransmitter interacts. Presynaptic receptors may also exist and regulate the release of one or both neurotransmitters. Preliminary studies have addressed the relationship between presynaptic GABA immunoreactivity and postsynaptic gly receptor immunoreactivity (67). Several combinations of labeling are seen, but there is a population of synapses with presynaptic terminals containing GABA or GAD im-

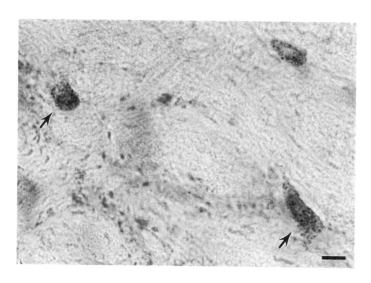

FIG. 5. Double labeled neurons (*arrows*) in the ventral nucleus of the trapezoid body of the guinea pig. Horseradish peroxidase was injected into the contralateral cochlear nucleus, and after retrograde transport, tissue was processed for gly immunocytochemistry. Retrogradely transported horseradish peroxidase appears as granules, while gly immunoreactivity shows a diffuse reaction product.

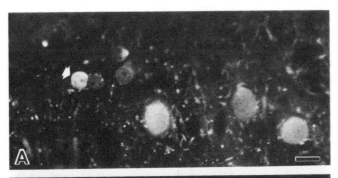

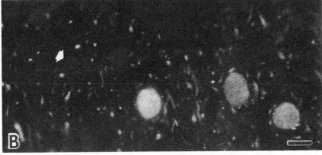

FIG. 6. Colocalization of GABA (**A**) and gly (**B**) immunoreactivities in the guinea pig DCN. *Arrowhead* shows a small cell that is GABA immunoreactive but not gly immunoreactive. Bars = 15 μm. (From ref. 107, with permission.)

munoreactivity and with postsynaptic gly receptor immunoreactivity. In the spinal cord, similar results were reported in which all GAD-positive presynaptic terminals were associated with postsynaptic gly receptor immunoreactivity (99). In the cochlear nucleus, only a subpopulation of GABA- or GAD-immunoreactive presynaptic terminals appears to have postsynaptic gly receptor immunoreactivity. These studies must be extended to include gly and GABA receptor localization. Since immunocytochemical and ligand-binding studies suggest that GABA_A receptors are not abundant in the VCN, gly may be the predominant neurotransmitter in the VCN terminals where both GABA and gly are contained.

Excitatory Amino Acid Neurotransmitters in the Cochlear Nucleus

There is compelling evidence that EAAs are major neurotransmitters throughout the mammalian central nervous system. While the group of EAA neurotransmitters includes glu and asp, as well as small peptides, and possibly additional small molecules, glu is usually considered the most likely neurotransmitter candidate, but the data supporting this are not compelling. Different EAAs may be active at different synapses, and the combined action of two or more EAAs at a single synapse cannot be ruled out.

Evidence supporting an EAA as an auditory nerve neurotransmitter includes (a) a high concentration of glu and asp in auditory nerve terminals, (b) enrichment of glutaminase and asp aminotransferase in spiral ganglion cell bodies and auditory nerve terminals, (c) release of endogenous and exogenous glu and asp from auditory nerve terminals, (d) retrograde transport of D-asp in the auditory nerve, and (e) pharmacological demonstration of EAA receptors at auditory nerve synapses in the cochlear nucleus (21,48,57,103,105,110). A quisqualate or kainate subtype of an EAA receptor is probably used at the auditory nerve synapse (47,66), although *N*-methyl-D-aspartate (NMDA) receptors may also be involved (57).

Cochlear nucleus granule cells also may use an EAA neurotransmitter. The evidence for this is the uptake and retrograde transport of D-asp (69) as well as the high concentration of glutaminase in granule cell bodies (10). There is also indirect support for an EAA being the neurotransmitter of cochlear nucleus granule cells. These cells are anatomically similar to cerebellar granule cells (56,63) for which there are several lines of evidence that they release an EAA (86).

Several studies using antibodies against conjugates of glu and asp and gamma-L-glutamyl-L-glutamate have reported immunoreactive neurons in the cochlear nucleus or spiral ganglion (12,43,53), but identification of immunoreactive neurons in the cochlear nucleus has not been done. Receptors for EAAs have also been reported in the cochlear nucleus using autoradiographic localization (37,39,58).

Other Cochlear Nucleus Neurotransmitters

Survey analyses have shown that most putative neurotransmitters are present in the cochlear nucleus, but detailed studies have not been done in most cases. Considerable information is available on ACh, including the distribution of acetylcholinesterase (70) and origins of cholinergic inputs based on lesion studies (33). Recent lesion studies have provided information concerning the origin of cholinergic fibers in the cochlear nucleus. Most originate outside the nucleus since cutting all descending inputs reduces cholinergic enzyme activities in the cochlear nucleus almost entirely. In the rat the olivocochlear bundle contributes only a minor part of the cholinergic enzymes in the cochlear nucleus (34,35), but a larger part in the cat, suggesting a possible species relationship. In the rat most cholinergic fibers originate from the vicinity of the SOC and enter the cochlear nucleus from the trapezoid body (35).

Catecholamines and serotonin are present in the cochlear nucleus. Based on dopamine-beta-hydroxylase immunocytochemical localization (59,96) and the Falck-Hillarp histochemical method for catecholamine localization (51,52), catecholamines are found throughout the cochlear nucleus. Lesion studies indicate that catecholamine-containing fibers originate in the locus coeruleus (52,53). Fluorescence studies also suggest that serotonin is present in the cochlear nucleus and some neurons in the cochlear nucleus are excited by local application of serotonin (29,114).

Several neuroactive peptides, including enkephalin, neurotensin, substance P, somatostatin, cholecystokinin, and neuropeptide Y, are found in the cochlear nucleus. Several groups have reported enkephalin-immunoreactive cell bodies in the cochlear nucleus (3,7,101), and preproenkephalin mRNA is also present in some neuronal cell bodies in the cochlear nucleus (40). Cholecystokinin-immunoreactive cell bodies are also present in the cochlear nucleus (3) and are found in the VCN within and caudal to the eighth nerve bifurcation. In some cases these peptides may coexist with other neurotransmitters (6); glycinergic cells in the deep layers of the DCN appear to also stain for enkephalin and neuropeptide Y. Somatostatin immunoreactivity is present throughout the cochlear nucleus with positive neuronal cell bodies found in the VCN. Binding sites for somatostatin are reported to be high in the VCN (24). Binding sites for calcitonin gene-related peptide have been localized in the DCN by autoradiography (89).

Relationship Between Neurotransmitter and Synaptic Terminals in the Anteroventral Cochlear Nucleus

The morphology of synaptic terminals in the AVCN has been characterized in the cat (17,18,20,38) and guinea pig (38,68,87). Four types of terminals are reported. The most abundant are the primary afferent terminals, the end-bulbs of Held, which contain large, round synaptic vesicles and make multiple asymmetric contacts. The second terminal type contains oval/pleomorphic synaptic vesicles and makes symmetric contacts on cell bodies and dendrites. The third type contains flattened synaptic vesicles and also makes symmetric synaptic contacts. Finally, there is a small number of terminals that contain small, round synaptic vesicles and asymmetric synaptic contacts. These populations of terminals appear to originate from different populations of neurons, and the data indicate that they contain different neurotransmitters. Available data suggest that EAAs are present in primary afferent terminals, gly is present in terminals with flattened synaptic vesicles, and ACh is present in terminals with small, round synaptic vesicles. However, terminals with oval/pleomorphic synaptic vesicles are associated with at least two major neurotransmitters, GABA and gly. As discussed above, this may be related to the colocalization of these neurotransmitters. Since there are only four morphologically defined terminal types and many more neurotransmitters in the AVCN, it can be expected that other neurotransmitters, which may be classified as minor neurotransmitters, will also be found in these terminals, either alone or coexisting with other neurotransmitters.

SUPERIOR OLIVARY COMPLEX

The remaining auditory nuclei of the brainstem are not as thoroughly characterized with respect to their neurotransmitters as is the cochlear nucleus. GAD values are moderate and rather uniform throughout the lateral superior olive (LSO), medial nucleus of the trapezoid body (MNTB), medial superior olivary nucleus (MSO), and the VNTB (110). Immunocytochemical analyses have been done for GABA or GAD in the SOC of the rat, guinea pig, cat,

and gerbil. GAD-positive cell bodies are found throughout the LSO in the rat (60), cat (5), and gerbil (83), and GABA-positive cell bodies are reported in the guinea pig (41,76,98) and cat LSO (5,85). The distributions and sizes of immunoreactive cells appear similar in all cases and suggest that similar populations of cells are labeled in the three species. The identifications of these cell types and their projections remain to be determined. A possible projection is to the cochlea, since a population of efferents contains GABA and GAD and some efferents originate in the LSO.

GAD-positive cell bodies are not found in the MSO of the rat and gerbil, but a few GABA-immunoreactive cells are reported in the MSO of the guinea pig (41,76,98). Terminal labeling, reported to be heavy in the gerbil (83) and cat (5), is found in the MSO. Neither GAD- nor GABA-immunoreactive cell bodies are found in the MNTB in the species studied, but in all cases heavy terminal labeling is reported. The VNTB and lateral nuclei of the trapezoid body (LNTB) contain the most intensely immunoreactive neurons in the SOC labeled with either antibodies against GAD or GABA (41,98). Heavy terminal labeling is also reported.

The neurotransmitter role of gly in the SOC has received considerable attention. Moore and Caspary (61) were first to suggest that the pathway originating in the MNTB and terminating in the ipsilateral LSO was glycinergic, based on pharmacological studies in the chinchilla. This is supported by the high levels of ^{3}H-strychnine binding to the LSO demonstrated autoradiographically (31,116) and intense gly receptor immunoreactivity in the LSO (8). Several studies using antibodies against gly have demonstrated intense immunoreactivity in the MNTB (5,13,16,45,76,81,107) (Fig. 7); in fact, these neurons are the most intensely staining gly-immunoreactive neurons found in the brainstem.

Gly-immunoreactive cell bodies are also abundant in the LSO (107). In the cat these

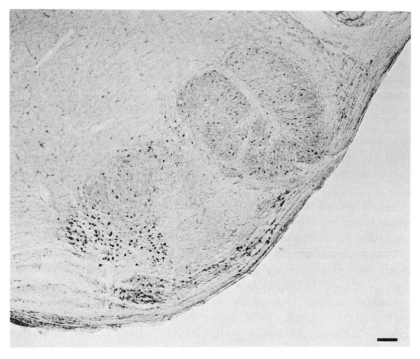

FIG. 7. Gly immunoreactive labeling in the guinea pig SOC. Heavy labeling of cell bodies is apparent in the MNTB, while heavy punctate labeling is seen in the LSO. Bar = 150 μm. (From ref. 107, with permission.)

neurons have been shown to project to the ipsilateral IC using retrogradely transported HRP and immunocytochemistry (85). ³H-gly injected into the IC is retrogradely transported to the contralateral LSO adding additional support that gly is the neurotransmitter of this pathway (46). The crossed projection from the LSO to the IC does not appear to be glycinergic. Since this pathway is not GABAergic, it has been suggested that this crossed pathway from the LSO to the IC uses an excitatory neurotransmitter (85).

Gly-immunoreactive neurons are also present in the VNTB and LNTB (5,76,107). Some of these neurons may project to the cochlear nuclei as discussed above.

Cholinergic neurons have been studied in the SOC by measuring ChAT enzymatic activity and with acetylcholinesterase histochemistry and ChAT immunocytochemistry. ChAT activity is moderate in the SOC with highest levels in the LSO (111). Acetylcholinesterase-containing cells have been described in the rat, mouse, chinchilla, and cat (70). ChAT immunoreactivity is present in the cells of origin of the medial and lateral cochlear efferent system (9,25). Some of these cells also contain enkephalin immunoreactivity.

OTHER NUCLEI

GAD immunoreactivity has been studied in the lateral lemniscus by Adams and Mugnaini (1) in the cat and by Moore and Moore (60) in the rat. Intense cell body and terminal labeling is found in the dorsal nucleus of the lateral lemniscus, and these neurons may represent one source of GABAergic input to the IC. It is reported that nearly all neurons in the dorsal nucleus of the lateral lemniscus may be GAD immunoreactive in the cat (1), rat (64), and gerbil (83), while another study on the rat using the same anti-GAD antibody (60) shows only a fraction of neurons in this nucleus being GAD immunoreactive.

Very high GAD levels are reported in the IC of the rat, cat, and guinea pig (27). Analyzing subdivisions of the IC of the cat showed that the GAD levels varied more than threefold with the highest enzyme activity in the dorsal medial and dorsal lateral central subdivisions (6). Lesions of the auditory cortex and dorsal and intermediate acoustic stria did not change the GAD activity in the IC. Subsequent immunocytochemical studies have supported the earlier biochemical results showing high levels of GAD and GABA immunoreactivities in the IC. Heavy cell body and terminal labeling is present throughout the IC (60,64,83).

Gly has a very distinct distribution in the IC of the cat with concentrations varying more than fivefold (6). Highest levels are in the ventral and ventral medial central subdivisions. Immunocytochemical analyses with anti-gly antibodies show immunoreactivity confined to terminals and fibers in the rat (13) and guinea pig (76) IC, but a thorough analysis has not yet been done.

CONCLUSION

As is apparent from this review, much information is available concerning the distributions of neurotransmitters in the auditory system. This progress is largely due to immunocytochemistry. With the increased research being done in this area and the fact that antibodies to neurotransmitters and their receptors are becoming readily available, it is certain that the distribution of most neurotransmitters will soon be known for auditory system pathways. Such information will provide an important basis for future studies addressing the function of neurotransmitters in the auditory system. Questions such as those concerning the functional role of coexisting neurotrans-

mitters in the cochlear nucleus, factors regulating the expression of postsynaptic receptors, and the roles of various neurotransmitters in processing information in the central auditory system will be addressed. Areas that appear to be only remotely related to neurotransmission, for example, questions addressing development, degeneration, and plasticity in the auditory system, will also encompass neurotransmitters and receptors in several ways. There are suggestions from other systems that neurotransmitters can act as neurotrophic factors and that functioning receptors are necessary for proper synapse development during development. Furthermore, neurotransmitters may be excellent markers for detecting changes in a particular population of neurons. Localization of neurotransmitters and their receptors will be central to these questions and others, but quantitative analyses will likely be necessary to assess responses in most cases. In this regard, quantitative immunocytochemistry provides a technique that allows the measurement of antigens in specific neurons in a system as complex as the central auditory system. Other techniques, such as *in situ* localization of mRNA, will be useful in further characterizing neurotransmitters and receptors in the auditory system.

REFERENCES

1. Adams JC, Mugnaini E. Dorsal nucleus of the lateral lemniscus: a nucleus of GABAergic projection neurons. *Brain Res Bull* 1984;13:585–590.
2. Adams JC, Mugnaini E. GAD-like immunoreactivity in the ventral cochlear nucleus. *Neurosci Abst* 1984;10:393.
3. Adams JC, Mugnaini E. Patterns of immunostaining with antisera to peptides in the auditory brainstem of cat. *Neurosci Abst* 1985;11:32.
4. Adams JC, Mugnaini E. Patterns of glutamate decarboxylase immunostaining in the feline cochlear nucleus complex studied with silver enhancement and electron microscopy. *J Comp Neurol* 1987;262:375–401.
5. Adams JC, Mugnaini E. Immunocytochemical evidence for inhibitory and disinhibitory cir-

cuits in the superior olive. *Hear Res* 1990;49: 281–298.

6. Adams JC, Wenthold RJ. Immunostaining of GABA-ergic and glycinergic inputs to the anteroventral cochlear nucleus. *Neurosci Abst* 1987;13:1259.

7. Altschuler RA. Met-enkephalin positivity in the small cells of the deep dorsal cochlear nucleus and posteroventral cochlear nucleus of the rat. *Neurosci Abst* 1979;5:15.

8. Altschuler RA, Betz H, Parakkal MH, Reeks KA, Wenthold RJ. Identification of glycinergic synapses in the cochlear nucleus through immunocytochemical localization of the postsynaptic receptor. *Brain Res* 1986;369:316–320.

9. Altschuler RA, Fex J, Parakkal MH, Eckenstein F. Colocalization of enkephalin-like and choline acetyltransferase-like immunoreactivities in olivocochlear neurons of the guinea pig. *J Histochem Cytochem* 1984;32:839–843.

10. Altschuler RA, Wenthold RJ, Schwartz AM, et al. Immunocytochemical localization of glutaminase-like immunoreactivity in the auditory nerve. *Brain Res* 1984;29:173–178.

11. Aoki C, Joh TH, Pickel VM. Ultrastructural localization of beta-adrenergic receptor-like immunoreactivity in the cortex and neostriatum of rat brain. *Brain Res* 1987;437:264–282.

12. Aoki E, Semba R, Kato K, Kashiwamata S. Purification of specific antibody against aspartate and immunocytochemical localization of aspartergic neurons in the rat brain. *Neuroscience* 1987;21:755–765.

13. Aoki E, Semba R, Keino H, Kao K, Kashiwamata S. Glycinelike immunoreactivity in the rat auditory pathway. *Brain Res* 1988;442:63–71.

14. Barber RP, Saito K. Light microscopic visualization of GAD and GABA-T in immunocytochemical preparations of rodent CNS. In: Roberts E, Chase TN, Tower DB, eds. *GABA in nervous system function*. New York: Raven Press, 1976;113–132.

15. Bergman M, Staatz-Benson C, Potashner SJ. Amino acid uptake and release in the cochlear nucleus after inferior colliculus ablation. *Hear Res* 1989;42:283–291.

16. Bledsoe SC, Snead CR, Helfert RH, Prasad V, Wenthold RJ, Altschuler RA. Immunocytochemical and lesion studies support the hypothesis that the projection from the medial nucleus of the trapezoid body to the lateral superior olive is glycinergic. *Brain Res* 1990;517: 189–194.

17. Brawer JR, Morest DK. Relations between auditory nerve endings and cell types in the cat's anteroventral cochlear nucleus seen with the Golgi method and Nomarski optics. *J Comp Neurol* 1975;160:491–506.

18. Cant NB. The fine structure of two types of stellate cells in the anterior division of the anteroventral cochlear nucleus of the cat. *Neuroscience* 1981;6:2643–2655.

19. Cant NB, Gatson KC. Pathways connecting the right and left cochlear nuclei. *J Comp Neurol* 1982;212:313–326.

20. Cant NB, Morest DK. The structural basis for

stimulus coding in the cochlear nucleus of the cat. In: Berlin C, ed. *Hearing science: recent advances*. San Diego: College-Hill Press, 1984;371–421.

21. Caspary DH, Rybak LP, Faingold CL. The effects of inhibitory and excitatory neurotransmitters on the response properties of brainstem auditory neurons. In: Drescher DG, ed. *Auditory biochemistry*. Springfield, IL: Charles C Thomas, 1985;198–226.

22. Chagnaud JL, Mons N, Tuffet S, Grandier-Vazeilles X, Geffard M. Monoclonal antibodies against glutaraldehyde-conjugated dopamine. *J Neurochem* 1987;49:487–494.

23. Davies WE. GABAergic innervation of the mammalian cochlear nucleus. *Inner Ear Biol* 1977;68:155–164.

24. Epelbaum J, Dussaillant M, Enjalberg A, Kordon C, Rostene W. Autoradiographic localization of a non-reducible somatostatin analog (125I-CGP 23996) binding sites in the rat brain: comparison with membrane binding. *Peptides* 1985;6:713–719.

25. Fex J, Altschuler RA. Neurotransmitter-related immunocytochemistry of the organ of Corti. *Hear Res* 1986;22:249–263.

26. Fex J, Wenthold RJ. Choline acetyltransferase, glutamate decarboxylase and tyrosine hydroxylase in the cochlea and cochlear nucleus of the guinea pig. *Brain Res* 1976;109:575–585.

27. Fisher SK, Davies WE. GABA and its related enzymes in the lower auditory system of the guinea pig. *J Neurochem* 1976;27:1145–1155.

28. Frostholm A, Rotter A. Autoradiographic localization of receptors in the cochlear nucleus of the mouse. *Brain Res Bull* 1986;16:189-203.

29. Fuxe K. Evidence for the existence of monoamine neurons in the central nervous system. IV. Distribution of monoamine terminals in the central nervous system. *Acta Physiol Scand* 1965;64(suppl 247):39–85.

30. Geffard M, McRae-Degueurce A, Souan ML. Immunocytochemical detection of acetylcholine in the rat central nervous system. *Science* 1985;229:77–79.

31. Glendenning KK, Baker BN. Neuroanatomical distribution of receptors for three potential inhibitory neurotransmitters in the brainstem auditory nuclei of the cat. *J Comp Neurol* 1988; 275:288–308.

32. Godfrey DA, Carter JA, Berger SJ, Lowry DH, Matschinsky FM. Quantitative histochemical mapping of candidate transmitter amino acids in the cat cochlear nucleus. *J Histochem Cytochem* 1977;25:417–431.

33. Godfrey DA, Park JL, Dunn JD, Ross CD. Cholinergic neurotransmissions in the cochlear nucleus. In: Drescher DG, ed. *Auditory biochemistry*. Springfield, IL: Charles C Thomas, 1985;163–183.

34. Godfrey DA, Park-Hellendall JL, Dunn JD, Ross CD. Effect of olivocochlear bundle transection on choline acetyltransferase activity in the rat cochlear nucleus. *Hear Res* 1987;28: 237–251.

35. Godfrey DA, Park-Hellendall JL, Dunn JD,

Ross CD. Effects of trapezoid body and superior olive lesions on choline acetyltransferase activity in the rat cochlear nucleus. *Hear Res* 1987;28:253–270.

36. Godfrey DA, Parli JA, Biavati MJ, Dunn JD, Ross CD. Effects of surgical lesions upon amino acid concentrations in cat cochlear nucleus. *Neurosci Abst* 1988;13:545.

37. Greenamyre JT, Young AB, Penney JB. Quantitative autoradiographic distribution of L-(^{3}H) glutamate-binding sites in rat central nervous system. *J Neurosci* 1984;4:2133–2144.

38. Gulley RL. Changes in the presynaptic membrane of the synapses of the anteroventral nucleus with different levels of acoustic stimulation. *Brain Res* 1978;146:373–379.

39. Halpain S, Wieczorek CM, Rainbow TC. Localization of L-glutamate receptors in rat brain by quantitative autoradiography. *J Neurosci* 1984;4:2247–2258.

40. Harlan RE, Shivers BD, Romano GJ, Howells RD, Pfaff DW. Localization of preproenkephalin mRNA in the rat brain and spinal cord by in situ hybridization. *J Comp Neurol* 1987; 258:159–184.

41. Helfert RH, Bonneau JM, Wenthold RJ, Altschuler RA. GABA and glycine immunoreactivity in the guinea pig superior olivary complex. *Brain Res* 1989;501:269–286.

42. Hepler JR, Toomim CS, McCarthy KD, et al. Characterization of antisera to glutamate and aspartate. *J Histochem Cytochem* 1988:36:13–22.

43. Herkenham M, McLean S. Mismatches between receptor and transmitter localizations in the brain. In: Boast CA, Snowhill WE, Alter CA, eds. *Quantitative receptor autoradiography*. New York: Alan R Liss, 1986;137–171.

44. Hökfelt T, Johansson O, Goldstein M. Central catecholamine neurons as revealed by immunohistochemistry with special reference to adrenaline neurons. In: Björklund, Hökfelt T, eds. *Handbook of chemical neuroanatomy. Volume 2. Classical transmitters in the CNS.* Amsterdam: Elsevier, 1984;157–276.

45. Hunter C, Chung E, Pasik P, Van Woert MH. Glycinergic pathways in the auditory system of the rat. *Neurosci Abst* 1987;13:544.

46. Hutson KA, Glendenning KK, Masterton RB. Biochemical basis for the acoustic chiasm. *Neurosci Abst.* 1987;13:548.

47. Jackson H, Nemeth EF, Parks TN. Non-N-methyl-D-aspartate receptors mediating synaptic transmission in the avian cochlear nucleus: effects of kynurenic acid, dipicolinic acid and streptomycin. *Neuroscience* 1985;16: 171–179.

48. Jarlstedt J, Karlsson B, Hamberger A. In vivo studies on amino acid transmitters in the central auditory system of the guinea pig. *Otolaryngol Head Neck Surg* 1985;93:27–30.

49. Juiz JM, Helfert RH, Wenthold RJ, De Blas AL, Altschuler RA. Immunocytochemical localization of the GABA$_A$/benzodiazepine receptor in the guinea pig cochlear nucleus: evidence for receptor localization heterogeneity. *Brain Res* 1989;504:173–179.

50. Kimura H, McGeer PL, Peng JH. Choline acetyltransferase containing neurons in rat brain. In: Björklund A, Hökfelt T, Kuhar MJ, eds. *Handbook of chemical neuroanatomy. Volume 3. Classical transmitters and transmitter receptors in the CNS.* Amsterdam: Elsevier, 1984; 51–67.

51. Kromer LF, Moore RY. Cochlear nucleus innervation by central norepinephrine neurons in the rat. *Brain Res* 1976;118:531–537.

52. Kromer LF, Moore RY. Norepinephrine innervation of the cochlear nuclei by locus coeruleus neurons in the rat. *Anat Embryol (Berl)* 1980;158:227–244.

53. Levitt P, Moore RY. Organization of brainstem noradrenaline hyperinnervation following neonatal 6-hydroxydopamine treatment in rat. *Anat Embryol (Berl)* 1980;158:133–150.

54. Luetje CW, Brumwell C, Norman MG, Peterson GL, Schimerlik MI, Nathanson NM. Isolation and characterization of monoclonal antibodies specific for the cardiac muscarinic acetylcholine receptor. *Biochemistry* 1987;26: 6892–6896.

55. Madl JE, Larson AA, Beitz AJ. Monoclonal antibody specific for carbodiimide-fixed glutamate: immunocytochemical localization in the rat CNS. *J Histochem Cytochem* 1986;34:317–326.

56. Martin MR. Morphology of the cochlear nucleus in the normal and reeler mutant mouse. *J Comp Neurol* 1981;197:141–152.

57. Martin MR. The pharmacology of amino acid receptors and synaptic transmission in the cochlear nucleus. In: Drescher DG, ed. *Auditory biochemistry*. Springfield, IL: Charles C Thomas, 1983;184–197.

58. Monaghan DT, Cotman CW. Distribution of N-methyl-D-aspartate-sensitive L-^{3}H-glutamate-binding sites in rat brain. *J Neurosci* 1985;5: 2909–2919.

59. Moore JK. Cholinergic, GABAergic and noradrenergic input to cochlear granule cells in the guinea pig and monkey. *Neurosci Abst* 1988;13:545.

60. Moore JK, Moore RY. Glutamic acid decarboxylase-like immunoreactivity in brainstem auditory neuclei of the rat. *J Comp Neurol* 1987;260:157–174.

61. Moore MJ, Caspary DM. Strychnine blocks binaural inhibition in lateral superior olivary neurons. *J Neurosci* 1983;3:237–242.

62. Mugnaini E. GABA neurons in the superficial layers of the rat dorsal cochlear nucleus: light and electron microscopic immunocytochemistry. *J Comp Neurol* 1985;235:61–81.

63. Mugnaini E, Morgan JI. The neuropeptide cerebellin is a marker for two similar neuronal circuits in rat brain. *Proc Natl Acad Sci USA* 1987;84:8692–8696.

64. Mugnaini E, Oertel WH. An atlas of the distribution of GABAergic neurons and terminals in the rat CNS as revealed by GAD immunohistochemistry. In: Björklund A, Hökfelt T, eds.

Handbook of chemical neuroanatomy. Volume 4. GABA and neuropeptides in the CNS. Amsterdam: Elsevier, 1985;436–621.

65. Mugnaini E, Osen KK, Dahl AL, Friedrich VL, Korte G. Fine structure of granule cells and related interneurons (termed Golgi cells) in the cochlear nucleus complex of cat, rat and mouse. *J Neurocytol* 1980;9:537–570.

66. Nemeth EF, Jackson H, Parks TN. Evidence for the involvement of kainate receptors in synaptic transmission in the avian cochlear nucleus. *Neurosci Lett* 1985;59:297–301.

67. Oberdorfer MD, Parakkal MH, Altschuler RA. Colocalization of glycine and GABA in the cochlear nucleus. *Neurosci Abst* 1988;13:544.

68. Oberdorfer MD, Parakkal MH, Altschuler RA, Wenthold RJ. Ultrastructural localization of GABA-immunoreactive terminals in the anteroventral cochlear nucleus of the guinea pig. *Hear Res* 1988;33:229–238.

69. Oliver DL, Potashner SJ, Jones DR, Morest DK. Selective labeling of spiral ganglion and granule cells with D-aspartate in the auditory system of cat and guinea pig. *J Neurosci* 1983;3:455–472.

70. Osen KK, Mugnaini E, Dahl AL, Christiansen AH. Histochemical localizations of acetylcholinesterase in the cochlear nucleus and superior olivary nuclei. A reappraisal with emphasis on the cochlear granule cell systems. *Arch Ital Biol* 1984;122:169–212.

71. Osen KK, Ottersen OP, Storm-Mathisen J. Colocalization of glycine-like and GABA-like immunoreactivities: a semiquantitative study of individual neurons in the dorsal cochlear nucleus of cat. In: Ottersen OP, Storm-Mathiesen J, eds. *Glycine neurotransmission.* New York: Wiley, 1990;417–451.

72. Ostapoff EM, Morest DK, Potashner SJ. Uptake and retrograde transport of [³H]GABA from the cochlear nucleus to the superior olive in guinea pig. *J Chem Neuroanat* 1990;3:285–295.

73. Ottersen OP, Storm-Mathisen J. Neurons containing or accumulating transmitter amino acids. In: Björklund A, Hökfelt T, Kuhar MJ, eds. *Handbook of chemical neuroanatomy. Volume 3. Classical transmitters and transmitter receptors in the CNS,* part II. Amsterdam: Elsevier, 1984;141–246.

74. Ottersen OP, Storm-Mathisen J. Differential neuronal localizations of aspartate-like and glutamate-like immunoreactivities in the hippocampus of rat, guinea pig and senegulese baboon (Papio Papio), with a note on the distribution of γ-aminobutyrate. *Neuroscience* 1985;16:589–606.

75. Ottersen OP, Storm-Mathisen J, Somogyi P. Colocalization of glycine-like and GABA-like immunoreactivities in Golgi cell terminals in the rat cerebellum: a postembedding light and electron microscopic study. *Brain Res* 1988; 450:342–353.

76. Peyret D, Campistron G, Geffard M, Aran JM. Glycine immunoreactivity in the brainstem auditory and vestibular nuclei of the guinea pig. *Acta Otolaryngol (Stockh)* 1987;104:71–76.

77. Pfeiffer F, Graham D, Betz H. Purification by affinity chromatography of the glycine receptor of rat spinal cord. *J Biol Chem* 1982;257:9389–9393.

78. Pfeiffer F, Simler R, Grenningloh G, Betz H. Monoclonal antibodies and peptide mapping reveal structural similarities between the subunits of the glycine receptor of rat spinal cord. *Proc Natl Acad Sci USA* 1984;81:7224–7227.

79. Pickel VM, Joh TH, Reis DJ. A serotonergic innervation of noradrenergic neurons in nucleus locus coeruleus: demonstration by immunohistochemical localization of transmitter specific enzymes tyrosine and tryptophan hydroxylase. *Brain Res* 1977;131:197–214.

80. Potashner SJ, Lindberg N, Morest DK. Uptake and release of gamma-aminobutyric acid in the guinea pig cochlear nucleus after axotomy of cochlear and centrifugal fibers. *J Neurochem* 1985;45:1558–1566.

81. Pourcho RG, Goebel DG. Immunocytochemical demonstration of glycine in retinas. *Brain Res* 1985;348:339–342.

82. Richards JG, Schoch P, Haring P, Takacs B, Mohler H. Resolving GABAₐ/benzodiazepine receptors: cellular and subcellular localization in the CNS with monoclonal antibodies. *J Neurosci* 1987;7:1866–1886.

83. Roberts RC, Ribak CE. GABAergic neurons and axon terminals in the brainstem auditory nuclei of the gerbil. *J Comp Neurol* 1987;258: 267–280.

84. Saint Marie RL, Ostapoff EM, Morest DK. The form and distribution of GABAergic synapses on the principal cell types in the ventral cochlear nucleus of the cat. *Hear Res* 1989;42: 97–112.

85. Saint Marie RL, Ostapoff EM, Morest DK, Wenthold RJ. Glycine-immunoreactive projection of the cat lateral superior olive: possible role in midbrain ear dominance. *J Comp Neurol* 1989;279:382–396.

86. Sandoval ME, Cotman CW. Evaluation of glutamate as a neurotransmitter of cerebellar parallel fibers. *Neuroscience* 1978;3:199–206.

87. Schwartz AM, Gulley RL. Non-primary afferents to the principal cells of the rostral anteroventral cochlear nucleus of the guinea pig. *J Anat* 1978;153:489–508.

88. Schwartz IR, Yu S-M, DiCarlantonic G, Wenthold RJ. A comparison of GABA and glycine immunoreactivity in the gerbil dorsal cochlear nucleus. *Neurosci Abst* 1987;13:544.

89. Sexton PM, McKenzie JS, Mason RT, Moseley JM, Martin TJ, Mendelsohn FA. Localization of binding sites for calcitonin gene-related peptide in rat brain by in vitro autoradiography. *Neuroscience* 1986;19:1235–1245.

90. Shiraishi T, Senba E, Tohyama M, Wu JY, Kubo T, Matsunaga T. Distribution and fine structure of neuronal elements containing glutamate decarboxylase in the rat cochlear nucleus. *Brain Res* 1985;347:183–187.

91. Spangler KM, Cant NB, Henkel CK, Farley GR, Warr WB. Descending projections from the superior olivary complex to the cochlear nucleus of the cat. *J Comp Neurol* 1987;259: 452–465.

92. Staatz-Benson C, Potashner SJ. Uptake and release of glycine in the guinea pig cochlear nucleus. *J Neurochem* 1987;49:128–137.

93. Staatz-Benson C, Potashner SJ. Uptake and release of glycine in the guinea pig cochlear nucleus after axotomy of afferent or centrifugal fiber. *J Neurochem* 1988;51:370–379.

94. Steinbusch HWM. Serotonin-immunoreactive neurons and their projections in the CNS. In: Björklund A, Hökfelt T, Kuhar MJ, eds. *Handbook of chemical neuroanatomy. Volume 3. Classical transmitters and transmitter receptors in the CNS.* Amsterdam: Elsevier, 1984; 68–125.

95. Storm-Mathisen J, Leknes AK, Bore AI, et al. First visualization of glutamate and GABA in neurons by immunocytochemistry. *Nature* 1983; 301:517–520.

96. Swanson LW, Hartman BK. The central adrenergic system. An immunofluorescence study of the locations of cell bodies and their afferent connections in the rat utilizing dopamine-beta-hydroxylase as a marker. *J Comp Neurol* 1975;163:467–506.

97. Swanson LW, Simmons DM, Whiting PJ, Lindstrom J. Immunohistochemical localization of neuronal nicotinic receptors in the rodent central nervous system. *J Neurosci* 1987;7:3334–3342.

98. Thompson GC, Cortez AM, Lam DM. Localization of GABA immunoreactivity in the auditory brainstem of guinea pigs. *Brain Res* 1985;339:119–122.

99. Triller A, Cluzeaud F, Korn H. Gamma-aminobutyric acid containing terminals can be apposed to glycine receptors at central synapses. *J Cell Biol* 1987;104:947–956.

100. Triller A, Cluzeaud F, Pfeiffer F, Betz H, Korn H. Distribution of glycine receptors at central synapses: an immunoelectron microscopy study. *J Cell Biol* 1985;101:683–688.

101. Uhl GR, Goodman RR, Kuhar MJ, Childers SR, Snyder SH. Immunohistochemical mapping of enkephalin containing cell bodies, fibers and nerve terminals in the brain stem of the rat. *Brain Res* 1979;166:75–94.

102. Verhofstad AAJ, Steinbusch HWM, Joosten HWJ, Penke B, Varga J, Goldstein M. Immunocytochemical localization of noradrenalin, adrenalin and serotonin. In: Polak JM, Van Noordon S, eds. *Immunocytochemistry.* Bristol: Wright PSG, 1983;143–168.

103. Wenthold RJ. Release of endogenous glutamic acid, aspartic acid and GABA from cochlear nucleus slices. *Brain Res* 1979;162:338–343.

104. Wenthold RJ. Evidence for a glycinergic pathway connecting the two cochlear nuclei: an immunocytochemical and retrograde transport study. *Brain Res* 1987;415:183–187.

105. Wenthold RJ, Altschuler RA. Immunocytochemistry of aspartate aminotransferase and glutaminase. In: Hertz L, Kvamme E, McGeer EG, Schousboe A, eds. *Glutamine, glutamate and GABA in the central nervous system.* New York: Alan R. Liss, 1983;33–50.

106. Wenthold RJ, Hampson DR, Wada K, Hunter C, Oberdorfer MD, Dechesne CJ. Isolation, localization, and cloning of a kainic acid binding protein from frog brain. *J Histochem Cytochem* 1990;38:1717–1723.

107. Wenthold RJ, Huie D, Altschuler RA, Reeks KA. Glycine immunoreactivity localized in the cochlear nucleus and superior olivary complex. *Neuroscience* 1987;22:897–912.

108. Wenthold RJ, Hunter C. Immunocytochemistry of glycine and glycine receptors in the central auditory system. In: Ottersen OP, Storm-Mathisen J, eds. *Glycine neurotransmission.* New York: Wiley, 1990;391–416.

109. Wenthold RJ, Hunter C, Wada K, Dechesne CJ. Antibodies to a C-terminal peptide of the rat brain glutamate receptor subunit, GluR-A, recognize a subpopulation of AMPA binding sites but not kainate sites. *FEBS Lett* 1990; 276:147–150.

110. Wenthold RJ, Martin MR. Neurotransmitters of the auditory nerve and central auditory system. In: Berlin C, ed. *Hearing science: recent advances.* San Diego: College-Hill Press, 1984; 341–369.

111. Wenthold RJ, Morest DK. Transmitter related enzymes in the guinea pig cochlear nucleus. *Neurosci Abst* 1976;2:28.

112. Wenthold RJ, Parakkal MH, Oberdorfer MD, Altschuler RA. Glycine receptor immunoreactivity in the ventral cochlear nucleus of the guinea pig. *J Comp Neurol* 1988;276:423–435.

113. Wenthold RJ, Zempel JM, Parakkal MH, Reeks KA, Altschuler RA. Immunocytochemical localization of GABA in the cochlear nucleus of the guinea pig. *Brain Res* 1986;380:7–18.

114. Whitfield IC, Comis SD. The role of inhibition in information transfer: the interaction of centrifugal and centripetal stimulation of neurones of the cochlear nucleus. Final Report (Part 2) European Office of Aerospace Research. U.S. Air Force Grant 63-115, 1966.

115. Wu SH, Oertel D. Inhibitory circuitry in the ventral cochlear nucleus is probably mediated by glycine. *J Neurosci* 1986;6:2691–2706.

116. Zarbin MA, Wamsley JK, Kuhar MJ. Glycine receptor: light microscopic autoradiographic localization with tritiated strychnine. *J Neurosci* 1981;1:532–547.

Neurobiology of Hearing: The Central Auditory System, edited by
R. A. Altschuler et al.
Raven Press, Ltd., New York © 1991.

7

Superior Olivary Complex: Functional Neuropharmacology of the Principal Cell Types

Donald M. Caspary and Paul G. Finlayson

*Department of Pharmacology, Southern Illinois University School of Medicine,
Springfield, Illinois 62794-9230*

The goal of this chapter is to present evidence regarding the identity and function of neurotransmitters that subserve important coding mechanisms within specific circuits of the auditory brainstem. Historically, studies associating neurotransmitters to specific superior olivary complex (SOC) cell groups have focused on the cells of descending systems such as the olivocochlear system (which projects bilaterally to both cochlea and cochlear nuclei) and ipsilateral pathways to the cochlear nucleus (CN) (for review, see refs. 55,112; Spangler and Warr, Chapter 2). This chapter presents the functional pharmacology of circuits involving the major ascending projection neurons of the SOC that receive information from both ears through direct and indirect pathways from the respective CN. Animal and human behavioral as well as psychophysical data provide strong support for the involvement of these neurons in circuits that not only code for the localization of sound in space but may also be important in the detection of signals in noise and in speech intelligibility (53,60). Specifically, anatomic, cytochemical, and pharmacologic data on one important binaural circuit are examined. This circuit includes neurons within two major subnuclei of the SOC, the medial nucleus of the trapezoid body (MNTB) and the lateral superior olivary nucleus (LSO).

Neurons of the CN that provide input to the SOC also need to be considered. Neurotransmitters of the medial superior olivary nucleus (MSO), the other major ascending output cell group within the SOC, are considered only briefly.

The seminal question that this chapter begins to address is: What are the neurotransmitters in the SOC that subserve binaural localization? The identity of neurotransmitters related to other cell groups within the SOC is presented only in passing. Functionally, it is important to consider that injury, age-related, and/or environmentally induced changes in transmitter function (e.g., transmitter metabolism, receptor turnover, neuronal loss) can alter normal physiological function, especially in circuits that compare two distinct inputs. Thus any developmental or age-related changes affecting neurotransmission at SOC principal cells could affect not only binaural localization but also the ability to make speech intelligible in a cluttered acoustic environment.

In attempting to establish a substance as a neurotransmitter at a particular synapse, several criteria need to be satisfied (118). These criteria include the presence in the presynaptic terminal of neurotransmitter synthetic enzymes, precursor substances, and the substance (putative neurotransmitter) itself. In addition, one should be able to demonstrate release of the substance from the terminal as well as the presence of a mechanism for inactivation of the substance. Finally, pharmacologic techniques such as iontophoresis can be utilized to establish the additional criteria of mimicry (identity of action) and pharmacologic identity. Even if the accepted criteria are satisfied, they may still provide only strong circumstantial evidence that a particular substance is a neurotransmitter at a specific synaptic site. These factors should be kept in mind when evaluating data supporting a particular substance as a neurotransmitter at any synapse. Evidence for the identity of a particular substance(s) as the neurotransmitter at specific synapses within the SOC is presented in this context.

The LSO is an important binaural structure and has been extensively studied. Principal cells of the LSO project bilaterally to the inferior colliculus (IC) representing a major output of the SOC (2,38,90,100,108). These neurons are exquisitely sensitive to interaural differences in intensity, displaying decreasing discharge rates as the stimulus moves from directly lateral to the ipsilateral ear to directly in front or in back of the subject (10,11,17,41,42,106). A number of excellent studies describes the single cell physiology of the LSO principal cell, and detailed ultrastructural studies have described the distribution and types of synaptic endings of the neurons in this circuit.

Thus because the synaptic morphology, response properties, and projection anatomy of the LSO principal cell are known, this circuit is exceptionally well suited to serve as a model for the study of neuropharmacology in the auditory system.

EXCITATORY AND INHIBITORY PROJECTIONS TO LATERAL SUPERIOR OLIVARY NUCLEUS PRINCIPAL CELLS

Principal cells of the LSO receive a direct excitatory input from spherical bushy cells located in the anterior ventral cochlear nucleus (AVCN) (Fig. 1, shaded area). Spherical bushy cell axons project via the trapezoid body and end as boutons on the proximal and distal dendrites of LSO principal cells (Cant, Chapter 5; 16,20,21,48, 50,51,100,109). These AVCN cells comprise the major ipsilateral projection to the LSO. Neurons in the AVCN have been studied using extracellular recording techniques to classify and categorize response properties (12,14,22,85). Intracellular recordings followed by dye injection have been used to correlate response types with cellular morphology types (22,87,89) (see also ref. 23 for review). In response to ipsilateral tone-burst stimuli at characteristic frequency (CF), spherical bushy neurons display response properties that are similar to those observed when recording from

---

FIG. 1. Anatomy and physiology of the binaural circuit involving the right lateral superior olivary (LSO) nucleus. Each schematic brainstem section highlights a particular key projection neuron from four brainstem auditory nuclei, which is part of the binaural circuit terminating on LSO principal cells. Representative physiological data from each of the highlighted neurons are displayed to the right of the drawing. An example of a temporal response pattern for each neuron is displayed as a poststimulus-time histogram (25–35 dB above CF threshold) on a representative rate-intensity plot at characteristic frequency. The direct inputs to LSO neurons, the spherical bushy cells in anteroventral cochlear nucleus (AVCN), and bushy (principal) cells in the medial nucleus of the trapezoid body both display primary-like temporal response patterns, while the globular bushy cells from the posterior portion of the AVCN display notch-primary-like patterns. LSO principal cells show chopper temporal response patterns. All these neurons display monotonic response patterns. The ear stimulated to evoke the responses displayed is indicated for each panel.

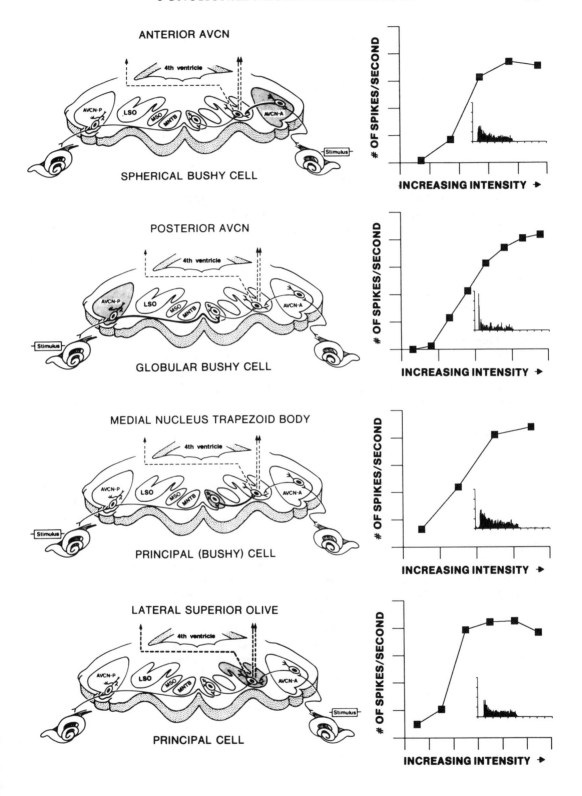

acoustic nerve fibers; monotonic rate-intensity functions and "primary-like" temporal response patterns in poststimulus-time histograms (PSTHs) (12,85,87) (Fig. 1). This excitatory limb of the circuit to the right LSO and the physiology of these neural elements are schematically represented in Fig. 1.

The inhibitory limb of this circuit begins its central projection in the contralateral CN, the CN opposite the LSO being discussed, and consists of two neural elements (Fig. 1). Globular bushy cells located primarily within the caudal AVCN and also within the rostral posterior ventral cochlear nucleus (PVCN) send thick axons into the trapezoid body that terminate as end-bulbs (calyces) of Held onto the principal cells of the MNTB (47,62,76,79,110,111). Unlike the spherical bushy cells, which respond with primary-like temporal response patterns, globular bushy cells are thought to respond with "notch-primary-like" temporal patterns (12,22,39,58,87,89) (Fig. 1).

The second element in the inhibitory limb to the LSO is the MNTB principal or bushy cells. Their projections terminate as boutons containing flattened vesicles on the somata and proximal dendrites of LSO principal cells (Fig. 1) (20,21,37,50,51,99,122). These MNTB principal cells display monotonic rate-intensity functions and primary-like response patterns (44,45,102). Other MNTB neurons receive small nerve terminals from a similar population of contralateral CN neurons (76). The stellate or elongate cells may be responsible for a second temporal response type in the MNTB, the "off" responder (44,45,102). We confine our present discussion to the principal or bushy cells of the MNTB since they appear to comprise the dominant projection onto LSO principal cells (99).

Although the inhibitory contralateral limb of the circuit is longer and has an additional synapse when compared to the ipsilateral pathway, conduction time to the LSO is apparently similar. Transmission time is likely minimized by the large-diameter, fast-conducting axons from the globular bushy cells in the CN to the calyceal endings that encase the postsynaptic MNTB neurons and form multiple synaptic contacts. This would insure quick, reliable transmission across this synapse (62,105; Cant, Chapter 5; Tsuchitani and Johnson, Chapter 8).

Figure 1 describes this circuit, highlighting the inhibitory and excitatory input to the LSO principal cells. Principal cells of the LSO respond to ipsilateral CF toneburst stimuli with phasic "chopper" temporal response patterns in PSTHs (Fig. 1) (103,104). Ipsilaterally evoked neuronal activity generally displays nearly total suppression when like binaural stimuli (similar frequency and intensity in both ears) are presented (Figs. 2 and 8) (11,17,44,45, 105). In Fig. 2, interaural intensity difference was varied by decreasing a contralateral stimulus from 20 dB more intense to 30 dB less intense than an ipsilateral stimulus presented at a constant intensity. This simulates the change in intensity associated with a sound source moving toward the ipsilateral ear. Only the parameter of interaural intensity was varied in this case. The discharge rate of this LSO neuron is nearly totally suppressed by a more intense contralateral stimulus, whereas when the ipsilateral stimulus becomes more intense, the rate approaches the ipsilateral alone condition (Fig. 2). Ipsilaterally evoked inhibition of spontaneous activity has also been observed in the unanesthetized cat (15). Thus these neurons show binaural inhibition and contralateral inhibition of ipsilaterally evoked activity and have been termed EI neurons. It should be noted that both the EI and IE nomenclature has been used to describe this binaural response pattern in the LSO. Although, as illustrated in Fig. 2, these cells are primarily sensitive to differences in interaural intensity, LSO principal cells are also sensitive to interaural time (see also Fig. 8) and interaural phase differences (17,42,73).

An important role for LSO neurons in the

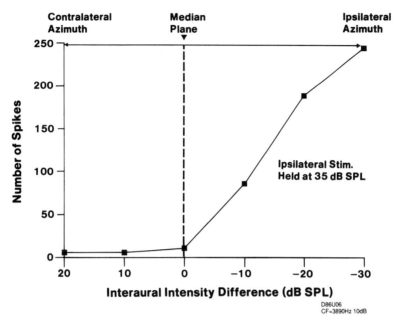

FIG. 2. An interaural intensity function recorded from a lateral superior olivary nucleus principal cell showing the effect of reducing the contralateral (inhibitory) stimulus intensity relative to a fixed ipsilateral (excitatory) stimulus. Note that for equal intensity binaural stimuli (the median plane) these neurons are frequently totally inhibited.

localization of sound in space is suggested by these electrophysiological findings. These findings are supported by behavioral studies in which selective lesioning of midline inputs to the SOC results in major deficits in the ability to localize sound in space (56,69,101).

BRIEF REVIEW OF METHODS

Intracellular and extracellular recordings and iontophoretic data were obtained from chinchilla (*Chinchilla Laniger*) weighing between 300 and 600 g and anesthetized with either or both pentobarbital and ketamine-HCl (see refs. 27,74 for details of surgical and stereotaxic procedures).

Extracellular recording and iontophoretic techniques used in this laboratory have been previously described (24,26,34,49,74). A brief description of the procedures used for extracellular iontophoretic studies in

LSO and MNTB follows. Single-barrel micropipettes were beveled to a 0.5 to 1.0-μm outer diameter and filled with 2.0 M potassium acetate. Five-barrel blanks (H-configuration) were pulled and broken back (5.0–10.0 μm) by drawing the micropipette across a ground glass surface. The single-barrel micropipette was then positioned at an angle of approximately 20° to the five-barrel pipette and glued (cyanoacrylic) with the single-barrel tip protruding 3 to 10 μm (49). The balancing (sum channel) was filled with filtered 4% Sigma Type VI horseradish peroxidase (HRP) in 0.5 M potassium chloride-Tris-HCl, and the remaining barrels were filled with selected putative neurotransmitters, agonists, and/or antagonists (Table 1). For intracellular recording, single-barrel blanks were pulled on a Brown-Flaming (Model P-77 Sutter) micropipette puller and filled with either 2.0 M potassium acetate or 4% Lucifer yellow-CH (Sigma) dissolved in either 1.0 M lithium chloride or

TABLE 1.

Agent	Conc.	pH	Source	Function
N-Methyl-D-aspartate (NMDA)	10 mM	7.0	Sigma	NMDA receptor agonist
Quisqualate (QUIS)	10 mM	7.0	Tocris	Non-NMDA, nonkainate receptor agonist
cis-2,3-Piperidine-dicarboxylic acid (PDA)	100 mM	7.0	Tocris	Low selectivity excitant amino acid antagonist
Kynurenic acid (Kyn)	5 mM	8.0	Sigma	Nonspecific (endogenous) excitatory amino acid receptor antagonist
D(–)-2-Amino-4-phosphonobutyric acid (APB)	5 mM	7.0	Cambridge Research Biochemicals	NMDA receptor antagonist
DL-2-Amino-5-phosphonovaleric acid (APV)	10 mM	3.5–8.0	Sigma	NMDA receptor antagonist
Glycine	500 mM	3.5–4.0	Sigma	Inhibitory neurotransmitter agonist
Strychnine HCl	10 mM	3.0	Sigma	Glycine receptor antagonist
Gamma-amino-N-butyric acid	500 mM	3.5–4.0	Sigma	Inhibitory neurotransmitter agonist
Bicuculline methiodide	10 mM	3.0	Sigma	GABA-receptor antagonist

1.0 M lithium acetate (50–150 mOhm). For all binaural studies, search stimuli were unramped noise bursts of 5 msec with the right stimulus delayed by 20 msec. Neurons were initially classified using 50 or 100 coherent tone bursts at CF (50-msec duration, 5-msec rise/fall) presented at the rate of 4/sec. During studies of interaural time differences and during intracellular recordings 3 msec unramped, 4/sec CF tone pips were utilized. All stimuli were delivered through TDH-49 or TDH-50 earphones (Telephonics) and calibrated off-line using a 0.3-cc coupler (chinchilla artificial ear) and corrected to dB SPL (re 0.0002 dyn/cm^2).

SYNAPTIC POTENTIALS

Fast synaptic potentials are usually mediated by transmitter-receptor complex activation of specific ionophores, which can be identified by examining their reversal potentials, conductance changes, and ions involved. Therefore, clues as to the possible identity and function of neurotransmitters can be obtained from the nature of the synaptic potentials. Intracellular recordings from LSO principal cells reflect the segregated nature of the excitatory ipsilateral and inhibitory contralateral inputs. Ipsilateral acoustic/electrical stimuli evoke large excitatory postsynaptic potentials (EPSPs), while contralateral stimuli evoke equally large inhibitory postsynaptic potentials (IPSPs) (Fig. 3) (19,34,119). When simultaneous/like binaural stimuli are presented during intracellular recordings from LSO principal cells, the IPSP is the predominant synaptic potential observed (Fig. 3). This intracellular finding reflects what is observed during extracellular recordings obtained from LSO neurons during presentation of like binaural stimuli (Figs. 2, 7, and 8). The dominance of the inhibitory input may reflect that the inhibition is near the recording site, i.e., somatic, whereas the excitation occurs more distally (20). Properties of these synaptic potentials relevant to transmitter/receptor identification are discussed in the appropriate sections.

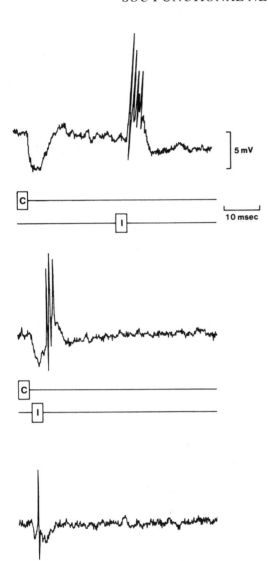

5 mV

10 msec

FIG. 3. Synaptic potentials recorded from a typical EI lateral superior olivary nucleus neuron in response to like dichotic stimuli (55 dB, characteristic frequency [CF] 4,134 Hz) presented at two ipsilateral time delays (top and middle trace) and simultaneously (0.0 msec delay) (bottom trace). Contralateral CF (C) stimuli result in a large inhibitory postsynaptic potential (IPSP), while ipsilateral CF (I) stimuli evoked a sustained excitatory postsynaptic potential (EPSP) with action potentials arising from the plateau. The IPSP and EPSP amplitudes were proportional to stimulus intensity, while the simultaneous condition generally resulted in near-total suppression of the ipsilateral excitatory response (bottom trace). The IPSP predominated during simultaneous binaural stimulation. Resting potential $= Em = RP\bullet - 37$ mV.

WHAT IS THE NEUROTRANSMITTER MEDIATING IPSILATERAL EXCITATION AT LATERAL SUPERIOR OLIVARY NUCLEUS PRINCIPAL CELL SYNAPSES?

Unfortunately, the identity of the neurotransmitter(s) released by spherical bushy cells onto the dendrites of LSO principal cells has not been extensively studied. The need for reliable transfer of coded auditory information (especially the onset of signals, phase, and other temporal information) suggests that a neurotransmitter(s) that can be rapidly released, inactivated, and reutilized is released at many auditory synapses, including the excitatory synapse onto LSO neurons. Low molecular weight neurotransmitters such as excitant amino acids (EAAs) fit this description (30). Although acetylcholine also fits this description, ascending auditory systems do not appear to use this transmitter (29,46). A number of studies suggest that an EAA or similar substance is a likely neurotransmitter candidate at the hair cell, eighth nerve synapse, and several sites along the auditory neuraxis including onto CN neurons (for review, see refs. 4,28,29,116). Preliminary data (33; see Faingold et al., Chapter 10) also suggest that an EAA may also be an excitatory neurotransmitter in the IC. In the LSO, a role for EAAs is suggested by recent immunocytochemical studies using affinity purified antibodies to fixative conjugated aspartate and glutamate, which show a number of immunoreactive neurons in AVCN (4,18,67). These studies, although suggestive, must

be viewed with caution since acidic amino acids are involved with numerous metabolic reactions, and staining specificity with conjugated EAA antibodies has been variable. Neurons in the SOC are also fragile to kainate injection (70), the toxicity of which may be mediated through non-*N*-methyl-D-aspartate (NMDA) EAA receptors (71).

The presence of EAA receptors has been further studied using iontophoretic application of EAA agonists and antagonists while recording the responses of LSO principal cells (25). Quisqualate (QUIS) and NMDA were selected as agonists, while the selective NMDA receptor antagonist DL-2-amino-5-phosphonovaleric acid (APV) and the nonselective EAA receptor antagonist *cis*-2,3-piperidine-dicarboxylic acid (PDA) were chosen as potential blockers of ipsilaterally evoked neuronal responses. Ionto-

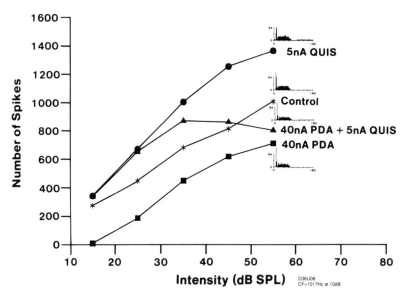

FIG. 4. Effects of non-NMDA agonists and antagonists on the rate-intensity function of lateral superior olivary nucleus neuron to ipsilateral stimuli. Iontophoretic application of 5 nA quisqualate (QUIS) shifts the control ipsilateral rate-intensity function to the left, while 40 nA of the nonselective excitatory amino acid antagonist *cis*-2,3-piperidine-dicarboxylic acid (PDA) partially blocks the ipsilateral tone-evoked responses, shifting the rate-intensity function to the right. Simultaneous application of PDA and QUIS results in a blocking of the QUIS-evoked responses at intensities between 40 and 60 dB SPL. Representative poststimulus-time histograms are displayed for each paradigm for stimuli at 55 dB.

phoretic application of the agonist QUIS was found to excite LSO neurons and shift rate-intensity functions to the left (Fig. 4). This shift could be partially blocked by PDA, while application of the antagonist PDA alone shifted the ipsilaterally evoked rate-intensity functions to the right (Fig. 4). The partial blockade of ipsilateral excitation and reduction of spontaneous activity were greater with PDA than the effect with the NMDA receptor antagonist APV (25). A recently developed, specific non-NMDA receptor antagonist 6,7-dinitroquinoxaline-2,3-dione (DNQX) effectively blocked ipsilateral excitation at LSO principal cells (25). Similarly, tone-evoked and spontaneous activity was enhanced to a greater extent by iontophoretic application of QUIS than of NMDA. These findings suggest the presence of EAA receptors on LSO principal cells. Furthermore, based on the relative potencies of the antagonists in blocking tone-evoked activity, if an EAA mediates the rapid ipsilateral excitatory responses from ventral CN (VCN) spherical bushy cells, it is likely to release an EAA that serves as a ligand for QUIS or kainate receptors rather than NMDA receptor types. In other sensory systems including the spinal cord and the visual system, rapid transmission is mediated by EAAs acting at non-NMDA receptors (13,57,61,68).

Receptors of the NMDA and non-NMDA types may also be differentiated by their actions. Non-NMDA receptors appear to mediate fast synaptic potentials, while NMDA receptors mediate slow potentials, and the reversal potential of these EPSPs appears to be different (for review, see ref. 65). Intracellular recordings from LSO neurons show fast ipsilaterally evoked EPSPs, which is consistent with the possibility that non-NMDA receptors mediate ipsilateral excitation in these neurons. Further examination of these synaptic potentials, especially reversal potentials, should aid in the identification of the transmitter at this synapse.

WHAT IS THE CONTRALATERAL EXCITATORY NEUROTRANSMITTER TO PRINCIPAL CELLS OF THE MEDIAL NUCLEUS OF THE TRAPEZOID BODY?

Less is known regarding the identity of the neurotransmitter at the synapse between the globular bushy cell and the MNTB principal cell than the ipsilateral input to the LSO neurons described above. Published micrographs of VCN sections from studies that utilized affinity purified antibodies to either aspartate or glutamate display some immunolabeled neurons, but identification of specific immunolabeled cell types within the VCN is not yet possible (4,66,67). In one study that examined glutamate-like immunoreactivity in the VCN, it was shown that no immunoreactive neurons appear in the VCN globular cell area (80). Although Ottersen and Storm-Mathisen (80) describe a lack of glutamate-like immunoreactivity in the caudal brainstem, they point out that end-bulbs, presumably those ending on MNTB principal cells, do show moderately intense glutamate-like immunoreactivity and that "thick, intensely labelled fibers cross the midline ventrally in the trapezoid body." The source of the glutamate-like positive end-bulbs and fibers is likely the globular bushy cells in the CN. In preliminary iontophoretic studies, chinchilla MNTB neurons displaying either primary-like or off temporal discharge patterns were sensitive to EAA agonists and antagonists (Fig. 5). Both NMDA and non-NMDA receptor antagonists reduced contralaterally evoked discharges, while QUIS and NMDA excited these neurons. Thus only very preliminary observations exist regarding the identity of the neurotransmitter released at this synapse. The presence of EAA receptors and sparse immunocytochemical evidence suggest that EAAs or a similar molecule are possible candidates, but convincing support for this hypothesis is at present lacking.

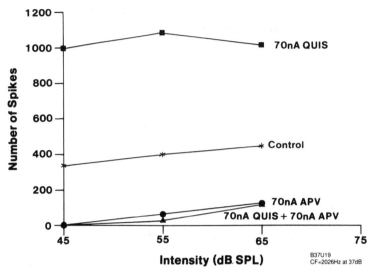

FIG. 5. Effects of quisqualate (QUIS) and an NMDA antagonist, DL-2-amino-5-phosphono-valeric acid (APV), on a short rate-intensity function of a neuron with a primary-like temporal response pattern recorded from within the medial nucleus of the trapezoid body. Iontophoretic application of QUIS (70 nA) more than doubles the discharge rate of this unit, whereas the antagonist APV markedly suppressed spontaneous activity, tone-evoked activity, and the combined excitation of QUIS and characteristic frequency tones.

WHAT IS THE NEUROTRANSMITTER MEDIATING BINAURAL INHIBITION IN THE LATERAL SUPERIOR OLIVARY NUCLEUS?

Unlike the uncertainty regarding the nature of the excitatory neurotransmitter at the other two synapses in the LSO binaural circuit, considerable data now exist supporting the hypothesis that glycine is the neurotransmitter of the MNTB principal cells mediating inhibition in the LSO. Convincing immunocytochemical evidence from studies using affinity purified fixative conjugated antibodies to glycine shows intense immunoreactivity of the MNTB principal cells (Fig. 6, kindly provided by Dr. Richard Saint Marie) (5,19,52,83,90,114, 115). Intense glycine immunoreactivity also labels axons coursing to the LSO, and dark-staining puncta, presumably immunolabeled boutons, are seen surrounding LSO principal cells (Fig. 6) (5,52,90,115). Kainic acid lesions of the homolateral MNTB abolish punctate labeling surrounding LSO neu-

rons (8), puncta that have been shown by electron microscopy to be glycine-immunoreactive boutons (52). Bouton endings surrounding LSO principal cells have also been shown to take up [³H]glycine (96). Glycine receptors located on LSO principal cells have also been observed. Using several monoclonal antibodies to the glycine receptor, somatic and proximal dendritic sites are labeled on principal cells opposite boutons containing flattened vesicles (3, 114). Binding studies using [³H]strychnine as a ligand for glycine receptors display autoradiographs showing high grain densities in the LSO in several different species (35,36,92,93,121).

Binaural inhibition recorded from LSO neurons during like binaural stimuli can be blocked by iontophoretic application of the glycine antagonist strychnine and is mimicked by application of the inhibitory amino acid glycine (Fig. 7) (29,74). Iontophoretic application of glycine during ipsilateral CF stimulation at different intensities suppresses the responses of LSO neurons in a

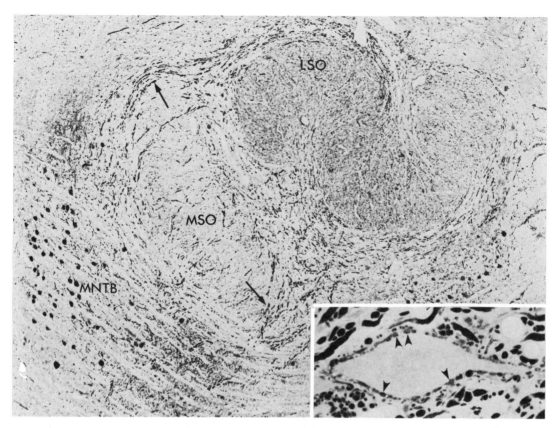

FIG. 6. A low magnification (45×) photomicrograph of a 1.4-μm plastic section through the right superior olivary complex of the cat. This section has been immunostained with a glutaraldehyde-conjugated, affinity-purified antibody to the inhibitory amino acid neurotransmitter glycine. Strongly glycine-immunoreactive cells can be seen in the medial nucleus of the trapezoid body (MNTB). Thick glycine-immunoreactive axons are seen to emerge from the MNTB and course toward the lateral superior olivary nucleus (LSO). Stained axons can be seen entering and surrounding the LSO, and darkly glycine-immunoreactive puncta can be seen surrounding the LSO principal cells (inset, 790×). The puncta primarily contact the somata and proximal dendrites of these neurons. Courtesy of Dr. Richard Saint Marie.)

manner similar to that observed when like binaural stimuli are presented at different intensities (Fig. 7). Application of strychnine onto LSO principal cells blocks binaural inhibition, resulting in a rate-intensity function similar to that recorded during ipsilateral stimulation (Fig. 7). Application of the gamma-amino-butyric acid (GABA) antagonist bicuculline does not block binaural inhibition (74). Iontophoretic application of strychnine also blocks contralateral inhibitory input during other dichotic paradigms including interaural delay and interaural

phase (74). As interaural time delays are increased from coincident binaural stimuli (0-msec delay) to ipsilateral delays of up to 100 msec, discharge rates gradually increase from near-total suppression to rates approximating the monaural ipsilateral condition (Fig. 8; see also Fig. 3). When strychnine is iontophoretically applied during this paradigm, the discharge rate is not suppressed by coincident tones but remains at the monaural ipsilateral rate, indicating complete blockage of the inhibitory input for all interaural delays examined (Fig. 8).

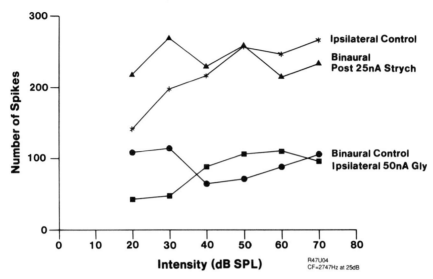

FIG. 7. Effects of glycinergic agents on binaural inhibition and tone-evoked activity in a lateral superior olivary nucleus neuron. Iontophoretic application of glycine (50 nA Gly) suppresses the ipsilateral rate-intensity response of this neuron to a level similar to rates observed with simultaneous presentation of equal intensity binaural stimuli (Binaural Control). Iontophoretic application of the glycine receptor antagonist strychnine (Strych) (immediately after 25 nA of Strych was applied [Post 25 nA Strych]) blocks binaural inhibition, resulting in a rate-intensity function similar to that observed when ipsilateral tones are presented alone (Ipsilateral Control).

The role of glycine in LSO is further supported by evidence that intravenous administration of strychnine blocks the binaural interaction component of the auditory brainstem evoked potential, a potential thought to originate from near the LSO (7).

Intracellular recordings show that contralateral stimuli evoke IPSPs from LSO principal neurons, which have similar characteristics to IPSPs recorded from spinal neurons known to receive inputs from glycinergic interneurons (34,119). These IPSPs dramatically reverse upon injection of chloride ions and when these cells are hyperpolarized (34). This is also the case with putative glycine IPSPs recorded from spinal cord neurons (120). Micromolar concentrations of strychnine reversibly block contralaterally induced IPSPs in LSO slices (119).

Considerable and compelling evidence exists supporting glycine as the inhibitory transmitter of the MNTB principal cells that project onto the somata and proximal dendrites of LSO principal cells. Therefore, glycine most likely mediates binaural inhibition in the LSO and as such shapes the binaural code that is projected to the IC from this structure (24) (Fig. 9).

FIG. 8. Iontophoretic application of 50 nA of the glycine receptor antagonist strychnine is seen to block binaural inhibition observed at ipsilateral delays between 0 and 4.8 msec. The duration of the fixed contralateral tone is 3.0 msec as indicated by the *arrow*. The discharge rate of this lateral superior olivary nucleus principal cell, which is 0 spikes/sec for simultaneously presented like binaural stimuli, is seen to recover to near ipsilateral control value (see mark at right of graph) as the ipsilateral stimulus is delayed beyond the contralateral stimulus. Note that iontophoretic application of strychnine has no effect on the control ipsilateral condition (see mark at right of graph). Stimuli (100) were presented at 4/sec and were unramped 3.0-msec tone-bursts at characteristic frequency (CF) (CF = 4,820 Hz at 43 dB SPL).

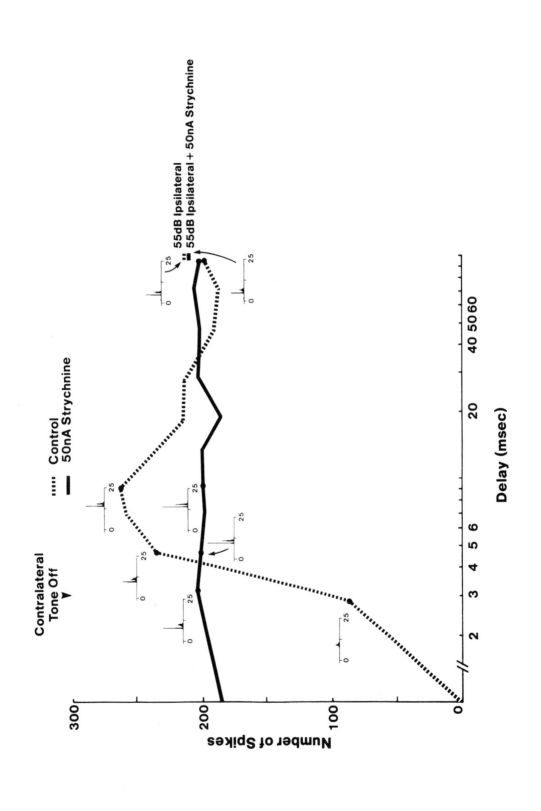

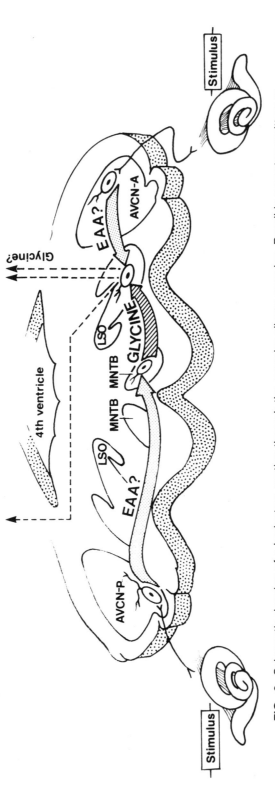

FIG. 9. Schematic drawing of a brainstem section through the superior olivary complex. Possible neurotransmitters released by the major projection neurons in the binaural lateral superior olivary nucleus (LSO) circuit for the right side (as shown in Fig. 1) are presented. Only the inhibitory glycinergic projection from the medial nucleus of the trapezoid body (MNTB) to the LSO has been well established. AVCN-P, anteroventral cochlear nucleus, posterior area; EAA, excitatory amino acid; AVCN-A, anteroventral cochlear nucleus, anterior area.

WHAT ARE THE NEUROTRANSMITTERS OF THE LATERAL SUPERIOR OLIVARY NUCLEUS PROJECTION NEURONS TO THE INFERIOR COLLICULUS?

Principal cells of the LSO send equal bilateral projections to the IC (31,38,90,100, 109). Recent neurotransmitter studies suggest that the ipsilateral projection may possess both an excitatory and inhibitory component, while the contralateral projection may be excitatory (90). Little evidence is available regarding the identity of the excitatory neurotransmitter(s) to either IC. Iontophoretic application of EAAs and their antagonists significantly alters the response properties of IC neurons (33,113; Faingold et al., Chapter 10). Although EAAs could be excitatory transmitters in this pathway, there is little additional evidence to support this contention. The ipsilateral inhibitory projection may be glycinergic since one population of LSO principal cells is immunolabeled with conjugated glycine antibodies and displays ipsilateral retrograde transport of [^{3}H]glycine injected into the homolateral IC (Figs. 6 and 9) (90,115). Neurons in the IC of several species display moderate levels of strychnine binding, and calcium-dependent, potassium-evoked release of glycine has been demonstrated in the rat IC (64,86,121). Discharge rates recorded from neurons in the IC were suppressed by iontophoretic application of glycine, responses that were blocked by strychnine and that required higher doses and were less specific than responses to GABA and bicuculline (32; Faingold et al., Chapter 10).

Although a population of neurons that label with GABA markers has been demonstrated in the LSO using glutamic acid decarboxylase (GAD) and conjugated-GABA antibodies, the targets of these neurons are uncertain (72,78,117). These neurons could be the source of the GABAergic input projecting via the trapezoid body to the AVCN, which is reduced by sectioning inputs to the CN (40) and/or the GABAergic input to the cochlea (97).

PUTATIVE NEUROTRANSMITTERS OF THE MEDIAL LATERAL SUPERIOR OLIVARY NUCLEUS

Little is known about neurotransmitters acting on MSO neurons. Cells of this nucleus are binaurally sensitive to low frequencies, with the majority of neurons displaying excitation to binaural stimuli (41,42,44,54). These same authors find that certain MSO neurons can also be inhibited by one ear and excited by the other, while some MSO neurons are responsive only to monaural stimuli. Many of these neurons display phase-locked temporal response patterns and are sensitive to differences in interaural phase (77).

Ipsilateral and contralateral inputs onto MSO neurons may originate from the same population of VCN neurons as the ipsilateral input to LSO neurons. Discrete lesions of the VCN lead to degeneration of terminals in both MSO and LSO, suggesting that the ipsilateral LSO and the MSO may receive projections from the same VCN cells (47,109,110). Discrete injections of wheat germ agglutinin-HRP into the LSO result in labeling of terminals in the MSO (21,98), strengthening but not confirming this suggestion. Gray's (43) type I endings, which contain spherical vesicles and are generally considered to be excitatory (107), make multiple asymmetric contacts with MSO neurons. These endings degenerate upon destruction of the CN (59,63). One could therefore advance the hypothesis that the excitatory neurotransmitter in MSO might be the same as the excitatory neurotransmitter in the LSO, possibly an EAA.

Inhibitory inputs to MSO neurons are suggested by the presence of boutons containing flattened or pleomorphic vesicles and making symmetric contacts onto several cell types within the MSO (82,94). Tritiated GABA and glycine are taken up by boutons that display morphology associated with inhibitory endings in other systems (96). These boutons contact MSO neurons with the distribution consistent with that of the type 2 and 3 bouton endings described by Schwartz (95). These data suggest that both GABA and glycine may be involved in determining the response properties of MSO neurons.

OTHER TRANSMITTERS IN THE SUPERIOR OLIVARY COMPLEX

The pharmacology of neurotransmission at other synaptic sites in the SOC has not been studied systematically. However, transmitter candidates at many of these contacts can be suggested based on morphological, immunocytochemical, and histochemical studies.

As indicated in the section on neurotransmitters of the MSO, common inputs and/or collaterals to different SOC nuclei could be expected to release the same transmitter. For example, collaterals of fibers, which form calyceal endings in the MNTB and are the excitatory input onto MNTB principal cells, terminate on other MNTB neurons and on neurons in the dorsomedial periolivary nucleus (DMPO) (76). These endings would probably release the same excitatory neurotransmitter as that released onto MNTB principal cells, possibly an EAA (see above). Similarly, MNTB principal neurons, in addition to innervating LSO principal cells, apparently send glycinergic collaterals to within the MNTB and to the DMPO (76,99). Such an intrinsic inhibitory glycinergic input could underlie the off-response pattern observed in nonprincipal MNTB neurons. MNTB principal cells may also send glycinergic projections to the ventral nucleus of the lateral lemniscus (VNLL) (99). While it is likely that SOC neurons provide inhibitory amino acid input to the CN, it should be noted that although unlikely, certain glycinergic inputs to the SOC could conceivably arise from the VCN (5,6,40,115).

Receptor binding and neurotransmitter localization studies also provide an indication of possible neurotransmitters involved at other synapses in the SOC. However, caution is advised since both binding and immunocytochemical studies are prone to both false positives and negatives and only provide an indication of possible candidates at specific synapses. Guth and Melamed (46) and Wenthold and Martin (116) have recently reviewed some of these binding studies.

Based on such studies, the other major inhibitory amino acid, GABA, also appears to be an important neurotransmitter in the SOC (84). GAD-immunoreactive terminals have been demonstrated on LSO and MSO dendrites. They are also found clustered around MNTB principal cell somas and scattered about periolivary nuclei and are more dense in a ventral region of the SOC (72,88). The origins of these projections are unknown, but Moore and Moore (72) suggest an intrinsic source that could be the GAD-positive neurons in the LSO and/or the few GAD-positive neurons scattered in periolivary areas.

Studies examining the olivocochlear systems indicate that acetylcholine and peptide transmitters may also be present in the SOC. Lateral olivocochlear neurons may send recurrent collaterals onto other SOC neurons and may release a number of different transmitters (acetylcholine, enkephalins, dynorphins, calcitonin gene-related peptide) onto other lateral olivocochlear neurons (1). In addition, lateral olivocochlear neurons may receive substance P, neuropeptide Y, and GAD-immunoreactive terminals.

Of the aminergic transmitters, there is no catecholaminergic fluorescence staining in the SOC (75). There is, however, moderate binding of the histamine H_2-receptor antagonist mepyramine in the SOC (81).

No further information on the function of these putative transmitters in the SOC, including binaural coding, is available at present.

CONCLUSION

Identification of neurotransmitters involved in major circuits in the SOC will enable us to understand how these circuits function in the coding of binaural signals and the possible involvement of these circuits in the discrimination of complex signals and signals in noise.

Certainly, additional work needs to be done to establish and confirm the identity of the excitatory neurotransmitters of both the LSO and MSO circuit. Quantitative receptor binding studies at the electron microscopic level as well as studies using receptor antibodies should help to establish the identity and functional nature of neurotransmitters or modulators acting at specific sites. Physiological characterization of tone-evoked synaptic potentials should also provide valuable information on the identification of the neurotransmitter(s) acting at these and other inputs. Immunocytochemical studies will also enable identification of the neurotransmitters of the projection neurons to the SOC and both the ascending and descending projections from SOC neurons. Finally, *in vitro* and *in vivo* intracellular and extracellular studies, in conjunction with pharmacologic investigations, can eventually provide the functional link for the correlation with developmental and age-related changes observed behaviorally.

Once the identity of a neurotransmitter is determined, such as the glycinergic input to LSO principal cells, its function can be tested in a number of different physiological paradigms. The effects of known pharmacologic agents such as neurotransmitter agonists, antagonists, and uptake blockers can also be examined in physiological and behavioral tests. Finally, the role of a particular neurotransmitter or neurotransmitter abnormality in communicative disorders of development or aging can be assessed in the context of future pharmacologic therapy.

ACKNOWLEDGMENTS

Maurus Moore and Carl Faingold participated in some of the experiments presented here, while our colleagues, Drs. Rybak and Walsh, provided valuable comments on early drafts. Excellent artistic and technical support was provided by B. Lawhorn Armour, S. Yuscius, J. Pippin, and C. Dodson. These studies were supported by NIH grant DC 00151-10, the Deafness Research Foundation, and funds from the Central Research Committee of the Southern Illinois University School of Medicine.

REFERENCES

1. Abou-Madi L, Pontarotti P, Tramu G, Cupo A, Eybalin M. Coexistence of putative neuroactive substances in lateral olivocochlear neurons of rat and guinea pig. *Hear Res* 1987;30:135–146.
2. Adams JC. Ascending projections to the inferior colliculus. *J Comp Neurol* 1979;183:519–538.
3. Altschuler RA, Betz H, Parakkal MH, Reeks KA, Wenthold RJ. Identification of glycinergic synapses in the cochlear nucleus through immunocytochemical localization of the postsynaptic receptor. *Brain Res* 1986;369:316–320.
4. Aoki E, Semba R, Kato K, Kashiwamata S. Purification of specific antibody against aspartate and immunocytochemical localization of aspartergic neurons in the rat brain. *Neuroscience* 1987;21:755–765.
5. Aoki E, Semba R, Keino H, Kato K, Kashiwamata S. Glycine-like immunoreactivity in the rat auditory pathway. *Brain Res* 1988;442:63–71.
6. Benson CG, Potashner SJ. Retrograde transport of [³H] glycine from the cochlear nucleus to the superior olive in the guinea pig. *J Comp Neurol* 1990;296:415–426.
7. Bledsoe SC, Shore SE. Intravenous strychnine affects the binaural interaction component of the auditory brainstem response (ABR). *Assoc Res Otolaryngol Abstr* 1984;7:63.
8. Bledsoe SC, Snead CR, Helfert RH, Prasad V, Wenthold RJ, Altschuler RA. Immunocyto-

chemical and lesion studies support the hypothesis that the projection from the medial nucleus of the trapezoid body to the lateral superior olive is glycinergic. *Brain Res* 1990;517:189–194.

9. Bobbin RP, Bledsoe SC, Jenison GL. Neurotransmitters of the cochlea and lateral line organ. In: Berlin C, ed. *Hearing science*. San Diego: College-Hill Press, 1984;159–180.

10. Boudreau JC, Tsuchitani C. Binaural interaction in the cat superior olive s-segment. *J Neurophysiol* 1968;31:442–454.

11. Boudreau JC, Tsuchitani C. Cat superior olive S-segment cell discharge to tonal stimulation. In: Neff WD, ed. *Contributions to sensory physiology*. New York: Academic Press, 1970; 143–213.

12. Bourk TR. Electrical responses of neural units in the anteroventral cochlear nucleus of the cat. Doctoral thesis, Department of Electrical Engineering and Computer Science, Massachusetts Institute of Technology, 1976.

13. Brodin L, Christenson J, Grillner S. Single sensory neurons activate excitatory amino acid receptors in the lamprey spinal cord. *Neurosci Lett* 1987;75:75–79.

14. Brownell WE. Organization of the cat trapezoid body and the discharge characteristics of its fibers. *Brain Res* 1975;94:413–433.

15. Brownell WE, Manis PB, Ritz LA. Ipsilateral inhibitory responses in the cat lateral superior olive. *Brain Res* 1979;177:189–193.

16. Browner RH, Webster DB. Projections of the trapezoid body and the superior olivary complex of the kangaroo rat (*Dipodomys Merriami*). *Brain Behav Evol* 1975;11:322–354.

17. Caird D, Klinke R. Processing of binaural stimuli by cat superior olivary complex neurons. *Exp Brain Res* 1983;52:385–399.

18. Campistron G, Buijs RM, Geffard M. Specific antibodies against aspartate and their immunocytochemical application in the rat brain. *Brain Res* 1986;365:179–184.

19. Campistron G, Buijs RM, Geffard M. Glycine neurons in the brain and spinal cord. Antibody production and immunocytochemical localization. *Brain Res* 1986;376:400–405.

20. Cant NB. The fine structure of the lateral superior olivary nucleus of the cat. *J Comp Neurol* 1984;227:63–77.

21. Cant NB, Casseday JH. Projections from the anteroventral cochlear nucleus to the lateral and medial superior olivary nuclei. *J Comp Neurol* 1986;247:457–476.

22. Caspary DM. Classification of sub-populations of neurons in the cochlear nuclei of the kangaroo rat. *Exp Neurol* 1972;37:131–151.

23. Caspary DM. Cochlear nuclei: functional neuropharmacology of the principal cell types. In: Altschuler RA, Hoffman W, Bobbin RP, eds. *Neurobiology of hearing: the cochlea*. New York: Raven Press, 1986;303–332.

24. Caspary DM. Electrophysiological studies of glycinergic mechanisms in auditory brainstem structures. In: Ottersen OP, Storm-Mathisen J,

eds. *Glycine neurotransmission*. West Sussex: John Wiley and Sons, 1990;3–32.

25. Caspary DM, Faingold CL. Non-N-methyl-D-aspartate receptors may mediate ipsilateral excitation at lateral superior olivary synapses. *Brain Res* 1989;503:83–90.

26. Caspary DM, Havey DC, Faingold CL. Effects of microiontophoretically applied glycine and GABA on neuronal response patterns in the cochlear nuclei. *Brain Res* 1979;172:179–185.

27. Caspary DM, Pazara KE, Kössl M, Faingold CL. Strychnine alters the fusiform cell output from the dorsal cochlear nucleus. *Brain Res* 1987;417:273–282.

28. Caspary DM, Rybak LP, Faingold CL. Baclofen reduces tone-evoked and spontaneous activity of cochlear nucleus neurons. *Hear Res* 1984;13:113–122.

29. Caspary DM, Rybak LP, Faingold CL. The effects of inhibitory and excitatory amino acid neurotransmitters on the response properties of brainstem auditory neurons. In: Drescher DG, ed. *Auditory biochemistry*. Springfield, IL: Charles C Thomas, 1985;198–226.

30. Collingridge GL, Bliss TVP. NMDA receptors—their role in long-term potentiation. *TINS* 1987;10:288–293.

31. Elverland HH. Ascending and intrinsic projections of the superior olivary complex in the cat. *Exp Brain Res* 1978;32:117–134.

32. Faingold CL, Gehlbach G, Caspary DM. On the role of GABA as an inhibitory neurotransmitter in inferior colliculus neurons: iontophoresis studies. *Brain Res* 1989;500:302–312.

33. Faingold CL, Hoffman WE, Caspary DM. Effects of iontophoresis of agents affecting the action of excitant amino acids on the acoustic responses of neurons in the inferior colliculus. *Hear Res* 1989;40:127–136.

34. Finlayson PG, Caspary DM. Synaptic potentials of chinchilla lateral superior olivary neurons. *Hear Res* 1989;38:221–228.

35. Frostholm A, Rotter A. Glycine receptor distribution in mouse CNS: autoradiographic localization of [^{3}H] strychnine binding sites. *Brain Res Bull* 1985;15:473–486.

36. Glendenning KK, Baker BN. Neuroanatomical distribution of receptors for three potential inhibitory neurotransmitters in the brainstem auditory nuclei of the cat. *J Comp Neurol* 1988;275:288–308.

37. Glendenning KK, Hutson KA, Nudo RJ, Masterson RB. Acoustic chiasm II: anatomical basis of binaurality in lateral superior olive of cat. *J Comp Neurol* 1985;232:261–285.

38. Glendenning KK, Masterton RB. Acoustic chiasm: efferent projections of the lateral superior olive. *J Neurosci* 1983;3:1521–1537.

39. Godfrey DA, Kiang NYS, Norris BE. Single unit activity in the posteroventral cochlear nucleus of the cat. *J Comp Neurol* 1975;162:247–268.

40. Godfrey DA, Parli JA, Dunn JD, Ross CD. Neurotransmitter microchemistry of the co-

chlear nucleus and superior olivary complex. In: Syka J, Masterton RB, eds. *Auditory pathway: structure and function.* New York: Plenum Press, 1988;107–122.

41. Goldberg JM, Brown PB. Functional organization of the dog superior olivary complex: an anatomical and electrophysiological study. *J Neurophysiol* 1968;31:639–656.

42. Goldberg JM, Brown PB. Response of binaural neurons of dog superior olivary complex to dichotic tonal stimuli: some physiological mechanisms of sound localization. *J Neurophysiol* 1969;32:613–636.

43. Gray EG. Axo-somatic and axo-dendritic synapses of the cerebral cortex; an electron microscope study. *J Anat* 1959;93:420–433.

44. Guinan JJ, Guinan SS, Norris BE. Single auditory units in the superior olivary complex. I. Responses to sounds and classifications based on physiological properties. *Int J Neurosci* 1972;4:101–120.

45. Guinan JJ, Norris BE, Guinan SS. Single auditory units in the superior olivary complex. II. Locations of unit categories and tonotopic organization. *Int J Neurosci* 1972;4:147–166.

46. Guth PS, Melamed B. Neurotransmission in the auditory system: a primer for pharmacologists. *Annu Rev Pharmacol Toxicol* 1982;22:383–412.

47. Harrison JM, Irving R. Ascending connections of the anterior ventral cochlear nucleus in the rat. *J Comp Neurol* 1966;126:51–64.

48. Harrison JM, Warr WB. A study of the cochlear nuclei and ascending auditory pathways of the medulla. *J Comp Neurol* 1962;119:341–379.

49. Havey DC, Caspary DM. A simple technique for construction of "piggy-back" multibarrel microelectrodes. *Electroencephalogr Clin Neurophysiol* 1980;48:249–251.

50. Helfert RH, Schwartz IR. Morphological evidence for the existence of multiple neuronal classes in the cat lateral superior olivary nucleus. *J Comp Neurol* 1986;244:533–549.

51. Helfert RH, Schwartz IR. Morphological features of five neuronal classes in the gerbil lateral superior olive. *Am J Anat* 1987;179:55–69.

52. Helfert RH, Bonneau JM, Wenthold RJ, Altschuler RA. GABA and glycine immunoreactivity in the guinea pig superior olivary complex. *Brain Res* 1989;501:269–286.

53. Herman GE, Warren LR, Wagener JW. Auditory lateralization: age differences in sensitivity to dichotic time and amplitude cues. *J Gerontol* 1977;32:187–191.

54. Inbody SB, Feng AS. Binaural response characteristics of single neurons in the medial superior olivary nucleus of the albino rat. *Brain Res* 1981;210:361–366.

55. Irvine DRF. Superior olivary complex: anatomy and physiology. In: Ottoson D, ed. *Progress in sensory physiology: the auditory brainstem.* New York: Springer-Verlag, 1986.

56. Jenkins WM, Masterton B. Sound localization:

effects of unilateral lesions in central auditory system. *J Neurophysiol* 1982;47:987–1016.

57. Jessell TM, Yoshioka K, Jahr CE. Amino acid receptor-mediated transmission at primary afferent synapses in rat spinal cord. *J Exp Biol* 1986;124:239–258.

58. Kiang NYS. Stimulus representation in the discharge patterns of auditory neurons. In: Tower DB, ed. *The nervous system. Human communication and its disorders.* New York: Raven Press, 1975.

59. Kiss A, Majorossy K. Neuron morphology and synaptic architecture in the medial superior olivary nucleus. *Exp Brain Res* 1983;52:315–327.

60. Konkle DF, Beasley DS, Bess FH. Intelligibility of time-altered speech in relation to chronological aging. *J Speech Hear Res* 1977;20:108–115.

61. Langdon RB, Freeman JA. Antagonists of glutaminergic neurotransmission block retinotectal transmission in goldfish. *Brain Res* 1986;398:169–174.

62. Lenn NJ, Reese TS. The fine structure of nerve endings in the nucleus of the trapezoid body and the ventral cochlear nucleus. *Am J Anat* 1966;118:375–389.

63. Lindsey BG. Fine structure and distribution of axon terminals from the cochlear nucleus on neurons in the medial superior olivary nucleus of the cat. *J Comp Neurol* 1975;160:81–104.

64. Lopez-Colome AM, Tapia R, Saleda R, Pasantes-Morales H. K$^+$-stimulated release of labeled gamma-aminobutyrate, glycine and taurine in slices of several regions of rat central nervous system. *Neuroscience* 1978;3:1069–1074.

65. MacDermott AB, Dale N. Receptors, ion channels and synaptic potentials underlying the integrative actions of excitatory amino acids. *TINS* 1987;10:280–284.

66. Madl JE, Beitz AJ, Johnson RL, Larson AA. Monoclonal antibodies specific for fixative-modified aspartate: immunocytochemical localization in the rat CNS. *J Neurosci* 1987;7:2639–2650.

67. Madl JE, Larson AA, Beitz AJ. Monoclonal antibody specific for carbodiimide-fixed glutamate: immunocytochemical localization in the rat CNS. *J Histochem Cytochem* 1986;34:317–326.

68. Massey SC, Miller RF. Excitatory amino acid receptors of rod- and cone-driven horizontal cells in the rabbit retina. *J Neurophysiol* 1987;57:645–659.

69. Masterton B, Jane JA, Diamond IT. Role of brainstem auditory structures in sound localization. I. Trapezoid body, superior olive, and lateral lemniscus. *J Neurophysiol* 1967;30:341–359.

70. Masterton B, Glendenning KK, Hutson KA. Preservation of trapezoid body fibers after biochemical ablation of superior olives with kainic acid. *Brain Res* 1979;173:156–159.

71. McGeer P, McGeer EG, Hattori T. Kainic acid

as a tool in neurobiology. In: McGeer EG, Olney JW, McGeer PL, eds. *Kainic acid as a tool in neurobiology.* New York: Raven Press, 1978;161–176.

72. Moore JK, Moore RY. Glutamic acid decarboxylase-like immunoreactivity in brainstem auditory nuclei of the rat. *J Comp Neurol* 1987; 260:157–174.

73. Moore MJ, Caspary DM. Binaural properties of neurons in the chinchilla lateral superior olivary nucleus. *J Acoust Soc Am* 1982;71:99.

74. Moore MJ, Caspary DM. Strychnine blocks binaural inhibition in lateral superior olivary neurons. *J Neurosci* 1983;3:237–242.

75. Moore RY, Bloom FE. Central catecholamine neuron systems: anatomy and physiology of the norepinephrine and epinephrine systems. *Annu Rev Neurosci* 1979;2:113–168.

76. Morest DK. The collateral system of the medial nucleus of the trapezoid body of the cat, its neuronal architecture and relation to the olivocochlear bundle. *Brain Res* 1968;9:288–311.

77. Moushegian G, Rupert AL, Whitcomb MA. Brain-stem neuronal response patterns to monaural and binaural tones. *J Neurophysiol* 1964; 27:1174–1191.

78. Mugnaini E, Oertel WH. An atlas of the distribution of GABAergic neurons and terminals in the rat CNS as revealed by GAD immunohistochemistry. In: Bjorklund A, Hökfelt T, eds. *Handbook of chemical neuroanatomy: GABA and neuropeptides in the CNS.* Amsterdam/ New York: Elsevier, 1985;436–608.

79. Osen KK. Cytoarchitecture of the cochlear nuclei in the cat. *J Comp Neurol* 1969;136:453–484.

80. Ottersen OP, Storm-Mathisen J. Glutamate- and GABA-containing neurons in the mouse and rat brain, as demonstrated with a new immunocytochemical technique. *J Comp Neurol* 1984;229:374–392.

81. Palacios JM, Wamsley JK, Kuhar MJ. The distribution of histamine H1-receptors in the rat brain: an autoradiographic study. *Neuroscience* 1981;6:15–37.

82. Perkins RE. An electron microscopic study of synaptic organization in the medial superior olive of normal and experimental chinchillas. *J Comp Neurol* 1973;148:387–416.

83. Peyret D, Campistron G, Geffard M, Aran JM. Glycine immunoreactivity in the brainstem auditory and vestibular nuclei of the guinea pig. *Acta Otolaryngol* 1987;104:71–76.

84. Peyret D, Geffard M, Aran JM. GABA immunoreactivity in the primary nuclei of the auditory central nervous system. *Hear Res* 1986; 23:115–121.

85. Pfeiffer RR. Classification of response patterns of spike discharges for units in the cochlear nucleus: tone-burst stimulation. *Exp Brain Res* 1966;1:220–235.

86. Probst A, Cortes R, Palacios JM. The distribution of glycine receptors in the human brain.

A light microscopic autoradiographic study using [³H] strychnine. *Neuroscience* 1986;17: 11–35.

87. Rhode WS, Oertel D, Smith PH. Physiological response properties of cells labeled intracellularly with horseradish peroxidase in cat ventral cochlear nucleus. *J Comp Neurol* 1983;213: 448–463.

88. Roberts RC, Ribak CE. GABAergic neurons and axon terminals in the brainstem auditory nuclei of the gerbil. *J Comp Neurol* 1987;258: 267–280.

89. Rouiller EM, Ryugo DK. Intracellular marking of physiologically characterized cells in the ventral cochlear nucleus of the cat. *J Comp Neurol* 1984;225:167–186.

90. Saint Marie RL, Ostapoff E-M, Morest DK, Wenthold RJ. Glycine-immunoreactive projection of the cat lateral superior olive: possible role in midbrain ear dominance. *J Comp Neurol* 1989;279:382–396.

91. Sanes DH. An *in vitro* analysis of sound localization mechanisms in the gerbil lateral superior olive. *J Neurosci* 1990;10:3494–3506.

92. Sanes DH, Geary WA, Wooten GF, Rubel EW. Quantitative distribution of the glycine receptor in the auditory brainstem of the gerbil. *J Neurosci* 1987;11:3793–3802.

93. Sanes DH, Wooten GF. Development of glycine receptor distribution in the lateral superior olive of the gerbil. *J Neurosci* 1987;7:3803–3811.

94. Schwartz IR. The differential distribution of synaptic terminal on marginal and central cells in the cat medial superior olivary nucleus. *Am J Anat* 1980;159:25–31.

95. Schwartz IR. The differential distribution of label following uptake of [³H] labelled amino acids in the dorsal cochlear nucleus of the cat. *Exp Neurol* 1981;73:601–617.

96. Schwartz IR. Autoradiographic studies of amino acid labeling of neural elements in the brainstem. In: Drescher DG, ed. *Auditory biochemistry.* Springfield, IL: Charles C Thomas, 1985;258–277.

97. Schwartz DWF, Schwartz IE, Hu K, Vincent SR. Retrograde transport of [³H]-GABA by lateral olivocochlear neurons in the rat. *Hear Res* 1988;32:97–102.

98. Shneiderman A, Henkel CK. Evidence of collateral axonal projections to the superior olivary complex. *Hear Res* 1985;19:199–205.

99. Spangler KM, Warr WB, Henkel CK. The projections of principal cells of the medial nucleus of the trapezoid body in the cat. *J Comp Neurol* 1985;238:249–262.

100. Stotler WA. An experimental study of the cells and connections of the superior olivary complex of the cat. *J Comp Neurol* 1953;98:401–423.

101. Thompson GC, Masterton RB. Brain stem auditory pathways involved in reflexive head orientation to sound. *J Neurophysiol* 1978;41: 1183–1202.

102. Tsuchitani C. Lower auditory brain stem structures of the cat. In: Naunton RF, Fernandez C, eds. *Evoked electrical activity in the auditory nervous system.* New York: Academic Press, 1978;373–401.

103. Tsuchitani C. Discharge patterns of cat lateral superior olivary units to ipsilateral tone-burst stimuli. *J Neurophysiol* 1982;47:479–500.

104. Tsuchitani C. The inhibition of cat superior olive unit excitatory responses to binaural tone bursts. I. The transient chopper response. *J Neurophysiol* 1988;59:164–183.

105. Tsuchitani C. The inhibition of cat lateral superior olive unit excitatory responses to binaural tone bursts. II. The sustained discharges. *J Neurophysiol* 1988;59:184–211.

106. Tsuchitani C, Boudreau JC. Stimulus level of dichotically presented tones and cat superior olive S-segment cell discharge. *J Acoust Soc Am* 1969;46:979–988.

107. Uchizono K. *Excitation and inhibition: synaptic morphology.* New York: Elsevier, 1975.

108. van Noort JV. *The structure and connections of the inferior colliculus. An investigation of the lower auditory system.* Netherlands: Van Gorcum and Comp. N.V., 1969.

109. Warr WB. Fiber degeneration following lesions in the anterior ventral cochlear nucleus of the cat. *Exp Neurol* 1966;14:453–474.

110. Warr WB. Fiber degeneration following lesions in the multipolar and globular cell areas in the ventral cochlear nucleus of the cat. *Brain Res* 1972;40:247–270.

111. Warr WB. Parallel ascending pathways from the cochlear nucleus: neuroanatomical evidence of function specialization. In: Neff WD, ed. *Contributions to sensory physiology.* New York: Academic Press, 1982;700–764.

112. Warr WB, Guinan JJ, White JS. Organization of the efferent fibers: the lateral and medial olivocochlear systems. In: Altschuler RA, Hoffman DW, eds. *Neurobiology of hearing: the cochlea.* New York: Raven Press, 1986;333–348.

113. Watanabe T, Simada Z. Pharmacological properties of cat's collicular auditory neurons. *Jpn J Physiol* 1973;23:291–308.

114. Wenthold RJ, Hunter C. Immunocytochemistry of glycine and glycine receptors in the central auditory system. In: Ottersen OP, Storm-Mathisen, eds. *Glycine neurotransmission.* West Sussex: John Wiley and Sons. 1990; 391–416.

115. Wenthold RJ, Huie D, Altschuler RA, Reeks KA. Glycine immunoreactivity localized in the cochlear nucleus and superior olivary complex. *Neuroscience* 1987;22:897–912.

116. Wenthold RJ, Martin MR. Neurotransmitters of the auditory nerve and central auditory system. In: Berlin C, ed. *Hearing science.* San Diego: College-Hill Press, 1984;341–370.

117. Wenthold RJ, Zempel JM, Parakkal MH, Reeks KA, Altschuler RA. Immunocytochemical localization of GABA in the cochlear nucleus of the guinea pig. *Brain Res* 1986;380:7–18.

118. Werman RA. A review criteria for identification of a central nervous transmitter. *Comp Biochem Physiol* 1966;18:745–766.

119. Wu SH, Kelly JB. Physiological properties of neurons in the mouse superior olive: membrane characteristics and postsynaptic responses studied *in vitro. J Neurophysiol* 1991;65:230–246.

120. Young AB, Macdonald RL. Glycine as a spinal cord neurotransmitter. In: Davidoff RA, ed. *Handbook of the spinal-cord.* New York: Marcel Dekker, 1983;1–44.

121. Zarbin MA, Wamsley JK, Kuhar MJ. Glycine receptor: light microscopic autoradiographic localization with [³H]-strychnine. *J Neurosci* 1981;1:532–547.

122. Zook JM, DiCaprio RA. Intracellular labeling of afferents to the superior olive in the bat, Eptesicus fuscus. *Hear Res* 1988;34:141–148.

Neurobiology of Hearing: The Central Auditory System, edited by
R. A. Altschuler et al.
Raven Press, Ltd., New York © 1991.

8

Binaural Cues and Signal Processing in the Superior Olivary Complex

*Chiyeko Tsuchitani and †Don H. Johnson

*Sensory Sciences Center, Graduate School of Biomedical Sciences, The University of Texas
Health Sciences Center, Houston, Texas 77030; †Department of Electrical and Computer
Engineering, Rice University, Houston, Texas 77001*

The superior olivary complex (SOC) is a pontine nuclear group interposed between the cochlear nuclear complex and the inferior colliculus. The SOC was first considered to be an acoustic reflex center that provided afferent input to motor nuclei controlling head and eye movements (1). More recent studies indicate that the SOC nuclei are involved in an efferent system controlling the transmission of acoustic information from the cochlea and cochlear nuclei and in acoustic signal processing.

The SOC contains neurons that provide efferents to the cochlear nuclear complex and the cochlea. Papez (2) described a small fiber bundle that originated in medial areas of the SOC, crossed the midline superiorly, and joined the vestibular nerve. Rasmussen (3,4) reported that this bundle was formed by the axons of periolivary neurons that surround the main SOC nuclei. He called it the olivocochlear fiber bundle and described it as projecting bilaterally back to the cochlear nuclear complex and cochlea. The physiology, connectivity, and histochemistry of the olivocochlear neurons were described in the first volume of this series (5,6) and is not presented in this chapter.

The SOC sends most of its axons in the lateral lemniscus to "higher" auditory structures (2). The demonstration of Stotler

(7) that the medial superior olivary nucleus (MSO) received symmetrical input from the ipsilateral and contralateral cochlear nuclear complex suggested that the SOC might be important in binaural processing (Fig. 1). The single unit electrophysiological study of Galambos et al. (8) confirmed that units in the MSO and lateral superior olive (LSO) are binaurally responsive. Rasmussen (4) later described the binaural input to the LSO; the ipsilateral input originates in the homolateral cochlear nuclear complex and the contralateral input originates in the homolateral medial nucleus of the trapezoid body (MNTB), which, in turn, receives input from the contralateral ear. Numerous anatomical and physiological studies have since confirmed that the MSO and LSO receive inputs from both ears (see Cant, Chapter 5). As the vast majority of MSO and LSO axons ascend in the lateral lemniscus to the nuclei of the lateral lemniscus and the central nucleus of the inferior colliculus (7,9,10), the MSO, MNTB, and LSO are considered to play a major role in binaural signal processing.

CUES FOR BINAURAL PROCESSING

It has long been recognized that binaural hearing provides a distinct advantage over

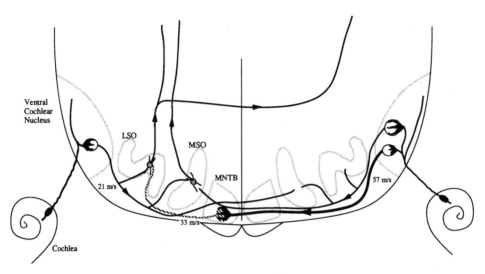

FIG. 1. Schematic diagram illustrating the major connections of the main superior olivary complex nuclei: the lateral superior olive (LSO), the medial superior olive (MSO), and the medial nucleus of the trapezoid body (MNTB). The first-order afferent—the spiral ganglion cells—send their axons to the cochlear nuclear complex. Within the cochlear nuclear complex, collaterals terminate as end-bulbs of Held on the spherical cells and globular cells of the ventral cochlear nucleus. The spherical cells send their axons to the ipsilateral LSO and to the ipsilateral and contralateral MSO. These axons are myelinated, medium-diameter nerve fibers with a conduction velocity of approximately 21 m/sec. The axons of the globular cells are myelinated, large-diameter fibers that conduct at approximately 57 m/sec. These axons travel to the contralateral MNTB where they form large calyces of Held terminals that envelope the cell soma of MNTB principal neurons. The MNTB principal neuron sends its axon to the ipsilateral LSO. This axon is a myelinated, large-to-medium diameter fiber that has a conduction velocity of approximately 33 m/sec. The cochlear nuclear inputs to the LSO, MSO, and MNTB are believed to be excitatory and primary-like in discharge pattern. The MNTB input to the LSO is believed to be inhibitory and primary-like in discharge pattern. The LSO sends its axons bilaterally into the lateral lemniscus, while the MSO axons enter the ipsilateral lateral lemniscus. Many of the LSO and MSO axons terminate in the central nucleus of the inferior colliculus.

monaural hearing in detecting and localizing a sound source in space and in detecting and discriminating signals in noise. The binaural advantage depends on the comparison of the signals at the two ears that are disparate because of differences in the sound propagation paths to the two ears. As each ear is located approximately perpendicular to the midsagittal plane, a sound generated from a source directly opposite one ear (at 90° azimuth in Fig. 2) must travel around the head to reach the opposite ear. Therefore, the onset of the acoustic signal reaches the radiated ear before reaching the opposite ear (Fig. 3A) with an *interaural time of arrival difference* that is determined

by the distance between the ears and the speed of sound. *Interaural phase differences* (Fig. 3B) also occur as a result of the difference in the distance traveled by a given point in the acoustic signal (e.g., the crest of a sinewave) to reach the two ears. These interaural phase differences provide cues for frequencies with wavelengths greater than the head diameter, e.g., less than about 1,600 Hz for an adult human.[1]

---

[1] A classic equation relates the wavelength λ, frequency f, and speed c of a propagating sinusoid: $\lambda f = c$. Taking λ to be the diameter of the head—roughly 20 cm—and c to be the speed of sound—330 m/sec, the frequency of a propagating wave corresponding to these dimensions is 1,650 Hz.

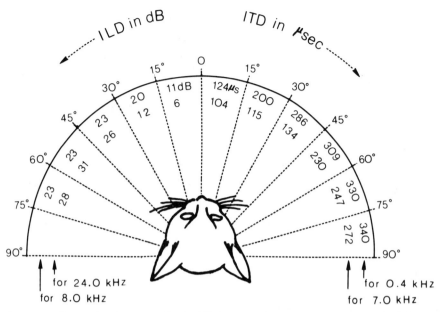

FIG. 2. A cartoon illustrating interaural level difference (ILD) and interaural time difference (ITD) as a function of sound-source deviation from the cat's midsagittal plane in azimuthal angle. The ILDs (left) were derived from Irvine (30). The outer ILDs were estimated from responses to an 8-kHz signal and the inner ILDs were estimated from responses to a 24-kHz signal. The ITDs (right) were based on the measures of Roth and co-workers (21). The outer ITDs were estimated from responses to a 400-Hz signal and the inner ITDs were estimated from responses to a 7-kHz signal.

The head and pinna are solid objects that function as sound barriers. At higher frequencies, the wavelength of sound is smaller than the dimensions of the head and it can *shadow* sound. The head thus creates an acoustic shadow opposite the sound source that is measurable as a decrease in sound pressure level at the ear opposite the radiated ear, i.e., as an *interaural level difference* (Fig. 3C). Acoustic signals with wavelengths greater than the head diameter travel around the head with little attenuation of the signal. Therefore, the level cue is available only at frequencies above 1,600 Hz for the adult human. When the acoustic signal is complex in form, such as the amplitude-modulated signal in Fig. 3D, interaural level differences and interaural time differences are both produced that vary with time. As the wavelength of sound decreases with increasing frequency, objects having dimensions comparable to the wavelength begin to reflect sound waves. The deflection and reflection of sound by the surfaces of the body, head, and pinna interact, producing a complex series of paths that sound waves can take before they reach the tragus (the entrance to the external auditory canal). These interactions spectrally transform the acoustic signal at the tragus. The resulting *interaural spectral difference cues* (Fig. 3E) may be used in the localization of a high-frequency, free-field sound source.

Neural processing of each of these binaural cues involves the comparison of neural activities resulting from stimulation of the two ears. The neuroanatomical organization of the auditory systems of mammalian and nonmammalian species differ significantly. The binaural cues available also differ for mammals and nonmammals. Much of neurophysiological research on binaural processing has been carried out in the cat. Therefore, the following section concentrates on the binaural processing ca-

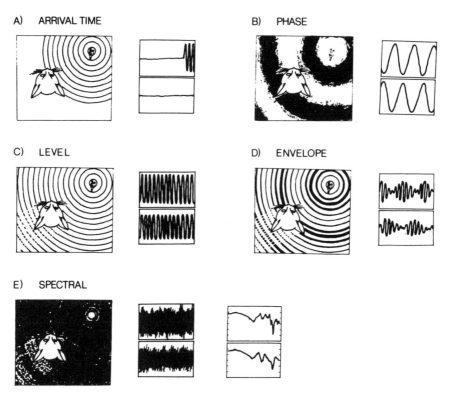

FIG. 3. A cartoon illustrating the types of interaural differences that occur when the signal source is located off the midsagittal plane of the cat's head. **A:** The drawing on the left illustrates the peaks of the sinusoidal signal as it travels from the source toward the cat. The first peak reaches the ear nearest the source before it reaches the ear farthest from the source. On the right, the pressure changes at the two ears as a function of time following the signal onset are illustrated for the near ear (top) and far ear (bottom). **B:** Illustration of the interaural phase difference that occurs with a low-frequency (<3 kHz) signal. **C:** Illustrations of the shadowing effects of the head and pinnae with a high-frequency (>3 kHz) signal. **D:** Illustrations of the interaural level and time differences that occur with a high-frequency signal that varies in level over time. **E:** Illustrations of the interaural spectral differences that occur with a high-frequency complex signal. Illustration on the far right is of the power spectra of the pressures measured at the near (top) and far (bottom) ears.

pabilities of the cat and compares them to those of the human.

Interaural Time Differences

The value of the interaural time difference (ITD) is related to the position of the sound source relative to the ears; the kind of ITD is related to the type of acoustic signal (11). For a sound source rotated in the horizontal plane (Fig. 2), the ITD increases as the signal source is moved from the midsagittal plane (0° azimuth) to the midfrontal plane (approximately 90° azimuth) and decreases as the source moves behind the head back toward the midsagittal plane. Three kinds of ITD differences can be specified for an acoustic signal such as a tone burst with a 2.5-msec rise/fall time and a 100-msec duration: the leading edge ITD (ITD_t), the phase-derived ITD (ITD_p), and the group ITD (ITD_g) (12).

Leading Edge Time Differences

The ITD_t is the difference in the times of arrival of the leading edge or onset of an acoustic signal at the two ears (Fig. 3A). The ITD_t of an acoustic signal is determined by the distance between the two ears, the speed of sound, and the angular distance of the sound source from the midsagittal plane (12,13). For wideband clicks, there is close agreement between the predicted ITD_t and the measured ITD_t for human subjects: When a click source is located at 90° azimuth, they both are 0.65 msec (13,14).[2] The ITD_t of the leading edge of a high-frequency tone or noise burst with a rapid onset time is similar to that of the leading edge of the click stimulus (12). Psychophysical studies have indicated that the ITD_t of tone-burst stimuli will dominate localization judgments when the burst rise time is less than 25 msec and the burst duration is less than 200 to 300 msec (15,16). Binaural signals that are separated by an ITD_t much greater than that resulting from the travel time between the two ears can produce a single, fused acoustic image that is localized to one side. Human subjects report that earphone-delivered clicks with ITD_t as great as 1.5 to 5 msec produce a single, fused lateralized image (17). Cats responded as if a single click were lateralized to the ear receiving the leading signal when clicks were delivered through earphones with an ITD_t less than 1.6 msec (18). At the opposite end of the continuum, well-trained human subjects can detect an ITD_t as small as 0.010 msec between wideband clicks, with most subjects exhibiting thresholds of 0.02 to 0.03 msec (19). According to Masterton et al. (18), cats can detect ITD_t as short as 0.02 to 0.05 msec for earphone-delivered clicks generated by 0.030 msec square-wave pulses. Thus, the range of click ITD_t that produces an acoustic image of a single lateralized click is approximately 0.02 to 1.6 msec for cats and 0.01 to 5 msec for humans. The effects of introducing ITD_t between earphone-delivered tone and noise bursts are more complex as ITD_t may also produce interaural phase differences (IPD) that can be used as binaural cues.

Phase-Derived Time Differences

While the ITD_t is an effective binaural cue for all types of acoustic signals, steady-state ITD in a signal's microstructure may dominate as a binaural cue when the duration of a signal tone burst exceeds 300 msec (15). For example, a phase difference may exist between the pressure waves at the two ears at any given instant of time during steady-state acoustic stimulation (Fig. 3B). This IPD is related to interaural travel time and can be converted into a time difference, the ITD_p.[3] The ITD_p is dependent on the azimuth, the frequency of the signal, and the head-pinna size. Off the midsagittal plane, signals with wavelengths greater than the head-pinna size produce IPD within a cycle of the signal. For example, the maximum interaural time delay for an adult human head with diameter of 18 cm would be about 0.680 msec (the cycle period of a 1,470 Hz sinusoid) (13). For a tone with a frequency less than this frequency, an ITD_p should occur when the signal source is located anywhere off the midsag-

---

[2]The propagation delay of an acoustic wave Δ is given by the ratio of the distance traveled d and the speed of sound c: $\Delta = d/c$. For $\Delta = 0.65$ msec and $c = 330$ m/sec, the distance traveled is about 21.5 cm, which matches the diameter of the average human head. The ears on a cat are separated by about 7 cm; the time sound takes to travel that distance is about 0.2 msec.

[3]A phase shift corresponds to a time delay normalized to the period of the sinusoid. The period of a sinusoid equals $1/f$: the reciprocal of its frequency. Taking the phase ϕ to be expressed in degrees, a phase shift is converted to a time delay by the formula $(\phi/360) \cdot (1/f)$.

ittal plane, with a specific value of ITD_p associated with a specific azimuth displacement. The ITD_p becomes ambiguous as a binaural cue when the half-wavelength of the signal is less than the efficient interaural distance, e.g., when the frequency of the sound is greater than 735 Hz. A 735- to 1,500-Hz signal source located opposite one ear produces waveforms at the two ears that are opposite in phase, i.e., greater than 180° out of phase: With phase difference as the only interaural cue, it is difficult for a listener to determine whether the signal at the irradiated ear is leading or lagging the signal at the opposite ear, and reversals in lateralization judgments may occur. When an acoustic signal has a frequency cycle period shorter than the head diameter, an IPD for a *specific* cycle of a steady-state signal would not exist at any given instant of time. That is, when an acoustic signal has a cycle period shorter than 0.680 msec, the signal at the irradiated ear has passed through one or more cycles before the signal at the opposite ear has passed through the first cycle. Consequently, the ITD_p cannot serve as a reliable cue of a high-frequency source location since the source can produce the identical IPD at a number of different azimuthal locations.

The ITD_p would serve as an unambiguous cue for signal source location only if it were unchanged with source position for all stimuli producing the ITD_p. However, the ITD_p determined from pressure measurements made on the "head surface" near the tragus of a mannequin head (with no torso) exhibited a frequency dependency at all azimuths (20). At displacement angles less than 60° azimuth, the ITD_p remained fairly constant for frequencies below 500 Hz, decreased to lower values as frequency was increased to 2,000 Hz, and remained fairly constant at frequencies above 2,000 Hz. At higher displacement angles, the ITD_p decreased less with increases in frequency but was constant only below 340 Hz and above 3,000 Hz. At 90° azimuth, the ITD_p was approximately 0.8 msec for frequencies below

340 Hz and 0.65 msec for frequencies above 3,000 Hz. The addition of a torso reduced the ITD_p values for frequencies below 700 Hz at all displacement angles and introduced greater fluctuations in ITD_p at the higher frequencies. Roth et al. (21) determined phase-derived ITDs for cats by comparing the waveforms of the sound pressure levels measured at the entrance of the ears. The low-frequency signals (between 400 and 2,500 Hz) consisted of 25-msec duration tone bursts with rise-fall times of 3.9 msec. The ITD estimates were determined as the *averaged* difference between the positive zero-crossing times of corresponding cycles in the first 6-msec sample of the measured signals. The averaged ITDs cannot be considered accurate measures of ITD_t or ITD_p, as the measured periods were nonstationary during the 6-msec sample time. However, the results do resemble those obtained from the mannequin studies of Kuhn (20). At any sound location off the midsagittal plane, the ITD decreased with increases in frequency. With tone bursts presented at 90° azimuth, the ITD ranged from a high of approximately 0.358 msec to a 500-Hz tone to a low of 0.3 msec to a 2,500-Hz tone. At any given azimuth, the measure of ITD fluctuated considerably as a function of frequency. These fluctuations, which were greater at higher azimuthal displacements, were considered to result in part from reflections from supporting structures. Retraction of the pinna reduced the ITD for all frequencies and at all azimuths, with a greater reduction in ITD at the higher frequencies. The measured ITDs were greater than the ITD_t predicted by the Woodworth model of the head as a rigid sphere; these differences were attributed to the more cone-like shape of the cat's head.

While the physical constraints of the interaural distance appear to limit the usefulness of ITD_p between high-frequency signals as a binaural cue, psychophysical and neurophysiological studies with earphone-delivered tones indicate that there is another limiting factor—the ability of the auditory system to process certain temporal features of high-frequency signals. For example, human subjects are unable to detect an ITD_p between earphone-delivered tones with frequencies above 1,500 Hz (22). Cats are unable to detect an ITD_p between earphone-delivered tones with frequencies above 3,000 Hz (23). The smallest detectable ITD_p between earphone-delivered signals is related to the signal frequency. For human subjects, it decreases from 0.056 msec for a 125-Hz tone to 0.011 msec for a 1,000-Hz tone and increases to 0.024 msec for a 1,300-Hz tone (22). Cats are less sensitive to ITD_p than humans (by approximately 0.01 msec) but utilize ITD_p cues at higher stimulus frequencies: They can lateralize a 2,000-Hz tone with an ITD_p of 0.08 msec (23). For human subjects, the maximum ITD_p producing a single, fused lateralized acoustic image is also related to stimulus frequency and is approximately one-quarter to one-third the period *(T)* of the frequency (24,25). As the ITD_p is increased to *T*/4, the position of the sound image is perceived to move toward the ear receiving the signal with the leading phase. When the ITD_p is increased further, the lateral position changes little beyond that perceived at *T*/4 and the sound image becomes diffuse and often splits as the ITD_p approaches *T*/2. If there were no species differences, a 125-Hz tone should produce a fused lateralized image with a maximum ITD_p of approximately 2 to 2.67 msec for cats. For the cat, the range of ITD_p producing a lateralized, single image would be approximately 0.03 to 0.33 msec for a 1,000-Hz tone.

Psychophysical studies have demonstrated that for earphone-delivered, low-frequency signals (i.e., less than 1,500 Hz for the human), judgments of lateral position correspond more closely to the IPD than to the ITD_p (25,26). With IPD held constant at less than 90°, there is only a slight shift in image position toward the midsagittal plane when tone frequency is increased. For example, binaurally presented tone bursts with identical onset times and IPD of 30° were lateralized to similar positions for tone frequencies of 200, 500, and 1,000 Hz despite large ITD_p differences; i.e., 0.417 msec for 200 Hz, 0.167 msec for 500 Hz, and 0.083 msec for 1,000 Hz. Although the ITD_p that results with free-field stimulation is related to signal frequency and source position, the time differences are not sufficient to account for the finding that lateralization is based on IPD (20). For example, the signal source must be at approximately 30° azimuth to produce an ITD_p of 0.4 msec for 200 Hz, at 15° to produce an ITD_p of 0.16 msec for 500 Hz, and at less than 15° to produce an ITD_p of 0.1 msec for 1,000 Hz. As human subjects are sensitive to less than a 2° change in azimuth when the signal source with a frequency between 200 and 1,000 Hz is moved anywhere between 0° and 30° azimuth (27), they would not confuse the location of a 200-Hz source at 30° azimuth with the location of a 500-Hz source at 15° azimuth. It has been argued that since the binaural system utilizes IPD to lateralize low-frequency signals, it must compare ITD_p between matched frequency components to localize a signal source (25).

Group Time Differences

The third ITD, the group delay or ITD_g, is the interaural delay between the envelopes of acoustic signals that vary in amplitude over time (Fig. 3D). For example, an interaural delay, ITD, between steady-state, complex waveform signals presented through earphones produces an IPD for each frequency component of the complex signal that is proportional to the ITD and to the frequency of the component. The relationship between IPD and the frequency is linear and has a slope that describes the ITD_g and that is equal to the ITD (IPD = ITD$\cdot f$) (28). Free-field presentation of a steady-state, pure tone signal may also produce an ITD_g. Acoustic signals that are reflected off the surfaces of the body, head, and pinna produce a compound wave as the incident wave combines with its time-delayed replications. The compound wave travels along the surface of the head at a velocity that is frequency dependent (12). For pure tone burst signals delivered free field to mannequins, the ITD_g is identical to the ITD_t and ITD_p at high frequencies (i.e., at greater than 2,000 Hz for the adult human) (12). According to the analysis of Roth et al. (21), the ITD_g is equal to the ITD_p for free-field delivered, low-frequency tone bursts (i.e., below 500 Hz for the adult human) and only influences measures of the ITD_p for frequencies between 500 and 2,000 Hz. It is in this frequency range that the largest shifts in ITD_p are measured for the mannequin without a torso (20). As the stimulus conditions that produce ITD_g also produce interaural envelope differences and/or interaural spectral differences, binaural processing under these stimulus conditions are examined in the sections covering the interaural envelope and spectral differences.

Interaural Level Difference

When a sound source is located off the midsagittal plane, sound waves may be reflected off the side of the head and pinna at the radiated ear, creating a sound shadow at the opposite ear and an interaural level difference or ILD (Fig. 3C). The effectiveness of the head and pinna as a sound barrier depend on the head-pinna size and the wavelength of the acoustic signal. In the case of the human, the head-pinna size is large compared to the wavelengths of signals with frequencies greater than 1,500 to 2,000 Hz. For the cat, signals with frequencies greater than 2,500 to 3,000 Hz should be attenuated by the head and pinna. At frequencies below 1,000 Hz, the head-pinna is small compared to the wavelength of the signal, and the signal will tend to travel around the head with little attenuation.

The cat has relatively large pinnae that are located on the dorsal surface of the head and are mobile. Their physical prominence is indicative of their important role in binaural hearing in the cat. In addition to its sound shadowing effect, the pinna has a directional pressure-gain effect that contributes to the ILD (29,31). For example, when the signal source is located anywhere in the frontal plane, the ratio of the pressure measured at the tympanic membrane of one ear to the pressure measured in the free field is greater than one. With the signal source at 0° azimuth, the gain at one ear (expressed as a pressure ratio in dB) increases with frequency from approximately 5 dB below 1,000 Hz to approximately 20 dB at 4,000 Hz and decreases to less than 5 dB at 12,000 Hz for anesthetized cats (29). While the gain is produced by both the pinna and external auditory canal, the contribution of the pinna is especially important to binaural hearing because its gain effect is directionally dependent. For example, a signal source with a frequency greater than 6,000 Hz located at 30° to 60° azimuth will produce a pressure gain in the cat of 10 to 20 dB above that produced when the signal source is located at 0° azimuth (30). The directional gain properties of the human pinna, as determined from mannequins, are greatest for frequencies above 2,500 Hz and at 40° to 60° azimuth (12).

The pinna gain effect is counteracted by its shadowing effect when a sound source is directed toward the opposite ear. Consequently, when the sound source is directed toward one ear of a cat, pressure measurements at the tympanic membrane of the opposite ear indicate that (a) at the opposite ear, there is no or little pressure gain to signals with frequencies below 1,000 Hz; (b) a gain of less than 10 dB occurs with signal frequencies between 1,000 and 5,000 Hz; and (c) a loss of 10 dB occurs with signal frequencies at and above 8,000 Hz (29). The sound shadow effect also varies with signal location and is greatest in cats for signals with frequencies at and above 14,000 Hz (30). For the cat, the external parts of the pinna appear to increase pressure at the tympanic membrane for frequencies above 1,000 Hz when the source is directed toward the ear and to decrease pressure for frequencies above 3,000 Hz when the source is directed toward the opposite ear (29). Thus, the pinna contributes to the ILD by producing a gain in pressure at the ear facing the sound source and by decreasing the pressure at the opposite ear through its sound shadowing effect.

At all azimuth locations in the frontal plane, the ILD is minimal and changes little with signal position for steady-state, low-frequency signals, i.e., below 1,500 Hz for humans and below 3,000 Hz for cats (30,31). At higher frequencies, the ILD increases with azimuth but in a complex manner. For some high-frequency signals, the ILD may increase monotonically as the signal source moves from 0° azimuth and may reach a maximum value at approximately 40° to 60° azimuth (Fig. 2, left). For other high-frequency signals, the ILD may exhibit large variations with small shifts in azimuth and produce multiple peaks and valleys in the ILD/azimuth functions (30). At these frequencies, the ILD would provide unreliable cues for signal source localization. For cats, the ILD at 90° azimuth is less than 5 dB at frequencies below 2,000 Hz, increases to a maximum of approximately 25 dB at 8,000 Hz, drops to approximately 15 dB at 16,000 Hz, and fluctuates between 20 and 30 dB at higher frequencies (29,30). For humans, the ILD at 90° azimuth is less than 5 dB at frequencies below 500 Hz, increases to a maximum of approximately 20 dB at 6,000 Hz, drops slightly at 8,000 Hz, and increases back up to 20 dB at 12,000 Hz (31).

The relationships between the ILD and the perceived lateral position of *earphone-delivered* signals are reported to be similar over a considerable range of signal frequencies (200–5,000 Hz), levels (30, 50, and 70 dB above threshold), and durations (20, 100, and 500 msec) (32). Thus, unlike the ITD_p, the ILD can serve as a binaural cue in sound lateralization for low- and high-frequency signals. The range of ILDs that can be used as a binaural localization cue is similar to that normally produced by the head and pinna. The minimum detectable ILD is less than 1 dB for cats and humans (23). For humans, the maximum ILD that produces a fused lateralized image is between 10 and 30 dB (33). Beyond this maximum ILD, the acoustic image may become diffuse and split into multiple images (11).

Interaural Envelope Differences

In recent years, research from many laboratories has demonstrated that although human listeners cannot lateralize on the basis of ITD_p between high-frequency stimuli, they can lateralize on the basis of ITD between comparable peaks of complex signals such as high-frequency clicks, amplitude-modulated, high-frequency tones (Fig. 2D), and high-frequency bandpass noise (22,34–37). Interaural disparities produced by time-varying signals are often termed interaural envelope differences (IED). The sinusoidal amplitude-modulated (SAM) tone is an example of a signal that produces time-varying interaural disparities. The signal is a carrier tone of frequency, f_c, that has its amplitude varied at a modulator frequency, f_m. The formula for this signal is $(1 + a\cos2\pi f_m t)\cos2\pi f_c t$. The waveform consists of three components, the f_c, and two sidebands, $f_c + f_m$ and $f_c - f_m$.[4] When the depth of modulation is one, the sidebands have half the amplitude of the carrier. When only the carrier is delayed, the

---

[4]This statement is easily proven using trigonometric identities. Because $\cos\alpha\,\cos\beta = \frac{1}{2}[\cos(\alpha+\beta) + \cos(\alpha-\beta)]$, we have $(1+\alpha\cos2\pi f_m t)\cos2\pi f_c t = \cos2\pi f_c t + \frac{\alpha}{2}[\cos2\pi(f_c+f_m)t + \cos2\pi(f_c-f_m)t]$.

phases of the three components of the signal are delayed by the same amount (28).[5] The phase shift, IPD, is determined by the time delay and frequency of the carrier. When only the modulator is delayed, the carrier phase is not shifted while the phases of the two sidebands move in opposition, the lower sideband is advanced (i.e., a leading IPD for $f_c - f_m$), and the upper sideband is delayed (i.e., a lagging IPD for $f_c + f_m$). Consequently, a modulator delay produces a phase difference spectrum (phase difference as a function of frequency) with a slope that is equal to the time delay and is termed the group delay ITD_g. When the entire signal is delayed, the effect is the sum of delaying the carrier and modulator; all components are phase shifted to produce both ITD_p and ITD_g. The interaural disparities generated by filtered clicks or filtered noise can also be described in terms of ITD_p and ITD_g (38). Since the binaural system is insensitive to ITD_p between high-frequency sinusoids, it should only be sensitive to the ITD_g of modulator and signal delay of complex high-frequency signals. Note that these two delays—modulator (envelope) and signal—also produce a time-varying ILD (ILD_t) during the period of the time delay. Most psychoacoustical studies of binaural lateralization based on IED between high-frequency signals have been carried out on highly trained human subjects as the IED are often very difficult to detect. Therefore, the following describes the abilities of humans, rather than of cats, to use IED cues in binaural lateralization experiments.

Comparison of lateralization performance

with time-varying, low-frequency and high-frequency signals illustrates the relative importance of the ITD_p and ITD_g/ILD_t cues. The threshold ITD_t required to localize a low-frequency filtered click is less than half that of a high-frequency filtered click when both are presented with a wideband noise, i.e., 0.07 and 0.157 msec, respectively (39). Presumably, low-frequency clicks elicit shorter ITD_t thresholds because they produce ITD_ps that dominate as binaural cues. The high-frequency clicks, even in the presence of a wideband masker, also produced low-frequency ITD_p cues: The addition of a lowpass noise masker to the high-frequency click increased their threshold ITD_t to 0.263 msec. These results suggest that there may be more than one system processing ITD_t cues: one that is low frequency, IPD sensitive, and responsive to short ITD_ts and one that is high frequency and ILD sensitive and requires longer ITD_ts than the low-frequency system. Henning (38) has argued that because introducing ITD_g between low-frequency clicks did not result in lateralization, the auditory system is insensitive to ITD_g in low-frequency signals. However, when the ITDs in a modulator and a SAM low-frequency carrier were in opposition, i.e., the modulator lagging ($-ITD_g$) and the carrier leading ($+ITD_p$), the signal was lateralized toward the ear receiving the leading carrier signal, but not as far lateral as when the ITD is between the entire signal (37). That is, the ITD_p was the strongest binaural cue for low-frequency signals, but other interaural disparities, e.g., ITD_g/ILD_t, also affected binaural perceptions.

Introducing an ITD between complex high-frequency signals of long duration also resulted in lateralization of the signal. However, the ITD required for lateralizing high-frequency bandpass noise was much longer than that required for lateralizing low-frequency bandpass noise; i.e., 0.062 msec for a 3,056 to 3,344 Hz bandpass noise and 0.014 msec for a 425 to 600 Hz bandpass noise (22). These noise signals were 1.4 sec

---

[5]This result is easily shown using the trigonometric identity approach. To delay a signal by Δ means replacing t by $t - \Delta$ in its formula. For a sinusoid, this time delay becomes a phase shift: $\cos 2\pi f(t - \Delta) = \cos(2\pi f t - 2\pi f \Delta)$. The phase shift is therefore $2\pi f \Delta$. To delay only the carrier means the amplitude-modulated signal becomes $[1 + a\cos 2\pi f_m t]\cos 2\pi f_c(t - \Delta)$. Expanding this expression, as in the previous footnote, shows that the delay corresponds to the same phase shift in each component.

in duration, with slow (300 msec) rise/fall times and presented with a signal delay that produced interaural disparities in the signal microstructure (ITD_p) and macrostructure (ITD_g). Low-frequency noise was not used to mask possible low-frequency distortion products in the high-frequency bandpass noise. The shorter threshold ITD for low-pass noise indicates that ITD_p served as the main interaural disparity cue for low-frequency noise and that the ITD_g may have served as the main cue for high-frequency noise. The difference between the ITD_t thresholds to high-frequency clicks (0.157 msec) and high-frequency noise (0.062 msec) may be related to differences in signal duration (11). For SAM high-frequency carriers, a modulator delay resulted in lateralization over a limited range of modulator frequencies (40). When a carrier frequency of 3,000 to 5,000 Hz was amplitude-modulated at 50 Hz, a modulator delay greater than 0.6 msec was required for lateralization. Because the component frequencies of high-frequency carriers that were amplitude-modulated at 50 Hz were above 2,000 Hz (e.g., with f_c at 3,000 Hz, $f_c - f_m$ is 2,950 Hz and $f_c + f_m$ is 3,050 Hz), the binaural system could not have detected an IPD between individual components of the signal. The length of the threshold modulator delay (approximately 0.6 msec) indicates that the ITD_g must be of fairly long duration to produce a detectable IED at low modulator frequencies. Increasing the modulator frequency to 100 Hz produced lateralization with a modulator delay of 0.2 msec. The shortest modulator delay to produce lateralization was 0.083 msec when the carrier frequency was 4,017 Hz and the modulator frequency was 250 Hz. Above 250 Hz, the threshold delay increased as modulator frequency was increased, with threshold increases occurring at lower modulator frequency for lower carrier frequency. For example, with a modulator of 450 Hz, the modulator delay required to lateralize a SAM tone was nearly 1 msec for a 3,017-Hz carrier and less than

0.3 msec for a 5,017-Hz carrier. The binaural processes involved in lateralizing these SAM signals apparently did not involve low-frequency binaural processing; intense low-frequency masking did not eliminate lateralization and introducing time delays between a SAM high-frequency signal in one ear and a pure tone at the modulator frequency in the opposite ear did not result in binaural lateralization (36).

It has been suggested that the interaural disparities occurring during the rising edges of transient segments in a time-varying, high-frequency signal could be considered transient ILD (39). For example, the ITD_t between high-frequency signals may be an ILD_t that lasts the duration of the onset delay. Presumably, the threshold ITD_ts to high-frequency signals are longer than those to low-frequency signals because the binaural system requires a longer sample time to process ITD_t or ITD_g than to process ITD_p. In addition, the magnitude of the high-frequency signal presumably influences the ITD_g threshold such that a shorter sample time is required for signals with greater magnitude (17). The relationship between the threshold ITD of a SAM high-frequency carrier signal and the modulator frequency support this view: If the modulator frequency is very low, a large ITD is required to produce an ILD_t of sufficient magnitude and duration for the signal to be lateralized. Whereas, if the modulator frequency is higher, a shorter delay will produce an ILD_t of sufficient magnitude and duration for lateralization. However, if the modulator frequency is too high, the delay required to produce a ILD_t of sufficient magnitude may be too short in duration for the binaural system to process. One difficulty with this argument is that if the ILD_t were the only basis for lateralization of modulator-delayed, SAM high-frequency signals, all high-frequency carriers should exhibit similar upper modulation frequency limits. According to Nuetzel and Hafter (36), lower carrier frequencies exhibit lower modulation frequency limits.

Interaural Spectral Differences

Psychophysical and neurophysiological studies of binaural processing have primarily used signals delivered through earphones. If the ITD or ILD of earphone-delivered signals are within "normal range," the sensation produced is one of a sound source localized within or near the head that is "lateralized" toward the left or right depending on the values of the interaural cues. When an acoustic signal is delivered in the free field, a number of additional cues result that produce a sensation of a signal generated by an externalized source localized somewhere in space. For example, the shoulders, head, and pinna reflect and diffract the acoustic signal, creating time-delayed replications of the acoustic signal. The scattered waves interact with the incident waves to produce gains, losses, and time shifts in the signal that modify the effective spectrum reaching the ears (41). The geometry of the pinna indicates that it would be most effective at reflecting higher frequency signals, i.e., those with frequencies greater than 3,000 to 6,000 Hz (42,43). Based on measures from mannequins, it has been determined that the body torso is primarily responsible for the reflection of signals with frequencies below 2,000 Hz, while the pinna reflections occur predominantly for signals with frequencies above 4,000 Hz (12). Pinna reflection in the cat occurs at frequencies greater than 1,000 Hz and are maximal near 4,000 Hz (29,44).

It has been argued that pinnae asymmetries produce interaural spectral differences (ISD) that play a role in binaural processing. For example, when differences in spectra were introduced between earphone-delivered signals, the signals were "externalized" and perceived as produced by a free-field sound source (42). If the two ears were symmetrical, binaural difference cues would not be produced with a sound source located in the median vertical plane, i.e., located at, above, or below the horizontal plane at 0° azimuth. However, binaural localization is more accurate than monaural localization in the median vertical plane (42) and is most effective for wideband signals containing high frequencies (42,45). For cats, the smallest detectable displacement of a tone source (the minimum audible angle [MAA]) in the median vertical plane was nearly five times that of noise, i.e., MAA of 16° for a 2,000-Hz tone versus 3.4° for a broadband noise (46). For humans, binaural localization in the median vertical plane is most accurate to complex signals with energy in the 8,000- to 16,000-Hz range (47). The greater sensitivity to changes in the spatial location (i.e., the smaller MAA) of noise signals compared to low-frequency and high-frequency signals is considered to be due in part to the greater availability of spectral cues in noise signals (46). An ISD created by introducing an ITD between earphone-delivered complex signals can also be used as a binaural cue. For example, with earphone delivery the threshold ITD of wideband noise (0.006 msec) is nearly half that of low-frequency tones (the shortest at 0.011 msec for 1,000 Hz) (22,48).

BINAURAL PROCESSING IN THE SUPERIOR OLIVARY COMPLEX

Neural Models of Binaural Processing

Numerous theoretical models have been developed to describe binaural phenomena (49). Rayleigh (50) identified two basic cues utilized in binaural sound localization, the IPD for low-frequency sinusoids and the ILD for high-frequency sinusoids, and thus was one of the earliest proponents of the *duplex theory of sound localization*. According to this theory, two separate systems operate in binaural hearing: The low-frequency system utilizes the IPD, which results when the signal has a wavelength that is greater than the distance between the two ears (Fig. 3B). The high-frequency system operates on the ILD created by the acoustic shadowing effects of the head and pinna (Fig. 3C). Early neural models of sound localization dealt primarily with specifying the characteristics of the neural processing of IPD. These models hypothesized interaction in the central nervous system that was dependent on stimulus-related neural discharges whose timing was critical to IPD processing (24,51,52). According to these models, an IPD processor receives excitatory inputs from the two ears (Ex/Ex)[6] that elicit a discharge from the processor only when the input discharges are coincident in their times of arrival at the processor. A basic assumption in these models is that the timing of the inputs to the IPD central processor is related to the periodicity or frequency of the stimulus. That is, the input neurons must generate discharges that are synchronized to a certain phase of the tonal stimulus. Consequently, the IPD is represented as a time difference between the discharges originating from the two ears. The timing of the discharges from the ear providing the leading input must be offset by a time delay—a neural time delay—to provide coincident inputs at the IPD processor neuron. Thus, some IPD neurons receive a time-delayed ipsilateral input to compensate for the ITD_p that results when signals are directed toward the ipsilateral ear, while other IPD neurons receive a time-delayed contralateral input to compensate for the ITD_p that results when the signals are directed toward the contralateral ear. Presumably, for each detectable IPD there exists a specific set of central

processor neurons that receive an input with a fixed neural time delay that is similar to the ITD_p. When a match occurs between the ITD_p and a neural time delay, the inputs from the two ears arrive simultaneously (or within a short period of time) at an IPD processor neuron, and the IPD neuron discharges. Thus, the IPD processor is basically a coincidence detector or cross-correlator that operates on the phase-locked discharge of its low frequency sensitive inputs (49). The IPD, which is determined "computationally" by matching the ITD_p to a neural time delay, is represented spatially in the IPD processor nucleus by the location of the neuron with a neural time delay matched to the ITD_p.

There is a neurophysiological basis for the hypothesis that the binaural inputs to the IPD central processor are carrying temporal information that can be used in coincidence detection or cross-correlation. The discharges of cat auditory nerve fibers and of certain cat cochlear nuclear neurons occur with greater probability during one half cycle of a sinusoid provided the sinusoid frequency is below 7,000 Hz (53–55). The degree of this "phase-locking" is strong (i.e., the distribution of interspike intervals with respect to a given phase of the sinewave is narrow) to sinusoids with frequencies below 2,000 Hz. The phase-locking decreases with increases in frequencies up to 5,000 to 7,000 Hz. The ability to phase-lock to low-frequency sinusoids is not related to the tuning characteristics of neurons, i.e., auditory nerve fibers maximally sensitive to high-frequency tones will phase-lock to low-frequency tones provided the stimulus level is sufficient to excite the fiber. With low-frequency stimuli, the rate of discharge and the degree of phase-locking increase with increases in stimulus level (56). These phase-locked discharges may provide the inputs necessary for determining the IPD of signals with frequencies less than 3,000 Hz that cats use in binaural lateralization (23). Following the report of Galambos and co-workers that the discharges of MSO units

---

[6]A standard notation for binaurally responsive neural units has been defined to describe general response characteristics. If stimulation of either ear causes an increase in rate of discharge, the unit is said to be Ex/Ex (Excitatory/Excitatory). The first letter pair denotes the response induced by stimulation of the ipsilateral ear, the second the contralateral. If one side excites while stimulation of the other ear causes a decrease in the rate of discharge (inhibits), the unit is categorized an Ex/In unit or an In/Ex unit, depending on which side inhibits the response.

were related to ITD_t between click stimuli, models of binaural processing have attributed the initial site of the detection and encoding of interaural time/phase differences to the MSO (8,57–59). The mechanisms producing the hypothesized neural time delay in the leading input channel have not been identified.

The theories that equate sound localization to the detection of time differences between the phase-locked discharges of binaural inputs have difficulty in dealing with the observation that there is also a binaural advantage over monaural detection and localization of high-frequency stimuli (60). It is generally accepted that the ILD and the ITD (i.e., the ITD_t and ITD_g) are used in the binaural processing of high-frequency signals. Theories of binaural hearing account for the utilization of these high-frequency binaural cues (49) by hypothesizing a second central processor that detects differences between the latency and/or magnitude of the responses of its binaural inputs. The latency and magnitude of the input responses are related to the stimulus level at each ear and can be compared to determine the ILD and ITD. If the ITD_t and ITD_g can be described in terms of transient ILD, only an ILD processor is required to utilize both ILD and ITD high-frequency cues (61). The inputs to the ILD processor must be Ex/In or In/Ex opponent types (62); that is, the input from one ear excites the ILD processor neurons, while the input from the opposite ear inhibits these neurons. The ILD processor neurons discharge when the excitatory input is greater than the inhibitory input (i.e., when an ILD exists) or when the excitatory input leads the inhibitory input (i.e., when an ITD_t or ITD_g exists). Because the LSO consists predominantly of Ex/In neurons sensitive to ILD, it is assumed to be the ILD central processor nucleus for high-frequency (i.e., >1,000–3,000 Hz) signals (62–64).

The neural processing of binaural information plays an important role not only in the localization of sound sources but also in the extraction of signals out of noise. In fact, binaural hearing provides significant advantages in signal detection and speech intelligibility in a noisy background, especially in a normal listening environment. This binaural advantage is considered by some to result from the neural processing of binaural cues, especially those produced by acoustic defraction effects in reverberant environments that result in the spatial separation of the signal and noise sources. Stimulus conditions that optimize performance in spatial localization and signal-in-noise detection produce a single fused sound image that is externalized, i.e., involve ISD cues. Those stimulus conditions that decrease performance produce a diffuse, fluctuating image or multiple images. According to the localization theory of binaural hearing, the neural processing of acoustic signals used in binaural sound localization is considered to be similar to those functioning in the binaural extraction of a signal from a noisy background (65). No other central processors need be proposed: For example, the IPD and ILD processors receive input from two separate groups of input neurons. Each of the input neurons responds to a limited band of stimulus frequencies and is maximally sensitive to a specific frequency of sound, the characteristic frequency (CF). Each of these neurons provide input to specific IPD or ILD processor neurons that are, in turn, tonotopically organized, i.e., spatially with respect to CF, within the IPD and ILD processor nuclei. Thus, the spatial distribution of the responding binaural neurons represents both the frequency components in the ISD and the IPD of the low-frequency components, while the level of activity and the number of active neurons represent the ILD. In the binaural extraction of a signal-in-noise, an organism may orient its head and ears to minimize interaural disparities in the signal of interest while maximizing interaural disparities in the background noise or vice versa. There is some controversy over whether the subjective perception of lateral position is a necessary part of binaural signal-in-noise detection and discrimination (66–68). Not all agree that the acoustic and sensory cues used in binaural signal detection and binaural sound localization are identical and are processed by the same or different neural mechanisms.

Neural Processing in the Superior Olivary Complex

The question of how interaural disparities are determined and represented by putative ITD and ILD processor neurons can be best answered by examining the responses of the neurons to interaural disparities. At the level of the SOC these responses have been measured extracellularly, most commonly by recording single-unit action potentials with metal electrodes. The responses to monaural and binaural stimulation are routinely determined. SOC units may be excited by stimulation of either ear (Ex/Ex), excited by stimulation of the ipsilateral ear only (Ex/No), excited by stimulation of the contralateral ear only (No/Ex), excited by stimulation of the ipsilateral ear and inhibited by stimulation of the contralateral ear (Ex/In), etc. Binaural stimulation may result in a discharge rate greater than that elicited by stimulating one ear alone (Ex/Ex:Sum or Ex/No:Fac) or in a discharge rate less than that resulting from stimulating one ear alone (Ex/In:Sub). The tuning curves (the signal frequencies and levels necessary to elicit a response) with monaural and binaural stimulation are determined to ascertain the degree of match between the tuning of the binaural inputs and the complexity of the binaural interaction, e.g., the contralateral input may have excitatory and inhibitory effects depending on stimulus frequency and/or level.

The latency of the response to monaural and binaural stimulation may be measured at different signal levels to determine whether the latency shifts with monaural signal level, with ILD, and with ITD_t. The

coefficient of variation (the standard deviation divided by the mean) (CV) of the latency of the first spike to repeated monaural stimuli has been used as an indicator of the ability of a neuron to measure signal onset time and thus encode ITD_t (69). Rate-level functions relating the discharge rate (spikes/sec) to signal level are also measured under monaural and binaural stimulus conditions to determine whether discharge rate can be used to encode ILD. The temporal pattern or statistical properties of the discharges to monaural and binaural stimuli are also important features of the neural response that may be related to stimulus conditions. The period histogram describes the timing of discharges relative to the positive zero-crossing times of the individual cycles in the tonal stimulus and is used to provide a graphic illustration of phase-locked discharges. The mean period is the average time between the positive zero-crossing time of the tone and the time of occurrence of a discharge. The synchronization index is a scalar measure of the strength or degree of phase-locking and is measured from the period histogram (56). The synchronization index is zero when the period histogram is flat (i.e., when there is no phase-locking) and is one when all discharges are contained in one bin of the period histogram. The association of a maximal discharge rate and a maximal synchronization index with a specific ITD_p for a group of SOC units has been interpreted as evidence that these SOC units are capable of detecting and encoding IPD (64). As similar first-spike latencies and discharge rates may be elicited under monaural and binaural conditions, other graphic and statistical measures are used to examine the relationship between neural responses and stimulus conditions. The poststimulus onsets-time (PST) histogram illustrates the relationship between the timing of stimulus-elicited discharges and the stimulus onset time (Fig. 4). It may be used to describe the relationship between the time course of neural discharges and the time course of in-

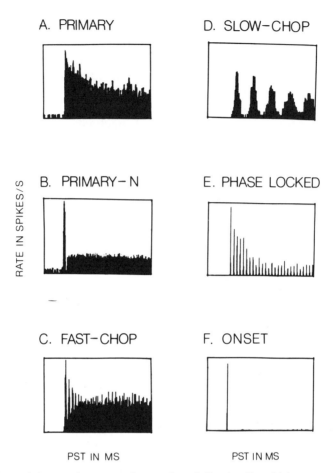

A. PRIMARY

D. SLOW-CHOP

B. PRIMARY-N

E. PHASE LOCKED

C. FAST-CHOP

F. ONSET

RATE IN SPIKES/S

PST IN MS   PST IN MS

FIG. 4. Illustrations of the most common types of poststimulus time histograms generated by the discharges of cat superior olivary complex units to tone-burst stimuli. The instantaneous rate of discharge is plotted as a function of the time relative to the tone-burst onset. The primary-like histograms (**A** and **B**) are similar to those generated by the first-order afferents of the auditory system. The chopper-type (**C** and **D**) histograms first appear in the cochlear nuclear complex. The intervals between the peaks in the histograms are not related to the stimulus frequency. They represent discharges that are time-locked to the tone-burst onset. The initial discharges in the fast-chopping histogram occur at a higher rate than those in the slow-chopping histogram and produce narrower chopping peaks with shorter interpeak intervals. The interpeak periods in phase-locked (**E**) histograms are related to the tone frequency. Phase-locked histograms are produced by discharges to low-frequency (<2–5 kHz) tones. The onset (**F**) histograms are characterized by a transient high rate of discharge that cannot be sustained beyond the first 10 to 15 msec of the response. In the lateral superior olive, an onset histogram is indicative of cell injury.

teraural disparities between high-frequency signals, such as pure tones with ILD and high-frequency bandpass noise bursts and high-frequency clicks with ITD. In the case of the SAM signals, the PST histograms could be generated relative to the positive, zero-crossing time of the individual cycles of the modulating sinusoid, creating a SAM period histogram. A SAM synchronization index may be determined from the SAM period histogram and used as a measure of discharge synchronization to monaural amplitude modulation and of the ability to detect/encode interaural disparities in the

SAM signals. Other measures of the interspike intervals in discharges to monaural and binaural signals may also reveal some aspects of the neural processes involved in binaural hearing. The interval histogram describes the distribution of interspike interval times between successive spikes in a response. The interval histograms of some SOC neurons have been described to be related to monaural and binaural stimulus conditions: They are unimodal with monaural stimulation and can be bimodal with binaural (ILD) stimulation (70). The CV of the interspike intervals is often used as a measure of the regularity of the discharges, e.g., discharges with interspike interval CV less than 0.3 are described to be regular in occurrence (71,72). The ILD-sensitive SOC neurons produce similar discharge rates to monaural and binaural stimuli but exhibit differences in interspike interval CVs between monaurally elicited discharges (e.g., less than 0.3) and binaurally elicited discharges (e.g., greater than 0.5) with similar discharge rates (70). These measures indicate that the timing of the discharges of the ILD processor neurons may be very regular when elicited by monaural stimulation and irregular when elicited by binaural (ILD) stimulation.

Binaural Processing in the Medial Superior Olive

Because the MSO was one of the first auditory brainstem nuclei to be identified as receiving bilateral inputs and as sending its axons to "higher auditory centers," it has long been considered an integral part of the binaural information processing system (Fig. 1). It has been suggested that it is the first stage of the IPD processing system that compares the times of arrival of the discharges from the ipsilateral and contralateral ears (57). As the morphology of the MSO plays a major role in determining its response characteristics and our ability to record single-unit activity within it, salient

structural features will be described. In the cat, the cell soma of these neurons are arranged in two to four layers. Their dendrites are oriented perpendicular to the laminae and extend dorsolaterally and ventromedially from the cell soma. Each neuron's axon arises more often from a proximal dendrite than from the cell soma (73). The spherical/bushy cells of the most rostral portion of the anteroventral cochlear nucleus (AVCN) provide the principal input to the MSO (74–76). Axons from the AVCN are myelinated and of medium diameter (3–4 μm) with an estimated conduction velocity of 21 m/sec (77,78). The terminals of the ipsilateral AVCN end on the dorsolateral aspect of the neuron, while the terminals of the contralateral AVCN end on the ventromedial aspect of the neuron (7). The terminals appear as elongated (20 μm long and 1–2 μm thick) endings and as small (2-μm diameter) *boutons en passant* that originate from the elongated endings (79). Both types of terminal are found on the cell soma and dendrites, with broader elongated endings in the region of the cell soma. The elongated endings contain multiple areas of synaptic contact that are separated by areas ensheathed in glia (80–82). Finger-like terminals containing multiple sites of synaptic contact on cell soma (the end-bulbs or calyces of Held) have been associated with high fidelity between input and output events (one to one in the MNTB) and are believed to achieve this fidelity by a synchronized release of neurotransmitter from multiple sites when an action potential invades the terminal (83). AVCN neurons that feature this type of synaptic organization exhibit response characteristics and upper frequency limits in phase-locking that are similar to those of auditory nerve fibers and are termed *primary-like* (55,84). However, there is no evidence that MSO neurons phase-lock as well as AVCN primary-like units or that they produce action potentials characteristic of AVCN and MNTB neurons receiving the large terminals of Held. MSO neurons differ from these AVCN and MNTB neurons in possessing large dendritic fields and in receiving smaller endings that are distributed on soma and dendrites. Also, the interdigitation of myelin sheath between the sites of synaptic contact of the elongated endings on MSO neurons have not been observed in the AVCN or MNTB terminals of Held (85). Lindsey has argued that the myelin sheath between synapses indicate a sequential rather than a simultaneous activation of the synaptic sites that may help to maintain the temporal features of an input that is distributed in small packets over a relatively large space (82).

There may be an anatomical basis for a delay between the times of arrival of the ipsilateral and contralateral inputs to the MSO. No differences have been noted between the axon diameters of the ipsilateral and contralateral inputs to the MSO and both inputs are believed to end on cell soma and dendrites. If the axons were of the same diameter, the contralateral input, which must travel a greater distance (by approximately 5.5–7 mm) than the ipsilateral input, would arrive approximately 0.26 to 0.33 msec *after* the ipsilateral input. Unfortunately this delay is opposite to that required by the coincidence detector/cross-correlator model of the IPD processor neuron: The ipsilateral input (which would be stimulated first by a low-frequency signal source directed toward the ipsilateral ear) should be delayed to overcome the ITD.

It is extremely difficult to record single-unit discharges extracellularly from the MSO (86,87). The MSO generates a large extracellular field potential that consists of a fast component that resembles the cochlear microphonic and follows the waveform of the acoustic stimulus and a slow component that resembles the summating potential of the inner ear and produces a sustained shift in potential for the duration of the stimulus (8,88). The polarity of the slow component of the evoked potential and the phase difference between the fast

component and the sinusoidal stimulus are determined by the ear stimulated and the location of the recording electrode. Polarity and phase reversals occur in the cell layer, indicating that the potentials reflect a depolarizing current flow into MSO dendrites during acoustic stimulation (8,89). The level of background activity (the discharges of surrounding cells, fibers, and terminals) is also quite high within the MSO when recording with metal electrodes. The amplitudes of the evoked potential and background activity increase with stimulus level, making it extremely difficult to isolate the stimulus-evoked activity of single MSO units. While recording with high-impedance, fluid-filled micropipettes reduces the evoked potential and background noise levels, it also increases the probability of cell injury and of recording from axons of unknown origin (90). The difficult recording conditions and the anatomical features of the MSO (e.g., the thin laminar arrangement of the MSO, the close proximity of other SOC nuclei and the ventral nucleus of the lateral lemniscus, and the presence of scattered cells in the neuropil surrounding the MSO) require that extreme care be taken in identifying a recorded unit as an MSO neuron. Most studies purporting to have recorded from MSO units used no or faulty methods (the waveform of auditory evoked potentials and/or depth measures) in localizing units and failed to determine histologically the site of recordings marked by the recording electrodes. The results of the few studies that provided adequate descriptions of unit localization methods will be described (8,86,87,91,92).

Most units in the cat MSO are binaurally excited and produce narrow tuning curves with matching CF for Ex/Ex units (87). The units are tonotopically organized within the MSO, with a larger area representing low CF (<4 kHz) units compared to the area representing high CF (>10 kHz) units. A similar tonotopic organization and disproportionate representation of low CF units have been reported for the dog (93). The bat

MSO is considerably different from the cat and dog MSO in that it consists predominantly of units with CF between 20,000 and 90,000 Hz (92). There may be species differences in the response properties of the MSO as nearly equal proportions of Ex/Ex and In/Ex units were encountered in the albino rat and bat MSO (91,92). Few In/Ex units were found in the cat MSO; most In/Ex units were located rostrally in the ventral nucleus of the lateral lemniscus (87). According to the study of the dog SOC (which did not describe unit localization methods), approximately 90% of the "MSO" units ($n = 105$) were excited by stimulation of the contralateral ear and over 88% were binaurally responsive with 65% Ex/Ex, 17% In/Ex, and 8.5% Ex/In.

There is very little else known about the response characteristics of MSO units. The measures obtained from the albino rat may not be very representative of mammalian MSO unit responses since their unit thresholds were extremely high, i.e., 50 to 90 dB SPL, and since the sample included only units with CFs between 2,200 and 6,600 Hz (91). No discharge pattern measures were obtained from these units. The bat MSO is also unique in the predominance of high CF units (92). Some of these bat MSO units (7 of 31 units) responded with a phasic (onset) discharge to CF short (2- or 16-msec duration) tone bursts, while most (23 of 31 units) discharged tonically to the tone bursts. The latency of the first spike to the CF tone bursts (rise time of 0.5 msec) was similar to those of LSO units (i.e., 2–4 msec for 20 of 27 units) or slightly longer (i.e., 4–5 msec for 7 of 20 units). The discharge patterns of the few cat MSO units studied provide only examples of what may be representative of most mammalian MSO units (87,94): The distribution of the first-spike latency to click stimuli overlapped that of LSO units (i.e., was between 3–5 msec for four MSO units). Two MSO units produced irregular discharge patterns with interval histograms characterized as Poisson-like. One of these units phase-locked to low-frequency tones

and the second produced primary-like PST histograms to tone bursts (Fig. 4). The short tone-burst PST histograms of MSO units have also been described to be *primary-notch* type (94). Phasic discharge patterns are rarely (17 of 204 units) produced by cat SOC units and may be more typical of units in the caudal ventral nucleus of the lateral lemniscus, which also typically contain nearly equal proportions of Ex/Ex and In/Ex units (87,95).

The descriptions of MSO activity most often cited in the literature is that of dog SOC units that were attributed to the MSO (93). The discharge rates of high CF ($>1,500$ Hz) Ex/Ex units ($n = 4$) were related to the average binaural stimulus level and were little influenced by interaural phase or level differences. When the unit thresholds to ipsilateral and contralateral stimulation differed, the rate-level functions to binaural stimulation had greater dynamic range than the rate-level functions to monaural stimulation. The Ex/Ex units with CF below 1,000 Hz ($n = 6$) generated phase-locked discharges to tones with frequency between 277 and 629 Hz. There was a difference between the mean period of the ipsilateral discharges and that of the contralateral discharges (MPD) that was between 2.7% and 35% of the stimulus period, T. The MPD was assumed to result from a neural time delay that matched an ITD_p produced when the signal source is located off the midsagittal plane. The discharge rate and synchronization index of the binaurally elicited discharges varied systematically with ITD_p. The values of these measures were related to the stimulus frequency, the unit's MPD, and the direction of the ITD_p relative to the ear that produced the shortest mean period (i.e., the leading ear). In general, the discharge rate and synchronization index increased to maximum values as the delay of the tone at the leading ear approached the unit MPD and decreased to minimum values as this delay approached $MPD + T/2$. Increasing the delay of the signal at the ear that produced the longer mean period (i.e., the lagging ear) first decreased then increased the discharge rate and synchronization and produced maximum values at $T-$ MPD. Based on these results, it has been argued that low CF Ex/Ex units in the MSO are IPD-sensitive neurons that are driven maximally when the excitatory inputs from the two ears are coincident upon arrival and that are *inhibited* when the inputs arrive with a time difference that is equal to half of the period of the acoustic signal. The MPD is considered the neural time delay between the ipsilateral and contralateral inputs that, when matched with an ITD_p, results in the coincident arrival of the binaural inputs to the MSO Ex/Ex units. Accordingly, for each detectable ITD_p there would be within the MSO a specific group of low CF Ex/Ex neurons with an MPD that matched the ITD_p.

For half of the units, the MPD did not prove to be an accurate measure of the ITD_p necessary to maximize the binaural discharge rate and synchronization. The two Ex/Ex units with short MPD (0.07 and 0.098 msec) required no ITD_p and a third Ex/Ex unit required an ITD_p (0.2 msec) that was greater than the MPD (0.13 msec) to produce maximum rate and maximum synchronization. These three units had MPD within the range of ITD_p normally resulting in a fused binaural image in cat. None was as short as the threshold ITD_p for low-frequency signals. Assuming that the cat MAA is between 3° and 5° azimuth for tones below 1,000 Hz (46,96), the estimated threshold ITD_p is between 0.01 and 0.02 msec for a cat with a 5.2-cm head diameter (12). The shortest MPDs of Ex/Ex units (0.07 and 0.098 msec) correspond to ITD_p produced by low-frequency signal sources located at 17° and 25° azimuth (12). The three Ex/Ex units that produced maximal binaural response measures when the ITD_p nearly matched the MPD had MPD values (0.483–1.052 msec) that were similar to the ITD_p that results with a low-frequency signal source located beyond 90° azimuth. At 90° azimuth, the estimated ITD_p would be ap-

proximately 0.356 msec for low-frequency signals (12). However, for two of these three units the ITD_p producing the maximum binaural response was less than one-third of the period of the stimulus frequency. Based on human psychophysical studies, an ITD_p less than one-third of the frequency period should produce a fused sound image that is lateralized toward the ear receiving the leading signal (24,25). One of the units did require an ITD_p that was 39% of the period (IPD of 142.1°) of the stimulus frequency, i.e., an ITD_p that might produce a diffuse sound image difficult to lateralize.

With so few data available from low CF MSO units, it is difficult to conclude at this time whether the measures used to estimate the neural delay time (the MPD) and the match between the neural delay time and the ITD_p (the maximum rate and maximum synchronization index) are adequate indicators of IPD processor neuron function.

Binaural Processing in the Lateral Superior Olive

The LSO, which contains Ex/In units (Fig. 5), is considered to play a major role in ILD processing (62,63,93). In the cat, the LSO is an S-shaped nucleus located less than a millimeter from the MSO. Most neurons in the LSO are similar in shape to those within the MSO (97,98) but differ in the types and sources of terminals. The cell soma and dendrites of the LSO principal neurons are covered with smaller terminal boutons (7). Terminals containing small, flattened vesicles typical of inhibitory synapses are found on the cell soma, large dendrites, and proximal axon (99). Terminals containing large, round vesicles typical of excitatory synapses are located on the dendrites and appear to be the only type found on the most distal dendritic branches. Both types of terminals originate from myelinated axons and contain multiple points of synaptic specializations but are not invested with myelin. The input from the ip-

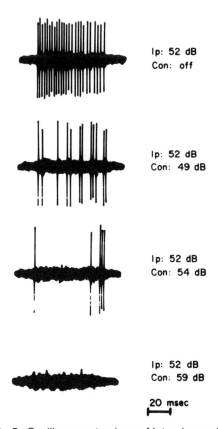

Ip: 52 dB
Con: off

Ip: 52 dB
Con: 49 dB

Ip: 52 dB
Con: 54 dB

Ip: 52 dB
Con: 59 dB

20 msec

FIG. 5. Oscilloscope tracings of lateral superior olive unit spike trains to monaural (ipsilateral) and binaural tone bursts. The stimulus levels (in dB SPL) for the ipsilateral (Ip) and contralateral (Con) ears are provided to the right of each trace. Increasing the contralateral stimulus level while holding the ipsilateral stimulus level constant produced a decrease in spike output. Note that at high contralateral stimulus levels the ipsilaterally elicited discharges can be completely inhibited during the tone burst. The characteristic frequency of the unit and the stimulus frequency were 35 kHz. The tone bursts were 60 msec in duration and were presented simultaneously to the two ears. (From ref. 109, with permission.)

silateral ear (Fig. 1) arises from the AVCN (74,76) and is carried primarily by medium-diameter (3–4 μm) myelinated axons (77, 78). The input from the contralateral ear is provided by the homolateral MNTB. The MNTB receives a contralateral input from the globular/bushy cells of the posterior AVCN (100) that is carried by large-diame-

ter (7–15 μm, mode of 9.5 μm) myelinated axons (77,78,101). These axons terminate as the large calyces of Held on the soma of MNTB principal neurons (102). These MNTB principal neurons are believed to correspond to the MNTB units that produce spike waveforms characterized by a positive potential that occurs 0.5 msec before each unit action potential and by primary-like discharge patterns (83,87,95). In the region of the LSO, the axons of the MNTB principal neurons are 3 to 9 μm (mode of 5.5 μm) in diameter (101).

The speed at which the ipsilateral and contralateral inputs travel to and influence LSO neurons is important in determining the ability of LSO units to process ITD_t and ITD_g. The contralateral input to the MNTB would be traveling over a slightly longer distance (approximately 7 mm) than the ipsilateral input to the LSO, but at nearly 2.7 times the conduction velocity of the ipsilateral input (57 m/sec : 21 m/sec). There is a synaptic delay at the MNTB of approximately 0.5 msec (83), however, the conduction velocity of the MNTB axon is approximately 1.6 times greater than that of the ipsilateral input to the LSO. Consequently, it is highly probable that the input from the contralateral ear reaches the LSO neurons at the same time as or before the input from the ipsilateral ear. It has been suggested that the terminals on the cell body, proximal dendrites, and proximal axon arise from the MNTB axons, while the terminals on the more distal dendrites arise from the medium-sized AVCN axons (99). If this were the case, the postsynaptic potentials produced by the MNTB (inhibitory) terminals closest to the spike generator site (presumably the axon hillock) would reach the spike generator sooner and with less degradation than the postsynaptic potentials produced by AVCN (excitatory) terminals located on the more distal dendrites. Consequently, the contralateral inhibitory input would have precedence over the ipsilateral excitatory input when no interaural time delay exists.

Electrophysiological recording conditions appear to be slightly better in the LSO than in the MSO. Although an extracellular field potential can be recorded in the cat LSO, it is smaller than that generated by the MSO (89). The dense packing of cell soma and terminal axons within the cat LSO results in a fairly high level of background noise, especially in low-frequency-sensitive areas. Therefore, there is considerable danger of injuring a neuron in attempting to isolate LSO single-unit activity from the background noise. The probability of injuring neurons and of recording from axons of unknown origin is much greater when recording with fluid-filled micropipettes than when recording with metal electrodes in the brainstem nuclei (90). Considerable care must be taken to establish the condition of units studied, especially in structures with unknown unit response characteristics. For example, fast adapting and transient (phasic or onset) type discharge patterns are associated with unit injury in the cat LSO (71). Because of the close proximity of surrounding SOC nuclei and the ventral nucleus of the lateral lemniscus, histological confirmation of marked recording sites is required to localize units. The few studies of the LSO that meet this requirement are included in this chapter (87,92,94,103,104).

All units in the cat LSO are excited by stimulation of the ipsilateral ear (87,103). Approximately half of those units with CFs between 1,000 and 3,000 Hz and virtually all units with CFs above 3,000 Hz are also inhibited by stimulation of the contralateral ear (105). Thus, in cats, who localize signals with frequencies above 3,000 Hz using ILD cues, most LSO units with CFs above 3,000 Hz are the Ex/In type. There appear to be species differences in the cell population of the LSO. Unlike the cat LSO, olivocochlear neurons comingle with afferent neurons in the rodent LSO (106–108). Also, in gerbils LSO units with CFs less than 1,000 Hz may be the Ex/In type (104). The cat LSO units produce excitatory tuning curves as narrow as those produced by cat

cochlear nuclear units and auditory nerve fibers (94). The LSO units are tonotopically organized with over two-thirds of the area of the cat LSO containing units with CFs greater than 3,000 Hz (103). The ipsilateral and contralateral inputs to the LSO Ex/In units are fairly well matched in their tuning characteristics: The CFs of the excitatory and inhibitory tuning curves are comparable. However, the tuning curve bandwidth of the inhibitory input is slightly wider than that of the ipsilateral (63,109).

The excitatory rate-level functions of cat LSO units are monotonic and reach maximum rates that range from approximately 80 spikes/sec to 700 spikes/sec to 200-msec duration CF tone bursts (109). The dynamic range of the excitatory rate-level functions (from threshold to the stimulus level producing the maximum rate) was between 15 and 50 dB, with the magnitude of the range related to the maximum rate, i.e., the lower the maximum rate the shorter the dynamic range (110). The maximum discharge rate and the slope of the excitatory rate-level functions were related to the stimulus frequency (110). While tones with frequencies below the unit ipsilateral/excitatory CF (CF_I) were capable of producing maximum rates similar to a tone at unit CF_I, tones with frequencies greater than the unit CF_I produced excitatory rate-level functions with lower maximum rates and lower slopes. The inhibitory rate-level functions generated by simultaneous binaural stimulation with 200-msec duration tone bursts set to the unit CF_I resembled the excitatory rate-level functions (63). The maximum rate inhibited, the dynamic range and slope of the inhibitory rate-level functions were determined by the stimulus level (i.e., the excitatory rate) at the ipsilateral ear (111). When the excitatory discharge was at or near the maximum rate, the contralateral stimulus often failed to totally inhibit the discharges: One or two spikes occurred at or following the termination of the tone bursts (63,112). Binaural stimulation with tones other than the unit CF_I produced similar results (109). In general, as the contralateral stimulus level was increased, the ipsilateral threshold increased, the maximum rate elicited decreased, and the slope of the inhibitory rate-function decreased (111). Consequently, when the ILD was held constant and the stimulus levels at the two ears increased, the discharge rate elicited did not remain constant. For example, when the ILD was held at 10 dB, the rate decreased by as much as 70% to 90% as the binaural stimulus level increased. As the LSO Ex/In unit discharge rates were related to the stimulus levels at the two ears, they did not provide an unambiguous clue to the ILD.

Since the presentation of an acoustic stimulus as simple as a monaural pure tone activates more than LSO units with CF_1 equal to the stimulus frequency, the spatial distribution of activity within the LSO was investigated by modeling the tuning curve and spike count measures to monaural and binaural (200-msec duration) tone-burst stimuli (109). When the monaural/ipsilateral tone burst was 10 dB above the threshold of units with CF_1 matched to the stimulus frequency, the simulated distribution of activity was centered over these units (Fig. 6). As the stimulus level was increased, the spike output of these units increased up to a limiting value, and units with CF_1 higher and lower than the stimulus frequency were activated. The spread of activity within the LSO was asymmetrical: a given increase in stimulus level exceeded the thresholds of more units with higher CF_1 (i.e., $CF_1 >$ the stimulus frequency) than units with lower CF_1. Also as the stimulus level was increased, the rate of increase in spike output was greater for higher CF_1 than for the lower CF_1 units. Increases in the monaural stimulus level produced broader and broader areas of units activated to maximum output. With binaural stimulation (ipsilateral level > contralateral level), the distribution of activity was dependent on the stimulus levels at the two ears and the ILD (Fig. 7). At moderate stimulus levels (ipsi-

lateral level <50dB), the distribution was flatter than that produced by a monaural stimulus at the same ipsilateral stimulus level. At higher stimulus levels, the activity of the units with CF_1 similar to the stimulus frequency was depressed while the activity of units with higher and lower CF_1 were not as severely depressed. Consequently, at the highest stimulus levels simulated, the model produced a bimodal distribution with very low levels of activity in the units that were maximally activated when the ipsilateral stimulus was presented alone (e.g., in Fig. 8 compare the spread of activity at Ip 20 Con 0 with the area of depressed activity at Ip 80 Con 60). This area of low activity was flanked by areas producing higher levels of activity.

The simulated distributions indicate that the stimulus level at the ipsilateral ear is related to the spread of activity in the LSO (i.e., the range of unit CF_1s activated) and that the ILD is related to the size of the depressed activity area. When the ILD was small, the spread of depressed activity was greater and only units with very high or low CF_1 were active at high stimulus levels (Fig. 8). With larger ILD, the spread of depressed activity was smaller and units with CF_1 nearer to the stimulus frequency produced higher levels of activity at high stimulus levels. The net result was that each pairing of ipsilateral and contralateral stimulus levels produced a unique distribution of activity. Although the distribution of activity might serve as a cue to indicate ILD and the ipsilateral and contralateral stimulus levels, this model ignores the possible role of the temporal pattern of LSO unit discharges in encoding binaural information.

The role of the temporal pattern of LSO unit discharges in binaural processing has been studied by examining the effect of the contralateral stimulus on the temporal pattern of the ipsilaterally elicited discharges. When the ipsilateral stimulus is at least 10 to 15 dB above unit threshold, LSO Ex/In units generated discharges that were sus-

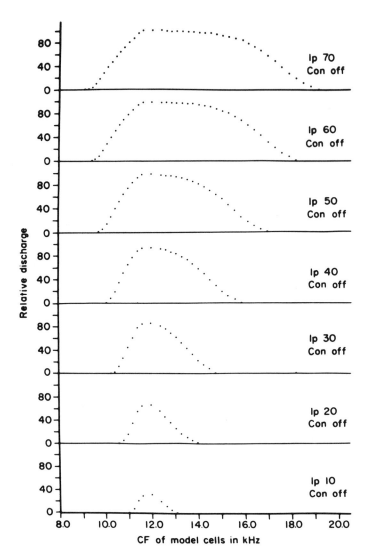

FIG. 6. The spatial distribution of lateral superior olivary unit responses to a monaural (ipsilateral) 12-kHz tone presented at different stimulus levels. The location in the lateral superior olive is indicated by the characteristic frequency (CF) of the unit. The magnitudes of the responses of units with similar CF are scaled relative to the maximum discharge elicited by a 12-kHz tone from units with CFs of 12 kHz. This distribution was simulated using models derived from the tuning curves and rate-level functions of the lateral superior olivary units. (From ref. 109, with permission.)

tained for the duration of the monaural stimulus (103) and that produced *chopper*-type PST histograms (Fig. 3C and D) (109). The sustained discharges of chopper units producing slow chopper-type PST histograms (Fig. 4D, characterized by wide peaks separated by interpeak intervals greater than 2 msec) occurred at rates less than 300 spikes/sec and generated symmetrically shaped interval histograms with interspike interval CVs less than 0.3 (70,71). Units that were capable of sustaining higher discharge rates produced a fast chopper

pattern characterized by an initial discharge that was tightly time-locked to the stimulus onset (Fig. 3C): The means of the interspike intervals of the first five spikes were less than 2 msec with standard deviation less than 0.55 msec. The sustained discharges of the fast chopper units generated less symmetrically shaped interval histograms and interspike intervals with CV less than 0.4. The regularity of the discharges of both types of units appeared to be maintained by pairing the occurrence of a short interspike interval with a longer one and a

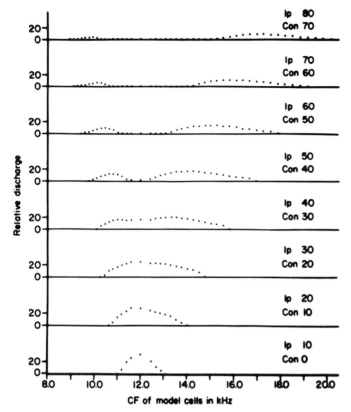

FIG. 7. The spatial distribution of lateral superior olivary unit responses to a binaural 12-kHz tone. The stimulus levels of the ipsilateral and contralateral tones are expressed in decibels above thresholds of the simulated units with characteristic frequency of 12 kHz. At all stimulus levels the interaural level difference was held to 10 dB. (From ref. 109, with permission.)

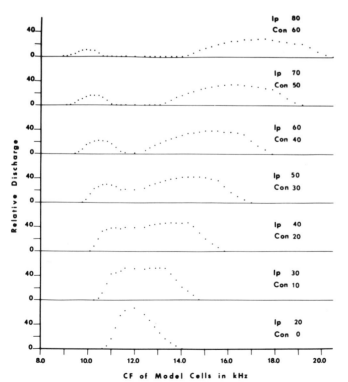

FIG. 8. The spatial distribution of lateral superior olivary unit responses to a binaural 12-kHz tone. At all stimulus levels the interaural level difference was held to 20 dB. (From ref. 109, with permission.)

long interspike interval with a shorter one. This type of serial dependence between successive interspike intervals produced conditional mean functions with a negative slope (71,113). Regularity in the discharge pattern of the fast chopper units appeared to be related to some degree to the ipsilateral stimulus level, while the discharge regularity of the slow chopper units did not appear to be as affected by stimulus level (113). The statistical measures of the discharge regularity and serial dependence of slow and fast chopper units fell along a continuum, indicating that these units may be considered as variations of a single population of LSO neurons. A third group of LSO Ex/In units, the *bimodal* units, generated sustained discharges to excitatory stimuli that were characterized by bimodal interval histograms and, in many cases, by a strong negative serial dependence. The CF tone burst-elicited discharges of the bimodal units were either the slow or fast chopper type. At moderate binaural stimulus levels with small ILD, the elicited discharges of all LSO units were observed to be less regular in pattern with many producing bimodal interval histograms. The first (short) mode in the interval histogram was related to the shortest intervals produced to the ipsilateral stimulus alone while the second mode was related to binaural stimulus levels.

The overall temporal pattern of the discharges to simultaneous binaural stimulation with CF_I tone bursts depended on the stimulus levels at the two ears (70,112). The gross time course of the inhibitory effect resembled that of the excitatory effect, i.e., the inhibition dropped off with time following stimulus onset. When the ipsilateral stimulus level was held constant and the contralateral level increased, the latency of inhibition decreased and the duration and magnitude of inhibition increased (Fig. 5). The shift in inhibitory latency with increases in contralateral stimulus level was manifested by the disappearance of successively earlier peaks in the PST histograms

of fast chopper units. Often high binaural stimulus levels with small ILD elicited phasic discharges to stimulus onset and offset, i.e., an *on-off* type response (e.g., Ip 52 dB Con 54 dB in Fig. 5). In many cases when the contralateral stimulus was of sufficient intensity, the first spike was inhibited, and, in some cases, only the discharge following the stimulus offset (an *off discharge*) remained. The gross temporal pattern of LSO Ex/In unit discharges to binaural tone bursts did not remain constant when the ILD was held constant and the binaural stimulus levels increased (112): As the binaural stimulus level was raised the discharge pattern shifted from a fast-adapting chopper type to an on-off type, and to an off type at the highest stimulus levels.

The LSO unit excitatory click latency has been described to be from 0.5 msec to over 1 msec longer than the click latency of primary-like MNTB units (94). The LSO unit excitatory latency to tone bursts with a 1-msec rise time was dependent on the stimulus frequency and level (105): It was shortest in response to CF tones and decreased with increases in stimulus level up to 15 to 20 dB above the unit's threshold. At stimulus levels between 15 and 35 dB above unit threshold, the standard deviation of the first-spike latency was less than 0.5 msec and the CV less than 0.3 (71), indicating that the first-spike discharge of LSO Ex/In units are strongly time-locked to the stimulus onset time. Stimulus level had a similar effect on the inhibitory response: Increasing the contralateral stimulus level decreased the latency of the inhibitory effect (112). Simultaneous stimulation of the two ears did result in inhibition of the first spike of the excitatory response of cat and gerbil Ex/In LSO units (63,104) but not of bat LSO Ex/In units (92). Stimulation of the contralateral ear at stimulus levels slightly below that required to inhibit the first-spike discharge to tone bursts did affect the timing (i.e., the CV) of the first-spike discharge of cat LSO Ex/IN units (112). Hence, in the cat and gerbil the presence, absence, or timing of the first-spike discharge of the excitatory response to binaural stimuli could be utilized to indicate ITD_t.

The effects of introducing an ITD_t between tone bursts (45 msec in duration, with 5-msec rise/fall times and with a repetition rate of 10 bursts/sec) on presumed LSO Ex/In unit responses have been studied in the cat (114). Unfortunately, the recording sites could not be marked with the fluid-filled micropipettes used in this study because of the small tips required to isolate single-unit discharges in the SOC. Most of these "LSO" units were the Ex/In type, although a few were the In/Ex type. The overall output (spikes/stimulus) of the Ex/In unit binaural response did not change when the stimulus levels were held constant and the ITD_t varied in 0.512-msec steps from a 2.048-msec lead to a 2.048-msec lag at the ipsilateral ear. However, the magnitude of the highest peak in the PST histogram of the binaural response increased as the ipsilateral lead time was increased from 0 msec. The peak magnitude at a given ITD_t was related to binaural stimulus levels: Increasing the binaural stimulus levels while holding the ILD constant (ipsilateral level > contralateral level) decreased the ITD_t necessary to produce an increase in peak response above that to an ITD_t of 0 msec. Consequently, the shortest ITD_t (0.512 msec) that produced a detectable increase in peak response occurred when the binaural stimulus levels were high. When the ITD_t was held constant and the ILD was increased by raising the ipsilateral stimulus level, the peak response increased in magnitude. Because increasing the ITD_t (ipsilateral leading) and increasing the ILD (ipsilateral greater) had similar effects on peak response magnitude, it was suggested that the magnitude of the peak response of "LSO" Ex/In units provided the basis for the phenomenon of time-intensity trading at high frequencies: For human subjects, the lateralization of highpass clicks with ITD_ts greater than 0.2 msec can be countered by increasing the level of the time-delayed signal (39). As the temporal features of the binaural responses to ITD_t and ILD stimuli were not examined in this study, it is unclear whether the time at which the peak response occurred shifted with ITD_t and/or ILD. Because the peak-response measures provided no evidence of a preference for ITD_t within "the physiological range" and exhibited inhibition even when the ipsilateral signal led the contralateral, it was concluded that neurons at higher levels of the auditory pathway would be required to sample from an array of "LSO" Ex/In units to determine the location of a signal source.[7]

Although the evidence that the LSO is involved in processing ILD is not in question, the involvement of this nucleus in processing ITD is not so clear. The initial time-locked discharges of LSO units may serve to encode ITD_t of high-frequency stimuli. If the relationship between the human threshold ITD_ts to high-frequency clicks with low-frequency masking and human threshold ITD_t to wideband clicks (0.263 and 0.01 msec, respectively) is similar in the cat, the cat threshold ITD_t to high-frequency clicks should be approximately 0.526 msec. Cat LSO units that produced a first-spike latency with standard deviation less than 0.5 msec should be capable of responding selectively to an ITD_t of 0.526 msec. The discharges of LSO units to SAM tones have not been studied. According to the data from human subjects, the ability of LSO units to respond to ITD_g produced by modulator delays should be related to the carrier and modulator frequencies. For humans, (a) carrier frequencies above 2,000 Hz produced shorter ITD_g thresholds than lower frequency carriers; (b) for a given carrier frequency, the ITD_g threshold first

---

[7]The shortest ITD_t used in the study (0.512 msec) was greater than the maximum ITD_t (0.435 msec) estimated to occur for a cat with an interaural distance of 7 cm (21). However, cats have been described to lateralize clicks with an ITD_t as great as 1.6 msec (18).

decreased and then increased as the modulator frequency was increased from 50 to 450 Hz; and (c) the modulation frequency at which the ITD_g threshold began to increase was related to the carrier frequency (i.e., the lower the carrier frequency, the lower the modulation frequency at which the threshold increased). In the LSO the unit CF would determine the carrier frequencies to which the unit will respond. What is not known is whether the LSO unit discharges will phase-lock to the modulation frequency of an ipsilaterally presented amplitude-modulated tone or whether such a phase-locked discharge is required for LSO unit encoding of modulator delays in binaurally presented amplitude-modulated tones.

CONCLUSIONS

The hypothesis that the low CF MSO units are spike-coincidence detectors is probably an oversimplification, as the synaptic organization of the MSO indicates that these neurons are not high fidelity units that produce one spike out for each spike in. The binaural interaction in MSO neurons probably involves the cross-correlation of intracellular potentials that are the sum of the individual excitatory postsynaptic potentials generated at each point of synaptic contact. If the extracellularly recorded MSO evoked potentials are summed dendritic potentials resulting from depolarizing current flow into MSO dendrites during synaptic activation (89), they reflect the waveform of the intracellular potential. The fast component waveform of the extracellular potential elicited by low-frequency stimuli resembles the waveform of the acoustic stimulus, i.e., it oscillates at the same frequency as the tonal stimulus (88). It is conceivable that during binaural stimulation the intracellular potential generated by stimulating one ear sum with that generated by stimulating the opposite ear when the potentials are in phase and subtract when they are out of phase. According to

this hypothesis, a spike is generated when the summed potentials exceed the membrane threshold.

The LSO does appear to fit the specifications for the ILD processor nucleus. The significance of the chopper discharge pattern and regularity of discharge to binaural processing may be as simple as regular discharge equals monaural/ipsilateral stimulation—irregular discharge equals binaural stimulation. While it is tempting to assign the initial time-locked discharges of LSO fast chopping units a role in ITD_t processing, the data have not been presented to support this hypothesis.

Many questions remain regarding the roles of MSO and LSO units in binaural processing. It is obvious that the population response to binaural stimuli must be reconstructed to understand the roles of these units in binaural processing. The difficulties encountered in recording from the MSO and LSO have impeded progress in this area. Much more is known about the response properties of low CF units in the inferior colliculus (115). However, it is unknown how much of what is observed at the level of the inferior colliculus is the result of processing in the superior olivary complex.

ACKNOWLEDGMENTS

This work was supported in part by grant NS20994 and NS20964 from the National Institutes of Health.

REFERENCES

1. Ramón y Cajal S. The acoustic nerve. In: *Histologie du système nerveux de l'homme et des vertébres*. Baltimore: Johns Hopkins Medical Institutions, 1967;774–838.
2. Papez JW. Superior olivary nucleus. Its fiber connections. *Arch Neurol Psychiatry* 1930;24: 1–20.
3. Rasmussen GL. The olivary peduncle and other fiber projections of the superior olivary complex. *J Comp Neurol* 1946;84:141–219.
4. Rasmussen GL. Efferent connections of the cochlear nucleus. In: Grahm AB, ed. *Sensori-*

neural hearing processes and disorders. Boston: Little, Brown, 1967;61–75.

5. Warr WB, Guinan JJ, White JS. Organization of the efferent fibers: the lateral and medial olivocochlear systems. In: Altschuler RA, Bobbin RP, Hoffman DW, eds. *Neurobiology of hearing: the cochlea.* New York: Raven Press, 1986;333–348.

6. Wiederhold ML. Physiology of the olivocochlear system. In: Altschuler RA, Bobbin RP, Hoffman DW, eds. *Neurobiology of hearing: the cochlea.* New York: Raven Press, 1986;349–370.

7. Stotler WA. An experimental study of the cells and connections of the superior olivary complex of the cat. *J Comp Neurol* 1953;98:401–423.

8. Galambos R, Schwartzkopff J, Rupert A. Microelectrode study of superior olivary nuclei. *Am J Physiol* 1959;197:527–536.

9. Adams JC. Ascending projections to the inferior colliculus. *J Comp Neurol* 1979;183:519–538.

10. Glendenning KK, Masterton RB. Afferent and efferent connections of the lateral superior olivary nucleus in cat. *Anat Rec* 1980;196:63–64.

11. Durlach NI, Colburn HS. Binaural phenomena. In: Carterette EC, Friedman MP, eds. *Handbook of perception, Volume IV: Hearing.* New York: Academic Press, 1978;365–466.

12. Kuhn GF. Physical acoustics and measurements pertaining to directional hearing. In: Yost WA, Gourevitch G, eds. *Directional hearing.* New York: Springer-Verlag, 1987;3–25.

13. Woodworth RS, Schlosberg H. *Experimental psychology.* New York: H Holt, 1954.

14. Fedderson WE, Sandel TT, Teas DC, et al. Localization of high-frequency tones. *J Acoust Soc Am* 1957;29:988–991.

15. Tobias JV, Schubert ED. Effective onset duration of auditory stimuli. *J Acoust Soc Am* 1959;31:1595–1605.

16. Abel SM, Kunov H. Lateralization based on interaural phase differences: effects of frequency, amplitude, duration, and shape of rise/decay. *J Acoust Soc Am* 1983;73:955–960.

17. Babkoff H, Sutton S. End point of lateralization for dichotic clicks. *J Acoust Soc Am* 1966;39:87–102.

18. Masterton B, Jane JA, Diamond IT. Role of brainstem auditory structures in sound localization. I. Trapezoid body, superior olive and lateral lemniscus. *J Neurophysiol* 1967;30:341–359.

19. Green DM. *An introduction to hearing.* New York: John Wiley, 1976.

20. Kuhn GF. Model for the interaural time differences in the azimuthal plane. *J Acoust Soc Am* 1977;62:157–167.

21. Roth GL, Kochhar RK, Hind JE. Interaural time differences: implications regarding the neurophysiology of sound localization. *J Acoust Soc Am* 1980;68:1643–1651.

22. Klumpp RG, Eady HR. Some measurements of interaural time difference thresholds. *J Acoust Soc Am* 1956;28:859–860.

23. Wakeford OS, Robinson DE. Lateralization of tonal stimuli by the cat. *J Acoust Soc Am* 1974;55:649–652.

24. Sayers BMcA, Cherry EC. Mechanism of binaural fusion in the hearing of speech. *J Acoust Soc Am* 1957;29:973–987.

25. Yost WA. Lateral position of sinusoids presented with interaural intensive and temporal differences. *J Acoust Soc Am* 1981;70:397–409.

26. Sayers BM. Acoustic-image lateralization judgements with binaural tones. *J Acoust Soc Am* 1964;36:923–926.

27. Mills AW. Auditory localization. In: Tobias JV, ed. *Foundations of modern auditory theory,* vol II. New York: Academic Press, 1972;303–348.

28. Henning GB. Some observations on the lateralization of complex waveforms. *J Acoust Soc Am* 1980;68:446–454.

29. Wiener FM, Pfeiffer RR, Backus ASN. On the sound pressure transformations by the head and auditory meatus of the cat. *Acta Otolaryngol* 1966;61:255–269.

30. Irvine DRF. Interaural intensity differences in the cat: changes in sound pressure level at the two ears associated with azimuthal displacements in the frontal horizontal plane. *Hearing Res* 1987;26:267–286.

31. Shaw EAG. Transformation of sound pressure level from the free field to the eardrum in the horizontal plane. *J Acoust Soc Am* 1974;56:1848–1861.

32. Yost WA, Dye RH. Discrimination of interaural differences of level as a function of frequency. *J Acoust Soc Am* 1988;83:1846–1851.

33. Yost WA, Hafter ER. Lateralization. In: Yost WA, Gourevitch G, eds. *Directional hearing.* New York: Springer-Verlag, 1987;49–84.

34. Henning GB. Detectability of interaural delay in high-frequency complex waveforms. *J Acoust Soc Am* 1974;55:84–90.

35. McFadden D, Pasanen EG. Lateralization at high frequencies based on interaural time differences. *J Acoust Soc Am* 1976;59:634–639.

36. Nuetzel JM, Hafter ER. Lateralization of complex waveforms. Effects of fine structure, amplitude, and duration. *J Acoust Soc Am* 1976;60:1339–1346.

37. Bernstein LR, Trahiotis C. Lateralization of low-frequency, complex waveforms: the use of envelope-based temporal disparities. *J Acoust Soc Am* 1985;77:1868–1880.

38. Henning GB. Lateralization of transient signals and types of delay. In: Klinke R, Hartmann R, eds. *Hearing—physiological bases and psychophysics.* New York: Springer-Verlag, 1983;196–201.

39. Yost WA, Wightman FL, Green DM. Lateralization of filtered clicks. *J Acoust Soc Am* 1971;50:1526–1531.

40. Nuetzel JM, Hafter ER. Discrimination of interaural delays in complex waveforms: spectral effects. *J Acoust Soc Am* 1981;69:1112–1118.

41. Blauert J. *Spatial hearing: the psychophysics of human sound localization.* Cambridge, MA: MIT Press, 1983.

42. Searle CL, Braida L, Cuddy D, et al. Binaural

pinna disparity: another localization cue. *J Acoust Soc Am* 1975;57:448–455.

43. Calford MB, Pettigrew JD. Frequency dependence of directional amplification at the cat's pinna. *Hearing Res* 1984;14:13–19.

44. Phillips DP, Calford MB, Pettigrew MB, et al. Directionality of sound pressure transformation at the cat's pinna. *Hearing Res* 1982;8:13–28.

45. Bilsen FA, Raatgever J. Spectral dominance in binaural lateralization. *Acoustica* 1973;28:131–132.

46. Martin RL, Webster WR. The auditory spatial acuity of the domestic cat in the horizontal and median vertical planes. *Hearing Res* 1987;30:239–252.

47. Roffler SK, Butler RA. Factors that influence the localization of sound in the vertical plane. *J Acoust Soc Am* 1968;43:1255–1259.

48. Tobias JV, Zerlin S. Lateralization threshold as a function of stimulus duration. *J Acoust Soc Am* 1959;31:1591–1594.

49. Colburn HS, Durlach NI. Models of binaural interaction. In: Carterette EC, Friedman MP, eds. *Handbook of perception, Vol. IV. Hearing.* New York: Academic Press, 1978;468–518.

50. Lord Rayleigh. On our perception of sound direction. *Philosophical Mag* 1907;13:214–232.

51. Jeffress LA. A place theory of sound localization. *J Comp Physiol Psychol* 1948;41:35–39.

52. Licklider JCR. Three auditory theories. In: Koch S, ed. *Psychology: a study of a science* New York: McGraw-Hill, 1959;41–44.

53. Kiang NY-S, Watanabe T, Thomas EC, et al. *Discharge patterns of single fibers in the cat's auditory nerve.* Cambridge, MA: MIT Press, 1965.

54. Rose JE, Brugge JF, Anderson DJ, et al. Phase-locked response to low-frequency tones in single auditory nerve fibers of the squirrel monkey. *J Neurophysiol* 1967;30:769–793.

55. Bourk TR. Electrical responses of neural units in the anteroventral cochlear nucleus of the cat. Ph.D. thesis, Massachusetts Institute of Technology, Cambridge, MA, 1976.

56. Johnson DH. The relationship between spike rate and synchrony in responses of auditory-nerve fibers to single tones. *J Acoust Soc Am* 1980;68:1115–1122.

57. van Bergeijk WA. Variation on a theme of Békésy: a model of binaural interaction. *J Acoust Soc Am* 1962;34:1431–1437.

58. Galambos R. Microelectrode studies on the auditory nervous system. *Ann Otol Rhinol Laryngol* 1957;66:503–505.

59. Hall JL. Binaural interaction in the accessory superior-olivary nucleus of the cat. *J Acoust Soc Am* 1965;37:814–823.

60. Hirsh IJ. The influence of interaural phase on interaural summation and inhibition. *J Acoust Soc Am* 1948;20:536–544.

61. Elfner LF, Tomsic RT. Temporal and intensive factors in binaural localization of auditory transients. *J Acoust Soc Am* 1968;43:746–751.

62. Colburn HS, Moss PJ. Binaural interaction models and mechanisms. In: Syka J, Aitkin L,

eds. *Neuronal mechanisms of hearing.* New York: Plenum Press, 1981;283–288.

63. Boudreau JC, Tsuchitani C. Binaural interaction in the cat superior olive S segment. *J Neurophysiol* 1968;31:442–454.

64. Goldberg JM, Brown PB. Response of binaural neurons of dog superior olivary complex to dichotic tonal stimuli: some physiological mechanisms of sound localization. *J Neurophysiol* 1969;32:613–636.

65. Zurek PM. Consequences of conductive auditory impairment for binaural hearing. *J Acoust Soc Am* 1986;80:466–472.

66. Carhart R, Tillman TW, Greetis ES. Release from multiple maskers: effect of interaural time disparities. *J Acoust Soc Am* 1969;45:411–418.

67. Cohen MF, Koehnke J. Detection and interaural time discrimination of a sinusoid masked by interaurally delayed white noise. *J Acoust Soc Am* 1982;72:1418–1420.

68. Stern RM, Slocum JE, Phillips MS. Interaural time and amplitude discrimination in noise. *J Acoust Soc Am* 1983;73:1714–1722.

69. Rhode WS, Smith PH. Encoding timing and intensity in the ventral cochlear nucleus of the cat. *J Neurophysiol* 1986;56:261–286.

70. Tsuchitani C. The inhibition of cat lateral superior olive unit excitatory responses to binaural tone bursts. II. The sustained discharges. *J Neurophysiol* 1988;59:184–211.

71. Tsuchitani C. Discharge patterns of cat lateral superior olivary units to ipsilateral tone-burst stimuli. *J Neurophysiol* 1982;47:479–500.

72. Walsh BT, Miller JB, Gacek RR, et al. Spontaneous activity in the eighth cranial nerve of the cat. *Int J Neurosci* 1972;3:221–236.

73. Kiss A, Majorossy K. Neuron morphology and synaptic architecture in the medial superior olivary nucleus. *Exp Brain Res* 1983;52:315–327.

74. Warr WB. Fiber degeneration following lesions in the anterior ventral cochlear nucleus of the cat. *Exp Neurol* 1966;14:453–474.

75. Osen KK. Afferent and efferent connections of three well-defined cell types of the cat cochlear nuclei. In: Anderson P, Jansen JKS, eds. *Excitatory synaptic mechanisms.* Oslo: Universitetsforlanget, 1970;295–300.

76. Cant NB, Casseday JH. Projections from the anteroventral cochlear nucleus to the lateral and medial superior olivary nuclei. *J Comp Neurol* 1986;247:457–476.

77. van Noort J. *The structure and connections of the inferior colliculus.* Assen, The Netherlands: Van Gorcum, 1969.

78. Brownell WE. Organization of the cat trapezoid body and the discharge characteristics of its fibers. *Brain Res* 1975;94:413–433.

79. Schwartz IR. Axonal organization in the cat medial superior olivary nucleus. In: Neff WD, ed. *Contributions to sensory physiology,* vol 8. New York: Academic Press, 1984;99–130.

80. Clark GM. The ultrastructure of nerve endings in the medial superior olive of the cat. *Brain Res* 1969;14:293–305.

81. Schwartz IR. Axonal endings in the cat medial

superior olive: coated vesicles and intercellular substance. *Brain Res* 1972;46:187–202.

82. Lindsey BG. Fine structure and distribution of axon terminals from the cochlear nucleus on neurons in the medial superior olivary nucleus of the cat. *J Comp Neurol* 1975;160:81–104.

83. Li RYS, Guinan JJ. Antidromic and orthodromic stimulation of neurons receiving calyces of Held. *MIT Q Prog Rep* 1971;100:227–234.

84. Rhode WS, Oertel D, Smith PH. Physiological response properties of cells labeled intracellularly with horseradish peroxidase in cat ventral cochlear nucleus. *J Comp Neurol* 1983;213:448–463.

85. Lenn NJ, Reese TS. The fine structure of nerve endings in the nucleus of the trapezoid body and the ventral cochlear nucleus. *Am J Anat* 1966;118:375–390.

86. Guinan JJ, Norris BE, Swift SH. A paucity of unit responses in the accessory superior olive of barbiturate anesthetized cats. *J Acoust Soc Am* 1967;41:1585.

87. Guinan JJ, Norris BE, Guinan SS. Single auditory units in the superior olivary complex. II. Locations of unit categories and tonotopic organization. *Int J Neurosci* 1972;4:147–166.

88. Tsuchitani C, Boudreau JC. Wave activity in the superior olivary complex of the cat. *J Neurophysiol* 1964;27:814–827.

89. Biedenbach MA, Freeman WJ. Click-evoked potential map from the superior olivary nucleus. *Am J Physiol* 1964;206:1408–1414.

90. Kiang NY-S. Stimulus coding in the auditory nerve and cochlear nucleus. *Acta Otolaryng* 1965;59:186–200.

91. Inbody SB, Feng AS. Binaural response of single neurons in the medial superior olivary nucleus of the albino rat. *Brain Res* 1981;210:361–366.

92. Harnischfeger G, Neuweiler G, Schlegel P. Interaural time and intensity coding in superior olivary complex and inferior colliculus of the echolocating bat *molossus ater*. *J Neurophysiol* 1985;53:89–109.

93. Goldberg JM, Brown PB. Functional organization of the dog superior olivary complex: an anatomical and electrophysiological study. *J Neurophysiol* 1968;31:639–656.

94. Kiang NY-S, Morest DK, Godfrey DA, et al. Stimulus coding at caudal levels of the cat's auditory nervous system: I. Response characteristics of single units. In: Moller AR, ed. *Basic mechanisms in hearing*. New York: Academic Press, 1973;455–478.

95. Guinan JJ, Guinan SS, Norris BE. Single auditory units in the superior olivary complex. I. Responses to sounds and classifications based on physiological properties. *Int J Neurosci* 1972;4:101–120.

96. Casseday JH, Neff WD. Localization of pure tones. *J Acoust Soc Am* 1973;54:365–372.

97. Scheibel ME, Scheibel AB. Neuropil organization in the superior olive of the cat. *Exp Neurol* 1974;43:339–348.

98. Helfert RH, Schwartz IR. Morphological evidence for the existence of multiple neuronal classes in the cat lateral superior olivary nucleus. *J Comp Neurol* 1986;244:533–549.

99. Cant NB. The fine structure of the lateral superior olivary nucleus of the cat. *J Comp Neurol* 1984;227:63–77.

100. Warr WB. Fiber degeneration following lesions in the multipolar and globular areas in the ventral cochlear nucleus of the cat. *Brain Res* 1972;40:247–270.

101. Spangler KM, Warr WB, Henkel CK. The projections of principal cells of the medial nucleus of the trapezoid body in the cat. *J Comp Neurol* 1985;238:249–262.

102. Tolbert LP, Morest DK, Yurgelun-Todd DA. The neuronal architecture of the anteroventral cochlear nucleus of the cat in the region of the cochlear nerve root: horseradish peroxidase labelling of identified cell types. *Neuroscience* 1982;7:3031–3052.

103. Tsuchitani C, Boudreau JC. Single unit analysis of cat superior olive S-segment with tonal stimuli. *J Neurophysiol* 1966;28:684–697.

104. Sanes DH, Rubel EW. The ontogeny of inhibition and excitation in the gerbil lateral superior olive. *J Neurosci* 1988;8:682–700.

105. Tsuchitani C. Functional organization of lateral cell groups of the cat superior olivary complex. *J Neurophysiol* 1977;40:296–318.

106. Strutz J, Bielenberg K. Efferent acoustic neurons within the lateral superior olivary nucleus of the guinea pig. *Brain Res* 1983;299:174–177.

107. White JS, Warr WB. The dual origins of the olivocochlear bundle in the albino rat. *J Comp Neurol* 1983;219:203–214.

108. Helfert RH, Schwartz IR. Morphological features of five neuronal classes in the gerbil lateral superior olive. *Am J Anat* 1987;179:55–69.

109. Boudreau JC, Tsuchitani C. Cat superior olive S-segment cell discharge to tonal stimuli. In: Neff WD, ed. *Contributions to sensory physiology*, vol 4. New York: Academic Press, 1970;143–213.

110. Tsuchitani C, Boudreau JC. Encoding of stimulus frequency and intensity by cat superior olive S-segment cells. *J Acoust Soc Am* 1967;42:794–805.

111. Tsuchitani C, Boudreau JC. Stimulus level of dichotically presented tones and cat superior olive S-segment cell discharge. *J Acoust Soc Am* 1969;46:979–988.

112. Tsuchitani C. The inhibition of cat lateral superior olive unit excitatory responses to binaural tone bursts. I. The transient chopper response. *J Neurophysiol* 1988;59:164–183.

113. Tsuchitani C, Johnson DH. The effects of ipsilateral tone burst stimulus level on the discharge patterns of cat lateral superior olivary units. *J Acoust Soc Am* 1985;77:1484–1496.

114. Caird D, Klinke R. Processing of binaural stimuli by cat superior olivary complex neurons. *Exp Brain Res* 1983;52:385–399.

115. Irvine DRF. *Progress in sensory physiology 7: the auditory brainstem*. New York: Springer-Verlag, 1986.

*Neurobiology of Hearing: The
Central Auditory System,* edited by
R. A. Altschuler et al.
Raven Press, Ltd., New York © 1991.

9

The Anatomy of the Inferior Colliculus: A Cellular Basis for Integration of Monaural and Binaural Information

Douglas L. Oliver and Amiram Shneiderman

*Department of Anatomy, The University of Connecticut Health Center,
Farmington, Connecticut 06032*

The inferior colliculus (IC) is critical for processing auditory information in the mammal. Virtually all ascending and descending auditory pathways make an obligatory synapse in the IC.[1] However, the colliculus is not merely a relay nucleus. The structure of the IC may determine how monaural and binaural information from the lower auditory system is integrated or sorted. Underlying this important function is the cellular anatomy of the IC. The cellular anatomy can specify how individual pathways synapse on single neuron types. The final outcome of integration in the IC is the response of these neurons to sounds. Neurons in the IC send their axons rostrally to the forebrain parts of the auditory system. Both the cellular anatomy of the colliculus and the intrinsic connections of the IC are important for the transfer of auditory information rostrally.

In this review, the cellular morphology of the IC in the mammal is discussed in the context of binaural information processing. A cellular approach emphasizes the components directly involved in shaping neural responses—the presynaptic axons, both the ascending and intrinsic, the dendrites, and the somata of postsynaptic neurons. Moreover, the cellular organization defines the structural matrix in the IC upon which the afferent pathways are superimposed and from which the efferent pathways depart.

In order to obtain cellular information on the IC and its intrinsic organization, recent neuroanatomical studies have turned to Golgi, axonal transport, electron microscopic, and intracellular injection methods. Studies in Golgi-impregnated material have redefined the subdivisions of the IC, so the presentation of the cellular basis for the subdivisions is the first topic of review. The second topic is raised by the question: Do the subdivisions share the same inputs? The relationship of the subdivisions to their inputs is termed the "nucleotopic organization" and defines the population of presynaptic axons present in each subdivision. Knowing the inputs available to a cell may help to predict its response to sound. Experimental studies of the major ascending inputs to the IC show that they condense to form bands in parallel to the principal cell

---

[1]Ramón y Cajal believed that many fibers from the lateral lemniscus continued past the IC to the medial geniculate body. He called these fibers the central acoustic tract. Cajal thought that some fibers from the lateral lemniscus terminated exclusively in the IC, while still others terminated in both midbrain and thalamic sites (see Chapter 22 in ref. 55).

types. This organization may be significant since there may be excitatory and inhibitory bands. The bands of afferents are the third topic of this chapter. The fourth section addresses the formation of functional zones or "synaptic domains" in the IC. Synaptic domains may be composed of predictable combinations of banded inputs. Ultimately, it may be possible to relate the responses of individual neurons to their morphology and their location within a specific type of synaptic domain. Finally, the intrinsic connections and efferent pathways of the IC are described. The effect of responses by IC neurons depends on whether the neurons are projection cells or interneurons. Thus, in the context of cellular anatomy, the subdivisions of the IC, the nucleotopic organization, the bands, and the synaptic domains may be used to show how information from the hindbrain auditory system is integrated and transmitted to the forebrain.

THE CELLULAR ORGANIZATION OF INFERIOR COLLICULUS DEFINES ITS SUBDIVISIONS

The three main divisions of the IC were first identified as distinct groups of neurons in Golgi impregnations by Ramón y Cajal (55). Cajal's nucleus of the IC, the dorsal or internuclear cortex (écorce superior), and the external cortex correspond largely to the central nucleus, the cortex, and the lateral nucleus (one of several paracentral nuclei) in recent studies (42,52). Despite the early work by Cajal, many studies of the IC use a second nomenclature based primarily on the packing density of cell bodies in Nissl-stained material. This scheme is illustrated in the atlas by Berman (8). The central nucleus of Berman includes both the nucleus and portions of the dorsal cortex identified by Cajal. Berman's pericentral nucleus corresponds to only the outer portion of the cortex, and his external nucleus

includes the lateral nucleus plus other structures between the IC and the superior colliculus. While the nomenclature of Berman is useful in its simplicity, it cannot resolve anatomically distinct groups of neurons that may have different functions. Thus, the need to identify the cellular components in the IC has led to a reestablishment of Cajal's parcellation by Morest and Oliver (42). Further refinements based on cellular organization in the IC (42,52) provide new definitions for the subdivisions and a basis for the following description.

Golgi Studies Reveal Unique Sets of Neuronal Types

Tectal Nuclei versus Tegmentum in the Auditory Midbrain

The nuclei of the auditory midbrain contain either tectal or tegmental neurons. Tectal neurons have rich dendritic arbors with frequent branches and, sometimes, frequent dendritic spines. Tectal cells typify the three main divisions of the IC proper: the central nucleus, the cortex, and the paracentral nuclei (Figs. 1 and 2). Tegmental neurons are typical of the reticular formation with far fewer dendrites, branches, and spines. Tegmental cells characterize the nuclei ventral to the IC (Figs. 1 and 2, SA, SB, CU) and the intercollicular tegmentum between the IC and the superior colliculus.

Central Nucleus

The central nucleus (Figs. 1–3) is defined by the presence of *disc-shaped cells* that form fibro-dendritic laminae together with the afferent axons (40,42,52). The disc-shaped cells represent 75% to 85% of the cells in the central nucleus and have dendritic fields that extend 200 to 800 μm in two dimensions but around 50 to 70 μm in the narrowest. All disc-shaped cells within

TABLE 1. *Abbreviations*

Inferior colliculus (IC) and midbrain tegmentum

B	brachium of inferior colliculus	M,pm	*pars medialis*, central nucleus
C,pc	*pars centralis*, central nucleus	RP	rostral pole nucleus
CG	central gray	SA	sagulum
CL	commissural nucleus	SB	subcollicular nucleus
CU	cuneiform nucleus	TM	mesencephalic trigeminal nucleus
DC	dorsal cortex	V,pi	*pars ventralis*, central nucleus
DM	dorsomedial nucleus		interstitial zone
L,pl	*pars lateralis*, central nucleus	VL	ventrolateral nucleus
LN	lateral nucleus	1,2,3,4	layers of dorsal cortex
		I,II,III,IV	

Cochlear nucleus

AVCN	anteroventral cochlear nucleus	DCN	dorsal cochlear nucleus
AA	anterior division, anterior part	PVCN	posteroventral cochlear nucleus
AP	anterior division, posterior part	A	anterior part
APD	anterior division, posterodorsal	O	caudal part (octopus cells)
PD	anterior division, dorsal part	G	granule cells
PV	anterior division, ventral part		

Lateral lemniscus

DNLL	dorsal nucleus	**Superior olivary complex**	
INLL	intermediate nucleus	LSO	lateral superior olive
VNLL	ventral nucleus	MSO	medial superior olive

Other

ARG	autoradiography	PAG	periaqueductal gray
HRP	horseradish peroxidase	SC	superior colliculus
WGA-HRP	wheat germ agglutinin conjugated to horseradish peroxidase		

the same subdivision of the central nucleus are oriented in parallel arrays. Although the dendrites of the disc-shaped cells share a collateral branching pattern where daughter branches are unequal in size, several varieties are evident. Large, medium, medium-large, and small disc-shaped cells are distinguished by the size of the somata and dendritic field, by their dendritic branching patterns, and by their dendritic appendages.

Stellate cells (Fig. 3, d, e) have oval or spherical dendritic fields that usually cross several fibro-dendritic laminae (52,59). Although they constitute around 20% of the cells, they include several types that vary in size and in the complexity of their dendritic branching. Most have dichotomous branching patterns with equal-sized daughter branches. Simple stellate cells have large, ovoid fields. Complex stellates are more medium sized but have more frequent

branches and numerous appendages. Small stellates have dendritic fields less than 200 μm in diameter.

The fibro-dendritic laminae (Fig. 3) formed by parallel arrays of disc-shaped neurons may provide a structural basis for tonotopic organization in the IC (37,66). The laminae also create four characteristic patterns within the central nucleus (Figs. 1, 2, and 4). Each pattern corresponds to one of the subdivisions of the central nucleus (52). The *pars centralis* (C in Figs. 1, 2, and 4) contains fairly linear laminae, running from ventrolateral to dorsomedial. These laminae are most easily observed in the transverse plane of section. This is the largest part of the central nucleus and contains the greatest number of large disc-shaped cells. The *pars medialis* (M) is smaller and its laminae parallel the general orientation of those in the *pars centralis*. However, the laminae are somewhat more curved as they

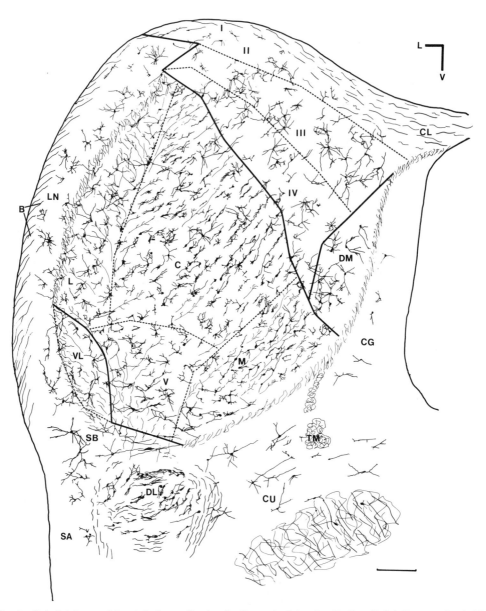

FIG. 1. Subdivisions of the inferior colliculus in the cat stained with the Golgi-Cox method. This transverse section is in the middle of the colliculus, just caudal to the commissure. This plane of section (anatomical transverse) is perpendicular to the floor of the fourth ventricle. Age 2 months. (For abbreviations, see Table 1.) (From ref. 42, with permission.)

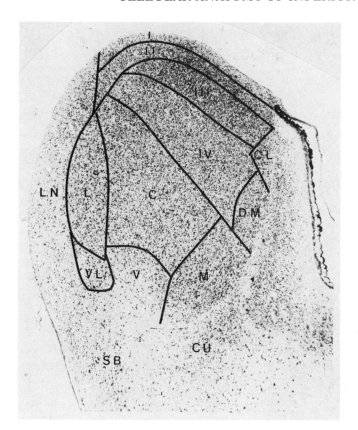

FIG. 2. Subdivisions of the inferior colliculus in the cat stained with thionin and cut in the anatomical transverse plane of section. This level is similar to that shown in Fig. 1 and represents the middle of the inferior colliculus in this plane of cut. Age 11 months. (For abbreviations, see Table 1.)

abut the medial edge of the IC. Neurons are smaller and more densely packed. The *pars lateralis* (L) contains laminae that are oriented orthogonal to the contiguous laminae centrally. The laminae are oblique in transverse sections but are easily seen in the sagittal plane. There is an irregular packing density in the *pars lateralis* due in part to the many efferent fibers passing through. In the *pars lateralis,* the packing density is somewhat higher than in the *pars centralis,* and medium-sized neurons predominate. The *pars ventralis* (V) has few cells and lacks distinct laminae. It occupies the ventrolateral remainder of the central nucleus and represents an interstitial zone where fibers of the lateral lemniscus enter.

Cortex

In contrast to the central nucleus, the cortex of the IC is a laminar structure dominated by stellate cells (Figs. 1 and 2). Its layers follow the contours of the dorsal and caudal surface of the IC, and its laminar pattern is more a product of the intrinsic axonal plexus than the arrangement of dendrites or somata. Afferent axons in the dorsal cortex from the telencephalon and the lateral lemniscus run perpendicular to the intrinsic layers to form a dense meshwork of neuropil quite distinct from that of the central nucleus. The orientation of the afferent fibers is similar to that in the *pars medialis* and *lateralis.* Although stellate cells are the most common types, some mediolaterally oriented and rostrocaudally oriented cells also are found. These latter cells can be quite similar to the disc-shaped cells in the central nucleus.

The dorsal cortex (Figs. 1 and 2) has four layers that are compact laterally and expand medially. The ventral-most, *layer IV,* is a lens-shaped structure whose axis is per-

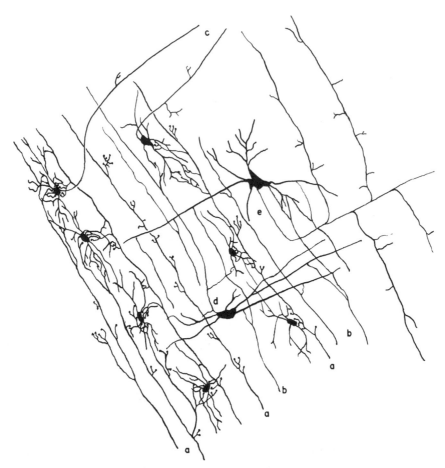

FIG. 3. Cell types and intrinsic organization of the central nucleus. Neurons with disc-shaped dendritic fields are oriented with the long axes parallel to the laminar afferents (a,b). Disc-shaped cells may emit sparse axon collaterals (c). Simple stellate (d) and complex stellate cells (e) have dendritic fields that cross the laminar stria, and their axons have more branches that extend over a wider area. (From ref. 52, with permission.)

pendicular to the laminae in the central nucleus. Filled with stellate cells of all sizes, layer IV also has limited numbers of rostrocaudally oriented or mediolaterally (horizontal) oriented cells. The latter type is most obvious at the border of the central nucleus where their dendrites are oriented perpendicular to the laminae. *Layer III* lies atop layer IV with its concave surface ventrally. A prominent fascicle of fibers delimits the dorsolateral surface of layer III and marks where the fibers enter and exit the brachium of the IC. At rostral levels, the

medial part of layer III abuts the commissure of the IC. Layer III has cells ranging from large to small that may be distinguished by size, by branching pattern, and by the number of dendritic spines. *Layer II* is filled with small to medium-sized stellate cells, and, together with the fibrous capsule *layer I*, forms most of the pericentral region of Berman (8). Different types of small and medium-sized cells are found in layer II. The few cells in layer I usually have flattened dendritic fields that parallel the surface of the IC and could represent more

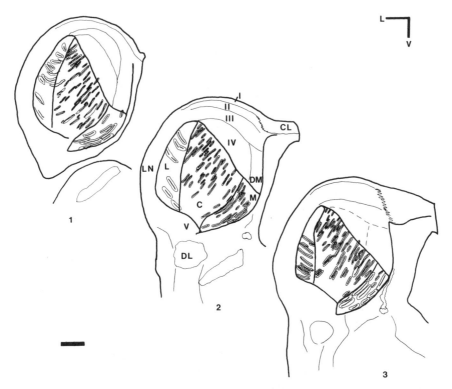

FIG. 4. Reconstruction of the laminar pattern formed by dendritic fields of disc-shaped cells in the adult central nucleus, transverse plane. Dendritic fields of single cells or groups of cells are represented as ovals surrounding a line. Each drawing is a composite of two 100-μm thick, Golgi-Cox impregnated sections. (For abbreviations, see Table 1.) (From ref. 52.)

than one cell type. The cortex also is found on the caudal surface of the IC where it is thinner and the deep layers may be incomplete.

Paracentral Subdivisions

The remaining subdivisions in the IC share the common feature of surrounding the central nucleus and the dorsal cortex (Figs. 1, 2, and 4). The paracentral nuclei include the *commissural, dorsomedial, lateral,* and *ventrolateral nuclei* as well as the *nucleus of the rostral pole* (42). For the most part, these nuclei contain tectal neurons. However, the lateral nucleus contains a mixture of tectal and tegmental cells. But, it is easily distinguished from the pure pop-

ulation of tegmental cells in the intercollicular tegmentum, rostrally.

Subdivisions in Inferior Colliculus Based on Cell Morphology Are Consistent Across Species

The IC has been investigated with Golgi techniques in a number of other mammalian species. Perhaps, the most important outcome of these studies is the remarkable similarity of the cellular anatomy. For example, the same cell types are present in the central nucleus (22,23,25,36,52,59,81). When studies use similar methods and criteria, numerous similarities in subdivisions and the overall organization emerge for the entire IC (25,36,42,49,52). All of the same subdivisions are present in roughly the same location. In the cat and the mouse (36,52), fibro-dendritic laminae are present in the same orientation in all four subdivisions of the central nucleus. Only the lateral extent of the dorsal cortex, which is greater in the mouse, distinguishes it from the cat.

Some species differences may exist. Other differences may reflect the interpretation of the observer. For example, important species differences have been observed in the laminar pattern and the extent of the central nucleus. The laminar pattern of the central nucleus in the primate is different from that in the cat, and the laminae are flatter, possibly more tilted toward horizontal (23,25). In the rat, the fibro-dendritic laminae have a uniform ventromedial to dorsolateral orientation, but, surprisingly, only one subdivision of the central nucleus is identified (22). The central nucleus extends quite dorsally, close to the surface of the IC in the rat, but it is truncated rostrally and laterally.[2]

Some apparent species differences could merely represent a shift or rotation of one or more subdivisions within the IC. This is plausible due to findings in an insectivore, the tree shrew (49). Each subdivision of the IC observed in the cat also was found in the tree shrew (*Tupaia glis*). However, the laminae of the central nucleus were rotated so that the layers in the central part were parallel to the frontal stereotaxic plane instead of perpendicular as in the cat. A partial explanation for this finding is in the relationship of the IC to the superior colliculus.

---

[2]The prominence of the external cortex in the rat (10) is somewhat puzzling. It is large where the central nucleus is reduced. The third layer of the external cortex is lateral to the central nucleus and the incoming fibers of the lateral lemniscus. Its location is identical to the *pars lateralis* in the central nucleus of the cat. The ventrolateral nucleus also may be included in this part of the rat's external cortex. Rostral to the central nucleus, the external cortex in the rat could include parts of the intercollicular tegmentum defined in the cat. If a homolog to the rostral pole nucleus is present, it too might be rostral to the central nucleus.

Most of the IC lies ventral to the superior colliculus, which is very large in the tree shrew, and the entire IC has been displaced and has rotated caudally. Despite the changes in the relative locations of the subdivisions, the definitions of the subdivisions based on cellular morphology are not different.

Undoubtedly, some species differences in the IC may reflect unique specializations related to behavior or habitat. The best example of a potentially specialized IC is found in the mustache bat (81). The laminar pattern of the central nucleus is disrupted in the 60 to 64 kHz region and may correspond to hypertrophied fibro-dendritic laminae. In other mammals, less dramatic differences in the IC may be evident. For example, there is a predictable variation in the size of the dorsal cortex related to the amount of neocortex devoted to auditory processing. Animals with the largest telencephalon also appear to have the largest dorsal cortex in the IC.

NUCLEOTOPIC ORGANIZATION: EACH SUBDIVISION HAS A UNIQUE COMBINATION OF INPUTS

Each subdivision in the IC, defined as a distinct group of neurons, may have a specific combination of inputs. The pattern of inputs to each subdivision may be termed its nucleotopic organization. In the case of the ascending pathways to the IC, the nucleotopic organization of a subdivision may be related to its role in binaural processing. The organization of afferents may provide important clues to the responses of neurons in the subdivisions.

Types of Inputs to the Inferior Colliculus

It will be useful, at this point, to outline the broad categories of inputs to the IC. Each input can be identified by the cells of origin in the cochlear nucleus and by the number of synapses en route to the IC. Ascending pathways to the IC all share a common origin from cells in the cochlear nucleus that receive inputs from type I spiral ganglion cells in the cochlea (for reviews, see refs. 15,39). *Direct, monaural pathways* carry information to the IC and emerge from the stellate, fusiform, and giant cells of the cochlear nuclei (1,9,45,48,54,61,62). In contrast, *indirect, binaural pathways* originate from bushy and globular cells in the anteroventral cochlear nucleus (AVCN) (14). Axons from these cells synapse in the main nuclei of the superior olivary complex, which, in turn, project to the IC (11,26,30,60,71,77). Indirect projections to the IC also arise from the periolivary nuclei (2,14,77). The *multisynaptic pathways* to the IC may be monaural or binaural and include projections from the cochlear nucleus, the superior olivary complex, a synapse in the lateral lemniscal nuclei, and lemniscal outputs to the IC (10,11,16,17, 20,26–28,33,43,45,48,54,60,65,72,74–76,78,

80). Ascending pathways to the IC terminate as either a *focused* or *diffuse* plexus of axons. Focused inputs are certainly related to *tonotopic organization* and terminate in discrete terminal fields or *bands,* described below. In contrast, diffuse projections lack the focused characteristics and terminate widely within one or more subdivisions of the IC. *Descending pathways* and *commissural pathways* represent the final types of inputs to the IC (5,7,17,18,24,50,56). The former originate in the auditory cortex, while the latter are from the opposite IC.

Central Nucleus Receives All Types of Ascending Inputs But Projections to the Parts of the Central Nucleus Differ

The central nucleus is the only subdivision to receive inputs from all three types of ascending pathways (Table 2) (11,20,30, 33,45,48,59,71,76,78,80). Direct pathways

TABLE 2. *Sources of the projections to the central nucleus and dorsal cortex[a]*

Projections to contralateral central nucleus		Projections to ipsilateral central nucleus		Projections to dorsal cortex[b]
Focused	Diffuse	Focused	Diffuse	
Cochlear nucleus				
AVCN	•	AVCN (low)	•	AVCN, layers 3, 4
PVCN	•	•	PVCN (rostral)	•
DCN	•	•	DCN	DCN, layer 4
Superior olive				
LSO	•	LSO	•	•
•	MSO (high)	MSO (low)	MSO (high)	•
•	Periolivary	•	Periolivary	Periolivary[c]
Lateral lemniscus				
DNLL	•	•	DNLL	DNLL, layer 4
•	•	•	INLL	INLL, layers 3, 4
•	•	•	VNLL	•
Neocortex				
•	•	•	•	A1, layers 3, 4
•	•	•	•	A2, layers 1, 2

For abbreviations, see Table 1.
[a]Projections are defined as either focused or diffuse. The focused projections exhibit a banding pattern in both the central nucleus and dorsal cortex.
[b]Projections to the dorsal cortex follow the same laterality and density as those to central nucleus. For example, the projection from AVCN to the dorsal cortex is focused and bilateral for the low frequencies, while it is contralateral only for the middle and high frequencies.
[c]Data on the laminar distribution of periolivary projections are not complete.

to the central nucleus are from the AVCN (Fig. 5), the posteroventral (PVCN), and the dorsal cochlear nuclei (DCN) (Table 2; Fig. 6A–D). Each of these focused projections terminate primarily in the contralateral IC and is tonotopically organized. Indirect pathways to the central nucleus include projections from the medial superior olive (MSO), the lateral superior olive (LSO), and the periolivary nuclei (Table 2) (Figs. 7 and 8A and A′) (25). Projections from the LSO and the periolivary nuclei are bilateral, while the projection from the MSO is mostly unilateral. Both MSO and LSO inputs are focused, tonotopic projections, while the periolivary projections are diffuse (2). Both the MSO and LSO (21) inputs may be absent in the caudal-most part of the central nucleus (Fig. 9). Indirect pathways to the central nucleus are from the dorsal (DNLL) (Figs. 6F and G and 8B and C) (25), the intermediate (INLL), and the ventral nuclei of the lateral lemniscus (VNLL) (Table 2). Most projections from the lateral lemniscal nuclei are to the ipsilateral IC and diffuse except those from the

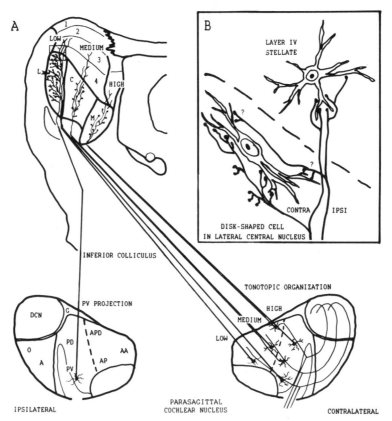

FIG. 5. Schematic of the projections from anteroventral cochlear nucleus to the inferior colliculus. **A:** The ipsilateral projection is restricted to the lateral colliculus. The contralateral projection covers the entire frequency range and forms bands in the central nucleus and the dorsal cortex. Bands are more distinct in the central and medial parts of the central nucleus due to the orientation of the laminae. **B:** Axons from AVCN terminate on the dendrites of disc-shaped cells in the central nucleus. Collaterals of these axons also synapse on cells in the deep layers of the dorsal cortex. (Modified from ref. 48, with permission.)

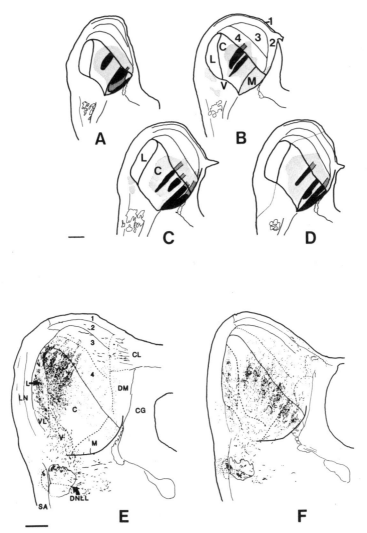

FIG. 6. Bands of afferents from the dorsal cochlear nucleus (**A–D**) and dorsal nucleus of the lateral lemniscus (**E** and **F**). Bands in the central nucleus are produced after small injections (A, B) and large injections (C, D) and extend into the fourth layer of the dorsal cortex (4). Labeling in the *pars lateralis* (L) of the central nucleus is common after injections in the dorsal nucleus of the lateral lemniscus (E, F, L) but are uncommon with projections from the dorsal cochlear nucleus. (For abbreviations, see Table 1.) (From refs. 45, 70, with permission.)

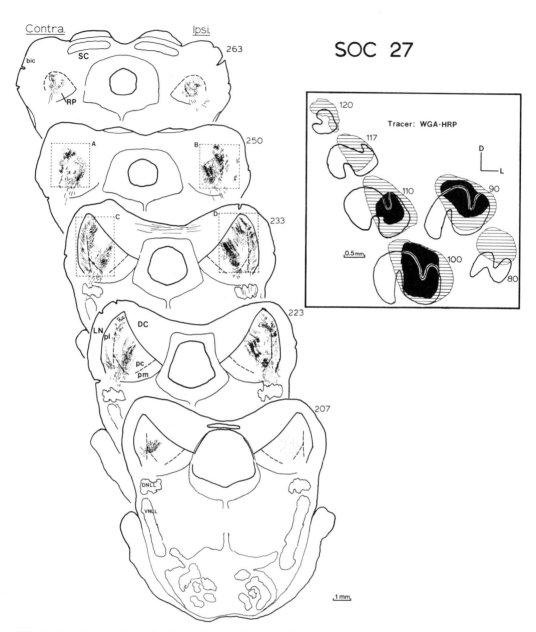

FIG. 7. Banding of afferents labeled in the inferior colliculus after an injection of wheat germ-HRP (WGA-HRP) into the lateral half of the lateral superior olive. The projection to the ipsilateral colliculus is banded, while the contralateral is less focused. (For abbreviations, see Table 1.) (From ref. 68, with permission.)

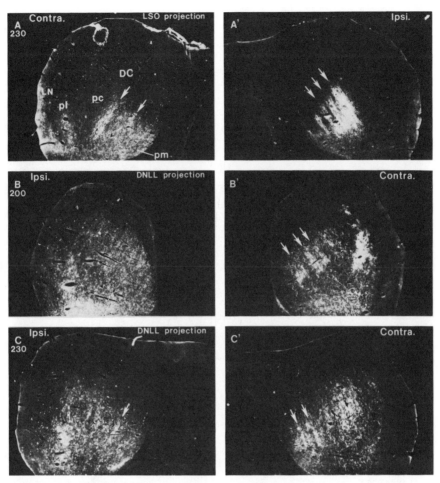

FIG. 8. Comparison of label bands in the inferior colliculus after injections in the lateral superior olive (A,A') and the dorsal nucleus of the lateral lemniscus (B,B';C,C'). Photomicrographs show that both projections from the lateral superior olive are banded with the contralateral projection slightly less so. In contrast, only the contralateral projection from the dorsal nucleus of the lateral lemniscus exhibits banding. (For abbreviations, see Table 1.) (From ref. 70, with permission.)

DNLL, which are bilateral. The contralateral projection of the DNLL is focused and tonotopically organized (70).

The inputs to the high- and low-frequency parts of the central nucleus are not the same and could contribute to features that distinguish neurons tuned to different frequency ranges. To a large degree, differences in these connections translate to a difference between the subdivisions of the central nucleus. For example, only the low-frequency AVCN has a bilateral projection to the lateral, low-frequency *pars lateralis* (48), but the AVCN projects to the entire frequency range in the contralateral IC (Fig. 5; Table 2). Likewise, the bulk of the projection from the MSO (30) is to the low- and mid-frequency parts of the *pars centralis* and the *pars lateralis* in the central nucleus (Fig. 9A and B). In contrast, the small, high-frequency part of the MSO exhibits only a sparse, bilateral projection to the *pars medialis,* the high-frequency part of the IC. A final example is the DCN pro-

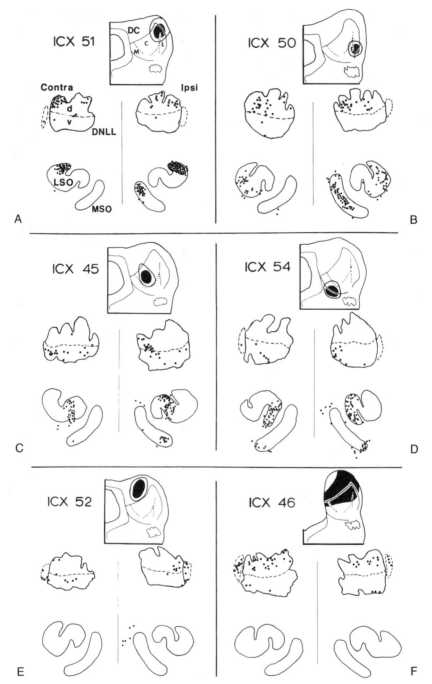

FIG. 9. Nucleotopic organization of projections from the dorsal nucleus of the lateral lemniscus (DNLL) and the superior olive after injections of wheat germ-HRP into the inferior colliculus. As the injections vary from dorsolateral to ventromedial in the central nucleus (**A–D**), there is a dorsal to ventral shift in the position of labeled cells in the DNLL and a lateral to medial shift in the lateral superior olive. Injections in the dorsal or the caudal cortex of the inferior colliculus (**E** and **F**) label neurons in the DNLL but not in the main nuclei of the superior olive. (For abbreviations, see Table 1.) (From ref. 70, with permission.)

jection to the *pars medialis* and the *pars centralis* of the contralateral central nucleus (23) (Fig. 6A–D). Inputs to the *pars lateralis* of the central nucleus from the DCN are sparse or absent as are inputs to the ipsilateral IC.

Dorsal Cortex Receives Descending Projections But May Lack Some Ascending Inputs

Unlike the central nucleus, the dorsal cortex receives a major descending input from the telencephalon (Table 2). Both primary auditory cortex (A1) and nonprimary belt regions (e.g., A2) project to the dorsal and caudal cortex of the IC (7,17,18,21,29). The primary auditory cortex contributes a banded, tonotopic projection that penetrates the full depth of the dorsal cortex (7,49). The projection from the nonprimary belt regions may terminate more superficially (7,21,24,50). The projection from the anterior auditory field in the cat (7) is similar to that of A1 but very weak. Each of the inputs from the neocortex are integrated with projections ascending in the lateral lemniscus.

A second difference that appears to distinguish the dorsal cortex from central nucleus is the absence of inputs from the MSO and the LSO (11,30,68,70). Small injections of horseradish peroxidase (HRP) or wheat germ conjugates of HRP in the dorsal cortex fail to label the main nuclei of the superior olivary complex (Fig. 9E and F). Likewise, small injections of anterograde tracers in the MSO and the LSO fail to reveal inputs to the deep layers of the dorsal cortex (Fig. 7). The absence of MSO and LSO projections is in contrast to the projection to layer IV from the DCN and the DNLL (Fig. 6) and the projections to layers III and IV from the AVCN (Fig. 5). One functional consequence of this nucleotopic organization is that the dorsal cortex may lack significant inputs from the binaural pathways. Thus, cells in the dorsal cortex

may be more influenced by the descending pathways from the telencephalon and the ascending monaural pathways.

Paracentral Nuclei Receive Different Patterns of Input

Although many of the paracentral nuclei can be distinguished on the basis of individual connections, a complete nucleotopic description of each nucleus is not available. The best known of the paracentral nuclei, the lateral nucleus, is the only part of the IC to receive afferents from the spinal cord and dorsal column nuclei and the neocortical regions between somatosensory cortex and primary auditory cortex (4,17,24,42, 49,64,65,68). However, it receives no direct lemniscal afferents, only efferent projections from the central nucleus (34). Likewise, the commissural nucleus does not receive lemniscal afferents, but it participates in the crossed connections of the commissure (5,42). In contrast, the other paracentral nuclei receive ascending projections via the lateral lemniscus. Only the dorsomedial nucleus receives inputs via the medial intercollicular tegmentum and the auditory cortex as well as the lemniscus (42,48). The rostral pole and the ventrolateral nuclei are distinguished more by their outputs than inputs. The rostral nucleus receives mostly high-frequency inputs but does not appear to be tonotopically organized or laminated (42,45,48). It has many neurons that project to the superior colliculus (e.g., 19). Neurons in the ventrolateral nucleus also receive nontonotopic inputs from the lemniscus and may project to the lateral tegmentum (51).

BANDS OF AFFERENTS MAY BE RELATED TO NEURAL RESPONSES

Although the nucleotopic organization of the IC suggests that single subdivisions may have unique collections of afferents, this level of organization may not be adequate to explain the responses of single cells. For example, many types of responses are found in the central nucleus, perhaps as a reflection of different combinations of its inputs. The partial segregation and clustering of binaural response types reported in the central nucleus (60,66) require a more refined mechanism than nucleotopic organization. Such a mechanism is suggested in studies that show that the afferents to the central nucleus are not organized as a homogeneous plexus. The focused inputs terminate as sheets or bands.

Bands of Preterminal Fibers Are Defined in Experimental Material

The heterogeneous nature of the afferents to the central nucleus of the cat was first demonstrated with lesions of the hindbrain nuclei or their ascending tracts (28, 40,52,59). A unilateral lesion of the superior olivary complex and adjacent structures produces a banded pattern of degeneration in the central nucleus, bilaterally. In frontal sections, the bands of thick, degenerating fibers are separated by areas of fine-fiber degeneration. The degenerating fibers are oriented in parallel to the fibro-dendritic laminae. Similarly, a lesion of the DNLL produces a fine, diffuse pattern of degeneration on the ipsilateral side and a more focused, coarse degeneration on the contralateral side (28).

Banded ascending projections to IC originate bilaterally from AVCN (Fig. 5) and LSO (Figs. 7 and 8A), the contralateral DCN and DNLL (Fig. 6), and the ipsilateral MSO (21,45,48,70). The pattern of afferents from individual nuclei can be demonstrated with the anterograde transport of tritiated amino acids, HRP, or wheat germ HRP. With these more sensitive methods, the bands are found both in the central nucleus and in the deeper layers of the dorsal cortex. Inputs to the dorsal cortex from the primary auditory cortex of the telencephalon are also banded (7). Typically, heavily labeled bands are 200 μm wide, although bands twice that size were found after AVCN injections. The projections from the LSO to the ipsilateral central nucleus illustrate typical, distinct, heavily labeled bands separated by interband areas of light labeling (Fig. 8A'). A second banding pattern after LSO injections is seen in the contralateral central nucleus (Fig. 8A). The fibers from the contralateral LSO are less heavily labeled, so the contrast between the bands and interbands is not sharp. The third pattern of labeling in the IC is diffuse labeling without obvious bands. One example that illustrates diffuse labeling is the projection from the DNLL to the ipsilateral IC (Fig. 8B and C). In contrast, the projections from the DNLL to the contralateral IC are distinctly banded (Fig. 8B' and C').

The bands are oriented in parallel to the fibro-dendritic laminae, an orientation similar to that observed with the degeneration techniques. Since the bands in the central nucleus follow the fibro-dendritic laminae, they have two components. The major, medial component is located in the *pars centralis* and the *pars medialis* where the bands are oriented from ventrolateral to dorsomedial. For some projections these bands extend into the dorsal cortex. The bands in the lateral component located in the *pars lateralis* are much shorter, but they still follow the fibro-dendritic laminae and are orthogonal to the laminae centrally. The number of bands that are labeled is determined by the size of the injection site. Small injections may label one or two bands, while larger injections may label several bands. When viewed in transverse sections, as many as 10 or 12 bands separated by interband regions may be possible in the central nucleus of the IC.

The three-dimensional organization suggests that each band is part of a longitudinal sheet that extends in the rostrocaudal dimension (Fig. 10). In the case of the LSO projections, bands are continuous at midlevels of the IC, while caudally the bands are discontinuous. When the tissue is sliced

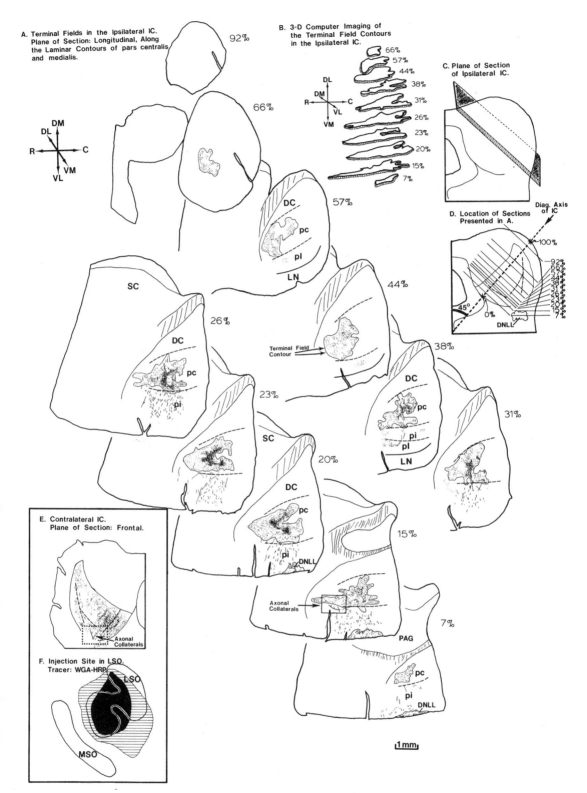

FIG. 10. Bands of afferents labeled in the inferior colliculus after an injection in the ipsilateral lateral superior olive (**F**). Sections through the ipsilateral colliculus were cut parallel to the laminae in the *pars centralis* (**C** and **D**). Plots of the labeling in individual sections (**A**) and reconstructed by computer (**B**) show that bands are discontinuous caudally. (For abbreviations, see Table 1.)

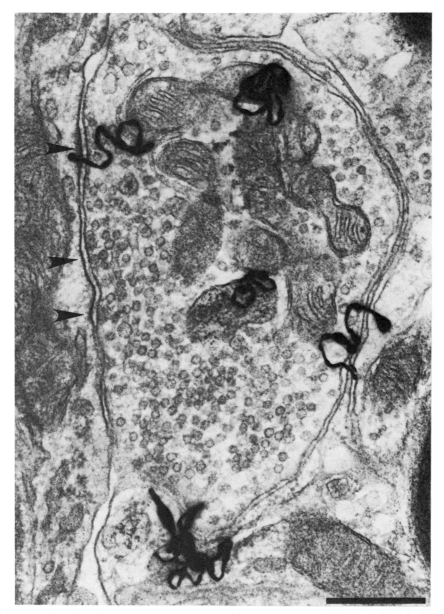

FIG. 11. Axonal ending from the anteroventral cochlear nucleus contains round synaptic vesicles and makes asymmetric synaptic contacts (*arrowheads*). Labeled with [³H]leucine, axonal transport, and electron microscopic autoradiography. Scale bar = 0.5 μm. (Adapted from ref. 48, with permission.)

parallel to the bands, it appears that the label has a Y-shaped configuration. At midlevels of the IC, the label is continuous, but caudally where the two limbs of the Y are located, it is discontinuous (Fig. 10). In serial sections, the bands from the LSO vary somewhat in their thickness. However, the difference in pattern between the ipsilateral and contralateral projections is always preserved, and the banding is always more fo-

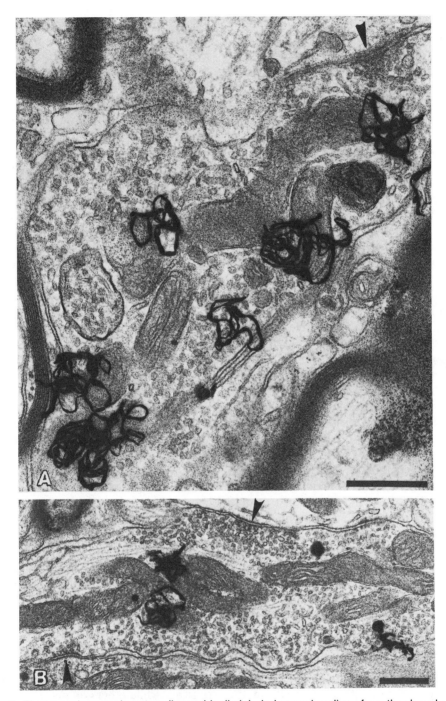

FIG. 12. Electron microscopic autoradiographically labeled axonal endings from the dorsal nucleus of the lateral lemniscus (DNLL) that synapse in the contralateral central nucleus. **A:** Labeled endings from the DNLL contain pleomorphic synaptic vesicles. **B:** Synaptic contacts (*arrowheads*) are symmetric and sometimes are formed on more than one postsynaptic process. Scale bars = 0.5 μm.

cused on the ipsilateral side. It is possible that bands from different sources will vary in their three-dimensional morphology. If so, differences in the bands may be related to the specific cell types and the axons that participate in the different pathways.

Excitatory and Inhibitory Bands for Binaural Processing

Bands from different sources may convey different types of information about sound. As discussed above, direct inputs to the IC from the cochlear nucleus are monaural, while indirect inputs through the superior olive convey binaural information. Axons from many of these brainstem nuclei will form *excitatory bands* and depolarize neurons in the IC. For example, when the banded inputs from the DCN are electrically stimulated at the dorsal acoustic striae, monaural units in the central nucleus are activated (67). Results from anatomical studies on the synaptic inputs to the IC from the DCN and the AVCN are consistent with excitatory activity (45,47,48). Axonal endings in bands from the cochlear nucleus contain round synaptic vesicles and make asymmetric synaptic junctions in the IC (Fig. 11). These endings synapse on dendrites and cell bodies and account for one-fourth to one-third of the endings with round synaptic vesicles in the central nucleus. While excitatory bands from the cochlear nucleus may provide monaural inputs to the IC, excitatory bands from the superior olivary complex are likely to supply binaural information to the IC.

Inhibitory bands may be created by the inputs from the DNLL and the ipsilateral LSO. Immunocytochemical studies show that most, if not all, of the cells in the DNLL contain gamma-aminobutyric acid (GABA), a putative inhibitory neurotransmitter (3,38,58,73). This suggests that the multisynaptic DNLL pathway could provide a banded, tonotopically organized, inhibitory input to the contralateral IC. The

DNLL receives inputs from both the cochlear nucleus and the superior olive, so it may process both monaural and binaural information (63). The fine structure of the DNLL projection to the IC is consistent with an inhibitory function (69). Axonal endings from the DNLL in the contralateral IC contain pleomorphic synaptic vesicles and make symmetric synaptic contacts, often on more than one postsynaptic structure (Fig. 12 A and B). Moreover, the projection from the DNLL is the source of about one-third of the endings with pleomorphic vesicles in the central nucleus.

An inhibitory function also is suggested for the ipsilateral projection from the LSO. At least 40% to 60% of the uncrossed projection from the LSO to the IC is immunoreactive with antibodies to glycine, a second putative inhibitory neurotransmitter (63). The remaining portion of the uncrossed projection and the entire projection to the opposite IC are not glycine immunoreactive. Cells in the LSO also have been labeled by retrograde transport after injections of [^{3}H]glycine in the ipsilateral IC (31). Since the projection from the ipsilateral LSO is distinctly banded and tonotopically organized, the glycinergic component of this projection could form inhibitory bands. The crossed projection from the LSO could form excitatory bands.

OVERLAPPING BANDS MAY CREATE SYNAPTIC DOMAINS RELATED TO DIFFERENT NEURAL RESPONSES

If banded inputs overlap in a predictable manner, they could form unique functional zones or *synaptic domains*. This premise requires that bands from some sources overlap, while others do not. If bands from all sources overlap, the result would be a homogeneous mixture of axonal endings. However, the original observations of bands in degeneration material suggested that the bands would interdigitate when superimposed (52). A better example of how bands may interdigitate is provided by an experiment in which the LSO was injected with different anterograde tracers on the two sides (21). The major observation is that the heavily labeled areas of the ipsilateral projection are complementary to the heaviest labeling in the contralateral projection (Fig. 13). This finding suggests that the potentially excitatory and inhibitory bands from the LSO do not overlap in the IC.

If there is a regular and predictable convergence of bands, this phenomenon could be directly related to some of the most common response types in the IC (see review by Irvine [32]). At least three types of synaptic domains are possible, and each could be dominated by a particular afferent pathway to the IC. One synaptic domain may be dominated by the contralateral LSO projection and account for responses where exci-

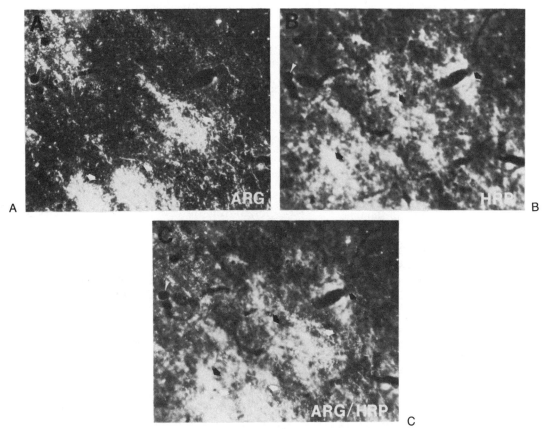

FIG. 13. Photomicrographs to illustrate the relationship of bilateral projections from the lateral superior olive (LSO) in a double-labeling experiment. The same field is shown in all three micrographs. *Arrows* point to three clusters of labeled processes in each frame. *Arrowheads* point to a blood vessel for the alignment of the frames. **A:** Bands from the ipsilateral LSO (*white arrows*) labeled with [³H]leucine after the section had been prepared as an autoradiograph (ARG). **B:** Bands from the contralateral LSO (*black arrows*) labeled by the anterograde transport of wheat germ-HRP (HRP) and photographed prior to the autoradiography procedure. **C:** ARG and HRP images superimposed through the use of a camera lucida. With few exceptions, the heavily labeled areas of the ipsilateral and contralateral projections are complementary. (From the experiment described in ref. 68. Photographs courtesy of Dr. C. K. Henkel.)

tation is produced by sounds in the contralateral ear and suppressed by sounds in the ipsilateral ear (EI). A second domain may be dominated by the MSO and could be related to cells in the IC that are excited by sounds in either ear (EE). A third domain in the central nucleus or the dorsal cortex may be dominated by monaural inputs from the contralateral cochlear nucleus. Monaural units (EO) where ipsilateral stimuli are ineffective could be related to this domain. For each domain, the likelihood of convergence of the ascending pathways is predicted by the response of the unit to sound in the ipsilateral ear. For example, the potentially inhibitory crossed projection of the DNLL is most compatible with the EI domain. The excitatory inputs from the ipsilateral AVCN are compatible with the EE domain. Although these relationships can be predicted, the specific features of synaptic domains in the IC remain to be established.

Disc-shaped Cells May Be Confined to a Single Synaptic Domain

If synaptic domains define functional zones within the central nucleus, then neurons within them may have similar response properties. This suggests that the dendritic orientation is an important factor in determining the response characteristics of a neuron. Disc-shaped cells are a major component of the fibro-dendritic laminae in the central nucleus and are quite likely to be confined to one type of synaptic domain or another. In the disc-shaped cell, the dendritic orientation parallels the afferent fibers in bands. However, the width of the dendritic field is invariably less than the 200-μm width of the band. Several disc-shaped cells, side by side, may be totally confined to a single synaptic domain. Anatomical evidence at the EM level shows that cells within a band receive numerous synaptic contacts on their dendrites (45,

48,69). Other disc-shaped cells nearby, outside that band but in another synaptic domain, could receive different synaptic inputs and display different response properties.

Stellate Cells May Enter More than One Synaptic Domain

In contrast to disc-shaped cells, the responses of stellate cells in the IC could reflect the synthesis of information from several synaptic domains. Stellate cells represent a significant second type of cell in the central nucleus and the main cell type outside of the central nucleus. Their dendritic fields are either spherical or ovoid and oriented perpendicular to the fibro-dendritic laminae and the bands. Because the dendritic field of a stellate cell is usually larger than 200 μm wide, it is likely that the dendrites will lie in two or more adjacent bands. If a single stellate receives synaptic inputs from more than one band or synaptic domain, its response properties may be different from those of a cell confined to a single synaptic domain.

Features Other than Dendritic Orientation May Effect Neural Responses

All neurons may not receive the same pattern of synaptic inputs on their surface. For example, large disc-shaped and stellate cells in the central nucleus receive many axosomatic synapses (46). Medium and small cells do not. Some of these numerous axosomatic inputs are presumed excitatory synapses from the cochlear nucleus. However, inputs from other sources may have different distributions. Even if the functional properties of a synaptic domain largely determine the response properties of a neuron, the synaptic distribution and other features may still be a factor in shaping the responses of individual cell types.

ORGANIZATION OF INTRINSIC CONNECTIONS AND EFFERENT PATHWAYS OF THE INFERIOR COLLICULUS

The IC plays a role as the interface between the hindbrain and the forebrain portions of the auditory system. The anatomy of the efferent projections of the IC suggests that they are not simply a continuation of the ascending pathways from the hindbrain. Unlike the ascending afferents that terminate primarily in the central nucleus, the efferent pathways originate in separate parts of the midbrain.

Types of Efferent Pathways

The efferent pathways of the IC are identified by their site of origin and their relation to targets in the medial geniculate body (6,12,34,44,49). The *central pathway* begins in the central nucleus of the IC, makes a synapse in the ventral division of the medial geniculate body, and terminates in the primary auditory cortex. The *pericentral pathways* begin in the cortical and paracentral parts of the colliculus. These terminate in the deep dorsal, dorsal, and ventrolateral nuclei in the medial geniculate. The *lateral tegmental system* (41) originates in the lateral midbrain tegmentum, primarily the sagulum, and in the posterior deep layers of the superior colliculus. These terminate primarily in the dorsal nucleus and supra-geniculate of the medial geniculate, respectively. Each pathway continues to a specific area of the auditory or temporal cortex. Pericentral pathways terminate in the belt cortex adjacent to the primary auditory cortex, and the lateral tegmental pathways terminate in a second tier of the belt cortex. Except for the central pathway, each efferent pathway is reciprocated by descending projections from the same parts of the cortex to the midbrain sites of origin.

In addition to these specific pathways, the *widespread pathway* originates from neurons distributed throughout the IC and the lateral tegmentum. This pathway has as its target the medial division of the medial geniculate body. That thalamic nucleus projects widely to all portions of the auditory cortex.

Intrinsic Connections of the Inferior Colliculus May Be Complex

Since only the central efferent pathway resembles a clear-cut continuation of the ascending inputs to the central nucleus, the intrinsic connections may be important for information processing within the IC. Intrinsic connections may distribute the integrated output of the neurons to other parts of the IC and to the adjacent midbrain tegmentum, which, in turn, contribute projections to the thalamus. The details of these intrinsic connections at the cellular level are just beginning to emerge.

Intracellular injections of HRP and Golgi impregnations show that neurons in the IC can have complex axonal arbors (35,52,59). For example, one stellate cell injected in the central nucleus has an axonal arbor with more than 2,000 terminal boutons (Fig. 14). Moreover, this axon continued into the brachium of the IC and is likely to be either an ascending or a descending efferent. This suggests that a cell may contribute to the intrinsic axonal plexus of the IC *and* also participate in efferent projections. Not all injected cells have axons this complex. Some are simpler but still distributed widely relative to the fibro-dendritic laminae (Fig. 3). Still other cells have axon collaterals that are more parallel to the laminae. It is probably reasonable to conclude that most neurons in the IC give off some type of axon collaterals within the colliculus.

Axons that branch within the IC may travel between subdivisions to form important intercollicular connections. For example, the central nucleus emits a heavy projection to the lateral nucleus as the efferent

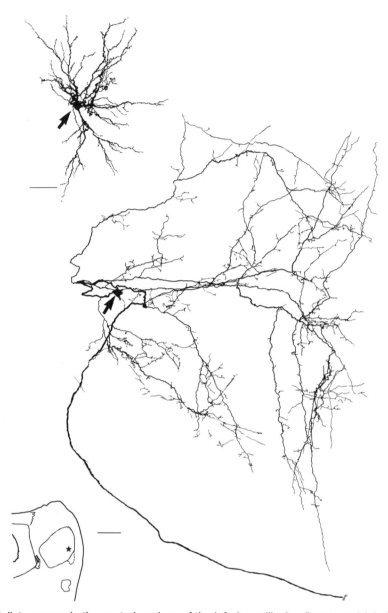

FIG. 14. Stellate neuron in the central nucleus of the inferior colliculus (inset, *star*) labeled by intracellular injection of HRP. *Arrows* indicate the position of the cell body in the drawings of the soma and the dendrites (upper left) and the axon (middle). The axon in this neuron makes extensive collateral branches and terminals within the central nucleus. Soma, dendrites, and axon drawn in sagittal plane of section. Location of cell (inset) shown in transverse computer reconstruction. (Modified from ref. 35, with permission.)

fibers travel toward the brachium (7,34). Axons from the central nucleus also travel dorsally to enter the commissure of the IC (5). Some of these are observed to emit collaterals in the dorsal cortex (34; Morest and Oliver, *unpublished observations*). However, many continue to the opposite IC and the medial geniculate body (5,49). Many cells in the dorsal cortex also may project to the opposite IC (49).

Some of these intercollicular connections in the IC may be involved in inhibitory circuits. Recent studies in the rat and cat show that many cells in the IC may use gamma-aminobutyric acid (GABA) as a neurotransmitter (53,57). In terms of the cell types defined in Golgi preparations, it is clear that some disc-shaped and stellate varieties can be labeled with glutamic acid decarboxylase (GAD) and GABA antibodies. However, further characterization of their cytological features is necessary. But, more important, this result suggests that intrinsic connections may include more than one type of inhibitory circuit.

Several Cell Types in the Inferior Colliculus May Project Rostrally

The ultimate consequence of information processing in the IC is the transmission of information about the auditory stimulus to the thalamus. Many of the cell types previously identified with Golgi methods may send their axons to the medial geniculate body (46). In the central nucleus, large, medium, and small disc-shaped as well as large stellate cells can be labeled after injections of HRP in the medial geniculate body. However, it is not known whether the different cell types have the same targets in the thalamus.

The presence of multiple cell types with efferent projections implies that some type of parallel processing is possible in this part of the auditory system. But the consequences of such processing are not well appreciated. It does seem likely that the neural responses of cells in the central nucleus of the IC could be dominated by synaptic domains. Disc-shaped cells could respond to sounds differently than do stellate cells because these types differ in their relationship with the fibro-dendritic laminae and the banded afferents. The responses of both cell types could be further shaped by intrinsic connections within the IC. Finally, the activity of both disc-shaped and stellate cells is conveyed to the medial geniculate body. Clearly, further research at the cellular level is necessary to discover how information about sound is transmitted rostrally in the central auditory pathway.

ACKNOWLEDGMENTS

This work includes the efforts of many individuals. We are indebted to Drs. D. K. Morest, W. C. Hall, and C. K. Henkel for their contributions. We especially wish to thank G. Beckius, C. Krevolin, N. Julian, L. T. Andrus, S. D. Flynn, and R. R. Morest for technical assistance. This work was supported by NIH grants DC00189 and NS18627.

REFERENCES

1. Adams JC. Ascending projections to the inferior colliculus. *J Comp Neurol* 1979;183:519–538.
2. Adams JC. Cytology of periolivary cells and the organization of their projections in the cat. *J Comp Neurol* 1983;215:275–289.
3. Adams JC, Mugnaini E. Dorsal nucleus of the lateral lemniscus: a nucleus of GABAergic projection neurons. *Brain Res Bull* 1984;13:585–590.
4. Aitkin LM, Kenyon CE, Philpott P. The representation of the auditory and somatosensory systems in the external nucleus of the cat inferior colliculus. *J Comp Neurol* 1981;196:25–40.
5. Aitkin LM, Phillips SC. The interconnections of the inferior colliculi through their commissure. *J Comp Neurol* 1984;228:210–216.
6. Andersen RA, Roth GL, Aitkin LM, Merzenich MM. The efferent projections of the central nucleus and the pericentral nucleus of the inferior colliculus in the cat. *J Comp Neurol* 1980;194:649–662.
7. Andersen RA, Synder RL, Merzenich MM. The topographic organization of corticocollicular

projections from physiologically identified loci in the AI, AII, and anterior cortical fields of the cat. *J Comp Neurol* 1980;191:479–494.

8. Berman AL. *A cytoarchitectonic atlas with stereotaxic coordinates.* Madison: The University of Wisconsin Press, 1968.

9. Beyerl BD. Afferent projections to the central nucleus of the inferior colliculus in the rat. *Brain Res* 1978;145:209–223.

10. Browner RH, Webster DB. Projections of the trapezoid body and the superior olivary complex of the Kangaroo rat (*Dipodomys merriami*). *Brain Behav Evol* 1975;11:322–354.

11. Brunso-Bechtold JK, Thompson GC, Masterton RB. HRP study of the organization of auditory afferents ascending to the central nucleus of inferior colliculus in cat. *J Comp Neurol* 1981; 197:705–722.

12. Galford MB. The parcellation of the medial geniculate body of the cat defined by the auditory properties of single units. *J Neurosci* 1983;3: 2350–2364.

13. Cant NB. Identification of cell types in the anteroventral cochlear nucleus that project to the inferior colliculus. *Neurosci Lett* 1982;32:241–246.

14. Cant NB, Casseday JH. Projections from the anteroventral cochlear nucleus to the lateral and medial superior olivary nuclei. *J Comp Neurol* 1986;247:447–476.

15. Cant NB, Morest DK. The structural basis for stimulus coding in the cochlear nucleus of the cat. In: Berlin CI, ed. *Recent developments in hearing science.* San Diego: College Hill Press, 1984;373–421.

16. Casseday JH, Covey E. Central auditory pathways in directional hearing. In: Yost WA, Gourvitch G, eds. *Directional hearing.* New York: Springer-Verlag, 1987;109–145.

17. Coleman JR, Clerici WJ. Sources of projections to subdivisions of the inferior colliculus in the rat. *J Comp Neurol* 1987;262:215–226.

18. Diamond IT, Jones EG, Powell TPS. The projection of the auditory cortex upon the diencephalon brain stem in the cat. *Brain Res* 1969;15: 305–340.

19. Edwards SB, Ginsburgh CL, Henkel CK, Stein BE. Sources of subcortical projections to the superior colliculus in the cat. *J Comp Neurol* 1979;184:309–330.

20. Elverland HH. Ascending and intrinsic projections of the superior olivary complex in the cat. *Exp Brain Res* 1978;32:117–134.

21. Faye-Lund H. The neocortical projection to the inferior colliculus in the albino rat. *Anat Embryol* 1985;173:53–70.

22. Faye-Lund H, Osen KK. Anatomy of the inferior colliculus in rat. *Anat Embryol* 1985;171: 1–20.

23. FitzPatrick KA. Cellular architecture and topographic organization of the inferior colliculus of the squirrel monkey. *J Comp Neurol* 1975;164: 185–208.

24. FitzPatrick KA, Imig TJ. Projections of auditory cortex upon the thalamus and midbrain in the owl monkey. *J Comp Neurol* 1978;177:537–556.

25. Geniec P, Morest DK. The neuronal architecture of the human posterior colliculus. *Acta Otolaryngol [Suppl]* 1971;295:1–33.

26. Glendenning KK, Brunso-Bechtold JK, Thompson GC, Masterton RB. Ascending auditory afferents to the nuclei of the lateral lemniscus. *J Comp Neurol* 1981;197:673–703.

27. Glendenning KK, Masterton RB. Acoustic chiasm: efferent projections of the lateral superior olive. *J Neurosci* 1983;3:1521–1537.

28. Goldberg JM, Moore RY. Ascending projections of the lateral lemniscus in the cat and monkey. *J Comp Neurol* 1967;129:143–156.

29. Gonzalez-Hernandez TH, Mayer G, Ferres-Torres R, Castañeyra-Perdomo A, Delgado MdMP. Afferent connections of the inferior colliculus in the albino mouse. *J Hirnforsch* 1987; 3:315–323.

30. Henkel CK, Spangler KM. Organization of the efferent projections of the medial superior olivary nucleus in the cat as revealed by HRP and autoradiographic tracing methods. *J Comp Neurol* 1983;221:416–428.

31. Hutson KA. Connections of the auditory midbrain: efferent projections of the dorsal nucleus of the lateral lemniscus, the nucleus sagulum, and the origins of the GABAergic commissure of Probst. Doctoral dissertation. Florida State University, Tallahassee, FL, 1988.

32. Irvine DRF. The auditory brainstem. In: Ottoson D, ed. *Progress in sensory physiology,* vol. 7. Berlin: Springer-Verlag, 1986.

33. Kudo M. Projections of the nuclei of the lateral lemniscus in the cat: an autoradiographic study. *Brain Res* 1981;221:57–69.

34. Kudo M, Niimi K. Ascending projections of the inferior colliculus in the cat: an autoradiography study. *J Comp Neurol* 1980;191:545–566.

35. Kuwada S, Yin TCT, Haberly LB, Wickesberg RE. Binaural interaction in the cat inferior colliculus: physiology and anatomy. In: Van Den Brink G, Bilsen FA, eds. *Psychophysical, physiological, and behavioral studies in hearing.* Delft: Delft University Press, 1980;401–411.

36. Meininger V, Pol D, Derer P. The inferior colliculus of the mouse. A Nissl and Golgi study. *Neuroscience* 1986;17:1159–1179.

37. Merzenich MM, Reid MD. Representation of the cochlea within the inferior colliculus. *Brain Res* 1974;77:397–415.

38. Moore JK, Moore RY. Glutamic acid decarboxylase-like immunoreactivity in brainstem auditory nuclei of the rat. *J Comp Neurol* 1987;260: 157–174.

39. Moore JK, Osen KK. The human cochlear nuclei. In: Creutzfeld O, Scheich H, Schreiner C, eds. *Hearing mechanisms and speech (Exp Brain Res [Suppl II]).* New York: Springer, 1979;36–44.

40. Morest DK. The laminar structure of the inferior colliculus of the cat. *Anat Rec* 1964;148:314.

41. Morest DK. The lateral tegmental system of the

midbrain and the medial geniculate body: study with Golgi and Nauta methods in cat. *J Anat (Lond)* 1965;99:611–634.55.

42. Morest DK, Oliver DL. The neuronal architecture of the inferior colliculus in the cat: defining the functional anatomy of the auditory midbrain *J Comp Neurol* 1984;222:209–236.

43. Nordeen KW, Killackey HP, Kitzes LM. Ascending auditory projections to the inferior colliculus in the adult gerbil, Meriones unguiculatus. *J Comp Neurol* 1983;214:131–143.

44. Oliver DL. A Golgi study of the medial geniculate body in the tree shrew (*Tupaia glis*). *J Comp Neurol* 1982;209:1–16.

45. Oliver DL. Dorsal cochlear nucleus projections to the inferior colliculus in the cat: a light and electron microscopic study. *J Comp Neurol* 1984;224:155–172.

46. Oliver DL. Neuron types in the central nucleus of the inferior colliculus that project to the medial geniculate body. *Neuroscience* 1984;11:409–424.

47. Oliver DL. Quantitative analyses of axonal endings in the central nucleus of the inferior colliculus and distribution of 3H-labeling after injections in the dorsal cochlear nucleus. *J Comp Neurol* 1985;237:343–359.

48. Oliver DL. Projections to the inferior colliculus from the anteroventral cochlear nucleus in the cat: possible substrates for binaural interaction. *J Comp Neurol* 1987;264:24–46.

49. Oliver DL, Hall WC. The medial geniculate body in the tree shrew, *Tupaia glis*. I. Cytoarchitecture and midbrain connections. *J Comp Neurol* 1978;182:423–458.

50. Oliver DL, Hall WC. The medial geniculate body of the tree shrew, *Tupaia glis*. II. Connections with the neocortex. *J Comp Neurol* 1978;182:459–494.

51. Oliver DL, Kuwada S, Batra R, Stanford TR, Henkel C. Structural components of binaural information processing in the auditory midbrain. Physiology and anatomy of HRP-injected cells in the cat and gerbil. *Soc Neurosci Abstr* 1986;12:1271.

52. Oliver DL, Morest DK. The central nucleus of the inferior colliculus in the cat. *J Comp Neurol* 1984;222:237–264.

53. Oliver DL, Nuding SC, Beckius G. Multiple cell types have GABA immunoreactivity in the inferior colliculus of the cat. *Soc Neurosci Abstr* 1988;14:490.

54. Osen KK. Projections of the cochlear nuclei on the inferior colliculus in the cat. *J Comp Neurol* 1972;144:355–372.

55. Ramón y Cajal S. Nerf acoustique: Sa branche cochléene ou nerf cochléaire. In: *Histologie de Système Nerveux de l'Homme et des Vertébrés*. Madrid: Instituto Ramón y Cajal (1972 reprint), 1909;774–838.

56. RoBards MJ. Somatic neurons in the brainstem and neocortex projecting to the external nucleus of the inferior colliculus: anatomical study in the opossum. *J Comp Neurol* 1979;184:547–566.

57. Roberts RC, Ribak CE. An electron microscopic study of GABAergic neurons and terminals in the central nucleus of the inferior colliculus of the rat. *J Neurocytol* 1987;16:333–345.

58. Roberts RC, Ribak CE. GABAergic neurons and axon terminal in the brainstem auditory nuclei of the gerbil. *J Comp Neurol* 1987;258:267–280.

59. Rockel AJ, Jones EG. The neuronal organization of the inferior colliculus of the adult cat. I. The central nucleus. *J Comp Neurol* 1973;147: 22–60.

60. Roth GL, Aitkin LM, Andersen RA, Merzenich MM. Some features of the spatial organization of the central nucleus of the inferior colliculus of the cat. *J Comp Neurol* 1978;182:661–680.

61. Ryugo DK, Willard FH. The dorsal cochlear nucleus of the mouse: a light microscopic analysis of neurons that project to the inferior colliculus. *J Comp Neurol* 1985;242:381–396.

62. Ryugo DK, Willard FH, Fekete DM. Differential afferent projections to the inferior colliculus from the cochlear nucleus in the albino mouse. *Brain Res* 1981;210;342–349.

63. Saint Marie RL, Ostapoff E-M, Morest DK, Wenthold RJ. A glycine-immunoreactive projection of the cat lateral superior olive: possible role in midbrain ear dominance. *J Comp Neurol* (*in press*).

64. Schroeder DM, Jane JA. Projection of dorsal column nuclei and spinal cord to brainstem and thalamus in the tree shrew, *Tupaia glis*. *J Comp Neurol* 1971;142:309–350.

65. Schweizer H. The connections of the inferior colliculus and the organization of the brainstem auditory system in the greater horseshoe bat (Rhinolophus ferrumequinum). *J Comp Neurol* 1981;201:25–49.

66. Semple MN, Aitkin LM. Representation of sound frequency and laterality by units in central nucleus of cat inferior colliculus. *J Neurophysiol* 1979;42:1626–1639.

67. Semple MN, Aitkin LM. Physiology of pathway from dorsal cochlear nucleus to inferior colliculus revealed by electrical and auditory stimulation. *Exp Brain Res* 1980;41:19–28.

68. Shneiderman A, Henkel CK. Banding of lateral superior olivary nucleus afferents in the inferior colliculus: a possible substrate for sensory integration. *J Comp Neurol* 1987;266:519–534.

69. Shneiderman A, Oliver DL. Inhibitory inputs to the inferior colliculus: an EM autoradiographic study of the projections from the dorsal nucleus of the lateral lemniscus (*submitted*).

70. Shneiderman A, Oliver DL, Henkel CK. The connections of the dorsal nucleus of the lateral lemniscus. An inhibitory parallel pathway in the ascending auditory system? *J Comp Neurol* 1988;276:188–208.

71. Stotler WA. An experimental study of the cells and connections of the superior olivary complex of the cat. *J Comp Neurol* 1953;98:401–432.

72. Tanaka K, Otani K, Tokunaga A, Sugita S. The organization of neurons in the nucleus of the lat-

eral lemniscus projecting to the superior colliculi in the rat. *Brain Res* 1985;341:252–260.

73. Thompson GC, Cortez AM, Lam DM. Localization of GABA immunoreactivity in the auditory brainstem of guinea pigs. *Brain Res* 1985;339:119–122.

74. Warr WB. Fiber degeneration following lesions in the anterior ventral cochlear nucleus of the cat. *Exp Neurol* 1966;14:453–474.

75. Warr WB. Fiber degeneration following lesions in the posteroventral cochlear nucleus of the cat. *Exp Neurol* 1969;23:140–155.

76. Warr WB. Fiber degeneration following lesions in the multipolar and globular cell areas in the ventral cochlear nucleus of the cat. *Brain Res* 1972;40:247–270.

77. Whitley JM, Henkel CK. Topographical organization of the inferior collicular projection and other connections of the ventral nucleus of the

lateral lemniscus. *J Comp Neurol* 1984;229:257–270.

78. Willard FH, Martin GF. The auditory brainstem nuclei and some of their projections to the inferior colliculus in the North American opossum. *Neuroscience* 1983;10:1203–1232.

79. Zook JM, Casseday JH. Origin of ascending projections to inferior colliculus in the mustache bat, Pteronotus parnelli. *J Comp Neurol* 1982;207:14–28.

80. Zook JM, Casseday JH. Convergence of ascending pathways at the inferior colliculus of the mustache bat, pteronotus parnelli. *J Comp Neurol* 1987;261:347–361.

81. Zook JM, Winer JA, Pollak GD, Bodenhamer RD. Topology of the central nucleus of the mustache bat's inferior colliculus: correlation of single unit properties and neuronal architecture. *J Comp Neurol* 1985;231:530–546.

Neurobiology of Hearing: The Central Auditory System, edited by R. A. Altschuler et al. Raven Press, Ltd., New York © 1991.

10

Functional Pharmacology of Inferior Colliculus Neurons

Carl L. Faingold, Greta Gehlbach, and Donald M. Caspary

Department of Pharmacology, Southern Illinois University School of Medicine, Springfield, Illinois 62794-9230

This chapter presents information concerning the identity of putative neurotransmitters of the inferior colliculus (IC), particularly data obtained utilizing microiontophoretic techniques. We attempt to identify possible functions of these transmitters in the physiology of this nucleus where possible, and pathological implications are also considered. This review concentrates on the central nucleus of the IC (ICc).

ANATOMICAL CONSIDERATIONS

The ICc receives axons from the lateral lemniscal tract that arise from several auditory structures. These include contralateral input from both the dorsal and ventral cochlear nucleus (CN) (68), ipsilateral input arising from the medial superior olive, and bilateral input ascending from the lateral superior olive (1,2,6,12,18,19,45,47,66,67, 70,91). The ipsilateral ventral nucleus of the lateral lemniscus, the dorsal nucleus of the lateral lemniscus (DNLL) of both sides, and the contralateral IC also project to IC (18). A descending pathway from the cortex has also been described (6). The number and complexity of these inputs, which may mediate both excitation and inhibition, make it difficult to define the exact sources

of particular inhibitory and excitatory components observed in the response patterns of IC neurons. Ascending afferent axons projecting from the CN, the superior olivary complex, and the nuclei of the lateral lemniscus to the ICc run in laminae formed by the cells of this nucleus and terminate on the principal cells (47). While the bitufted and fusiform principal cells contribute most to the formation of the laminae, multipolar cells are also observed (62,80,85). The cells in the ICc range from large (>25 μm) to small (10–15 μm), and the principal cells receive a dense plexus of terminals that forms symmetric synaptic contacts covering the soma and proximal dendrites of these neurons (80). Another dense plexus of terminals contacts the dendrites of these neurons, but most of the terminals of this plexus form asymmetric synaptic contacts.

PHYSIOLOGICAL CONSIDERATIONS

The acoustic response patterns of most IC neurons to tone burst stimuli display temporal periods of excitation, and, in many cases, periods of suppressed firing are also observed (8,13,19a,43,87). These suppressed periods may be subserved by inhibition. An excitatory response is evoked in many IC neurons upon contralateral acoustic stimulation. However, if a stimulus at the same frequency and similar intensity is simultaneously presented to the ipsilateral ear, this excitatory response is often suppressed (7,8,32). Frequency-selective firing suppression, "off," "on," nonmonotonic rate-intensity functions, postexcitatory suppression, and pauser responses are also observed in ICc neurons (see ref. 7 for review), and some or all of these phenomena may reflect inhibition at the level of the IC. Although patterns of firing suppression in the IC may reflect processing at lower levels, evidence has accumulated that supports the occurrence of direct neuronal inhibition in IC neurons as well. Important evidence for the occurrence of direct inhibition in IC neurons is provided by the observations of inhibitory postsynaptic potentials associated with and likely subserving binaural and ipsilateral inhibition as well as postexcitatory inhibition (54, 59,60,65). Excitatory responses observed in IC neurons are subserved by excitatory postsynaptic potentials (60,65). Electrical stimulation of the contralateral dorsal CN only results in excitation in IC neurons that exhibit binaural inhibition, suggesting that the inhibition originates from a different neuronal source (97). Direct bilateral projections from the anterior ventral CN to the IC have also been observed that may play a role in the binaural interactions observed in the IC (51a,69,103a). The region in the bat IC that contains predominantly binaurally inhibited neurons receives input primarily from the DNLL and the lateral superior olive (87a). The nature of binaural interactions in the ICc neurons has been shown to be qualitatively different from those occurring in the superior olivary complex, which also projects to the IC, indicating that additional binaural processing occurs in the IC (20,55). Many of the neurons of the lateral superior olive and nuclei of the lateral lemniscus that project to the IC contain inhibitory amino acids, and the reversal of ear dominance that occurs in many ICc neurons has been suggested to involve these inhibitory amino acid-containing projections (3,50,91).

NEUROTRANSMITTER NEUROCHEMISTRY AND LOCALIZATION

The identity of the neurotransmitters that mediate the complex acoustic response patterns of IC neurons has not been established. The variety of synaptic contacts as well as the vesicle sizes and shapes that have been observed in electronmicrographs of the IC (80,86) suggest that several different neurotransmitters may be present and may be released via acoustic stimulation onto IC neurons.

PUTATIVE INHIBITORY TRANSMITTERS

Gamma-Aminobutyric Acid Neurochemistry and Localization

Considerable neurochemical data support a role of the inhibitory amino acid gamma-aminobutyric acid (GABA) as a possible mediator of inhibition in the IC. GABA levels in the IC are reported to be quite high (42,99). High levels of the enzymes responsible for GABA synthesis (glutamic acid decarboxylase [GAD]) and degradation (GABA transaminase) are also observed in the IC (5,23,42,99). The IC has also been shown to contain a number of neurons that are strongly positive for mRNA that encodes for GAD (64a). Levels of GAD in the IC are reported to fall after cochlear but not CN lesions (5,27). The nonuniform distribution of the ascending pathways and the nonuniformity of GAD localization within the IC are consistent with a possible role of GABA as a transmitter in this nucleus (5,61). GABA can be released from IC slices and synaptosomes by calcium-dependent, potassium-mediated depolarization (57,81), and uptake of GABA in IC synaptosomes has also been reported (17a).

The IC is reported to show intense immunocytochemical staining for GABA transaminase, GAD, and GABA (19b,22a, 61,64,73,100). High levels of GABA$_A$ receptor and benzodiazepine receptor binding are also observed in the IC (15,45a,96). Benzodiazepine receptors are often found as accessory receptors in the GABA$_A$ receptor complex, and benzodiazepines are thought to act in large part by enhancing the action of GABA (72). GABA-immunoreactivity has been observed in somata, axons, and dendrites in the ICc (83). IC neurons also strongly label for the mRNA for the alpha-1 subunit of the GABA$_A$ receptor (48b). The dense plexus of GABA-immunoreactive nerve terminals that form symmetric synapses contains flattened or pleomorphic vesicles, covers the cell bodies and dendrites of the large neurons of ICc, and provides an anatomical basis for a strong GABAergic inhibition to these principal projection neurons (80). Many of the intrinsic multipolar or stellate cells in ICc are GAD-immunoreactive neurons with GAD-positive terminals that are reported to project onto the principal cells of IC (80, 83,103). It has been proposed that these GABAergic interneurons may be one important source of intrinsic GABA-mediated inhibition (80). Although a major portion of the GABAergic input to ICc principal cells appears to be intrinsic from these interneurons, an extrinsic GABAergic projection to the IC from the DNLL has also been demonstrated (3). Anatomical studies suggest that the contralateral DNLL may be a major source of ascending GABAergic inhibition (97a,b), and the DNLL is a major source of input to the IC region that contains binaurally inhibited neurons (87a). Recent preliminary studies in our laboratory with electrical stimulation or reversible blockade of the contralateral DNLL, which mimics or blocks binaural inhibition, respectively, support this hypothesis.

Glycine Neurochemistry and Localization

Low levels of glycine are present in the IC, especially in ventral regions, but the level of glycine is not affected by CN lesions (5). Low to moderate levels of receptor binding for glycine and the glycine antagonist strychnine are observed in the IC (11,45a,77,93,113). Calcium-dependent, potassium-evoked release of glycine from IC slices has also been reported (57). Glycine-immunoreactive lateral superior olivary principal neurons (108) may provide part of the glycinergic input to the IC (10,90,91). It has been reported that up to 50% of lateral superior olivary principal cells are glycine immunoreactive (91). The ipsilateral inhibitory projection to the IC from these olivary neurons has been suggested to explain the finding that contralateral stimulation is predominantly excitatory in IC, while ipsilateral stimulation is predominantly inhibitory, reversing the pattern observed in lateral superior olivary neurons (91).

Monoamine Neurochemistry and Localization

The IC is reported to receive noradrenergic innervation from the locus coeruleus (52). Low levels of norepinephrine, its synthetic enzyme (dopamine beta-hydroxylase), and its precursor (dopamine) are present in the IC (52,89,98,102). 5-Hydroxytryptamine is also reported to be present in the IC (26,44).

PUTATIVE EXCITATORY TRANSMITTERS

Excitant Amino Acid Neurochemistry and Localization

Considerably fewer data on putative excitatory transmitters of the IC are available than data regarding inhibitory transmitters. Significant levels of glutamate have been observed in the IC (5), and a small reduction of glutamate levels in extracentral regions of the IC occurs after lesions of the auditory cortex (5). Intermediate levels of glutamate-like immunoreactivity are observed in ICc with high levels in pericentral and external nuclei (73). Glutamate-like immunoreactivity is reported in the majority of cells in the IC (73). Receptor binding of excitant amino acids in the IC is readily observable (24). Quantitative studies indicate that glutamate binding levels in the IC are at an intermediate level (46). Intense immunoreactivity for the glutamate synthetic enzyme phosphate-activated glutaminase is observed in the IC (51b). Many IC neurons are also moderately positive for the mRNA that encodes for aspartate aminotransferase, a synthetic enzyme for aspartate (64a). A dense plexus of terminals contacts the proximal dendrites of the principal cells of the ICc, and most of these terminals are reported to form symmetric synapses, often associated with excitant amino acids (83).

Cholinergic Neurochemistry and Localization

The presence of the synthesizing enzyme for acetylcholine (choline acetyltransferase) and the degradative enzyme acetylcholinesterase has been observed in the IC (5,22,49). High concentrations of nicotinic and muscarinic acetylcholine binding have also been observed in the IC (45a,95), and binding of the nicotinic antagonist alphabungarotoxin, as well as muscarinic cholinergic ligands, is also extensive in this nucleus (63,88,104).

Cholecystokinin Neurochemistry and Localization

It has been suggested that cholecystokinin may play a role as a neuromodulator or neurotransmitter in the central nervous system (CNS) (51). Cholecystokinin is reported to be the most ubiquitous of putative peptide neurotransmitters in the CNS and has been localized by immunocytochemical and neurochemical analyses to brainstem auditory structures, including the IC (40). A detailed study of brainstem auditory structures indicated that many cholecystokinin-immunoreactive terminals and axons are observable in the IC, particularly in dorsal and caudal regions (4). The dorsal portion of the ICc contains a greater number of terminals than the ventral portion of this subnucleus.

Monoamines and peptides as well as other slower acting neurotransmitters may act to modify the action of amino acid rapidly acting transmitters (106). This concept may also be applicable in the IC, but this possibility has not been examined in this nucleus as yet.

IONTOPHORESIS STUDIES

The criteria of mimicry and pharmacological identity can be addressed using iontophoretic techniques most readily *in vivo* where synaptic inputs are intact and physiologically relevant stimuli can be readily presented and precisely controlled. Establishing that a specific neurotransmitter functions in coding of acoustic stimuli is a demanding task. First, the standard criteria that are necessary in other CNS systems must be satisfied. However, a combination of iontophoretic techniques with acoustic paradigms designed to evoke specific auditory response patterns is also needed. Only a small percentage of encountered neurons may exhibit a specific response component, and collecting a large enough neuronal population that exhibits such a response pattern is difficult. This degree of difficulty is compounded by the complexities of the response patterns observed in more rostral auditory nuclei. For example, less than 10% of ICc neurons exhibited a response pause in our studies, making the study of drug effects on this component possible in only a small number of experiments. Regardless of these limitations, the *in vivo* approach is the only way to examine these questions of acoustic coding. The use of the tissue slice approach currently being applied to brainstem auditory structures can also provide vital information on transmitter identification and is the best technique to examine intracellular events. Thus, inhibitory postsynaptic potentials observed in the IC slice are blocked by picrotoxin, an agent that blocks the action of GABA at the chloride channel (97c). However, the inability to utilize auditory stimuli limits the capacity of such *in vitro* studies to define acoustically evoked coding that is stimulus specific and vital for information transfer in this special sensory modality. Details on the techniques utilized in our *in vivo* studies for iontophoresis can be found in Salmoraghi and Weight (92) and Purves (78), and

specific details on the procedures utilized by this laboratory can be found in Faingold and co-workers (32). Our studies involved iontophoretic application of agents affecting the action of neurotransmitters in a total of 774 ICc neurons in 181 rats over a period of more than 5 years. This included 123 ICc neurons from rats with an inherited susceptibility to audiogenic seizures (AGS). Quantitative differences were noted between normal animals and AGS-susceptible rats (32), but the effects were qualitatively very similar. Briefly, the experiments were performed in Sprague-Dawley rats anesthetized initially with ketamine or pentobarbital. Following removal of the stereotaxic restraints the animal was maintained without the discomfort associated with conventional stereotaxic technique. The animal was then paralyzed utilizing a neuromus-

TABLE 1. *Drugs for iontophoretic application*

Agent	Concentration (mM)	pH	Source	Action
Gamma-amino-*N*-butyric acid (GABA)	500	3.5–4.0	Sigma	GABA agonist
Bicuculline methiodide	5	3.0	Sigma	GABA$_A$ antagonist
Nipecotic acid	200	3.0	Sigma	GABA uptake inhibitor
Flurazepam	100	4.0	Hoffman-LaRoche	Benzodiazepine agonist
Baclofen	10	7.0	Ciba	GABA$_B$ agonist
Glycine	500	3.5–4.0	Sigma	IAA (glycine) agonist
Strychnine	10	3.0	Sigma	Glycine antagonist
Norepinephrine	500	4.5–5.5	Sigma	Noradrenergic agonist
5-Hydroxytryptamine	50	3.5	Sigma	Serotoninergic agonist
L-Glutamic acid	1,000	7.0	Sigma	EAA agonist
L-Aspartic acid	500	8.0	Sigma	EAA agonist
NMDA	10	7.0	Tocris	EAA (NMDA) agonist
QUIS	10	5.0	Sigma	EAA (QUIS) agonist
D-alpha-aminoadipic acid	50	7.0	Sigma	EAA (NMDA) antagonist
APV	10	3.5–8.0	Cambridge	EAA (NMDA) antagonist
PDA	100	7.0	Cambridge	EAA (non-NMDA) antagonist
GDEE	200	3.5	Sigma	EAA (non-NMDA) antagonist
Streptomycin	50	5.0	Sigma	EAA (non-NMDA) antagonist
Carbachol	500	6.3	Sigma	Cholinergic agonist
Acetylcholine	1,000	4.0	Sigma	Cholinergic agonist
Cholecystokinin	0.1	8.0	Cambridge	Peptide agonist

APV, DL-2-amino-5-phosphonovaleric acid; EAA, excitant amino acid; GDEE, L-glutamic acid diethylester; IAA, inhibitory amino acid; NMDA, N-methyl-D-aspartate; PDA, *cis*-2,3-piperidine dicarboxylic acid; QUIS, quisqualate.

cular blocker, and all efforts were directed to monitor and maintain the animal in a pain-free condition (32). All experiments were performed under protocols that were approved by Institutional and National Institutes of Health panels, and paralyzed animals were not utilized after 1984. Additional studies were subsequently performed under ketamine/pentobarbital anesthesia in order to compare drug effects under anesthetized and unanesthetized conditions. Extracellular action potentials were recorded from neurons in the ICc using three-barrel twisted or "piggy-back" six-barrel glass microelectrodes (48). The drugs utilized in these studies and their proposed actions are listed in Table 1. Auditory stimuli were delivered through TDH-49 earphones and corrected to dB SPL re 0.0002 dyne/cm^2 (37). The tonal frequency to which the neuron responds at lowest intensity (characteristic frequency) (CF) was determined using an intensity-frequency scan with sculptured tone burst stimulation (9). Neuronal responses were analyzed on-line using poststimulus time histogram (PSTH) analysis (0.5 msec bin width). Acoustic stimulation consisted of 50 presentations of tone burst stimuli (at 2/sec, 100-msec duration with a 5-msec rise-fall) at CF. Electrode tracks and locations were verified by

examination of cresyl violet-stained frozen or paraffin sections.

IONTOPHORESIS OF PUTATIVE INHIBITORY NEUROTRANSMITTERS

Iontophoresis of Agents Affecting the Action of GABA

An early study indicated that IC neuronal firing is inhibited by iontophoretic application of GABA, and blockade of chloride ionophore of the GABA receptor by picrotoxin enhances neuronal responses to sound (105). We examined whether the inhibition observed in the firing patterns of IC neurons could be mimicked by application of GABA, prolonged by blockade of GABA uptake, or blocked by a GABA antagonist (33). The results of these studies attempted to help fulfill some of the additional criteria for establishing GABA as an endogenous inhibitory transmitter in IC neurons.

Iontophoretic application of GABA resulted in a 10% or greater reduction of firing in 99% of ICc neurons tested (see Table 2). During the application of GABA, the responses of these ICc neurons to acoustic stimuli at CF were reduced, as shown by the example in Fig. 1. This inhibitory effect

TABLE 2. *Agents affecting the action of inhibitory neurotransmitters: agents enhancing the action of inhibitory amino acids (IAAs)*

Agent	Number (%) of neurons			
	Total	Excited	Inhibited	No effect
GABA	261	1 (<1)	257 (98.5)	3 (1.1)
Baclofen	13	1 (7.7)	11 (84.6)	1 (7.7)
Flurazepam	58	6 (10.3)	46 (79.3)	6 (10.3)
Nipecotic acid	39	5 (12.8)	34 (87.2)	0 (0)
Glycine	42	1 (2.4)	41 (97.6)	0 (0)
IAA antagonists				
Bicuculline	351	320 (91.2)	10 (2.8)	21 (6.0)
Strychnine	19	12 (63.2)	6 (31.5)	1 (5.3)
Others				
NE	56	3 (5.4)	51 (91.1)	2 (3.6)
5-HT	6	0 (0)	6 (100)	

NE, norepinephrine; 5-HT, 5-hydroxytryptamine.

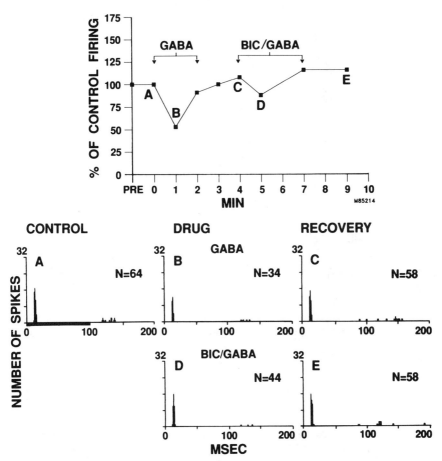

FIG. 1. An example of the inhibitory effect of GABA on the responses of an inferior colliculus (IC) neuron to acoustic stimuli and the reversal of the effect by application of a GABA$_A$ antagonist bicuculline (BIC). The top graph represents the time course of effects, and the bottom poststimulus time histograms (PSTHs) exemplify effects on the pattern of response at characteristic frequency (CF) in this and subsequent figures. The PSTHs were taken at the points on the graph corresponding to the letter designation for each histogram. The response in control before drug application is illustrated in A. The effect of GABA application (35 nA) alone is shown in B, and the effect of the same dose of GABA with simultaneous application of BIC (15 nA) is shown in D. Recovery from the effects of the drugs is shown in C and E. The *darkened line* at the bottom of histogram A shows the duration of the stimulus. N equals the total number of action potentials in the PSTH. (Stimulus: 100-msec tone bursts (5-msec rise-fall) 80 dB contralateral, 17.7 kHz (CF); threshold: 60 dB SPL; PSTHs: 50 stimulus repetitions, 1-msec binwidth.)

began within the first few seconds, most commonly lasted for the duration of the application, and ceased quickly after application was terminated in the vast majority of ICc neurons tested (see Figs. 1–3). In some cases, particularly in barbiturate-anesthetized animals or with prolonged GABA application times, some reduction in the effectiveness of inhibition was observed (31a).

The mean dose of GABA in nA required to produce a 50% decrease in firing of ICc neurons in nonanesthetized rats was not significantly different from that required in barbiturate-anesthetized animals. How-

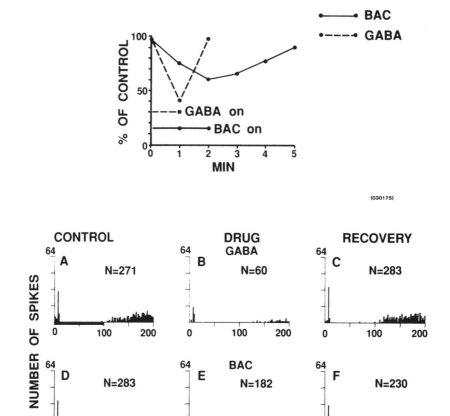

FIG. 2. An example of the comparative inhibitory effects of GABA and the GABA$_B$ agonist baclofen (BAC), on the responses of an inferior colliculus (IC) neuron to acoustic stimuli. The drug time course and poststimulus time histograms (PSTHs) are represented as in Fig. 1. The response in control before drug application is illustrated in column 1 (A and D). Column 2 (B and E) shows the effect of GABA application (35 nA) (in B) and the effect of BAC (75 nA) on the same neuron (in E). The BAC application period was twice that of GABA, it took longer to see the effect, and it tended to last longer. However, the degree of effect was less despite a higher current for application with BAC. Recovery from the effects of the drug is shown in the last column (C and F). The *darkened line* at the bottom of the histogram A shows the duration of the stimulus. N equals the total number of action potentials in the PSTH. (Stimulus: 100-msec tone bursts (5-msec rise-fall) 30 dB contralateral, 34.3 kHz (CF); threshold: 10 dB SPL; PSTHs: 50 stimulus repetitions, 1-msec binwidth.)

ever, the effectiveness of GABA in nonanesthetized animals was reduced in epileptic rats when compared to normal rats as measured by the amount of current required to produce the same degree of inhibition (32).

The effects of baclofen, a structural analog of GABA, which is reported to act via GABA$_B$ receptor activation (14) were also examined. Baclofen produced a reduction of tone-evoked responses, especially at lower stimulus intensities (Fig. 2). The onset of this effect was usually much slower, and the recovery was more gradual than that seen with GABA application. Thus, al-

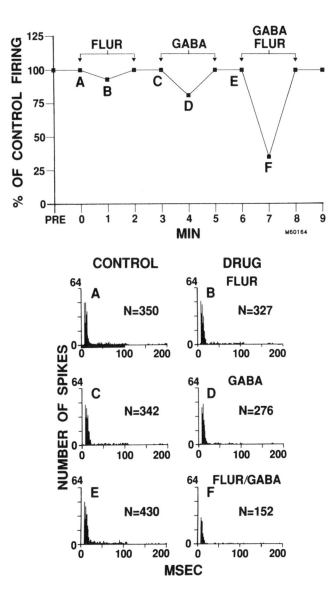

FIG. 3. An example of the inhibitory effects of GABA and a benzodiazepine, flurazepam (FLUR), on the responses of an inferior colliculus (IC) neuron to acoustic stimuli and the interaction of the agents applied simultaneously. The drug time course and post-stimulus time histograms (PSTHs) are represented as in Fig. 1. The response in control before drug application is illustrated in column 1 (A, C, and E). Column 2 (B and D) shows the effect of FLUR (200 nA, 2 min) alone, which was relatively ineffective in B, and the effect of GABA (40 nA, 1 min) in D. The action of combined application of GABA and FLUR is shown in F and is more than an additive effect. The *darkened line* at the bottom of histogram A shows the duration of the stimulus. N equals the total number of action potentials in the PSTH. (Stimulus: 100-msec tone bursts, 60 dB contralateral, 10.0 kHz (CF); threshold: 40 dB SPL.)

though baclofen application resulted in inhibition of ICc neuronal firing, the onset and offset of inhibition produced by this agent had longer latencies, and higher iontophoretic currents of baclofen were required than those needed to produce similar or greater effects with GABA. The effects of GABA could be partially or completely blocked by simultaneous application of the GABA$_A$ antagonist bicuculline, as shown by the example in Fig. 1. Bicuculline was effective in blocking the action of GABA in 15 of 17 neurons in which this interaction was examined.

Benzodiazepines depress neuronal firing, in part by enhancing the action of GABA (72). The firing of most (89%) of the ICc neurons examined was reduced by application of a benzodiazepine, flurazepam, as shown in Table 2. The onset of the depressant effect of flurazepam was generally delayed as compared to the onset of GABA, and it usually required longer periods of application to see effects. The effect of flurazepam was at least additive with the effect of GABA when both agents were applied simultaneously in most ICc neurons tested (see Fig. 3).

Nipecotic acid, which inhibits the uptake of GABA (53), was also applied iontophoretically in our studies. Nipecotic acid application produced a reduction of firing in 86% of the ICc neurons tested (see Table 2). The effects of this agent applied alone were generally not great in magnitude, as shown by the example in Fig. 4. However, in neurons that exhibited a major period of suppression in their response pattern to acoustic stimuli selective augmentation of

this inhibition was observed. The onset of the effect of nipecotic acid was delayed as compared to that seen with GABA application, and the effect generally required a longer duration of application in a fashion similar to that described above for baclofen. When nipecotic acid was applied in combination with GABA, the increase in inhibition was rather marked (see Fig. 4), consistent with its reported ability to block GABA uptake. In many ICc neurons application of nipecotic acid augmented the reduction in discharge rate induced by ipsilateral stimuli (31a). Application of nipecotic acid also reduced the response to monaural

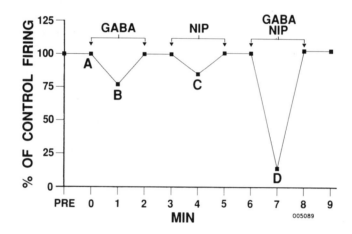

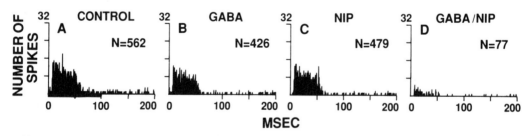

FIG. 4. An example of the effects of GABA and nipecotic acid (NIP), a GABA uptake inhibitor, and the interaction of the agents applied simultaneously on the responses of an inferior colliculus (IC) neuron to acoustic stimuli. The drug time course and poststimulus time histograms (PSTHs) are represented as in Fig 1. The response in control before drug application is illustrated in A. The effect of GABA (20 nA, 1 min) is shown in B, and the effect of NIP (80 nA, 1 min) is shown in C. The greater than additive effect of combined application of GABA and NIP is shown in D. The *darkened line* at the bottom of histogram A shows the duration of the stimulus. N equals the total number of action potentials in the PSTH. (Stimulus: 100-msec tone bursts, 20 dB contralateral, 13.8 kHz (CF); threshold: 0 dB SPL.)

stimulation, but the degree of firing reduction produced during application of nipecotic acid was greatest on responses that displayed extensive inhibition. A greater degree of nipecotic acid-induced decrease during binaural rather than monaural stimulation occurred in nearly two-thirds of ICc neurons examined (31a). Offset suppression in ICc neurons was also enhanced during the application of nipecotic acid in a number of ICc neurons. Thus, application of nipecotic acid resulted in a diminished overall tone-evoked response of neurons exhibiting offset suppression, but the spontaneous activity that followed the offset suppression was essentially abolished in many of these neurons (31a).

Many ICc neurons exhibited binaural inhibition in which the excitatory response to contralateral stimuli was considerably reduced by simultaneous stimulation of the ipsilateral ear with a like acoustic stimulus (e.g., Fig. 5A vs. 5D). This phenomenon was observed in 54% of 145 ICc neurons in which binaural inhibition and the effects of GABA application were both examined.

Application of a GABA$_A$ receptor antagonist, bicuculline, onto ICc neurons was tested in a large number of ICc neurons, and in 92% of cases the discharge rate of the neurons was increased (see Table 2). The firing increases following bicuculline application took many forms. Different portions of the IC neuronal response pattern were affected, depending on the initial response pattern displayed by the neuron. Thus, in neurons exhibiting onset responses only, the bicuculline-induced firing increase often occurred during this initial response (see Fig. 5B), or it could occur both during the onset period and in the 50 to 100-msec period following the onset period (Fig. 6H). In some cases the onset response became more sustained with bicuculline application (31a).

Bicuculline application also resulted in alterations of the response patterns of ICc neurons that exhibited binaural inhibition (see Fig. 5). Bicuculline frequently blocked binaural inhibition with minimal effects on the response to the contralateral stimulus (Fig. 5). This effect was observed most often when low iontophoretic currents were used. Thus, in a number of ICc neurons, bicuculline produced a relatively selective blockade of binaural inhibition without producing frank excitation. In addition to enhancing responses in neurons displaying binaural inhibition, application of bicuculline could also result in overcoming complete binaural inhibition in neurons displaying no excitatory response to binaural stimulation prior to application of this agent. These findings suggest that GABA may play an important role in the production of binaural inhibition in the IC. Bicuculline, as well as picrotoxin, which blocks the action of GABA at the chloride channel, also greatly increase the firing in IC neurons, block inhibitory postsynaptic potentials, and increase postsynaptic field potentials (primarily in dorsal cortex) in IC slices (75a,97c,112).

Many ICc neurons exhibit nonmonotonic rate-intensity functions that involve a reduction of the number of responses with continued increases in stimulus intensity (Fig. 6). Thus, in the example in Fig. 6, the response at highest intensity (Fig. 6D) contains fewer action potentials than the responses to moderate intensities (Fig. 6B and C). This phenomenon can be reversed by application of bicuculline, as shown in Fig. 6. After bicuculline application the response at highest intensity is selectively enhanced (Fig. 6H) with minimal effects on the responses at moderate intensities (Fig. 6F and G). This effect of bicuculline suggests that nonmonotonicity in IC neurons may also be partly subserved by GABA-mediated inhibition (31a).

Finally, bicuculline produced another effect on an inhibitory process in the IC: offset inhibition. Shortly after the tone burst ceases, a period of suppressed firing is observed in many ICc neurons displaying a sustained temporal firing pattern (see, for example, Fig. 8A). Bicuculline application

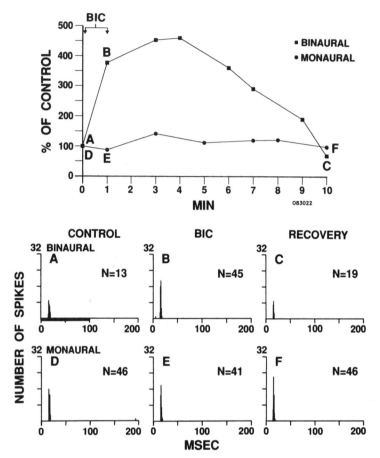

FIG. 5. An example of the effects of a GABA antagonist, bicuculline (BIC), on the responses of an inferior colliculus (IC) neuron to monaural and binaural acoustic stimuli at characteristic frequency (CF). The drug time course and poststimulus time histograms (PSTHs) are represented as in Fig. 1. The control response is shown in column 1 (A and D). The binaural inhibition produced in this neuron causes a reduction of over 70% (A vs D). After application of BIC (100 nA), the inhibitory effect of binaural stimulation is almost completely blocked (B vs D), but the monaural response at the same time point is essentially unaffected (E). Recovery of the binaural inhibition can be observed following the termination of BIC application as shown in the last column (C and F). The *darkened line* at the bottom of histogram A shows the duration of the stimulus. N equals the total number of action potentials in the PSTH. (Stimulus: 100-msec tone bursts, 50 dB contralateral or bilateral, 19.9 kHz (CF) threshold: 30 dB SPL.)

partially reversed this inhibition with the appearance in some neurons of an offset peak where only a valley had been observed prior to drug application (32).

ICc neurons that displayed a discontinuity in an otherwise sustained temporal response pattern (pause) were also affected by application of bicuculline. Moderate doses of bicuculline applied onto neurons displaying a pause resulted in significant decreases in pause duration in the vast majority of ICc neurons exhibiting this pattern (31a). The duration of the response discontinuity in most ICc neurons examined was increased during iontophoretic application of GABA and agents enhancing activation

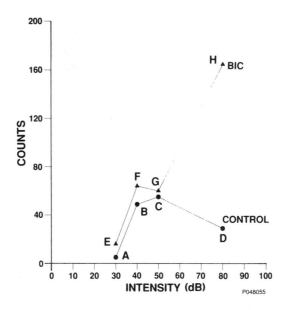

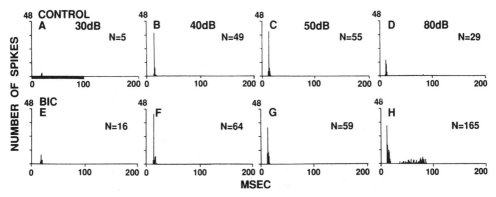

FIG. 6. An example of the effects of a GABA antagonist, bicuculline (BIC), on the responses of an inferior colliculus (IC) neuron to increasing stimulus intensity of the acoustic stimulus at characteristic frequency (CF). The top graph represents the effects of intensity on neuronal discharge rate in the absence and presence of BIC, and the bottom poststimulus time histograms (PSTHs) exemplify effects on the pattern of responses. The response before drug application is shown in the top row (A–D), and the responses after drug application are shown in the bottom row (E–H). Under control conditions, a nonmonotonic rate-intensity function is observed as the stimulus is raised above 40 dB. Following BIC application (50 nA, 4 min) the response to the 80-dB stimulus is greatly increased, suggesting that GABA may mediate the inhibition that results in the nonmonotonic rate-intensity function. The *darkened line* at the bottom of histogram A shows the duration of the stimulus. N equals the total number of action potentials in the PSTH. (Stimulus: 100-msec tone bursts, 2.76 kHz (CF) contralateral; threshold: 13 dB SPL.)

of GABA receptors. Thus, the application of GABA, nipecotic acid, or flurazepam increased the pause duration in most ICc neurons examined (31a). These data suggest a possible role for GABA in the generation of the response pause. Bicuculline iontophoresis also decreases the inhibitory effects of interaural time difference in ICc neurons in recent studies in the owl (43a).

Iontophoresis of Agents Affecting the Action of Glycine

An early study indicated that glycine could suppress IC neuronal firing, but in the same study the glycine antagonist strychnine did not enhance firing and in some cases suppressed IC responses (105). The former finding was confirmed in our studies, but the latter finding was not confirmed in our laboratory. Glycine application produced inhibition of neuronal firing in most ICc neurons examined (see Table 2), but strychnine consistently produced considerable firing increases (see Fig. 8). Glycine was quite effective in producing rapid onset inhibition of 98% of ICc neurons tested (Table 2). The effect of glycine was qualitatively similar to that seen with GABA. However, the degree of effectiveness of glycine was less than that of GABA. Thus, a smaller degree of firing reduction was observed despite higher iontophoretic currents of glycine in over two-thirds of the neurons ($N = 38$) in which GABA and glycine were applied sequentially, as shown in the example in Fig. 7. The mean dose (current) of glycine required to produce the same degree of reduction of firing was 33% greater than the mean dose of GABA in the same IC neurons.

Strychnine has been suggested to be relatively selective as an antagonist at glycine receptors, although there is evidence that this selectivity is not absolute. Blockade of receptors for GABA and other neurotransmitters along with nonselective excitatory effects have been reported under certain conditions (see ref. 37 for review). Strychnine increased the discharge rate of 63% of ICc neurons onto which this agent was applied (Table 2). Strychnine application onto certain ICc neurons could also act to block the effects of binaural inhibition. However, unlike the effects of bicuculline, it was rarely possible to find a dose of strychnine that selectively blocked binaural inhibition. The responses to monaural stimuli were also greatly enhanced following application of strychnine in most of the ICc neurons examined. Thus, before strychnine application in the example in Fig. 8, the number of action potentials in the PSTH from this ICc neuron was increased to over 200% of the monaural response. Both the contralateral excitatory response and the binaurally inhibited response were enhanced, but the degree of enhancement of the binaural response was actually less than that observed with the contralateral stimulus alone. This contrasts markedly with the effect of bicuculline application, which could readily produce a selective blockade of binaural inhibition (see Fig. 5). The reasons for the differences in the action of bicuculline and strychnine may imply that bicuçulline, at least in low doses, can produce a relatively specific blockade of GABA-mediated phenomena. However, strychnine has a broad spectrum of effects on the actions of several neurotransmitters as well as nonspecific excitatory effects that may account for the firing increases with this agent (28). In addition, kinetic factors involved in drug/receptor interactions may also play a role in this dichotomy, since a several-minute period of strychnine application was required before an effect was produced. When the response was enhanced after application of strychnine, this enhancement tended to be very long lasting, often lasting more than 30 min. This time course of action and recovery contrasts markedly with the effects of bicuculline, which most often were clearly visible within 1 min of application and which did not persist for more than 4 to 6 min in most neurons tested.

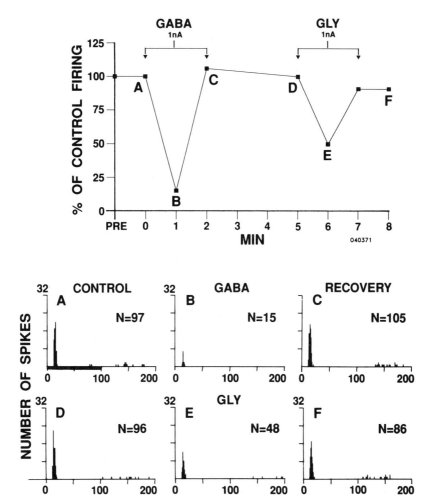

FIG. 7. An example of the sequential inhibitory effects of GABA and glycine (GLY) on the responses of an inferior colliculus (IC) neuron to acoustic stimuli. The drug time course and poststimulus time histograms (PSTHs) are represented as in Fig. 1. The response in control before drug application is illustrated in column 1 (A and D). Column 2 shows the effects of the same current of GABA (B) and GYL (E) (1 nA). The degree of inhibition was consistently greater with GABA, but the time course was similar for both agents. The *darkened line* at the bottom of histogram A shows the duration of the stimulus. N equals the total number of action potentials in the PSTH. (Stimulus: 100-msec tone bursts, 80 dB contralateral, 1.6 kHz (CF); threshold: 60 dB SPL.)

Iontophoresis of Agents Affecting Norepinephrine

Iontophoretic application of norepinephrine in IC neurons generally produced a reduction of spontaneous firing in an early study (25). The effects of norepinephrine on acoustically evoked firing were also examined in our laboratory (Table 2). Iontophoretic or pneumatic application of norepinephrine generally produced a modest decrease in ICc neuronal discharge with a

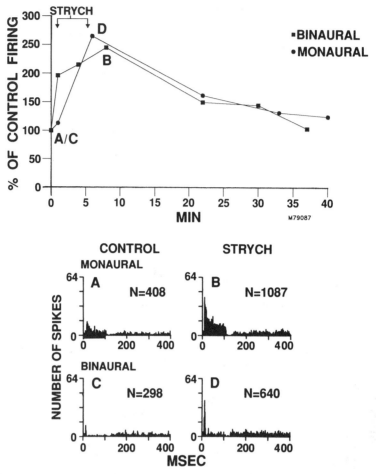

FIG. 8. An example of the effects of a glycine antagonist, strychnine (STRYCH), on the responses of an inferior colliculus (IC) neuron to monaural and binaural acoustic stimuli at characteristic frequency (CF). The drug time course and poststimulus time histograms (PSTHs) are represented as in Fig. 1. The control response is shown in column 1 (A and C). the binaural inhibition produced in this neuron causes a reduction of 27% (C vs A). After application of STRYCH (100 nA, 5 min) the responses to both monaural and binaural stimulation are enhanced (B and D). However, the monaural response is enhanced to about the same degree as the binaural response, suggesting a lack of selectivity of the effect of STRYCH for blockade of binaural inhibition unlike that seen with bicuculline, a GABA antagonist (see Fig. 4). The *darkened line* at the bottom of histogram A shows the duration of the stimulus. N equals the total number of action potentials in the PSTH. (Stimulus: 100-msec tone bursts, 50 dB contralateral or 50 contralateral with 70 dB ipsilateral, 9.2 kHz (CF); threshold: 20 dB SPL.)

slow onset (Fig. 9). However, it was rarely possible to completely block neuronal firing with norepinephrine, in contrast to the effects observed with application of inhibitory amino acids. The time course of the effects of norepinephrine was generally longer than that seen with flurazepam or ni-

pecotic acid. It has been reported in other brain regions that norepinephrine is able to modify the actions of other more rapidly acting neurotransmitters including GABA (106,107). This phenomenon was examined in our recent studies in ICc neurons, and the results indicate that the action of GABA

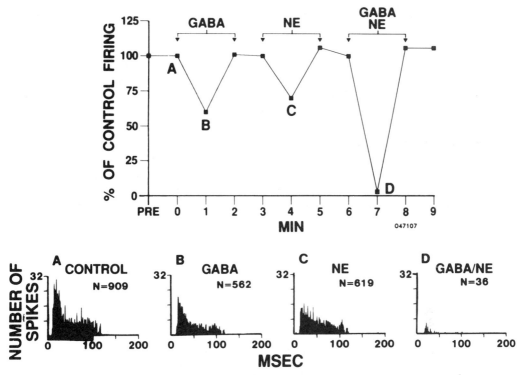

FIG. 9. An example of the action of norepinephrine (NE) and GABA and their interactive effects on the responses of an inferior colliculus (IC) neuron to acoustic stimuli (tone bursts) at characteristic frequency (CF). The drug time course and poststimulus time histograms (PSTHs) are represented as in Fig. 1. The response before drug application is shown in A, and the inhibitory effect of iontophoretic application of GABA (5 nA, 1 min) is shown in B. The effect of NE (80 nA) is shown in C, and the interactive effects of simultaneous application are shown in D illustrating a greater than additive inhibition of firing. N equals the total number of action potentials in the histogram. (Stimulus: 100-msec tone bursts, 50 dB contralateral, 40.2 kHz (CF); threshold: 30 dB SPL.)

is amplified by simultaneous application of norepinephrine. Thus, the inhibitory action of GABA was enhanced by simultaneous application of norepinephrine, as shown in Fig. 9. Increased GABA-mediated inhibition was also produced by doses of norepinephrine that did not produce a discernible effect when applied alone.

Iontophoresis of Agents Affecting 5-Hydroxytryptamine

Iontophoretic application of 5-hydroxytryptamine was only examined in a few ICc

neurons, but in each case this agent reduced the responsiveness to acoustic stimuli (Table 2). The onset and offset were slower than those seen with GABA. However, in ICc neurons with sustained response patterns, the onset portion of the response appeared to be selectively inhibited. This is unlike the effect of all of the other inhibitory agents that usually affected the sustained portion of the response pattern to a greater extent than the onset component or occasionally affected both portions of the response equally. The differential effect on different portions of the response that contrasts with the effects of other inhibitory agents suggests that further research into the functional implications of this phenomenon may be merited.

IONTOPHORESIS OF PUTATIVE EXCITATORY TRANSMITTERS

Iontophoresis of Agents Affecting the Action of Excitant Amino Acids

An early study examined the effect of glutamate on IC neurons and found that most of the cells examined were excited by iontophoresis of this agent (25). In our studies (35,35a), iontophoretic application of the naturally occurring excitatory amino acids aspartate and glutamate, as well as the receptor subtype-specific agonist *N*-methyl-D-aspartate (NMDA), enhanced the responses of ICc neurons (Fig.10). The discharge rate of 80% to 90% of ICc neurons was increased with application of glutamate, aspartate, or NMDA (Table 3), while inhibition was rarely observed (35,35a). Excitant amino acid application induced a reduction of the acoustic threshold in several ICc neurons in which it was examined.

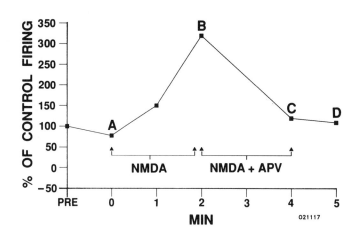

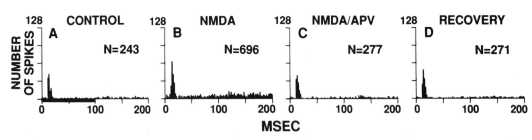

FIG. 10. An example of the effects of an excitant amino acid, *N*-methyl-D-aspartate (NMDA), the NMDA receptor antagonist 2-amino-5-phosphonovalerate (APV), and their interactive effects on the responses of an inferior colliculus (IC) neuron to acoustic stimuli at characteristic frequency (CF). The drug time course and poststimulus time histograms (PSTHs) are represented as in Fig. 1. The response before drug application is shown in A, and the excitatory effect of iontophoretic application of NMDA (160 nA) is shown in B. The application of NMDA was continued and then APV (180 nA) was applied simultaneously. The NMDA effect was blocked as shown in C. The *darkened line* at the bottom of histogram A represents the temporal characteristics of the stimulus. N equals the total number of action potentials in the histogram. (Stimulus: 100-msec tone bursts, 0 dB contralateral, 32.0 kHz (CF); threshold: −10 dB SPL.)

TABLE 3. *Agents affecting the action of excitatory neurotransmitters: excitant amino acids (EAA) agonists*

Agent	Number (%) of neurons			
	Total	Excited	Inhibited	No effect
NMDA	165	149 (90.3)	8 (4.8)	8 (4.8)
Glutamate	174	150 (86.2)	13 (7.5)	11 (14.8)
Aspartate	39	31 (79.4)	3 (7.7)	5 (12.8)
QUIS	11	8 (72.7)	1 (9.1)	2 (18.2)
EAA antagonists				
APV	98	13 (13.3)	82 (83.7)	3 (3.1)
DαA	21	3 (14.3)	17 (81.0)	1 (4.7)
GDEE	45	32 (71.1)	4 (8.8)	9 (20.0)
Agents affecting the action of acetylcholine (ACh): ACh agonists				
ACh	27	17 (62.9)	6 (22.2)	4 (14.8)
Carbachol	14	8 (57.1)	5 (35.7)	1 (7.1)
Others				
CCK	9	7 (77.7)	2 (22.2)	

APV, DL-2-amino-5-phosphonovaleric acid; CCK, cholecystokinin; DαA, D-alpha-aminoadipate; GDEE, L-glutamic acid diethylester HCl; NMDA, N-methyl-D-aspartate; PDA, cis-2,3-piperidine dicarboxylic acid; QUIS, quisqualate.

Iontophoretic application of the NMDA receptor-specific excitatory amino acid antagonists D-alpha-aminoadipate or 2-amino-5-phosphonovalerate (APV) blocked the excitatory effect of NMDA (Fig. 10). These antagonists often reduced the acoustically evoked and spontaneous firing of ICc neurons and were particularly effective in ICc neurons exhibiting only an onset response. The excitant amino acid antagonists also reduced the firing of IC neurons that had sustained firing patterns, but these responses rarely exhibited the complete suppression that could be induced in ICc neurons with only onset responses (Fig. 11). The receptor nonspecific excitant amino acid antagonists were much less effective in affecting the IC neuronal firing (Table 3). Thus, glutamic acid diethyl ester (as well as streptomycin and cis-2,3,piperidine dicarboxylic acid, which were examined in a few ICc neurons) was relatively unable to affect acoustically evoked firing, although they were generally effective in blocking the actions of exogenously applied glutamate. As noted previously, baclofen, a GABA_B agonist that is reported to decrease the release of excitant amino acids as one of its actions (71,76), produced a reduction of tone-

evoked responses of ICc neurons. These findings provide support for a role of an excitant amino acid as a candidate for the afferent excitatory transmitter in IC.

Iontophoresis of Agents Affecting Acetylcholine

An early iontophoretic study of the IC showed that about 10% of IC neurons were excited by glutamate in the absence of sound stimulation (25). Subsequently, Watanabe and Simada (105) reported that about two-thirds of IC neurons driven by acoustic stimuli exhibited enhanced firing after application of acetylcholine or the cholinesterase inhibitor physostigmine. In the latter study, muscarinic and nicotinic antagonists reduced acoustically driven responses in cases in which an effect was produced. Farley and co-workers (41) examined the effect of agents affecting the action of acetylcholine on the responses of ICc neurons to acoustic stimuli. They observed that 50% to 52% of ICc neurons exhibited enhanced firing after application of cholinergic agonists. Inhibitory effects were observed in 29% to 41% of cases with cholin-

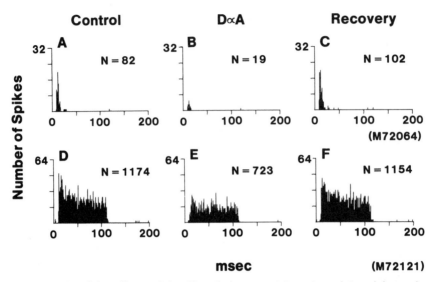

FIG. 11. An example of the effects of the *N*-methyl-ᴅ-aspartate antagonist ᴅ-alpha-amino-adipate (DαA), on the responses of two inferior colliculus (IC) neuronal response types to acoustic stimuli (tone bursts) at characteristic frequency (CF). The response before drug application is shown in column 1 (A and D), and the near blockade of the response to sound of the onset responder is shown in B following application of DαA (40 nA), while the sustained responder exhibited a 38% firing reduction (E) following application of this agent (135 nA). Recovery is shown in the last column (C and F). N equals the total number of action potentials in the histogram. (Top row stimulus: 100-msec tone bursts, 70 dB contralateral, 12.3 kHz (CF); threshold: 50 dB SPL. Bottom row stimulus: 20 dB contralateral, 26 kHz (CF); threshold: 0 dB SPL.)

ergic agonists in this study, while no effect was observed in 9% to 19% of ICc neurons (41).

In our studies we examined the effects of cholinergic agonists and compared these effects with those of excitant amino acids when possible on the same neuron. There was a dichotomy between the observed effects of these agents in terms of time course, magnitude, and degree of effects with the two types of putative transmitter. Application of the cholinergic agonists acetylcholine and carbachol resulted in firing increases in 68% of ICc neurons (Table 3). Nearly one-third (25%–35%) of ICc neurons exhibited reductions of neuronal discharge rate following application of these cholinergic agonists. These data contrast markedly with the percentage of neurons exhibiting increased discharge rates follow-ing application of excitant amino acids (80%–90%), and the percentage of cases of inhibitory effects of cholinergic agents was about five times that seen with the excitant amino acids (5%–7%). Cholinergic and excitant amino acid agonists were applied sequentially in 14 ICc neurons in our studies. The cholinergic agonist produced a reduction of discharge rate in 29% of these cases, while the excitant amino acid enhanced firing in each neuron. In cases where excitation was observed with both types of agonist, the degree of effect was greater with the excitant amino acids in 79% of cases, and both the onset and offset were faster with the excitant amino acid.

The effects of acetylcholine antagonists reported by Farley and co-workers (41) and NMDA-type excitant amino acid antagonists in our studies were quite dichotomous. Iontophoretic application of muscarinic receptor antagonists produced inhibition of the discharge rate of 14% to 65% of ICc neurons examined (41), which compares to the nearly 90% degree of effectiveness with the excitant amino acid antagonist APV observed in our studies (see Table 3). Nicotinic receptor antagonists, with the exception of a nicotinic ganglionic antagonist, were considerably less effective, and curare and atropine actually produced excitation in the vast majority of ICc neurons examined (41).

Iontophoresis of Agents Affecting the Action of Cholecystokinin

Iontophoretic application of cholecystokinin was quite effective in increasing the firing of ICc neurons. This effect was observed in 71% of the small number of ICc neurons on which it was tested (Table 3). The time course of effect was relatively rapid for a peptide and the effect was usually apparent within 1 to 2 min. The magnitude of effect of cholecystokinin was small relative to the magnitude of effects of excitant amino acids noted above. In several cases iontophoresis of cholecystokinin and an excitant amino acid was accomplished in the same ICc neuron sequentially. The effect of the excitant amino acids was greater in magnitude with a shorter onset period in most of the small number of ICc neurons examined. The cholecystokinin antagonist proglumide produced a reduction of firing in 67% of the small sample of ICc neurons onto which it was applied. This effect tended to be gradual in onset and offset.

Thus, of the agents with predominantly excitatory effects, excitant amino acids produced increased discharge rates in the greatest percentage of ICc neurons with the greatest magnitude of effect. The excitant amino acids also had the shortest latency of onset and the quickest offset consistent with the expected properties of a putative afferent transmitter in this nucleus.

Pathology of the Inferior Colliculus and Neurotransmitter Function

It has been a consistent tenet of neuroscience research that information about the function of a brain region can be obtained when it is affected by disease or is otherwise dysfunctional. The IC is strongly implicated in the initiation of AGS in both mice and rats with an inherited tendency to display this pathological condition (16,29, 101,109). A hearing deficit has been observed in both mice and rats subject to AGS (75,94). In the genetically epilepsy-prone rat (GEPR), which exhibits AGS, the hearing deficit is reported to involve loss of hair cells and deformation of the headplate (74,75). The auditory brainstem responses in the AGS-susceptible GEPR exhibit significantly elevated thresholds, and the latencies are prolonged (38,39). Surprisingly, there appears to be a critical window of hearing loss above which the rats show decreased seizure intensity. The response characteristics of IC neurons are altered in AGS (34,37,109). In the rat, the acoustic response thresholds are significantly elevated (37,75). An elevated incidence of onset-offset responses and a reduced efficacy of nonmonotonic rate-intensity functions are observed in ICc neurons of the AGS-susceptible GEPR (30,37). This may be related to the reduced efficacy of binaural inhibition observed in IC neurons of the GEPR (32). Binaural inhibition, nonmonotonic rate-intensity function, and offset inhibition may all be mediated by GABA, as noted above, since the $GABA_A$ antagonist bicuculline can regularly reverse the inhibition observed in each of these phenomena (see above and refs. 32,33). When GABA is applied iontophoretically onto ICc neurons of AGS-susceptible rats, a greater dosage (current) is required than that needed to produce the same degree (20%) of inhibition in IC neurons from normal animals, but the dose of bicuculline required to block offset inhibition is greater in ICc neurons of the normal rat (32).

These findings suggest that GABA is less effective in mediating inhibition in the IC of the AGS-susceptible rat, but evidence has been reported that more GABAergic neurons and a greater level of GABA is observed in the ICc of these animals (79,82). This suggests that a rise in inhibition in the IC may be a compensatory mechanism for the increased excitation of IC neurons induced by loud sounds, but the general response to increasing levels of a transmitter is down-regulation of the receptors for that neurotransmitter. Excess $GABA_A$ receptor activation results in desensitization to the effects of GABA (45b,84a). This could result in the decreased effectiveness of exogenously applied GABA and the endogenous GABA-mediated inhibition observed in the IC of these AGS-susceptible rats. Deficits of norepinephrine are observed in the IC and many other brain regions of the AGS-susceptible GEPR (56). In light of the increased effectiveness of GABA produced by norepinephrine in IC neurons (see Fig. 9), such a deficit of norepinephrine could also be involved in the reduced effectiveness of GABA in the GEPR IC. A greater than normal uptake of GABA in IC tissue of the GEPR has also been observed (17a). Any combination of these three mechanisms could reconcile an increase in GAD-immunoreactive neurons with a reduced efficacy of GABA. Further work will be needed to establish if any of these hypotheses are correct. Microinjection into the IC of a $GABA_A$ agonist, muscimol, or a GABA transaminase inhibitor, gabaculine, results in blockade of seizures in AGS-susceptible rats (17,31). Microinjection of a $GABA_A$ antagonist (bicuculline) into the IC of normal animals renders them susceptible to AGS (58). These findings of abnormalities in the GABA system in the IC of animals that exhibit sound-induced seizures

further support the role of GABA as an inhibitory transmitter, particularly involving binaural inhibition, in the neuronal response of normal IC neurons. Taken together, these data strongly suggest that GABA may be very important to the normal function of ICc neurons in mediating several inhibitory processes and that when the effectiveness of this neurotransmitter is compromised, it results in serious malfunction and the pathological state associated with AGS-susceptibility.

The increased excitation observed in IC neurons of the AGS-susceptible rats may also involve excitant amino acids. During AGS the levels of aspartate are elevated in the IC (21), and increased levels of glutamate are reported in the ICc of the AGS-susceptible rat not in seizure (79). The excitant amino acids in the IC are very important in initiating AGS in the rat, since blockade of excitant amino acid receptors (NMDA) by 2-amino-7-phosphonoheptanoate or blocking glutamate synthesis by microinjection of L-canaline into the IC will block AGS completely (31,36). In addition, microinjection of an excitant amino acid (NMDA) into the IC of normal rats renders them susceptible to AGS (58). Evidence for neuronal damage similar to that following administration of excitant amino acids (excitotoxicity) is also observed in the AGS-susceptible rats (84). These findings in the IC of animals susceptible to AGS support a role of an excitant amino acid as an afferent transmitter in the normal IC and indicate that serious pathology of the organism is associated with malfunction of excitant amino acid synapses in the IC.

The prominent role of GABA in mediation of the inhibitory phenomena in ICc neurons may be significant for hearing loss in aging. An extensive loss of GABA-like immunoreactivity and a decreased GABA release are observed in the IC of aged rats (11a,19c). Inhibitory function plays an important role in localization of sound in space (19c; for review, see ref. 7) and the ability to localize sound is diminished in human aging (48a). Binaural inhibition in the IC may be mediated, in part, by GABA, based on its selective blockade by bicuculline, and this finding is consistent with the suggested involvement of decreased GABA function in diminished ability to localize sound. Discrimination of signal-in-noise is decreased in presbycusis (57a). Nonmonotonic rate-intensity functions observed in most ICc neurons may be important in discrimination of signal-in-noise. The ability of bicuculline to block intensity-induced inhibition in ICc neurons noted above suggests that GABA may be involved in the ability to selectively distinguish specific communicative signals in noisy surroundings. The percentage of neurons exhibiting nonmonotonic rate-intensity functions declines significantly with aging in mice (110,111). These data, along with the putative mediation of this phenomenon by GABA, are consistent with the decline in GABA immunoreactivity in the IC in aged animals (19c). Thus, the decline of GABA levels with age implies that GABA-mediated inhibition is diminished, which would adversely affect the ability to discriminate signal-in-noise necessary for speech discrimination in a noisy environment.

SUMMARY AND CONCLUSION

This chapter has reviewed much of the currently available evidence on the identity and function of putative transmitters of the IC. The data strongly support a prominent role for GABA in the mediation of several important forms of inhibition of ICc neurons, as summarized below. The data supporting glycine, norepinephrine, and 5-hydroxytryptamine are less complete, and the specific roles of these transmitters in normal function cannot be accurately established with our current knowledge.

The possible role of an excitant amino acid as an excitatory transmitter is supported strongly by iontophoretic data, but several of the other criteria for establishing the function of these agents are more difficult to obtain, since glutamate is a metabolically important amino acid. The data on acetylcholine are not currently sufficient to support this agent as a good candidate for an afferent neurotransmitter in the IC. Clearly, considerably more work will need to be accomplished on release and the other criteria before the identity of afferent excitatory transmitter(s) can be established.

GABA appears to play a major role in inhibition in coding of the acoustic message in the IC. Thus, the phenomena of binaural inhibition, response pause, offset inhibition, and nonmonotonic rate-intensity functions each may be mediated, in part, by GABA acting directly on ICc neurons (31a). The extensive levels of GABA, the high GABA binding levels that are observed in IC, the release of GABA from the IC, and the sensitivity of ICc neurons to GABA and the GABA antagonist strongly suggest that GABA may be extremely influential in the inhibitory aspects of acoustic coding in this nucleus. Another aspect of response limitation observed in ICc neurons includes the "fatigability" observed in these neurons with increases in stimulus repetition rates (7), which exceeds that in lower brainstem auditory nuclei. This "fatigability" could be subserved, in part, by a pervasive offset suppression mediated by GABA. Consistent with this possibility is the finding that bicuculline application results in elevation of firing of nearly all ICc neurons, which may support the hypothesis of Brugge and Geisler (17b) that many features of the acoustic responses of brainstem auditory neurons are governed by inhibitory input. Thus, it has been proposed that the onset only response type, which is common in ICc neurons (7), may be caused by sustained inhibition during the remainder of the stimulus (17b). The ability of bicuculline to unmask a sustained component in ICc neurons that initially exhibit only an onset response (31a) suggests that in the ICc this sustained inhibition may be mediated, in part, by GABA.

As noted above, the pathways mediating the effects of GABA on ICc neurons include an important extrinsic pathway from the contralateral DNLL (3,97a). Recent preliminary studies in our laboratory with electrical stimulation or reversible blockade of the contralateral DNLL, which mimics or blocks binaural inhibition, respectively, are supportive of this concept. However, it is also well established that GABAergic interneurons are common within the ICc, and these neurons are a major potential source of intrinsic inhibition. Therefore, it is not currently clear which of the forms of GABA-mediated acoustically evoked inhibition are mediated by extrinsic or intrinsic pathways, and further experiments are needed to examine this important issue.

ACKNOWLEDGMENTS

The authors gratefully acknowledge the technical assistance of William E. Hoffman and the manuscript assistance of Catherine Copley, Jeffrey Pippin, and Dawn Melcher. The studies from this laboratory were supported by NIH grants NS 13849 and NS 21281 and the Deafness Research Foundation. The Division of Biomedical Illustration and Photography prepared the figures.

REFERENCES

1. Adams JC. Ascending projections to the inferior colliculus. *J Comp Neurol* 1979;183:519–538.
2. Adams JC. Multipolar cells in the ventral cochlear nucleus project to the dorsal cochlear nucleus and the inferior colliculus. *Neurosci Lett* 1983;37:205–208.
3. Adams JC, Mugnaini E. Dorsal nucleus of the lateral lemniscus: a nucleus of GABAergic projection neurons. *Brain Res Bull* 1984;13:585–590.
4. Adams JC, Mugnaini E. Distribution of cholecystokinin-like immunoreactivity in the brainstem auditory system (In: Vanderhaeghen J-J, Crawley JN, eds. *Neuronal cholecystokinin*). *Ann NY Acad Sci* 1985;448:563–565.
5. Adams JC, Wenthold RJ. Distribution of putative amino acid transmitters, choline acetyltransferase, and glutamate decarboxylase in the inferior colliculus. *Neuroscience* 1979;4:1947–1951.
6. Aitkin L. The inferior colliculus: nexus of the auditory pathway. In: *The auditory midbrain: structure and function in the central auditory pathway*. Clifton, NJ: Humana Press, 1986;75–100.
7. Aitkin L. Discharge characteristics of units in the auditory midbrain. In: *The auditory midbrain: structure and function in the central auditory pathway*. Clifton, NJ: Humana Press, 1986;101–128.
8. Aitkin LM, Irvine DRF, Webster WR. Central neural mechanisms of hearing. In: Brookhart JM, Mountcastle VB, Darian-Smith I, Geiger SR, eds. *Handbook of physiology. The nervous system*, vol III. Bethesda, MD: American Physiological Society, 1984;675–737.
9. Aitkin LM, Webster WR, Veale JL, Crosby DC. Inferior colliculus. I. Comparison of response properties of neurons in central, pericentral and external nuclei of adult cat. *J Neurophysiol* 1975;38:1196–1207.
10. Aoki E, Semba R, Keino H, Kato K, Kashiwamata S. Glycine-like immunoreactivity in the rat auditory pathway. *Brain Res* 1988;442:63–71.
11. Araki T, Yamano M, Murakami T, Wanaka A, Betz H, Tohyama M. Localization of glycine receptors in the rat central nervous system: an immunocytochemical analysis using monoclonal antibody. *Neuroscience* 1988;25:613–624.
11a. Banay-Schwartz M, Lajtha A, Palkovits M. Changes with aging in the levels of amino acids in rat CNS structural elements. II. Taurine and small neutral amino acids. *Neurochem Res* 1989;14:563–570.
12. Beyerl BD. Afferent projections to the central nucleus of the inferior colliculus in the rat. *Brain Res* 1978;145:209–223.
13. Bock GR, Webster WR, Aitkin LM. Discharge patterns of single units in inferior colliculus of the alert cat. *J Neurophysiol* 1972;35:265–277.
14. Bowery NG. Classification of GABA receptors. In: Enna SJ, ed. *The GABA receptors*. Clifton, NJ: Humana Press, 1983;177–213.
15. Bristow DR, Martin IL. Light microscopic autoradiographic localization in rat brain of the binding sites for the GABA$_A$ receptor antagonist [^{3}H]SR 95531: comparison with the [^{3}H]GABA$_A$ receptor distribution. *Eur J Pharmacol* 1988;148:283–288.
16. Browning RA. Neurobiology of seizure disposition—the genetically epilepsy-prone rat. VII. Neuroanatomical localization of structures responsible for seizures in the GEPR: lesion studies. *Life Sci* 1986;39:857–867.
17. Browning RA, Faingold CL. Effects on audiogenic seizures (AGS) in the genetically epilepsy prone rat (GEPR) of microinfusions into the inferior colliculus (IC) of noradrenergic (NA) and GABAergic agonists. *Pharmacologist* 1987;29:142.
17a. Browning RA, Marcinczyk M, Jobe PC. As-

sessment of GABA uptake and glutamic acid decarboxylase (GAD) activity in the genetically epilepsy-prone rat (GEPR) brain. *Soc Neurosci Abstr* 1989;15:1074.

17b. Brugge JF, Geisler CD. Auditory mechanisms of the lower brainstem. *Annu Rev Neurosci* 1978;1:363–394.

18. Brunso-Bechtold JK, Thompson GC, Masterton RB. HRP study of the organization of auditory afferents ascending to central nucleus of inferior colliculus in cat. *J Comp Neurol* 1981; 197:705–722.

19. Burne RA. Ascending projections to the inferior colliculus of the rat and bat. *Soc Neurosci Abstr* 1983;9:213.

19a. Carney LH, Yin TCT. Responses of low-frequency cells in the inferior colliculus to interaural time differences of clicks: excitatory and inhibitory components. *J Neurophysiol* 1989;62:144–161.

19b. Carr CE, Fujita I, Konishi M. Distribution of GABAergic neurons and terminals in the auditory system of the barn owl. *J Comp Neurol* 1989;286:190–207.

19c. Caspary DM, Raza A, Lawhorn Armor BA, Pippin J, Arneric SP. Immunocytochemical and neurochemical evidence for age-related loss of GABA in the inferior colliculus: implications for neural presbycusis. *J Neurosci* 1990;10: 2363–2372.

20. Chan JCK, Yin TCT. Interaural time sensitivity in the medial superior olive of the cat: comparisons with the inferior colliculus. *Soc Neurosci Abstr* 1984;10:844.

21. Chapman AG, Faingold CL, Hart GP, Bowker HM, Meldrum BS. Brain regional amino acid levels in seizure susceptible rats: changes related to sound-induced seizures. *Neurochem Int* 1986;8:273–279.

22. Cheney DL, LeFevre HF, Racagni G. Choline acetyltransferase activity and mass fragmentographic measurement of acetylcholine in specific nuclei and tracts of rat brain. *Neuropharmacology* 1975;14:801–809.

22a. Code RA, Burd GD, Rubel EW. Development of GABA immunoreactivity in brainstem auditory nuclei of the chick: ontogeny of gradients in terminal staining. *J Comp Neurol* 1989;284: 504–518.

23. Contreras NEIR, Bachelard HS. Some neurochemical studies on auditory regions of mouse brain. *Exp Brain Res* 1979;36:573–584.

24. Cotman CW, Iversen LL. Excitatory amino acids in the brain—focus on NMDA receptors. *Trends Neurosci* 1987;10:263–265.

25. Curtis DR, Koizumi K. Chemical transmitter substances in brain stem of cat. *J Neurophysiol* 1961;24:80–90.

26. Dahlstrom A, Fuxe K. Evidence for the existence of monoamine-containing neurons in the central nervous system. I. Demonstration of monoamines in the cell bodies of brainstem neurons. *Acta Physiol Scand* 1964;62(suppl 232):3–55.

27. Davies WE. The nature of neurotransmitters in the mammalian lower auditory system. *Assoc Res Otolaryngol Abstr* 1984;135.

28. Faingold CL. Seizures induced by convulsant drugs. In: Jobe PC, Laird II HE, eds. *Neurotransmitters and epilepsy.* Clifton, NJ: Humana Press, 1987;215–276.

29. Faingold CL. The role of the brain stem in generalized epileptic seizures. *Metab Brain Dis* 1987;2:81–112.

30. Faingold CL, Boersma Anderson CA. Inferior colliculus (IC) unit activity and audiogenic seizures (AGS) in behaving genetically epilepsy-prone rats (GEPRs). *Soc Neurosci Abstr* 1988; 14:253.

31. Faingold CL, Copley CA, Boersma CA. Blockade of audiogenic seizures (AGS) in genetically epilepsy-prone rats (GEPRs) by the microinjection into inferior colliculus (IC) of blockers of inhibitory and excitant amino acid (EAA) metabolism. *Soc Neurosci Abstr* 1987;13:1158.

31a. Faingold CL, Boersma Anderson CA, Caspary DM. Involvement of GABA in acoustically-evoked inhibition in inferior colliculus neurons. *Hear Res* 1991;201–216.

32. Faingold CL, Gehlbach G, Caspary DM. Decreased effectiveness of GABA-mediated inhibition in the inferior colliculus of the genetically epilepsy-prone rat. *Exp Neurol* 1986;93: 145–159.

33. Faingold CL, Gehlbach G, Caspary DM. On the role of GABA as an inhibitory neurotransmitter in inferior colliculus neurons: iontophoretic studies. *Brain Res* 1989;500:302–312.

34. Faingold CL, Gehlbach G, Travis MA, Caspary DM. Neurobiology of seizure disposition—the genetically epilepsy-prone rat. VIII. Inferior colliculus neuronal response abnormalities in genetically epilepsy-prone rats: evidence for a deficit of inhibition. *Life Sci* 1986;39:869–878.

35. Faingold CL, Hoffmann WE, Caspary DM. Effects of excitant amino acids on inferior colliculus neuronal responses to acoustic stimuli. *Soc Neurosci Abstr* 1984;10:1148.

35a. Faingold CL, Hoffmann WE, Caspary DM. Effects of excitant amino acids on acoustic responses of inferior colliculus neurons. *Hear Res* 1989;40:127–136.

36. Faingold CL, Millan MH, Boersma CA, Meldrum BS. Excitant amino acids and audiogenic seizures in the genetically epilepsy-prone rat. I. Afferent seizure initiation pathway. *Exp Neurol* 1988;99:678–686.

37. Faingold CL, Travis MA, Gehlbach G, et al. Neuronal response abnormalities in the inferior colliculus of the genetically epilepsy-prone rat. *Electroencephalogr Clin Neurophysiol* 1986;63;296–305.

38. Faingold CL, Walsh EJ, Maxwell JK. The auditory brainstem response in genetically epilepsy-prone rats susceptible to audiogenic seizures. *Epilepsia* 1987;28:583.

39. Faingold CL, Walsh EJ, Maxwell JK. Threshold and latency abnormalities of the auditory brainstem response of rats genetically suscep-

tible to audiogenic seizures. *Assoc Res Otolaryngol Abstr* 1988;77–78.

40. Fallon JH, Seroogy KB. The distribution and some connections of cholecystokinin neurons in the rat brain (In: Vanderhaeghen JJ, Crawley JN, eds. *Neuronal cholecystokinin*). *Ann NY Acad Sci* 1985;448:121–132.

41. Farley GR, Morley BJ, Javel E, Gorga MP. Single-unit responses to cholinergic agents in the rat inferior colliculus. *Hear Res* 1983;11:73–91.

42. Fisher SK, Davies WE. GABA and its related enzymes in the lower auditory system of the guinea pig. *J Neurochem* 1976;27:1145–1155.

43. Flammino F, Clopton BM. Neural responses in the inferior colliculus of albino rat to binaural stimuli. *J Acoust Soc Am* 1975;57:692–695.

43a. Fujita I, Konishi M. The role of GABAergic inhibition in processing of interaural time difference in the owl's auditory system. *J Neurosci* 1991;11:722–739.

44. Fuxe K. Evidence for the existence of monoamine neurons in the central nervous system. IV. The distribution of monoamine nerve terminals in the central nervous system. *Acta Physiol Scand* 1965;64(suppl 247):37–85.

45. Glendenning KK, Masterton RB. Acoustic chiasm: efferent projections of the lateral superior olive. *J Neurosci* 1983;3:1521–1537.

45a. Glendenning KK, Baker BN. Neuroanatomical distribution of receptors for three potential inhibitory neurotransmitters in the brainstem auditory nuclei of the cat. *J Comp Neurol* 1988;275:288–308.

45b. Gonsalves H, Gallager DW. Persistent reversal of tolerance to anticonvulsant effects and GABAergic subsensitivity by a single exposure to benzodiazepine antagonist during chronic benzodiazepine administration. *J Pharmacol Exp Ther* 1988;244:79–83.

46. Greenamyre JT, Young AB, Penney JB. Quantitative autoradiographic distribution of L-[^{3}H]glutamate-binding sites in rat central nervous system. *J Neurosci* 1984;4:2133–2144.

47. Harrison JM. Functional properties of the auditory system of the brain stem. In: Masterton RB, ed. *Handbook of behavioral neurobiology*. New York: Plenum Press, 1978;409–458.

48. Havey DC, Caspary DM. A simple technique for constructing 'piggy-back' multibarrel microelectrodes. *Electroencephalogr Clin Neurophysiol* 1980;48:249–251.

48a. Herman GE, Warren LR, Wagener JW. Auditory lateralization: age differences in sensitivity to dichotic time and amplitude cues. *J Gerontol* 1977;32:187–191.

48b. Hironaka T, Morita Y, Hagihira S, Tateno E, Kita H, Tohyama M. Localization of GABA$_A$-receptor α_1 subunit mRNA-containing neurons in the lower brainstem of the rat. *Mol Brain Res* 1990;7:335–345.

49. Hoover DB, Muth EA, Jacobowitz DM. A mapping of the distribution of acetylcholine, choline acetyltransferase and acetylcholinesterase in discrete areas of rat brain. *Brain Res* 1978;153:295–306.

50. Hutson KA. Connections of the auditory midbrain: efferent projections of the dorsal nucleus of the lateral lemniscus, the nucleus sagulum, and the origins of the GABAergic commissure of Probst. Doctoral dissertation. Florida State University, Tallahassee, 1988.

51. Innis RB, Aghajanian GK. Integrated anatomical and physiological studies of neuronal cholecystokinin receptors. *Ann NY Acad Sci* 1985;448:188–197.

51a. Irvine DRF, Gago G. Binaural interaction in high-frequency neurons in inferior colliculus of the cat: effects of variations in sound pressure level on sensitivity to interaural intensity differences. *J Neurophysiol* 1990;63:570–591.

51b. Kaneko T, Itoh K, Shigemoto R, Mizuno N, Glutaminase-like immunoreactivity in the lower brainstem and cerebellum of the adult rat. *Neuroscience* 1989;32:79–98.

52. Kobayashi RM, Palkovits M, Kopin IJ, Jacobowitz DM. Biochemical mapping of noradrenergic nerves arising from the rat locus coeruleus. *Brain Res* 1974;77:269–279.

53. Krogsgaard-Larsen P, Falch E, Larsson OM, Schousboe A. GABA uptake inhibitors: relevance to antiepileptic drug research. *Epilepsy Res* 1987;1:77–93.

54. Kuwada S, Yin TCT, Haberly LB, Wickesberg RE. Binaural interaction in the cat inferior colliculus: physiology and anatomy. In: Vander Brink G, Bilsen FA, eds. *Psychophysical, physiological and behavioral studies in hearing*. Delft: Delft University Press, 1980;401–408.

55. Kuwada S, Yin TCT, Syka J, Buunen TJF, Wickesberg RE. Binaural interaction in low-frequency neurons in inferior colliculus of the cat. IV. Comparison of monaural and binaural response properties. *J Neurophysiol* 1984;51:1306–1325.

56. Laird II HE, Jobe PC. The genetically epilepsy-prone rat. In: Jobe PC, Laird II HE, eds. *Neurotransmitters and epilepsy*. Clifton, NJ: Humana Press, 1987;57–94.

57. Lopez-Colome AM, Tapia R, Salceda R, Pasantes-Morales H. K$^+$-stimulated release of labeled gamma-aminobutyrate, glycine and taurine in slices of several regions of rat central nervous system. *Neuroscience* 1978;3:1069–1074.

57a. Maurer JF, Rupp RR. The aging auditory process: presbycusis. In: *Hearing and aging*. New York: Grune and Stratton, 1979;33–63.

58. Millan MH, Meldrum BS, Faingold CL. Induction of audiogenic seizure susceptibility by focal infusion of excitant amino acid or bicuculline into the inferior colliculus of normal rats. *Exp Neurol* 1986;91:634–639.

59. Mitani A, Shimokouchi M, Nomura S. Effects of stimulation of the primary auditory cortex upon colliculogeniculate neurons in the inferior colliculus of the cat. *Neurosci Lett* 1983;42:185–189.

60. Moiseff A. Intracellular recordings from owl inferior colliculus. *Soc Neurosci Abstr* 1985;11:735.

61. Moore JK, Moore RY. Glutamic acid decarboxylase-like immunoreactivity in brainstem auditory nuclei of the rat. *J Comp Neurol* 1987; 260:157–174.
62. Morest DK, Oliver DL. The neuronal architecture of the inferior colliculus in the cat: defining the functional anatomy of the auditory midbrain. *J Comp Neurol* 1984;222:209–236.
63. Morley BJ, Lorden JF, Brown GB, Kemp GE, Bradley RJ. Regional distribution of nicotinic acetylcholine receptor in rat brain. *Brain Res* 1977;134:161–166.
64. Nagai T, Maeda T, Imai H, McGeer PL, McGeer EG. Distribution of GABA-T-intensive neurons in the rat hindbrain. *J Comp Neurol* 1985;231:260–269.
64a.Najlerahim A, Harrison PJ, Barton AJL, Hefferman J, Pearson RCA. Distribution of messenger RNAs encoding the enzymes glutaminase, aspartate aminotransferase and glutamic acid decarboxylase in rat brain. *Mol Brain Res* 1990;7:317–333.
65. Nelson PG, Erulkar SD. Synaptic mechanisms of excitation and inhibition in the central auditory pathway. *J Neurophysiol* 1963;26:908–923.
66. Nordeen KW, Killackey HP, Kitzes LM. Ascending auditory projections to the inferior colliculus in the adult gerbil, Meriones unguiculatus. *J Comp Neurol* 1983;214:131–143.
67. Oliver DL. Dorsal cochlear nucleus projections to the inferior colliculus in the cat: a light and electron microscopic study. *J Comp Neurol* 1984;224:155–172.
68. Oliver DL. Projections to the inferior colliculus from the anteroventral cochlear nucleus in the cat: possible substrates for binaural interaction. *J Comp Neurol* 1987;264:24–46.
69. Oliver DL, Krevolin C. Anteroventral cochlear nucleus (AVCN) projections to the inferior colliculus (IC) in cat. Possible substrates for binaural interactions in the midbrain. *Soc Neurosci Abstr* 1984;10:1147.
70. Oliver DL, Morest DK. The central nucleus of the inferior colliculus in the cat. *J Comp Neurol* 1984;222:237–264.
71. Olpe H-R, Baudry M, Fagni L, Lynch G. The blocking action of baclofen on excitatory transmission in the rat hipocampal slice. *J Neurosci* 1982;2:698–703.
72. Olsen RW, Wamsley JK, Lee RJ, Lomax P. Benzodiazepine/barbiturate/GABA receptor-chloride ionophore complex in a genetic model for generalized epilepsy. In: Delgado-Escueta AV, Ward AA Jr, Woodbury DM, Porter RJ, eds. *Basic mechanisms of the epilepsies: molecular and cellular approaches* (Advances in Neurology, vol 44). New York: Raven Press, 1986;365–378.
73. Ottersen OP, Storm-Mathisen J. Neurons containing or accumulating transmitter amino acids. In: Björklund A, Hökfelt T, Kuhar MJ, eds. *Handbook of chemical neuroanatomy, vol 3. Classical transmitters and transmitter receptors in the CNS, part II.* Amsterdam: Elsevier, 1984;141–246.
74. Penny JE, Brown RD, Hodges KB, Kupetz SA, Glenn DW, Jobe PC. Cochlear morphology of the audiogenic-seizure susceptible (AGS) or genetically epilepsy prone rat (GEPR). *Acta Otolaryngol (Stock)* 1983;95:1–12.
75. Penny JE, Brown RD, Wallace MS, Henley CM. Neurobiology of seizure disposition—the genetically epilepsy-prone rat. X. Auditory aspects of seizure in the genetically epilepsy prone rat. *Life Sci* 1986;39:887–895.
75a.Pierson MG, Smith KL, Swann JW. A slow NMDA-mediated synaptic potential underlies seizures originating from midbrain. *Brain Res* 1989;486:381–386.
76. Potashner SJ. Baclofen: Effects on amino acid release and metabolism in slices of guinea pig cerebral cortex. *J Neurochem* 1979;32:103–109.
77. Probst A, Cortes R, Palacios JM. The distribution of glycine receptors in the human brain. A light microscopic autoradiographic study using [^{3}H]strychnine. *Neuroscience* 1986;17:11–35.
78. Purves RD. *Microelectrode methods for intracellular recording and ionophoresis.* New York: Academic Press, 1981.
79. Ribak CE, Byun MY, Ruiz GT, Reiffenstein RJ. Increased levels of amino acid neurotransmitters in the inferior colliculus of the genetically epilepsy-prone rat. *Epilepsy Res* 1988;2:9–13.
80. Ribak CE, Roberts RC. The ultrastructure of the central nucleus of the inferior colliculus of the Sprague-Dawley rat. *J Neurocytol* 1986;15:421–438.
81. Ring JB, Rigler-Daugherty SK, Jobe PC, Faingold CL, Browning RA. Release of ^{3}H-norepinephrine (NE) and ^{3}H-GABA from synaptosomes isolated from the genetically-epilepsy-prone rat (GEPR). *Pharmacologist* 1985;27:232.
82. Roberts RC, Ribak CE. GABAergic neurons and axon terminals in the brainstem auditory nuclei of the gerbil. *J Comp Neurol* 1987;258:267–280.
83. Roberts RC, Ribak CE. An electron microscopic study of GABAergic neurons and terminals in the central nucleus of the inferior colliculus of the rat. *J Neurocytol* 1987;16:333–345.
84. Roberts RC, Ribak CE. The ultrastructure of the central nucleus of the inferior colliculus of the genetically epilepsy-prone rat. *Epilepsy Res* 1988;2:196–214.
84a.Roca DJ, Rozenberg I, Farrant M, Farb DH. Chronic agonist exposure induced down-regulation and allosteric uncoupling of the gamma-aminobutyric acid/benzodiazepine receptor complex. *Mol Pharmacol* 1990;37:37–43.
85. Rockel AJ, Jones EG. The neuronal organization of the inferior colliculus of the adult cat. I. The central nucleus. *J Comp Neurol* 1973;147:11–60.
86. Rockel AJ, Jones EG. Observations on the fine

structure of the central nucleus of the inferior colliculus of the cat. *J Comp Neurol* 1973;147: 61–92.

87. Rose JE, Greenwood DD, Goldberg JM, Hind JE. Some discharge characteristics of single neurons in the inferior colliculus of the cat. I. Tonotopical organization, relation of spike-counts to tone intensity, and firing patterns of single elements. *J Neurophysiol* 1963;26:294–320.

87a. Ross LS, Pollak GD. Differential ascending projections to aural regions in the 60kHz contour of the mustache bat's inferior colliculus. *J Neurosci* 1989;9:2819–2834.

88. Rotter A, Birdsall NJM, Field PM, Raisman G. Muscarinic receptors in the central nervous system of the rat. II. Distribution of binding of [³H]propylbenzylcholine mustard in the midbrain and hindbrain. *Brain Res Rev* 1979;1:167–183.

89. St. Laurent J, Roizen MF, Miliaressis E, Jacobowitz DM. The effects of self-stimulation on the catecholamine concentration of discrete areas of the rat brain. *Brain Res* 1975;99:194–200.

90. Saint Marie RL, Ostapoff E-M, Morest DK, Wenthold RJ. The chemical acoustic chiasm: asymmetric glycine immunoreactivity in the bilateral projection from the lateral superior olive to the inferior colliculus in the cat. *Soc Neurosci Abstr* 1987;13:548.

91. Saint Marie RL, Ostapoff E-M, Morest DK, Wenthold RJ. Glycine-immunoreactive projection of the cat lateral superior olive: possible role in midbrain ear dominance. *J Comp Neurol* 1989;279:382–396.

92. Salmoraghi GC, Weight F. Micromethods in neuropharmacology: an approach to the study of anesthetics. *Anesthesiology* 1967;28:54–64.

93. Sanes DH, Geary WA, Wooten GF, Rubel EW. Quantitative distribution of the glycine receptor in the auditory brain stem of the gerbil. *J Neurosci* 1987;7:3793–3802.

94. Saunders JC, Bock GR, James R, Chen C-S. Effects of priming for audiogenic seizure on auditory evoked responses in the cochlear nucleus and inferior colliculus of BALB/c mice. *Exp Neurol* 1972;37:388–394.

95. Schwartz RD, McGee R Jr, Kellar KJ. Nicotinic cholinergic receptors labeled by [³H]acetylcholine in rat brain. *Mol Pharmacol* 1982;22:56–62.

96. Seighart W. Comparison of benzodiazepine receptors in cerebellum and inferior colliculus. *J Neurochem* 1986;47:920–923.

97. Semple MN, Aitkin LM. Physiology of pathway from dorsal cochlear nucleus to inferior colliculus revealed by electrical and auditory stimulation. *Exp Brain Res* 1980;41:19–28.

97a. Shneiderman A, Oliver DL. EM autoradiographic study of the projections from the dorsal nucleus of the lateral lemniscus: a possible source of inhibitory inputs to the inferior colliculus. *J Comp Neurol* 1989;286:28–47.

97b. Shneiderman A, Oliver DL, Henkel CK. Connections of the dorsal nucleus of the lateral lemniscus: an inhibitory parallel pathway in the ascending auditory system? *J Comp Neurol* 1988;276:188–208.

97c. Smith PH. Synaptic responses of neurons in brain slices of the guinea pig inferior colliculus. IUPS Satellite Symposium on Hearing, 1986; 82.

98. Swanson LW, Hartman BK. The central adrenergic system. An immunofluorescent study of the location of cell bodies and their efferent connections in the rat utilizing dopamine-beta-hydroxylase as a marker. *J Comp Neurol* 1975;163:467–505.

99. Tachibana M, Kuriyama K. Gamma-aminobutyric acid in the lower auditory pathway of the guinea pig. *Brain Res* 1974;69:370–374.

100. Thompson GC, Cortez AM, Lam DM-K. Localization of GABA immunoreactivity in the auditory brainstem of guinea pigs. *Brain Res* 1985;339:119–122.

101. Urban GP, Willott JF. Response properties of neurons in inferior colliculi of mice made susceptible to audiogenic seizures by acoustic priming. *Exp Neurol* 1979;63:229–243.

102. Versteeg DHG, Van Der Gugten J, De Jong W, Palkovits M. Regional concentrations of noradrenaline and dopamine in rat brain. *Brain Res* 1976;113:563–574.

103. Vetter DE, Mugnaini E. Immunocytochemical localization of GABAergic elements in rat inferior colliculus. *Soc Neurosci Abstr* 1984;10: 1148.

103a. Volman SF, Konishi M. Spatial selectivity and binaural responses in the inferior colliculus of the great horned owl. *J Neurosci* 1989;9:3083–3096.

104. Wamsley JK, Lewis MS, Young III WS, Kuhar MJ. Autoradiographic localization of muscarinic cholinergic receptors in rat brainstem. *J Neurosci* 1981;1:176–191.

105. Watanabe T, Simada Z-I. Pharmacological properties of cat's collicular auditory neurons. *Jpn J Physiol* 1973;23:291–308.

106. Waterhouse BD, Moises HC, Woodward DJ. Noradrenergic modulation of somatosensory cortical neuronal responses to iontophoretically applied putative neurotransmitters. *Exp Neurol* 1980;69:30–49.

107. Waterhouse BD, Moises HC, Yeh HH, Woodward DJ. Norepinephrine enhancement of inhibitory synaptic mechanisms in cerebellum and cerebral cortex: mediation by beta adrenergic receptors. *J Pharmacol Exp Ther* 1982; 221:495–506.

108. Wenthold RJ, Huie D, Altschuler RA, Reeks KA. Glycine immunoreactivity localized in the cochlear nucleus and superior olivary complex. *Neuroscience* 1987;22:897–912.

109. Willott JF. Comparison of response properties of inferior colliculus neurons of two inbred mouse strains differing in susceptibility to audiogenic seizures. *J Neurophysiol* 1981;45: 35–47.

110. Willott JF, Parham K, Hunter KP. Response properties of inferior colliculus neurons in middle-aged C57BL/6j mice with presbycusis. *Hear Res* 1988;37:15–27.

111. Willott JF, Parham K, Hunter KP. Response properties of inferior colliculus neurons in young and very old CBA/J mice. *Hear Res* 1988;37:1–14.

112. Yamauchi R, Amatsu M, Okada Y. Effect of GABA (gamma-aminobutyric acid) on neurotransmission in inferior colliculus slices from guinea pigs. *Neurosci Res* 1989;6:446–455.

113. Zarbin MA, Wamsley JK, Kuhar MJ. Glycine receptor: light microscopic autoradiographic localization with [^{3}H]-strychnine. *J Neurosci* 1981;1:532–547.

Neurobiology of Hearing: The Central Auditory System, edited by R. A. Altschuler et al. Raven Press, Ltd., New York © 1991.

11

Processing in the Colliculi

David Caird

Zentrum der Physiologie, 6000 Frankfurt am Main, Federal Republic of Germany

In writing this review, I have tried to give a general overview of auditory information processing in the mammalian colliculi. To characterize information processing in a structure, one must be able to compare the information input with the output. This is rather difficult for the inferior colliculus (IC) as, mostly due to its easy accessibility for single unit recording, more is known about cell responses here than in more caudal nuclei of the auditory pathway. In particular, there is a great deal more data available on the responses of IC cells to binaural signals than on those of cells in the superior olivary complex (SOC), the first structure where information from both ears is processed before being passed on to the colliculus. Therefore binaural responses in IC cells reflect both SOC and collicular interactions and it is not clear to what extent such responses are due to IC processing rather than "preprocessing" in the SOC. Similarly, a considerable amount of information is now available about the responses of cells in the deep layers of the superior colliculus, but the mechanism responsible for the considerable transformation in cell response characteristics between inferior and superior colliculus (SC) is not well understood. Consideration of processing in the colliculus has therefore been neglected in favor of descriptions of responses of collicular cells to various aspects of auditory stimulation.

The emphasis of this chapter is on general principles that are presumably applicable to all species. The most commonly studied species is the cat, but, unless explicitly stated to the contrary, it is assumed that the data from this and other species reflect basic principles common to all animals. Much of our information on collicular function comes from auditory specialists; the barn owl and various species of bats. A review of these data would exceed the space available in this chapter, and I use selected data from such species to illustrate aspects of collicular responses that have been studied in "normal" (i.e., nonspecialized) animals. When discussing these data, it is assumed that these highly specialized mechanisms are evolutionary developments of mechanisms common to all animals and can be used to illustrate particular aspects of collicular function.

ANATOMICAL SUBDIVISIONS OF THE INFERIOR COLLICULUS

The IC is a large and complex caudal midbrain auditory structure and is an obligatory relay for nearly all ascending auditory fibers (11). As different anatomical subdivisions of the IC have very different structures and afferent inputs, it is necessary to briefly consider its anatomy before discussing its function. Such a discussion is complicated by the fact that the original IC parcellation of Rockel and Jones (119), to which the majority of physiological studies refer, has been more recently considerably modified by Morest and Oliver (105,108). To briefly summarize, Rockel and Jones defined a large central nucleus, divided into a nonlaminated dorsomedial division and a laminated ventrolateral portion, which was capped by the pericentral nucleus, a thin sheet over dorsal and posterior central nucleus, and flanked laterally by the external nucleus. These divisions can be seen in the Nissl-stained sections that are used to follow up most physiological studies. In the parcellation of Morest and Oliver, only the

laminated ventrolateral part was considered to be central nucleus. The pericentral nucleus and dorsomedial division of the central nucleus were divided into layers I through IV of the dorsal cortex. The central nucleus is surrounded by the paracentral nuclei (equivalent to the "external nucleus" in earlier studies [119]). Although most physiological studies refer to the earlier classification, that of Morest and Oliver will be used here because it more closely agrees with the physiological data. For further details, see Chapter 9. The most significant structural distinction is between the laminated central nucleus and the other divisions. The central nucleus receives a

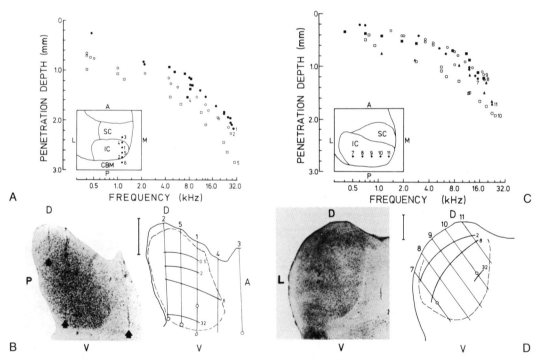

FIG. 1. Isofrequency contours in the ferret inferior colliculus. Reconstruction of isofrequency contours from single unit mapping data in the ferret in the sagittal (**A,B**) and medial (**C,D**) planes. For each penetration, the unit best frequency is plotted against penetration depth. The insets show the position of the penetrations on a dorsal view of the midbrain. In C and D the anatomical reconstructions of the tracks (*lines* in the drawings) and unit depth with respect to lesions (*circles*) are shown. The isofrequency lines connect the same best frequencies on adjacent tracks. In the medial plane (D), the orientation of these lines is the same as the 2DG contours in the gerbil (Fig. 2) and the fibrodendritic laminae in the cat (108). IC, inferior colliculus; SC, superior colliculus; CBM, cerebellum; L, lateral; M, medial; A, anterior; P, posterior; D, dorsal; V, ventral. (From ref. 103 with permission.)

heavy and highly structured auditory afferent projection. Auditory projections to the cortex and paracentral nuclei are less highly structured and they also receive somatosensory and descending cortical projections. The physiology of these structures is correspondingly different, and they are discussed separately in the following sections. The laminar organization of the central nucleus seen in anatomical studies suggests that a functional laminar organization is present. As will be seen in the next section, physiological studies show this to be the case.

THE CENTRAL NUCLEUS FREQUENCY MAP: SINGLE UNIT STUDIES

Many studies using single unit and multiunit recording have shown a tonotopic organization in the central nucleus. As recording depth in the central nucleus increases, neuronal best frequency increases in a graded manner (cat [13,95,120,122, 130], ferret [103], guinea pig [114], rat [33], opossum [4], mouse [51,142,155], rabbit [6,145], monkey [44,124]). Three-dimensional reconstructions from horizontal (130) and vertical (cat [95], mouse [142], monkey [44], ferret [103]) electrode penetrations show the representation of a given frequency to be a sheet of tissue extending through the central nucleus and tilting downward laterally and caudally (Fig. 1).

The laminae in the lateral part of the central nucleus are oriented differently to those in the main part (108). There are some physiological data that suggest that frequency mapping in the lateral central nucleus is not the same as that in central and medial portions. In the cat, Roth et al. (122) and Rose et al. (120), using lateral to medial horizontal penetrations, showed an initial very sharp best frequency decrease followed by a slower increase in best frequencies. A similar frequency mapping discontinuity was reported along an oblique lateral penetration by Clopton and Winfield

(rat [30]). Using vertical penetrations, Stiebler and Ehret (mouse [142]) found little or no change in best frequency with depth in this lateral region, as would be expected if the penetrations were passing along steeply inclined isofrequency contours. However, only these last authors (142) discuss their data with respect to the lateral division of the central nucleus. For the earlier studies, it is not certain that the recordings are from the lateral central nucleus and not the lateral paracentral nucleus.

THE CENTRAL NUCLEUS FREQUENCY MAP: DEOXYGLUCOSE STUDIES

Isofrequency contours in the IC can also be visualized with radioactive deoxyglucose (2DG) labeling. 2DG uptake increases with metabolic activity and the central auditory system, with its high metabolic rate, lends itself particularly well to 2DG studies (138). By stimulating with tones of different frequency, bands of 2DG uptake corresponding in orientation to the dendritic laminae have been demonstrated in several species (cat [135], monkey [151], mouse [155], gerbil [125], guinea pig [91]) (Fig. 2). The bands extend through the rostrocaudal IC axis as three-dimensional sheets (91, 135,151), as seen in Golgi studies (108) and the single unit mapping reconstructions quoted in the previous section. These intense labeling bands have been shown to correspond to neuronal best frequencies using simultaneous 2DG labeling and single unit recording (cats [135,152], monkeys [151]) and to bands of labeled cell bodies after small horseradish peroxidase (HRP) injections in the medial geniculate body (135).

In transverse sections, the labeling bands run through the central nucleus, thinning out dorsomedially in the cortex (135,151) (Fig. 2). This is as would be expected from the anatomical data of Oliver and Morest showing that the afferent axons forming the laminae in the central nucleus extend as

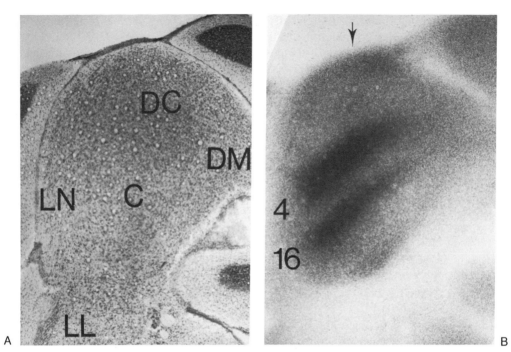

FIG. 2. 2DG uptake in gerbil inferior colliculus. **A:** Nissl-stained section through the colliculus. DC, dorsal cortex; C, central nucleus; *dotted line,* boundary between cortex and central nucleus. **B:** The same section. 2DG uptake after stimulating the awake, freely moving animal with 4- and 16-kHz tones. *Dark areas* show high 2DG uptake. The uptake occurs in bands parallel to the central nucleus laminae; the isofrequency bands continue into the medial cortical region but stop abruptly at the presumed boundary between lateral and central parts of the central nucleus. These stripes are continuous through serial transverse sections, i.e., they are three-dimensional sheets of tissue extending through both medial and sagittal axes of the colliculus (for more details, see ref. 25). Some physiological studies, however, suggest that there may be a reverse frequency map in more lateral parts of the cortex (*arrow*).

fine collaterals into the cortex. However, the continuation of isofrequency projections into the cortex appears at first sight to contradict the single unit studies showing a reversed frequency map in the dorsal cortex of cat and opossum (see dorsal cortex section). 2DG labeling reflects synaptic activity rather than cell body action potentials, i.e., the inputs to a structure, not the processing taking place there (107). The continuation of the tonotopic 2DG labeling stripes into the dorsal cortex shows that it receives a tonotopic input similar to that in the central nucleus. The apparent contradiction between this input and the single unit mapping data in the cortex are discussed in the section on dorsal cortex.

At the ventrolateral end of the isofrequency 2DG contours, the bands of labeling cease without changing orientation and no 2DG labeling correlate of the tilted laminae in the lateral central nucleus can be seen (Fig. 2) (135). The laminae in the lateral central nucleus are not only tilted with respect to the central laminae but twisted obliquely with respect to a transverse plane of section (108), rather than at right angles to it, and it may be that this twist blurs any isofrequency labeling bands that may be present in this region.

The 2DG bands to pure tone stimuli are wider than individual laminae in all studies cited above (a minimum of 2–3 laminae [135,152]). This is probably due to both limited resolution of the 2DG method and the spread of excitation across frequencies due to the use of suprathreshold stimulation levels. 2DG labeling may not be as precise as single unit studies with threshold or near-threshold stimulation levels, but it allows an elegant demonstration of activity patterns in an entire cell population—in this case isofrequency contours.

THE CENTRAL NUCLEUS FREQUENCY MAP: FINE STRUCTURE

More detailed examination of the single units in the central nucleus has shown the entire hearing range to be represented in the central nucleus but with an overrepresentation of higher frequencies (cat [95], rat [33], ferret [103], squirrel monkey [44]). Stiebler and Ehret (142) found that only the higher frequencies of the mouse hearing range were represented in the central nucleus and that the lower frequencies were found in the dorsal cortex. They also found an overrepresentation of the upper limit (>30 kHz) of the hearing range in the medial part of the central nucleus, often showing a sharp jump in unit best frequency as the electrode was advanced from the central to the medial part of the central nucleus.

The mouse may be an intermediate stage between nonspecialized animals and ultrasonic sensitive bats (141) in which such discontinuities in the frequency map are even more marked. In the colliculi of many bat species, the representation of echolocation frequencies is often so hypertrophied as to distort the whole structure of the colliculus. In the mustache bat, the 60-kHz echolocation frequency representation is as big as the rest of the colliculus (168). This dorsoposterior division resembles a hypertrophied lamina and, as will be discussed later, has provided insights into possible organization of binaural function within an isofrequency band.

Merzenich and Reid (95) reported that, as

an electrode descended through the cat central nucleus, neuronal best frequencies increased in a stepwise fashion. Instead of a graded increase with depth, best frequencies would remain constant for up to 200 to 300 μ and then increase by a fraction of an octave. Langner and Schreiner (88) reported that the neuronal best frequencies were not exactly the same all over an isofrequency contour but were graded so that increasing best frequencies were found more caudally. The variation across an isofrequency contour was similar to that found by Merzenich and Reid (95). Ehret and Merzenich (41), using bandpass noise masking, reported that individual cells in the cat central nucleus had an effective bandwidth similar to that of psychophysical critical bands. Taken together, these data suggest that the representation of frequency in each isofrequency lamina is the physiological substrate of psychophysical critical bands.

THE CENTRAL NUCLEUS FREQUENCY MAP: SUMMARY

Nearly all single unit recording studies use Nissl staining to locate the recording sites and indirectly compare the data with Golgi studies by other authors. However, the large body of indirect evidence discussed above strongly suggests that the anatomical laminae of the central nucleus do in fact represent isofrequency sheets. It is indeed somewhat difficult to imagine that different points along a lamina characterized by multiple collaterals from the same afferent axons could have different best frequencies. The data quoted here support the description of Oliver and Morest of lamination in the central nucleus (108) rather than that of Rockel and Jones (119). Similarly, the evidence available does suggest a significantly different frequency representation in lateral central nucleus. Detailed analysis of frequency tuning within isofrequency contours (41,88,95) also suggests that the anatomical laminae in IC central nucleus correspond not only to isofrequency sheets but also provide an anatomical substrate for psychophysical critical bands.

THE DORSAL CORTEX

In contrast to the central nucleus, the dorsal cortex receives heavy descending cortical and ascending somatosensory afference (8,34) and does not have structurally highly ordered auditory afferent input (108). This is reflected in the physiological studies of the cortex, which shows the cells to have broad or complex tuning curves, be responsive to somatosensory stimuli, and affected by anesthesia (3). In barbiturate-anesthetized cats, Merzenich and Reid (95) and Aitkin et al. (barbiturate or chloralose/urethane) (13) found cells in superficial cortex to be broadly tuned, sensitive to contralateral monaural stimulation, and to habituate to repeated presentations of the same stimulus. Although the cells were broadly tuned, they were nevertheless tonotopically organized with best frequencies decreasing with increasing penetration depth, i.e., the opposite of the frequency map in the central nucleus (13,95). Aitkin (3) stressed that the reversal point was quite deep in the "central nucleus" and stated that this "physiological boundary" was probably the real dorsal margin of the central nucleus. This probably corresponds to the deep cortex/central nucleus boundary of Morest and Oliver (105). It is not clear from the published data if this reverse frequency map is found throughout the deep cortex or just in more lateral areas.

In the medial cortex, Merzenich and Reid (95) (cat: barbiturate) found no response to auditory stimulation. Semple and Aitkin (130) (cat: barbiturate and ketamine), Moore et al. (103) (ferret: barbiturate), and Fitzpatrick (44) (squirrel monkey: barbiturate), on the other hand, found no clear physiological boundary between the central

nucleus and the medial cortex and stated that the central nucleus frequency map continued into this area. This is supported by more recent 2DG marking experiments (see central nucleus frequency map, fine structure section).

It may be that there are two tonotopic representations in the cortex: one in the medial region similar to that in the central nucleus and another, of opposite orientation, in the superficial and lateral layers. More data on single unit responses related to the subdivisions defined by Morest and Oliver are needed to resolve this problem.

There also appear to be species differences. In the mouse, Stiebler and Ehret (142) (barbiturate/Taractan, free-field stimulation) showed the dorsal cortex and central nucleus frequency maps to be continuous. The lowest frequencies of the mouse hearing range are represented in the dorsal cortex and not in the central nucleus. Single unit tuning curves in both these regions were mostly sharp. In the cortex, tuning curves had very steep flanks at both sides (i.e., no low-frequency tails were present) or were closed (no response at high stimulus intensities). Ehret and Moffat (43) found dorsal cortex neurons to be less sensitive to noise stimuli and synthetic calls than central nucleus cells. This sensitivity was affected by barbiturates in the cortex but not in the central nucleus. The structure of the mouse IC is similar to that of the cat (92,155), and the reason for these differences is unknown. Apart from these mouse studies, there is very little information on cortical responses in the colliculus, nearly all reports being brief statements in studies devoted to the central nucleus.

THE PARACENTRAL NUCLEI

The main auditory input to the paracentral nuclei is from the central nucleus, and they also receive ascending somatosensory and descending cortical afference (8,14, 34,79). Data on the responses of cells in the paracentral nuclei ("external nucleus") are also scarce. In the cat lateral paracentral nucleus, Merzenich and Reid (95) found no tone responses, whereas Aitkin and co-workers found mostly binaural cells with broad irregular tuning curves. The cell responses habituated to repeated stimulation and were often better to complex acoustic stimuli (8,13). Similar results have been found in other species (rabbit [6], opossum [4], mouse [149]). Aitkin (3) stated that low frequencies were underrepresented in the cat paracentral nuclei. In the mouse, Stiebler and Ehret (142) found that the entire hearing range was not represented in the lateral paracentral nucleus: units with high and low (outside the 3–30-kHz range) best frequencies were not found. Tonotopy was also different from that in the central nucleus. Neuronal best frequencies increased from dorsolateral to ventromedial and dropped at the boundary with the central nucleus. Similar loose tonotopic maps have been found in this area in the cat (13,120) and rat (33). However, Aitkin et al. (4,5) (opossum and cat) found no tonotopy in the main part of the paracentral nuclei and suggested that earlier reports of tonotopy were in fact from lateral cortical areas. In the cat, Aitkin et al. (5,8) showed lateral and ventral paracentral nucleus units to have spinal inputs. Fifty-four percent of the sample were bimodal, mostly sensitive to stimulation of either ear and inhibited by stimulation of the dorsal column. A few cells were responsive to stimulation of the skin. Receptive fields on the skin were large, and no somatotopic organization could be seen. The areas sampled are now known to be structurally quite different (105), but no more recent study has examined the responses in these nuclei in more detail.

As the paracentral nuclei receive input from the central nucleus (8,14,34,79), the cells here would be ideally situated to analyze the output of arrays of central nucleus cells across frequency bands. This has been shown to be the case in the barn owl (sec-

tion on space mapping in the colliculus of the barn owl), but the data on the mammalian paracentral nuclei are at present insufficient to allow a precise definition of its functions. Similarly, this part of the IC is obviously involved in the integration of somatic and auditory information, but at the present time one can only speculate about the exact mechanisms and functions involved.

At this level, there appears to be the first division between the "primary-like" auditory system with sharp tuning and strict tonotopic representation (central nucleus) and the "diffuse" auditory system (dorsal cortex, paracentral nuclei) with poor frequency selectivity and preference for complex acoustic stimuli (3). These two systems not only have different characteristics but also project separately to different areas in the medial geniculate body and auditory cortex (14,34,79).

DISTRIBUTION OF DIFFERENT CELL TYPES ON ISOFREQUENCY SHEETS IN THE CENTRAL NUCLEUS

The central nucleus receives inputs from many brainstem auditory structures, principally all three divisions of the contralateral cochlear nucleus, ipsilateral medial superior olive (MSO) and ventral nucleus of the lateral lemniscus, and bilateral projections from the lateral superior olive (LSO) and intermediate and dorsal nuclei of the lateral lemniscus (1,21,39,106,109,136,167). The frequency representations in these nuclei overlap considerably, i.e., a particular frequency cannot be assigned to a particular nucleus. The projections to a given frequency sheet in the central nucleus therefore come from a number of lower nuclei. As will be seen below, these projections are not diffusely mixed, but each nucleus appears to project to a different area or different areas on the isofrequency sheet. In addition, there is considerable overlap of the different projections so that a given cell may receive inputs from more than one lower nucleus. Each isofrequency sheet seems therefore to receive a patchwork of overlapping multiple projections from many different brainstem auditory nuclei. After small injections of HRP into the central nucleus, labeling can be detected in all the nuclei listed above. However, after each injection only some of the nuclei are marked (divergence), but even the smallest injections result in marking in more than one brainstem structure (convergence) (12, 92,122,136,137).

With single unit recording, divergence and convergence can be seen in the representation of each ear on the isofrequency sheets. Conventionally, the inputs from each ear are denoted as excitatory (E), inhibitory (I), or none (O) with the contralateral ear first. Although nearly all central nucleus cells respond to monaural stimulation of the contralateral ear, approximately 80% of them receive input from both ears (23,103,114,122,130). There are three main classes of cells in the central nucleus: EO, EI, and EE. At this level, contralateral excitation is dominant: OE and IE cells are conspicuous by their absence, and even the cells receiving excitatory input from both ears are mostly contralateral dominant: EE (23,103,132). This simple EO/EE/EI classification has two major flaws: Many, if not the majority, of binaural cells have mixed excitatory and inhibitory inputs from each ear and many studies use slightly different criteria for binaural classification. The first reservation is more fully discussed in the section on binaural cell responses in the IC. Where authors have used different criteria for cell classification than those described above is indicated. The differences are most evident in the case of EI and EE cells showing strong facilitation. The inhibitory input to EI cells can only be seen when there is some activity to inhibit. As there is little spontaneous activity in the colliculus of most anesthetized preparations, EI cells will only be seen when binaural stimulation is used to suppress the contralateral mon-

aural response. Monaural stimulation of the nondominant ear of an EE cell may evoke no spikes. The excitatory nature of the input may only be apparent when the response to the dominant ear is greatly increased by simultaneous stimulation of the nondominant ear (facilitation) or the cell may respond only to binaural stimulation (EO/F and OO/F cells). To further complicate matters, many binaural cells are sensitive to differences in the input to the two ears, and their responses may be suppressed by nonoptimal signal configurations (see section on binaural effects: binaural cues). There is some evidence that facilitation cells are a subset of the EE cell population, which is particularly important in binaural processing (see later), but this will not be considered at this point.

The distribution of these cell types shows that convergence of different inputs onto single central nucleus cells is present. The two superior olivary nuclei, MSO and LSO, are binaural; that is, they process inputs from both ears before passing it on to the colliculus. The MSO has an overrepresentation of low frequencies (50), and many cells are sensitive to interaural phase differences (IPD) in tones presented binaurally (22,49). The LSO, on the other hand, receives excitatory inputs from the ipsilateral ear and inhibitory inputs from the contralateral ear (IE cells) (20). The LSO cells are mostly high frequency, non-IPD sensitive (22). As the LSO projects bilaterally to the IC, one would therefore expect EI and IE cells to be found in roughly equal proportions. In fact, IE cells are rare (23,122,130). The ipsilateral LSO projections to the IC are mainly from the low-frequency region of the LSO (48). There is less inhibitory input to low-frequency LSO cells (20,47), i.e., many (but not all [22]) are classifiable as OE. However, OE cells are also rare in the colliculus. The evidence suggests that there is an appreciable IE and OE input from the ipsilateral LSO which is processed by IC cells that are not themselves IE or OE. In fact, this ipsilateral projection is probably inhibitory (126,137; see Chapters 7 and 9, *this volume*).

Physiological evidence was provided by Semple and Aitkin (131), who electrically stimulated the dorsal acoustic stria in the cat. Cells responding to such electrical stimulation were judged to receive inputs from the contralateral dorsal cochlear nucleus, and many of the cells could also be inhibited by ipsilateral acoustic stimulation (131). This evidence shows that inputs from different caudal brainstem nuclei converge onto individual cells in IC.

Separation of projections from different brainstem nuclei can be seen in the distribution of cell types in IC. In the cat central nucleus, Semple and Aitkin (130) studied the distribution of EO, EE (defined as cells sensitive to stimulation of each ear but IPD insensitive), EI, and IPD cells. As IPD sensitivity declines sharply above 2 kHz in the cat (23,83), it is not surprising that IPD cells were found to be confined to the dorsal central nucleus, particularly in the rostral and lateral parts. EO cells were found caudally and ventrally; EE cells were found throughout the central nucleus but were more numerous medially. The distribution of EI cells, which were mostly of higher best frequencies, (22,23,122,130) overlapped that of the EO cells ventrally and laterally but spread more rostrally. This agrees with the HRP studies of Aitkin and Schuck (12) and Maffi and Aitkin (90): MSO projections (IPD cells) were found to be to the rostrolateral part of the dorsal central nucleus, and, in the ventral high-frequency region, cochlear nucleus (EO) projections more medial, and SOC (EE and EI) projections tending to be more rostrolateral. Schreiner and Langner (127) found the distribution of EE cells to vary across frequencies. The EE cells formed a wedge covering about one-third of each lamina and extending away from the center. The orientation of this wedge was different for different frequencies, but it generally extended to the rostral margin of the central nucleus (Fig. 3). The distribution of EI cells appeared to

be in irregular clusters (127). Roth et al. (122) also stated that single unit types were clumped, i.e., units with different characteristics were grouped together in different parts of an isofrequency sheet (see also free-field studies in IC section).

The distribution of ipsilaterally inhibited inputs to the cat central nucleus was visualized with 2DG by Webster et al. (150, 152). Using anesthetized animals and a closed sound system, they delivered pure tone signals to one ear and noise to the other. In the IC contralateral to the tone stimulus, an isofrequency band could be seen in the central nucleus (section on the central nucleus frequency map: 2DG studies). Ipsilateral to the tone stimulus, the broad excitation induced by noise stimulation of the other ear was interrupted by a band of reduced labeling. This band was identical in configuration to the heavily labeled band on the other side, showing the excited and inhibited inputs from the ears to be congruent. However, little information about relative strength of excited and inhibited inputs along a band in either transverse of longitudinal directions could be gleaned: The inhibited bands were a little broader in caudal regions, but no mediolateral variations could be seen (150). It seems that the resolution of the 2DG method is insufficient to show the distribution of EE and EI inputs along an isofrequency band in the central nucleus. If the 2DG method reflects synaptic input (section on the central nucleus frequency map: 2DG studies), the inhibitory effects here must be already established at the inputs to the central nucleus, i.e., the IE cells of the contralateral LSO (20,22,48), rather than being due to interactions within the colliculus. The inhibited bands appeared somewhat wider than the excited bands, but it is not clear if this is the effect of the photographic method used to visualize 2DG uptake or represents a broader tuning of inhibitory inputs. Since the excitatory and inhibitory frequency characteristics of these inputs, the LSO cells, appear to be closely matched (22),

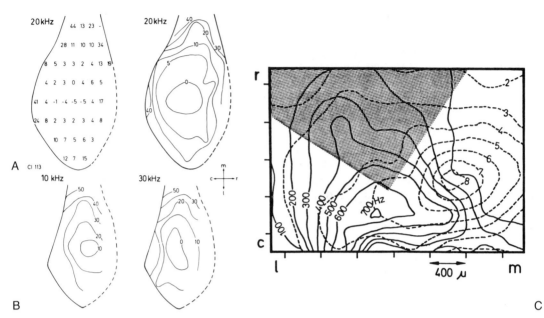

FIG. 3. Distribution of unit response characteristics on isofrequency contours. **A:** Dorsal view of a 20-kHz isofrequency contour in a mouse. Left: The numbers are the thresholds, in dB SPL, of the single units of 20 kHz best frequency recorded at each point. Isothreshold contours are plotted from these raw data on the right. **B:** 10 and 30 kHz best frequency isothreshold contours in one animal. (From ref. 140, with permission.) **C:** Representation of best modulation frequency (*solid lines*), Q_{10}dB (*dashed lines*) and EE binaural cell types (*shaded area*) on a 12-kHz isofrequency contour in the cat. The contours are computed from single and multiunit activity in parallel vertical penetrations. (Courtesy of G. Langner.)

the former possibility seems more likely. The inhibited bands extend dorsomedially into the cortex, as seen for the excited isofrequency bands in the contralateral IC.

More recent studies have addressed fine differences in cell characteristics such as threshold, latency, and modulation sensitivity. Stiebler (140,142), using free-field stimulation in mice, showed that unit threshold was correlated with position. Units with the lowest thresholds were found in the center of or slightly rostrolaterally to the center of an isofrequency sheet. Thresholds increased away from the center, resulting in an ovoid isothreshold contour map (Fig. 3). Similarly, Schreiner and Langner (87,88, 127) mapped unit best modulation frequency, Q_{10}dB, latency, and fine structure of best frequency across isofrequency sheets in the cat. They found best modulation frequency and Q_{10}dB to be concentri-

cally mapped (but around different centers) on each isofrequency sheet) (Fig. 3). A best frequency fine gradient from caudal (higher best frequency) to rostral (lower best frequency) and a roughly orthogonal latency (short/lateral to long/medial) was also found. Variations in binaural characteristics over isofrequency sheets are discussed in the section on topographic representation of binaural characteristics.

In summary, it seems to be well established that the isofrequency sheets in the central nucleus receive segregated but overlapping inputs from various auditory nuclei. The mapping of the fine structure of various unit response parameters such as threshold, fine tuning, best modulation frequency, and latency is a particularly interesting new development. The concept of independent maps of different parameters (e.g., frequency tuning and amplitude modulation sensitivity) suggests how complex neural response types within a given frequency band could be created by cross-mapping of different, simpler response type variations.

FREQUENCY, INTENSITY, AND TIME CODING IN THE CENTRAL NUCLEUS

Most central nucleus cells have sharply tuned response areas like those of primary auditory fibers (13,42,95,103,120). The frequency characteristics of the ipsi- and contralateral inputs to the EE cells are similar. Ipsilateral thresholds are, however, higher and the best frequency slightly lower (gerbil [133]). Broad or multipeaked tuning curves are found in some cases and probably correspond to the stellate cells, whose dendrites cross more than one lamina. Closed tuning curves (i.e., no response to high sound pressure levels [SPLs]) are found for cells with strongly nonmonotonic intensity functions (43) (see below). Little spontaneous activity is present in most anesthetized preparations, and few cells appear to have inhibitory side bands. However, the proportion of cells seen in inhibitory side bands is greater in unanesthetized prepara-

tions in which spontaneous activity is higher (19,124,156). Two studies in which inhibitory side bands were systematically searched for showed the majority of cells tested to have inhibitory areas away from their best frequency (barbiturate-anesthetized ferret [103], barbiturate/Taractan-anesthetized cat [41]). Side bands were also seen in one 2DG study. Webster et al. (152) showed that monaural stimulation with noise and a tone resulted not only in marking of an isofrequency band in the contralateral colliculus but also in a band of reduced marking just dorsolateral to it, i.e., corresponding to lower frequencies than that used for stimulation. These data show that inhibitory side bands are in fact common in central nucleus cells.

The rate intensity functions (RIFs) of central nucleus cells to monaural contralateral stimulation can be either monotonic or nonmonotonic. The dynamic range of most IC cells is small: Monotonic units usually reach a spike-rate plateau within 10 to 30 dB of threshold. Nonmonotonic functions reach a maximum and then decline with increasing stimulus intensity (3,42,114,118, 120,133,156) (Fig. 4). However, RIFs can be greatly affected by stimulus binaurality

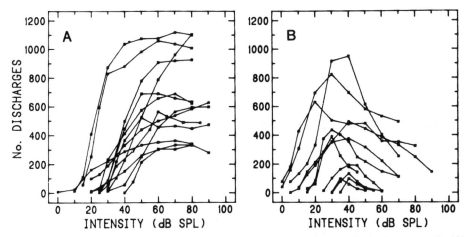

FIG. 4. Rate intensity functions (RIFs) in the gerbil inferior colliculus. Typical monotonic (**A**) and nonmonotonic (**B**) single unit RIFs with monaural contralateral best frequency stimulation in the gerbil. Spike rate is plotted on the Y axis. dB SPL on the X axis. (From ref. 133, with permission.)

and frequency content. For EI cells with strong inhibitory inputs, SPL may be irrelevant and only the difference between the ears may be coded. For other EI cells, the RIF is affected by both mean binaural SPL and level difference (134). Some EE cells are affected by both level differences and SPL, others only by SPL (134). RIFs can also be affected by spectral content of the signal. Addition of noise masking generally shifts monaural tone RIFs to the right and can, at low levels, increase the maximum spike rate (118). It is therefore not clear how monaural pure tone RIFs correlate with the reactions of the units under natural (binaural, mostly broad band signals) stimulation conditions.

Similarly, the functional role of the different temporal response patterns (poststimulus time histograms [PSTHs]) is not at all clear. Most units can be assigned to "on" or "sustained" types, discharging either at the onset of or throughout the stimulus. Many cells exhibit a combination of on and sustained responses, often separated by a pause (23,76,121). PSTH type can, however, be affected by stimulus level (42,83, 120,132,156), anesthesia (80), or bandwidth (23) and is not correlated with binaural interaction characteristics (23,83). It is therefore difficult to assign functional roles to the different types. An exception is found in various species of echolocating bats, in which "on" responders with step-like monotonic RIFs have been shown to be important for temporal coding of the locating call and echo. In some bats, units tuned to the call frequency can lock to small amplitude and frequency modulations around this frequency with sufficient accuracy to encode the reflections from the wings of flying insects (129).

In the rat IC, Rees and Møller (101,116) studied coding of best frequency tones or noise amplitude modulated (AM) with pseudorandom noise. Modulation transfer functions (MTFs) to the noise were calculated. At low intensities (within 15 dB of unit threshold), MTFs were low pass (6–200 Hz), becoming band pass type at higher intensities. AM sensitivity was only found in the central nucleus and declined steeply above 200 Hz in all cases (117). Compared with responses at lower levels in the auditory pathway, maximum AM locking frequencies were lower and the responses were significantly nonlinear (101, 116). Langner et al. (87) reported AM sensitivity up to 1 kHz in the cat with mostly multiunit recordings. This AM sensitivity has been interpreted by Langner in terms of pitch coding in the IC. In the midbrain of the guinea fowl, Langner (84–86) found units that appeared to have intrinsic oscillations. The oscillations were triggered by the start of a sound signal (carrier and modulation sinusoids switched on simultaneously at zero crossing) and, if the AM frequency was suitable, could lock to the AM cycles. The peak discharge occurred when a whole number of cycles of the carrier, a whole number of cycles of the AM sinus, and a whole number of synaptic delays (0.4 msec) coincided. A similar relationship was shown for human psychophysical perception of such signals: for a given modulation frequency the pitch perception did not increase smoothly with carrier frequency but in jumps corresponding approximately to 0.4-msec changes in the cycle length of a pure sinusoidal tone (84). Langner (85) proposed that these cells were acting as coincidence detectors between a phase-locked response and delayed oscillations of multiples of 0.4 msec. As pitch is determined by both carrier and AM frequencies, distribution of AM sensitivity across an isofrequency sheet in IC (Fig. 4) would imply a distribution of pitch representation (88, 127). The IC, with its multiple inputs with different synaptic delays, would be well suited to be the substrate for such a mechanism, but further details remain to be studied.

BINAURAL EFFECTS: BINAURAL CUES

As noted earlier, the majority of IC cells are binaurally sensitive. The binaural cues and terms used are outlined here (see also Chapters 8 and 15). Unlike the visual system, in which a given direction in space corresponds to a place on the retina, the direction of a sound source must be computed by the central nervous system (CNS). As a sound source moves away from midline in the horizontal plane (azimuth), the sound waves arrive earlier and are louder at one ear, giving rise to interaural time differences (ITDs) and interaural level differences (ILDs). Both ITDs and ILDs are dependent on signal frequency. This is true both of the physical cues and the CNS interactions responsible for their processing. At low frequencies, interaural phase differences (IPDs) are the main binaural localization cue. At high frequencies, IPD is no longer coded by the CNS, and delays in the signal envelope are used as the ITD cue (56). IPD and continuous amplitude modulation are classed as ongoing time delays (OTDs) (100) as opposed to transient time delays (TTDs), such as click or tone burst ramp ITDs. ILD coding becomes more dominant as frequency increases.

Binaural interactions can be divided into low-frequency and high-frequency systems. The terms "high-frequency" and "low-frequency" in this context relate to the turnover frequency, where IPD ceases to be processed by the auditory CNS of the animal in question (about 1.5 kHz for humans [56], 2.5 kHz for the cat [23,82], but up to 7–9 kHz for the barn owl [99,144]). The physiological characteristics of these binaural systems correspond to the physical cues available: The low-frequency system is highly sensitive to ITDs (in the form of IPD/OTD) and not to ILDs, and the high-frequency system is mainly ILD and, to a lesser extent, TTD/envelope OTD sensitive.

Measurements of ITD/azimuth values show that ITD is frequency dependent. ITD decreases with increasing carrier frequency so that a given ITD value does not represent one azimuth angle across all frequencies (although this effect of frequency is much less than that of the frequency on ILD/azimuth curves). The values are higher than those calculated using a simple spherical head model, reaching a maximum of 350 μsec in the cat (27,123; see also Chapter 8, *this volume*). The rate of change with azimuth angle is greatest near the midline and the effects of pinna position are negligible (27). In contrast to ITDs, where signal frequency mainly changes the type of ITD cue available to the CNS, ILDs are highly frequency dependent and affected by the position of the pinna. ILDs are significant only at high frequencies, where wavelength is short relative to head size, allowing sound shadowing by the head and pinna. As frequency increases, the pinna and meatus become more directionally selective up to about 20 to 30 kHz (wallaby [35], cat [26,27,31,53,104,113]) (Fig. 5). At high (8 kHz and above) frequencies, ILD/azimuth curves in the cat show large fluctuations in ILD with small changes in azimuth (60) (Fig. 5). ILDs are therefore maximal for sound sources located on the acoustic axis of one pinna, and, as they are highly frequency dependent, a given ILD cannot represent a given azimuth across frequencies. In addition, the sharp gain change effects with small changes in angle at high frequencies mean that, even for a single frequency, a given ILD does not necessarily correspond to a given angle. In contrast to maximum ILD, the rate of change of ILD with azimuth is, however, less frequency dependent. It is also highest (0.4 dB/° up to 10 kHz [27]) and monotonic across the midline (31,60).

Monaural effects, i.e., spectrum transformations due to reflections around the head and pinna (31,68), are also important cues for sound localization. Such effects are necessary for the judgment of elevation and allow, for example, monaural judgment of sound azimuth if broad band signals are presented (see Chapter 15). Monaural pinna effects are known to be important for the spatial selectivity of neurons in the superior colliculus (see section on superior colliculus auditory space map), but the physiological processing of pinna spectrum transformations is poorly understood.

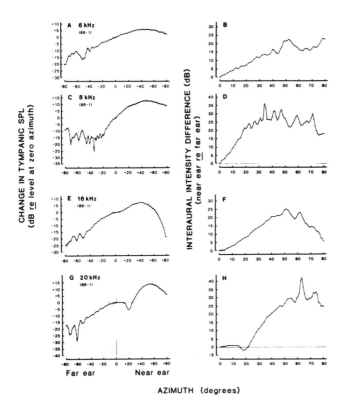

FIG. 5. Interaural level difference (ILD)/azimuth curves from the cat. In the left columns, the change in SPL measured in the ear canal of an anesthetized cat is plotted as a sound source is moved from 80° contralateral (far ear) to 80° ipsilateral (near ear) in small (1° and 2°) azimuth steps. The right columns show the corresponding ILD (near ear-far ear) ("interaural intensity difference") values at each stimulation frequency. At far azimuth values, where ILDs are maximal, sharp peaks and dips can be seen. Around the midline, on the other hand, the rate of change of ILD with azimuth is monotonic, less affected by the stimulation frequency and maximal at 8 kHz. (Modified from ref. 60, with permission.)

Such monaural spectrum cues may be sufficient to explain the superior localization performance to broad band signals. However, there are good reasons to believe that the binaural processing involved in sound localization is intrinsically a broad band phenomenon. The data presented above show that, for a single frequency, a given ITD or ILD can be caused by more than one angle of incidence. Accurate coding of sound source direction therefore needs comparison of information from more than one frequency. Physiological studies have found neurons appearing to be specifically sensitive to sound source direction to be broadly tuned (section on superior colliculus auditory space map), i.e., the spatial coding takes place in the diffuse rather than the primary (3) ascending auditory system.

BINAURAL CELL RESPONSES IN THE INFERIOR COLLICULUS

Binaural cells in the IC can be conveniently divided into three classes: high-frequency EI and EE cells and the low-frequency IPD cells. The effects of ILDs and ITDs, applied using dichotic stimulation, on these three cell types are shown in Fig. 6, based on data from our laboratory. The EI cells were found to be sensitive to ILDs (nearly all cells) and ITDs (some cells) favoring the contralateral ear. The ITD responses of the EI cells were rather labile, being often affected by signal type (tone burst ramp or click TTD or noise OTD) and, taken over the physiological range of approximately 0 to 350 μsec and 0–20 or 30 dB, were nearly always weaker than the ILD responses. Time intensity trading ratios for these cells were calculated by dividing the slope of the ILD/spike rate function by that of the ITD/spike rate function in this range (Fig. 6A). The mean time intensity trading ratios for the EI frequency cells that were ITD sensitive (i.e., excluding the non-ITD-sensitive cells with infinitely high trading ratios) were high (mean 122 μsec/dB). The EI cells are therefore sensitive to ILDs favoring the contralateral ear, and this ILD response can be complemented in some cases by ITD sensitivity. The strength of the inhibitory inputs to the EI cells shows considerable variation (23). This was also found in the gerbil IC by Semple and Kitzes (134), who found the most strongly inhibited EI cells to be sensitive to ILD but unaffected by SPL. Other EI cells were affected by both SPL and ILD (134).

IPD cells have cyclic ITD curves at one per stimulation frequency and are little affected by ILDs. Time intensity trading ratios were found to be the lowest of the three cell types (mean 9.1 μsec/dB [23], 5.8 μsec/dB [164]). Since the IPD cells often show facilitation at favorable delays and suppression at nonfavored delays (2,23,83,121), it is not helpful to classify them as EE or EI. IPD cells are mostly contralaterally dominant and have onset or sustained PSTHs (23,83) and monotonic or nonmonotonic RIFs (83). A small proportion of cells in this frequency range has been found to be the EI type, but their binaural responses (noncyclic delay curves and TTD sensitivity) seem to resemble those of the high-frequency EI rather than the IPD cells (82). The IPD cells are highly OTD sensitive but unaffected by envelope shifts (23,82). The peak of the OTD curve is mostly in the contralateral physiological range (23,82). IPD sensitivity declines rapidly above 2,500 Hz, and most IPD cells are not monaurally phase sensitive. Kuwada et al. (83) found that only 18% of IPD cells were monaurally phase locked, mostly to frequencies below 600 Hz. Palmer et al. (111) found IPD cells in the guinea pig to phase lock well to the fundamental frequency (100 Hz) of synthetic vowels but that, in contrast to cells in the cochlear nucleus, locking to higher frequency components was not present.

Many high-frequency EE cells were also sensitive to ITDs (presented as TTDs or noise burst OTDs) (23). In these cases, maximal response was at a given ITD value, which was often in the contralateral physiological range. Over the whole population, this ITD sensitivity was less strong than that of the IPD cells. The trading ratios from the ITD- (TTD or OTD) sensitive EE cells were between those of the IPD and EI cells (mean 22.4 μsec/dB).

The effects of ILDs were variable, but many EE cells had complementary peaked ILD and ITD curves (22). Similar peaked ILD curves were found in the kangaroo rat (143) and gerbil (134). Semple and Kitzes (134) found that many EE cells were ILD sensitive and showed peak discharge at zero ILD. Spike rate was generally affected by ILD and SPL, but the position of the peak of the ILD curve was SPL independent. Interestingly, they stated that the position of the peak discharge of those ILD-sensitive cells with a peak response at a nonzero value was not stable with changes in SPL.

The binaural characteristics of these cell types correspond to the psychophysical characteristics of the low- and high-frequency binaural systems. The IPD cells are highly OTD sensitive and ILD insensitive, and the high-frequency cells are ILD and, in some cases, ITD (envelope OTD and TTD) sensitive. High-frequency EE and EI cells have also been shown to be sensitive to AM OTDs (15,166) and noise OTDs (37) in other studies. As pointed out by Hirsch et al. (57,163), the ITD effects in these cells can be considered to be a secondary effect of an ILD/latency compensation mechanism. The IPD cells have a much lower weighting of intensity; this is presumably because their inputs—the phase-locked-CN octopus cell-MSO system—provide much more secure coding of time information (59).

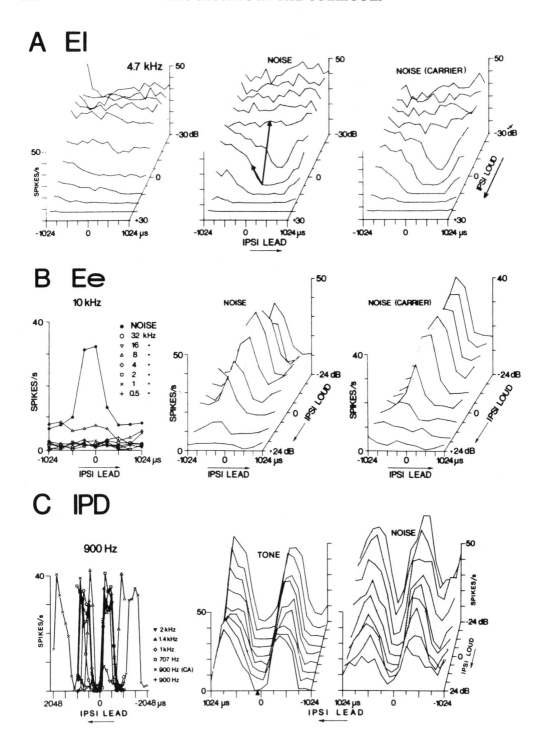

The boundary between the EI and EE cell categories is blurred. For example, the binaural response of many EE cells is less than the sum of the monaural responses, and their ITD or ILD peak responses can be outside the physiological range, making them functionally indistinguishable from EI cells (23,159). Monaural stimulation of one ear can evoke both excitation and inhibition (23,30), and the EI and EE categories are best regarded as an expression of the main input from each ear.

The data discussed above were obtained with dichotic stimulation via closed sound systems. One would expect the free-field directional characteristics of the three cell types to be as follows: EI cells would be maximally responsive along the pinna axis, whereas IPD and EE cells would be expected to be maximally sensitive to a particular direction. This in fact appears to be the case (see section on free-field studies in IC). The results of Semple and Kitzes (see above) imply that only those EE cells sensitive to midline sound sources (i.e., peak response at zero ILD, stable with SPL) would reliably code sound source direction. The EE and EI cell populations could be acting as crossed detectors (EI: lateral/ pinna axis, EE: midline) whose output could be compared to code sound source direction (89) (section on superior colliculus auditory space map). Before discussing the results of free-field experiments, the responses of the IPD cells, which have been most extensively studied in dichotic experiments, are discussed.

INTERAURAL PHASE DIFFERENCE CELLS: CHARACTERISTIC DELAYS

Rose et al. (121) showed that the IPD/ spike rate curves from single IC cells stimulated with different frequencies could coincide at one particular OTD. They introduced the concept of characteristic delay (CD) cells, i.e., they proposed that such cells had a fixed physiological delay between the inputs from each side, which could be compensated by equal and opposite ITDs in the sound signal. As long as the stimulus frequency was within the cell's response area, the cell would give the same response (e.g., a peak on the ITD/spike rate curve) to signals with this ITD, i.e., they would be selective for a particular sound source direction. The phenomenon of CD

FIG. 6. Binaural cell types: interaural time difference (ITD) and interaural level difference (ILD) responses. The reaction of the three main binaural cell types: high-frequency EI and EE and low-frequency interaural phase difference (IPD) to ITDs and ILDs presented dichotically is shown. **A:** EI cell, excited by input from the contralateral ear and inhibited by ipsilateral input. A series of ITD curves to best frequency tone bursts, noise bursts and carrier only shifted noise bursts (the stimulus envelope, 5-msec rise and fall times, 35 msec plateau, was the same at both ears and only the carrier was delayed) are shown. The vertical axis shows the total number of spikes evoked by each set of stimulus presentations, expressed as spikes/sec. The ITD series (*solid lines*, ±1,024 μsec in 128-μsec steps) were repeated at each ILD (±30 dB in 6-dB steps) shown on the diagonal axis. Around interaural zero, the response increases with ITDs or ILDs, favoring the contralateral ear (*arrows*). The cell is sensitive to noise burst OTDs but not to tone burst ramp TTDs. **B:** EE cell: The response to binaural stimulation is greater than the sum of monaural responses and the contralateral ear is dominant (EE cell). ITD curves to various signals show that this cell is also not very sensitive to tone burst ITDs (left). The ITD/ILD plots show this cell to be sensitive to OTDs in noise bursts, giving a peak response at about zero ITD, and to be little affected by ILDs. **C:** IPD cell: Left: IPD stimulation with tone bursts of different frequencies results in spike rates that fluctuate at one per stimulation frequency. The peaks of the curves coincide at about 300 μsec contra-lead, i.e., this appears to be a characteristic delay cell (but see ref. 165). The ITD (OTD)/ILD plots show a cyclic OTD response to both tone and noise bursts and little effect of ILD.

has been extensively investigated by Kuwada (82) and Yin and co-workers (164) using binaural beats. These are obtained by presenting different frequencies to each ear, e.g., 1,000 and 1,001 Hz. The IPD changes continuously at the beat frequency (1 Hz). The technique allows a large amount of IPD data to be rapidly gathered and direction and speed of IPD changed to be easily varied by changing the frequency difference between the two ears. CD itself was studied by means of analysis of IPD curves at various frequencies. For each cell, the IPD value giving the peak response was plotted against frequency. The slope of this graph gives the CD and the intercept (i.e., where frequency is zero) is the characteristic phase (CP) (165). The majority (60%) of IPD-sensitive cells had a CD that was mostly (71% of CD cells) in the physiological range of ±300 μsec. Surprisingly, for the majority of cells, the CD was on the flank of the delay curves and not at the peak or trough (i.e., CP was not 0 or 0.5). For these cells, therefore, the delay giving the maximal response will vary with signal frequency, as seen for some IPD cells in the guinea pig IC when stimulated with harmonic signals (111). The composite curve, produced by adding the IPD curves at all the frequencies tested, was found to be less sensitive to ILDs or changes in SPL. The peak of this composite curve ("best delay") may be the functional output of an IPD cell and CD and CP the mechanisms that produce it (81,165). The difference between CD and best delay may, however, be an artifact of barbiturate anesthetic as in the IC of the unanesthetized rabbit (81) and barn owl (146). CD is nearly always the same as the peak or trough of the IPD curve and barbiturate anesthesia can significantly affect CP in rabbit IPD cells (80).

Interestingly, the distribution of the peaks of the IPD curves in the guinea pig is the same as in the cat (111), despite the guinea pig's smaller head. For this animal, therefore, the peak responses of most IPD cells lie outside the physiological range. This suggests that the acuity of IPD sensitivity is defined by the physiology of the binaural pathway rather than adapted to the animal's acoustic environment. The extreme accuracy of the barn owl's IPD system seems to be achieved by extending the IPD system to higher frequencies, since the basic mechanisms appear to be the same as in other animals (165). For cells whose peak response is outside the physiological range, the rate of change of the spike rate (i.e., the steep flank of the IPD curve) may be the relevant cue, especially across the midline (161).

The wide band noise OTD curves from IPD cells in the cat IC are almost identical to the composite curves (161) and mostly show a peak in the contralateral physiological range. As OTD is increased, most cells show a cyclic modulation at a frequency near the best frequency, decreasing in amplitude with larger delays. Some cells show asymmetric peaks with sharp slopes across the midline or stable minima in their OTD curves: the position of the peak is determined by CD and its symmetry by CP (165). Stimulating with different, harmonically related tones to the two ears or noise with various degrees of interaural correlation (32,160) showed that these cells act as binaural cross-correlators as originally proposed by Jeffress (63). The response area where this cross-correlation is carried out is determined by filtering and phase locking in the peripheral auditory system (160). As already mentioned, IPD cells have both excitatory and inhibitory inputs and often show facilitation at favorable delays and suppression at nonfavorable delays (rabbit [2], cat [83,121], guinea pig [111]). The peak of the spike rate/signal delay curve is thus often flanked by troughs where the discharges are often completely suppressed (Fig. 7A–C). In some units, however, this suppression is not evident, giving only a peak (Fig. 7D) or, in other cells, only an inhibitory dip is seen (Fig. 7E) (32,111,161). Carney and Yin (30) studied the time course of these inhibitory effects in the cat IC using clicks as stimuli and showed that the ex-

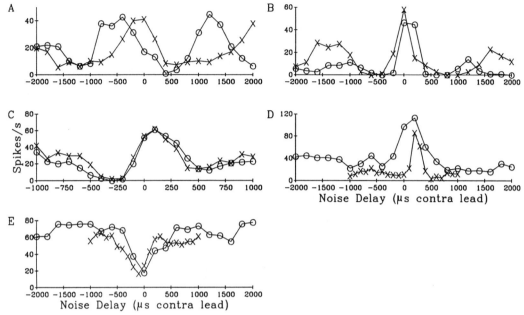

FIG. 7. Delay functions in guinea pig interaural phase difference (IPD) cells. Response as a function of the interaural delay of a wide band noise stimulus (*crosses*) or best frequency (600–1,500 Hz across this sample) tone burst (*circles*) for 10 different neurons in the inferior colliculus of the guinea pig to illustrate the different shapes of the delay functions. Typically, the peak was flanked by one (**C**) or two (**B**) inhibitory dips, although these could be absent (**D**, *circles*) or vary with stimulus (D, *crosses*). In **E**, the major response was a reduction of the discharge near zero delay with no corresponding facilitation. In most cases, best (or worst in E) delay was the same for noise and best frequency tone but there were exceptions (**A**), presumably where characteristic delay is not the same as best delay and the noise delay response is dominated by frequencies other than best frequency (see IPD cells: characteristic delays section). (From ref. 111: very similar curves are seen in the cat [32,161].)

citatory input from each ear was often preceded by an inhibitory component. For example, 44% of ipsilaterally driven cells showed an early contralateral inhibitory component. In such cells, this early inhibitory component sharpens the delay curve by suppressing the cell response at small ipsi-lead values (30).

An interesting species difference is seen in the owl IC. Here the noise OTD curves cannot be calculated by linearly summing the IPD curves at different frequencies, unlike the cat, in which such linear summation appears to be present (161,165). In the owl, peaks at long OTDs with noise stimulation are not a linear sum of the individual IPD functions for different frequencies and are

suppressed. This ties in neatly with the physics of sound localization in the owl: due to the high IPD frequency limit and the small head, phase ambiguities (OTDs greater than one cycle of the stimulus) are possible in this animal. This nonlinear suppression of peaks at longer delays is thus a physiological mechanism that suppresses phase ambiguities (146).

As pointed out by Yin and Kuwada (164), the IPD cells cannot unequivocally code sound source direction since the discharge rate is affected by both OTD and SPL. Comparison of the output of an array of IPD cells would be necessary for the coding of a sound source direction. Although low-frequency tones can be localized on the basis of IPD, recent studies have emphasized the role of high frequencies and EI cell interactions in the coding of auditory space (section on the SC auditory space map). The main role of the IPD cells may be rather to provide spatial channels so that in-

formation coming from a particular direction can be preferentially analyzed, e.g., the cocktail party effect. In our laboratory we have carried out experiments on the reaction of cat IC cells to the simplest such task: the binaural masking level difference.

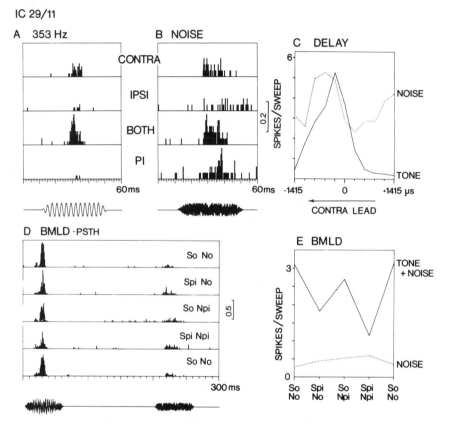

FIG. 8. The binaural masking level difference (BMLD). **A** and **B**: BMLD test for a typical interaural phase difference (IPD) neuron in the cat inferior colliculus. Poststimulus time histograms (PSTHs) for stimulation with best frequency tone bursts (A) or noise bursts (B) at the same rms signal level in the following configurations: monaural contralateral, monaural ipsilateral, binaurally in phase (0), and binaurally out of phase (signal inverted at one ear: π). **C**: Spike rate interaural time difference (ITD) curves for best frequency tones and noise bursts are shown. Note that the peak of both curves is nearer zero ITD, i.e., this is a 0 cell not a π cell. **D**: PSTHs to the BMLD test used. For each signal configuration, a tone (40 msec) and noise (60 msec) burst followed by the noise burst alone was presented. Each PSTH is the sum of 49 presentations. The configurations S_0N_0 (both signals in phase at the two ears), $S_\pi N_0$ (signal inverted at one ear), S_0N_π (noise inverted at one ear), and $S_\pi N_\pi$ (both signals inverted at one ear) were presented. Finally, S_0N_0 was presented again as a control for random spike rate fluctuations. The configurations S_0N_π and $S_\pi N_0$ are BMLD positive. **E**: Mean spike rate to the tone and noise burst for each configuration. Note that the spike rate decreases for both S_π and N_π, i.e., it is correlated with the amount of signal in phase at the two ears and not with the BMLD configuration.

INTERAURAL PHASE DIFFERENCE CELLS: THE BINAURAL MASKING LEVEL DIFFERENCE (BMLD)

If a low-frequency tone is presented over headphones and mixed with noise, the noise level that just masks perception of the tone is dependent on the binaural signal configuration. The signal (S) and the noise (N) masker can be presented with the same phase at each ear (S_0, N_0) or inverted at one ear. This latter condition, equivalent to a 180° shift in all frequency components of the signal and noise masker is here desig-

nated S_π or N_π. The masking level is lowest when both signals have the same binaural configuration: both in phase (S_0N_0) at the two ears or both inverted at one ear ($S_\pi N_\pi$). Binaural disparities such as inverting noise (S_0N_π) or signal ($S_\pi N_0$) at one ear allow the tone to be heard so that an increase in masking level of up to 12 dB is necessary to suppress perception of the tone. More details are given in Chapter 15. This effect has also been shown psychophysically in cats (36,149).

We have tested IPD cells in the cat IC with such signal configurations. The cells

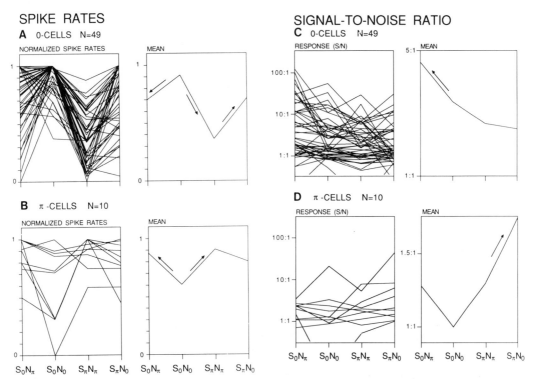

FIG. 9. Binaural masking level difference-cell population. **A** and **B:** The spike rate (fraction of the maximal value) is plotted for the four signal configurations for 50 0 cells (A) and 10 π cells (B). The individual values are plotted left and the mean curves right. The trend for each cell type is the same for signal and noise masker (i.e., greater response to S_0 and N_0 for the 0 cells, S_π and N_π for the π cells) and is not correlated with BMLD configuration. The BMLD-configurations (S_0N_0, $S_\pi N_\pi$) are in the middle and the BMLD+ conditions at the edges of the graph (*arrows*). **C** and **D:** Response signal/noise ratio. The response to the tone and noise burst divided by the response to the following noise burst for each BMLD signal configuration. The response S/N is plotted logarithmically on the Y axis. C: 0 cells; D: π cells. The S/N ratio is maximal for the favored signal configuration (S_0 for the 0 cells, S_π for the π cells) masked by the nonfavored noise configuration (N_π and N_0, respectively) (*arrows*).

were tested with alternate tone + noise and noise bursts in the configurations: S_0N_0 (BMLD−), $S_{\pi}N_0$ (BMLD+), S_0N_{π} (BMLD+), and $S_{\pi}N_{\pi}$ (BMLD−) (Fig. 8). Most cells responded better to in phase signals (0 cells) rather than out of phase signals (π cells). This would be expected from the IPD curves of these cells: the peak is more often nearer S_0 than S_{π} (Fig. 8). The $0/\pi$ response preference was always the same for noise and tone, and the tone response was usually dominant. For the 0 cells, the responses were therefore graded: $S_0N_0 > S_0N_{\pi} > S_{\pi}N_0 > S_{\pi}N_{\pi}$ (Fig. 9). The less numerous π cells had responses graded in the opposite direction: $S_{\pi}N_{\pi} > S_{\pi}N_0 > S_0N_{\pi} > S_0N_0$.

Cells that responded better, S_0N_{π} or $S_{\pi}N_0$, i.e, BMLD cells, were not found. The response of the cells was therefore correlated with the amount of acoustic signal (tone or masker) present in the favorable configuration and not with the BMLD situation.

A possible BMLD substrate was found in the signal/noise ratio of the cell responses. When the response to the tone + noise burst was divided by that to the noise burst for each signal configuration, the response to the favored signal (S_0 or S_{π} for 0 and π cells) was higher when the BMLD+ masker (N_{π} or 0 for 0 and π cells) was applied (Fig. 9). Similar results were obtained for some (70% of those tested) IPD cells in the guinea pig. In these experiments, the signal (a 500-msec best frequency tone burst or

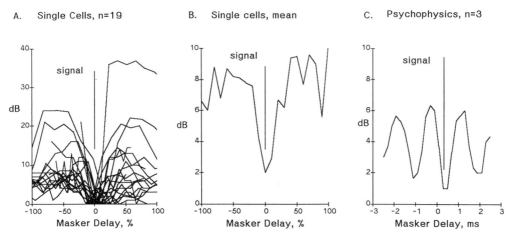

FIG. 10. Binaural masking in the guinea pig inferior colliculus (IC). **A:** The response of 19 interaural phase difference cells in the IC of the guinea pig to 500-msec segments of a signal (in this case the synthetic vowel /a/ [111]) in the presence of a continuous broad band noise masker. The signal was presented at the best delay of each cell and the delay of the noise varied, generally in the range ±1,000 μsec in 100-μsec steps. For each noise delay value, a masked threshold was obtained by comparing the response in the signal + noise and noise alone intervals. In most cases, threshold was defined as one spike more in the signal + noise interval. In these cells, masking was greatest when the noise was at the same delay as the signal and least at half of a cycle of the noise delay function away from this value, i.e., on the peak and dips of the delay curve as seen in Fig. 8. As the cells have different best frequencies and therefore noise delay functions, the plots have been normalized as a function of the noise delay function and superimposed by setting the best delay and lowest masking level as zero. **B:** The mean response from all the cells in A. **C:** The mean threshold curve for three human subjects (the experimenters) for the same signal and noise situation. The vowel was presented at 300 μsec right lead at 62 dB SPL, the lowest masking noise level was 34 dB. The oscillation period shows that the major determinant of ITD-related detectability are the components of the vowel near the first formant of 740 Hz. (From Caird, Palmer, and Rees, *in preparation*.)

segment of a synthetic vowel) was presented at best delay and in the presence of continuous masking noise. The delay of the masking noise was varied, and at each delay the noise level was changed until a given response signal/noise ratio (typically one spike more in the signal + noise period than in the noise period) was obtained. When the noise masker was also at best delay, the necessary level was at a minimum, reaching maxima at ±50% of the noise delay function, i.e., at the minima of the delay curve to noise alone (Fig. 10A). The mean response range of the sample illustrated (Fig. 10B) is very similar to that of the human psychophysical masking curves for the same stimulus (Fig. 10C). It seems, however, that, as for the coding of direction, single cells in the central nucleus cannot code BMLDs. This task would have to be carried out by other cells integrating the output of an array of 0 or π cells. Comparison of the signal/noise relationships in these two channels would allow the tone to be coded in either of the BMLD+ configurations (84).

INTERAURAL PHASE DIFFERENCE CELLS: OTHER PSYCHOPHYSICAL EFFECTS

Three other psychophysical effects, precedence, dichotic repetition pitch, and perceived width, can also be correlated with the responses of the IPD cells. Carney and Yin (30), using click stimuli, showed a long-lasting (up to 100 msec) inhibition in cat IC IPD cells. In the vast majority of cells, such long-lasting inhibition could be demonstrated after ipsilateral (87% of cells tested) or contralateral ear (100% of cells tested) stimulation. This slow inhibitory effect was in addition to the fast effects discussed previously and would be ideally suited to form a physiological basis for the precedence effect (Chapter 15).

Dichotic repetition pitch is heard when white noise is presented dichotically with a large OTD (16). For example, with an OTD of 4,000 μsec, a pitch of 250 Hz is perceived. Since the OTD modulation frequencies of the IPD cells are often the same as best frequency, one would expect such a delay to preferentially stimulate the secondary peaks of the 250-Hz IPD cells, giving rise to a 250-Hz tonal sensation (161).

The perceived width of a stimulus (spaciousness) is also correlated with the IPD cell responses. In dichotic listening experiments, the perceived width of a noise signal increases with the amount of low-frequency energy present (17). The OTD curves of the IPD cells are wider to noises with low-frequency components (32). Chan et al. (32) therefore suggested that spaciousness was correlated with excitation across arrays of IPD cells with different peak values: A signal with more low-frequency components would excite a larger number of cells—due to the broader OTD curves—than a higher frequency signal. If the peak of excitation across such an array is used to code direction, spreading of the peak should correspond to a sensation of greater width.

FREE-FIELD STUDIES IN THE INFERIOR COLLICULUS

A number of studies have addressed the free-field directional selectivity of neurons in the IC. Mostly this is done by moving a speaker along a hoop in the frontal sound field in an anechoic chamber (7,9,10) or using an array of speakers (89). When the speaker hoop is pivoted at each end, elevation can be also varied to allow a three-dimensional analysis of receptive fields (102,104,130). Analysis can either be made of receptive field size or spike rate/angle functions. Receptive fields are defined as the area where a given spike rate is exceeded for a stimulus at a fixed intensity. By plotting the SPL needed to evoke a given amplitude of the cochlear microphonic potential (iso-CM curves), they can be directly compared with the directional sensitivity of the ear in the same experiment. This allows an estimate of the contributions of peripheral directional sensitivity of the ear and central processing. Further detail may be obtained by plotting spike rate/angle curves. This shows not only where response is maximal ("best area") but the way the cell response changes away from the receptive field. This is an important distinction as this rate of change, particularly across the midline, may be an important cue for spatial coding (45,89). The two major direction-selective cell types in these studies correspond to the EI (high frequency, selective for the contralateral pinna axis) and IPD (low frequency with peaked azimuth/response functions) cell types studied in dichotic experiments.

The free-field properties of IC cells were examined by Aitkin et al. (7) in the central and paracentral nucleus of the cat and brush-tailed opossum. The results from the two species were so similar that they were pooled. Aitkin et al. used a hoop system to measure azimuth selectivity in an anechoic chamber at a constant elevation of 15° to 20° (the level of the pinna axis). When the azimuth sensitivity of cells at all best frequencies was analyzed, neurons with peaked azimuth functions were found to be mostly low frequency, i.e., IPD cells (7). A further study, confined to low (less than 3 kHz) best frequency neurons in the cat, found that 52% of the cells were azimuth selective (10). These were divided into peak response cells, with a maximum at a particular angle, and cells showing maximal discharge when the speaker was far contralateral, declining as it was moved across the midline (Fig. 11). Twenty-eight percent of the sample was directionally nonselective (omnidirectional) and 9% showed more than one peak in the frontal sound field. In general, maximal azimuth selectivity was shown by cells with best frequencies between 0.8 and 1.6 kHz; low (130–800 Hz) and high (1.6–3 kHz) best frequency cells were most likely to be omnidirectional. Plugging one ear showed binaural facilita-

tion at some points of the azimuth curve and inhibition at others, as shown for dichotic IPD curves. Removal of the pinnae had no effect on cell azimuth selectivity. Interpretation of data from receptive field studies is more difficult. Semple and Aitkin (130) found low-frequency neurons to be nonselective, but Moore et al. (103,104) and Calford et al. (26) found many such cells to have restricted receptive fields. At high sound intensities, many of these cells developed a second excitatory area (26,103, 104). Aitkin et al. (10) showed that the peak response of many cells could be shifted by up to 20° with changes in intensity, but some cells were not shifted. Similarly, some cells showed no change in the position of the medial border with increasing intensity. Although the shape of many of these curves was invariant with intensity, absolute spike rate was not. Receptive field size therefore increases with intensity (26,104), and these cells cannot directly code sound source direction. Furthermore, a limited number of tests with small changes in frequency suggested that frequency could also affect the shape of the azimuth response (10,89). The results of Yin et al. (161,165) indicate that this might be expected. In contrast to these low-frequency cells, the majority of high best frequency cells have their maximal response area opposite the contralateral pinna (7,9,24,103,104,129). Receptive field size decreased (i.e., increasingly sharp selectivity) with increasing frequency. Three-dimensional plots, coupled with CM measurements of the spatial selectivity of the ear (26,104,130), have shown that the spatial selectivity of these cells correlates very closely with that of the ear. Such receptive fields are therefore basically monaural, i.e., at high frequencies there is in principle no difference between the receptive field of an EI and an EO cell as the response is a combination of the RIF to stimulation of the contralateral ear and ear selectivity (26, 130). Since spike rate is affected by SPL, stimulus frequency, and azimuth, these cells also cannot code a given sound direc-

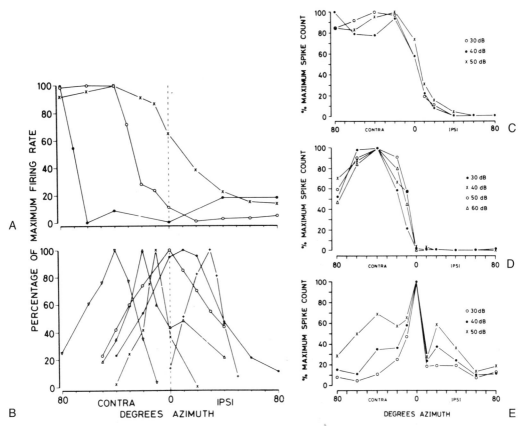

FIG. 11. Free-field responses of low- and high-frequency cells. **A** and **B:** Azimuth/spike rate functions for low frequency (0.8–1.4 kHz best frequency) azimuth selective units in the cat inferior colliculus. Stimulation was with best frequency tones at levels. The best frequency and threshold is shown to the right of each graph. The loudspeaker was moved around a track in an anechoic chamber with a constant 20° elevation. The functions can be either maximal at far contralateral sound source angles with a sharp medial border (A) or show a peak at a given azimuth angle (B). (From ref. 12, with permission.) **C–E:** Azimuth/spike rate functions for high (>4 kHz) best frequency neurons in the central nucleus of the cat inferior colliculus, noise stimulation. The units can have curves with fixed medial borders (C) or a peak response at a given azimuth angle (E). A gradation between the two types seems to be present (B). The spike rate curves (expressed as percentage of the maximum for that intensity) are SPL invariant. The stimulation level in dB above threshold (at the best angle) is shown to the right of each curve. (From ref. 9, with permission.)

tion with spike rate. Furthermore, since they are all basically maximally responsive to the same direction, higher order neurons looking at an array of such cells would also be unable to code sound direction on the basis of peak responses across an array of cells. However, two possible mechanisms whereby a population of EI cells could code direction are available. They both depend on graded strength of inhibitory inputs across the population varying two key response characteristics: medial border of the receptive field and sensitivity to mean binaural SPL.

The strength of the inhibitory inputs to EI cells varies greatly from cell to cell (134). EI cells with weak inhibitory inputs would resemble EO cells, i.e., the spike

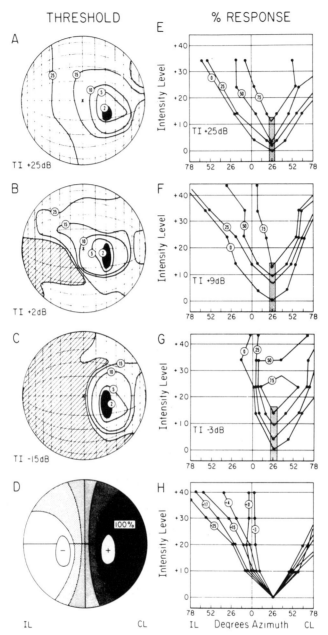

FIG. 12. EI cell response gradients in the dorsoposterior division (DPD) of the mustache bat. **A–D:** The responses of 60 kHz EI cells with different thresholds of inhibition. (TI-dB with respect to contralateral excitatory threshold) in the DPD of the mustache bat. The contour lines show the dB SPL stimulation necessary to evoke a spike response with the loudspeaker at that point in space. The *cross* indicates the midline; IL (ipsilateral) and CL (contralateral) to the recording side. **E–H:** The contours, isospike rate lines, and figures show the percentage of the maximal response that is obtained at the given azimuth angle (X axis) and SPL (Y axis). Note that the area of maximal response is always the same but that the size of the receptive field, in particular its medial boundary, decreases with increasing inhibitory strength. The characteristics of EI cells with different TIs are shown schematically in D and **H**. In H the threshold curves for EI cells of different TI (figures) are shown. These cells are topographically organized; TI decreases with increasing depth in the DPD. (From ref. 45, with permission.)

rate would increase with SPL following the rate intensity function of the cell. In cells with strong inhibitory inputs, inhibition would also increase with mean binaural SPL and these cells would be expected to be sensitive to ILD rather than SPL. There is evidence that this is indeed the case: Semple and Kitzes (134), using dichotic stimulation in the gerbil, found that about 18% of the EI cell population were not affected by mean binaural SPL. These cells were SPL insensitive, i.e., the spike rate was determined by ILD and not mean SPL. The receptive fields of these cells would be expected not to expand with increasing SPL and free-field mapping data show that such cells do exist. Moore et al. (103) and Aitkin and Martin (9) found that 20% and 12% of their samples had fixed medial receptive field borders at all intensities tested. Although these cells have the same receptive field orientation (pinna axis), nearer the midline they could code increasing sound laterality with increasing spike rate. Sound direction could also be coded by comparison of the outputs across a graded EI cell population. As SPL increases, the medial borders of the cells' receptive fields cells move ipsilaterally but at different rates for cells with different strength of ipsilateral inputs. This is clearly shown in the IC of the mustache bat. The main component of the echolocating call of this CF-FM bat is at 60 kHz, and the 60 kHz isofrequency representation is a massively hypertrophied lamina, the dorsoposterior division (DPD) (154,168). In the DPD, EE, EO, and EI cell populations are separated into blocks (154). In the EI cell block, there is a dorsoventral gradient of increasing inhibitory strength (or decreasing inhibitory threshold) with depth (168,154), so that the receptive medial borders move more laterally deeper in the DPD. Although the cells' spike rates are affected by SPL and the receptive field centers are all at the contralateral pinna axis, spike rates across the whole population would show graded change with stimulus azimuth (Fig. 12). Sound direction could also be coded by in-

tegrating information from EE and EI cells. The dichotic data predict that EE cells should in many cases have peak responses at a given sound source angle (23) or at the midline (134). Sound source direction could be coded by integration of outputs from cells with such midline receptive fields and EI cells with lateral receptive fields. Semple et al. (130) and Calford et al. (26) did not find high-frequency cells with restricted receptive fields (i.e., EE cells appeared to be omnidirectional), but Aitkin et al. (7,9) did find high-frequency cells with peak spike response/azimuth curves (Fig. 11). In the mustache bat, EE cells have midline receptive fields (45). The most selective cells were those showing strong facilitation (EE/ Fac or OO/Fac), i.e., inhibited at nonfavorable ILDs. Some of these cells were also insensitive to mean SPL (44). The free-field data therefore suggest that the high-frequency binaural cell types (EI cell/pinna axis, EE cell/frontal sound field) can have receptive fields as predicted from their ITD and ILD characteristics in dichotic experiments (23,134,143). Evidence that sound source direction is indeed represented in the superior colliculus across arrays of EI and EE cells with graded binaural dominance is presented in the section on the SC auditory space map.

Moore et al. (103) found that the effects of elevation in cat IC cells were less than that of azimuth. The only study of the mechanism of elevation sensitivity in IC cells is on the mustache bat. In this specialized echolocator, the pinna have different elevation sensitivities for the three main harmonics (30, 60, and 90 kHz) of the echolocating call (45). Comparison of unit responses across these frequency bands would allow elevation coding, but the exact mechanism for such coding is unknown.

TOPOGRAPHIC REPRESENTATION OF BINAURAL CHARACTERISTICS

If comparison of the output from an array of collicular cells is necessary before direction can be coded, there must be a physical substrate for these arrays. Yin et al. (162) noted that penetrations from caudal to rostral along isofrequency contours in the low-frequency region of the cat IC sometimes showed evidence of a binaural response gradient. In some tracks, the peak of the composite OTD curves was more medial from cells at more rostral recording locations (the CD values were graded in the opposite direction). This effect was, however, variable and not found in all penetrations. Our data from caudorostral penetrations obliquely crossing isofrequency contours in high-frequency regions are also inconclusive: some penetrations show an increase ipsilaterally of peaks or flanks of the ITD or ILD curves but most do not. EI and EE cells were intermingled in clumps; mostly several of one type would be recorded followed by several of the other (*unpublished data*). As noted by Yin et al. (162), these binaural parameters do not appear to be randomly distributed, but a clear spatial distribution cannot be seen. In free-field studies, Aitkin and Martin (9) could find no topological representation of azimuth sensitivity for high-frequency neurons. On the other hand, Aitkin et al. (10) found that peak response curves (measured with best frequency stimuli) from cells in the 1.1- to 1.4-kHz range were correlated with recording position. In the lateral and rostral part of the central nucleus, the azimuth angle giving peak response was correlated with rostrocaudal recording position: More rostrally situated cells had more peripheral azimuths. This agrees with the gradients for CD of Yin et al. (162) but not for the composite OTD curves. It seems that in the cat IC, there is no marked topological representation of peak azimuth or medial edge of the receptive field along each isofrequency contour. The topological organization of EI cells in the DPD of the mustache bat is an extreme case, and it is not clear how representative this hypertrophied three-dimensional structure is of a "normal" two-dimensional isofrequency lamina.

If there is a space map in IC, one would expect it to be in the paracentral region. This is because there is known to be a space map in the superior colliculus that receives its auditory inputs from this region (section on the SC auditory space map). The paracentral nucleus receives in turn its main auditory input from the central nucleus (section on the paracentral nuclei) and the broadly tuned cells here would be ideally suited to integrate information from arrays of central nucleus cells. Finally, such a space map is found in the equivalent structure in the barn owl, but not in the equivalent to the central nucleus (next section). The cat data are, however, not clear. Semple and Aitkin (130) and Aitkin et al. (7) found little difference between the spatial selectivity of paracentral and central nucleus cells in the cat and opossum. The only difference found was for the dorsal cortex, where the cells were more likely to be omnidirectional (7,10). High-frequency cells often had better selectivity to noise bursts (7,9), and the sharpest low-frequency azimuth function was from a cell that only responded to noise bursts (10). This preference for noise stimulation would be expected from the proposed directionally selective units comparing the outputs of an array of central nucleus cells. However, if there is a separate area in the cat IC where the cells are specifically sensitive to sound source direction, it is not very prominent. Such is, however, not the case in one animal that is very highly specialized for sound localization: the barn owl.

SPACE MAPPING IN THE COLLICULUS OF THE BARN OWL

The barn owl is a nocturnal predator that can locate its prey in total darkness. Suitable sound sources (broad band, frequency between 4 and 8 kHz) can be localized with less than 2° error near the midline in elevation and azimuth, a performance better than any animal tested (78). The structure equivalent to IC, the mesencephalis lateralis dorsalis (MLD) is divided into a frequency-mapped region (equivalent to the central nucleus) and, on the anterior and lateral border, a space-mapped region (equivalent to the paracentral nucleus) (77). The space-mapped cells are responsive to frequencies in the 4- to 8-kHz range and respond best to noise stimulation (76). Each cell in the space-mapped MLD has a receptive field limited in both azimuth (25°) and elevation (70°) (76), surrounded by an inhibitory area (77). The best areas, where spike response is maximal, are smaller (30 × 10° on average). The receptive fields and (more accurately) best areas of these MLD cells are topologically distributed: lateral to central azimuth is mapped caudorostrally and dorsoventral elevation is mapped dorsoventrally (76). There are important differences between the mechanisms of direction coding in the owl and in mammals. The owl uses ILDs and OTDs in the same frequency band to code elevation and azimuth. There is a vertical disparity in the position of the ear canals of the owl on each side, and this, combined with refractions around the facial ruff feathers, gives rise to elevation-dependent ILDs (78). The other owl "specialty" is coding IPDs up to much higher frequencies; MLD neurons are sensitive to OTDs at up to 8 kHz, and OTDs in this frequency range elicit head orientation movements (99). Since IPD curves are sharper at higher frequencies, this ensures that the OTD selectivity of such cells is much higher than those of the cat (161). Up to the level of the MLD, ILD and ITD are coded in separate brainstem structures (100,144). The inputs from these brainstem channels converge onto space-mapped MLD cells to give selectivity to elevation (ILD) and azimuth (OTD). These effects are not complementary, i.e., these cells show no time intensity trading with dichotic stimulation (99). Wagner et al. (148) have shown that there is a direct projection from arrays of cells with a common best OTD in the nonspace-mapped MLD to the corresponding area in

the space-mapped MLD. Electrode penetrations at right angles to the isofrequency contours record cells with increasing best frequency but similar best OTDs. Small injections of HRP in the space-mapped MLD result in stripes of cell body labeling with the same orientation as the physiologically recorded isodelay contours (148). The principal differences between the owl and mammals are therefore the high-frequency limit of IPD sensitivity and the coding of elevation with ILD. The IPD sensitivity in the owl MLD is different in degree but not in kind from that in cat IC IPD cells (161). On the other hand, elevation coding does appear to be fundamentally different from the situation in mammals. The similarities are that space mapping is not present in the central nucleus, but in broadly tuned cells that receive inputs from the central nucleus (73,148). In both owls and mammals, there is an orderly representation of auditory space in the superior colliculus (72,74) (section on SC auditory space map) and a strong projection (topological in the case of the owl [75]) to the superior colliculus from the paracentral nucleus (section on the dorsal cortex).

THE SUPERIOR COLLICULUS AUDITORY SPACE MAP

The deep layers of the SC receive auditory projections from the paracentral part of IC (34,39,40,79) and dorsal nucleus of the lateral lemniscus (39,40). The auditory cells in these layers cells respond best to broad band contralateral sound signals and there is no tonotopic representation (38,57, 71,97,157). Although most cells are broadly tuned, they are mostly sensitive to high frequencies and EI type (57,156,158). The second most common type is EO/Fac or OO/Fac (156,158). Spatial receptive fields have been plotted for SC cells in the guinea pig (70), cat (97), and ferret (69). Although the receptive fields are rather broad, the centers are topographically organized along the rostrocaudal axis so that lateral sound sources are represented more caudally and frontal sound sources more rostrally. Elevation is represented in the cat (97) and ferret (69) SC along the medial (up) to lateral (down) axis. Although most studies plot receptive fields, Middlebrooks and Knudsen (98) showed that unit receptive fields were a less reliable spatial mapping cue than the direction giving peak response (best area). Lateral receptive fields were often very large—many cells were excited by a sound source anywhere in the contralateral hemifield (Fig. 13) (38,70,97).

Best areas, on the other hand, were small and showed a much more accurate point-point representation of auditory space and a much closer agreement with receptive fields of visual cells in the same part of the SC (Fig. 13). As pointed out by King and Hutchings (69), visual receptive fields are also larger than saccadic accuracy. It seems that space is coded in the SC as a topographic representation of peak response across arrays of cells rather than as a point-point representation of discrete receptive fields.

Dichotic studies of single units in the SC have shown a graded caudorostral progression of EI inhibitory threshold (strongest inhibition found most caudal) through EO/Fac to OO/Fac (158,159). The EO/Fac and EE/Fac cells have peaked ILD response curves (57,157) and their topographic distribution fits nicely with that of the free-field receptive fields. The medial boundaries of the EI cell ILD curves shift more medially, giving way to peak ILD curves with progressively more medial peak positions as the recording site moves rostrally (Fig. 14) with a graded progression through one cell population (EI cells) and across cell populations (EI to EE/Fac cells) and emphasizes the limitations of the EE/EI cell classification discussed previously. This effect was studied by Middlebrooks (96) with free-field stimulation in the cat. Plugging the ipsilateral ear (contralateral to the sound source) gave an increase in receptive field size in 50% of the sample tested and a decrease in receptive field size and fewer spikes in 28% of the cases. The rest of the cells showed a decrease in response at the best area and an increase away from the best area. Middlebrooks suggested that these corresponded to EI, Fac, and mixed cells, respectively, and noted that these types corresponded to the position of the best area: EI lateral, Fac frontal, and mixed in between. The cells in the SC are broadly

FIG. 13. Free-field responses in the cat superior colliculus. **A** and **B:** Three-dimensional plots of the receptive fields (defined as the area where auditory stimulation with noise bursts gave an increase in spike rate) obtained with a three-dimensional speaker/hoop system. Two receptive field types are seen. Rostral units have sharp frontal receptive fields (A), while caudal units have diffuse receptive fields covering most of the hemisphere of auditory space contralateral to the recording side (hemifield, B). The *cross* marks the midline in both azimuth and elevation. **C–E:** Best area. Within the receptive field, the maximal spike rate is evoked by stimulation in a smaller and more sharply defined area, the best area (BA). **C:** The BA and receptive field (*shaded area*) are shown in three-dimensional coordinates. **D** and **E:** Spike counts for stimulus presentations varying in azimuth at the best elevation (D) and in elevation at the best azimuth (E) are shown. BA and the borders of the receptive field (*dotted lines*) are marked. **F–H:** Topological representation of azimuth selectivity. The location of the BA is plotted against position along the caudorostral axis of the superior colliculus in F. *Open circles* represent frontal units and *filled circles* hemifield. *Triangles* show units whose receptive field borders were not measured and *crosses* are nondirectionally selective cells. Note that the recording position/azimuth representation is virtually linear for BA but not for the receptive field center (**G**) or medial border of the receptive field (**H**). Similar relationships between recording position and elevation sensitivity were found along the medial axis of the superior colliculus. (From ref. 97, with permission.)

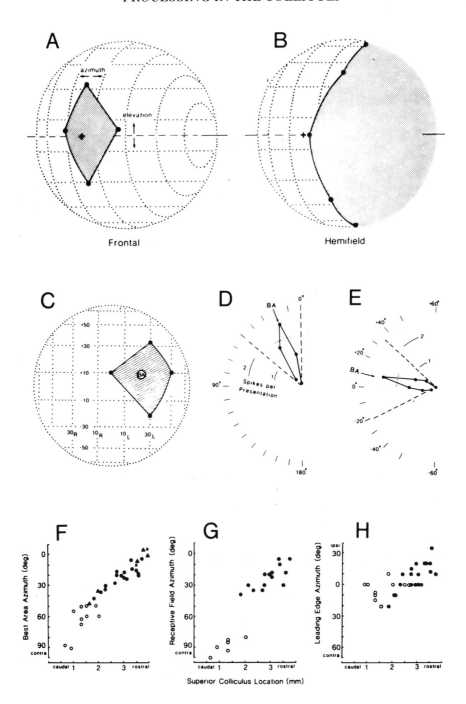

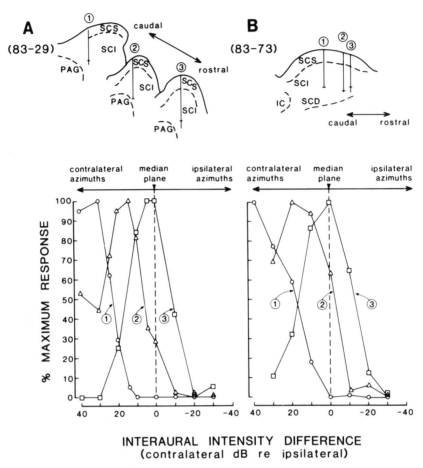

FIG. 14. Binaural cell response gradient in the cat superior colliculus. Topographic representation of EI and EE cell responses in the superior colliculus. In two experiments (**A** and **B**), auditory cell response, tested with dichotic stimulation ILDs (interaural level difference), shows a gradation from EI (1) to EE (OO/FAC) peak response (3) as the penetrations site progresses from caudal to rostral. At intermediate levels (2), peak response is at ILD values corresponding to azimuths between the rostral/median plane (3) and caudal/contralateral azimuth (1) units. SC, SCS, intermediate and superficial layers of the superior colliculus; IC, inferior colliculus; PAG, periaqueductal gray. (From ref. 159, with permission.)

tuned, and monaural cues are important for the space map. Palmer and King (110) blocked or destroyed the ear ipsilateral to the recording side (i.e., contralateral to the sound source) and showed that the (receptive field) space map was maintained for threshold stimuli. Removing the pinna and concha of the contralateral ear (ipsilateral to the sound source) destroyed the space map—all cells had receptive fields opposite the severed ear canal. At higher stimulus levels, blocking of the ipsilateral ear did reduce the selectivity of these cells (see also ref. 38). This suggests that the SC space map is basically monaural but stabilized by binaural interactions at higher levels. This would perhaps be expected for the caudal EI cells: The monaural E input pattern could be stabilized by the I inputs from the other ear as stimulus level increases—as seen in some IC EI cells (134). The equivalent effect of the Fac cells is not so obvious. The ear block studies of Middle-brooks (96) suggest, however, that these Fac cells receive substantial inhibitory in-puts—ear block increased the response away from the best area. These inputs may stabilize the receptive field or best area re-sponses at higher stimulus levels.

Frequency selectivity also plays a role in the spatial selectivity of SC cells. There is a tendency in the cat (96) and owl for higher frequency sensitivity to be found in more rostral units (74). Thus, caudal units with more lateral receptive fields tend to be sen-sitive to lower frequencies (but still in the high-frequency, non-IPD range) where the pinna acoustic selectivity is broader. Ros-tral units, with frontal, smaller (97) recep-tive fields, are sensitive to frequencies where directional selectivity of the external ear is highest. This would suggest that fre-quency and inhibitory strength could be combined to produce lateral EI cell recep-tive fields. The more caudal the cell, the stronger the inhibitory input and the more lateral the medial border of the receptive field (159). Similarly, for these cells the lower frequency sensitivity allows the lat-eral border of the receptive field to spread more laterally. The best area is presuma-bly where the cutoffs of the two mechan-isms coincide. More rostrally, increasing strength input from the ear would shift the receptive fields of the Fac cells further for-ward. It is, however, not at all clear how these effects could generate a monaural map. All published studies have shown the direction of maximal pinna sensitivity to be similar for all frequencies (only selectivity increases with frequency) (section on free-field studies in the IC).

An interesting comparative point is seen in the SC of the guinea pig where the frequency selectivity gradient, seen with acoustic evoked field potentials, is the op-posite of that in the cat. Best responses are obtained with 20-kHz stimulation caudally and 10-kHz stimulation rostrally (29). The functional gradient is, however, the same as that in the cat: In the guinea pig the ear se-lectivity is most lateral at higher (above 12 kHz) frequencies (28).

As the SC is best known for its map of visual space, it would be interesting to know if the visual and auditory maps coin-cide. Although early studies did find the vi-sual, somatosensory, and auditory maps to be coincident, the definition of the auditory receptive fields was not accurate enough to allow accurate comparison (70). More recent experiments, in which care was taken to fix the eye, show a good corre-spondence between auditory and visual re-ceptive fields (69,71). This applies to visual and auditory cells recorded at different depths in the same penetration as well as to bimodal cells (71). The best correspon-dence is seen in the barn owl, which cannot rotate its eyes in their orbits (72), and in the frontal, binocular area where visual and au-ditory receptive fields are smallest (97).

One of the major surprises of the mam-malian SC space map is the lack of IPD cells. Not only is this surprising given the high ITD sensitivity and azimuth selectivity of these cells, it also means that the space map is affected by pinna movements. Mid-dlebrooks and Knudsen (98) examined the effect of pinna movements in the cat by turning the ipsilateral or contralateral (to the recording side) ear to the side. Turning the contralateral ear shifted the best area laterally and up; ipsilateral ear turn shifted best area frontally. Units with more frontal best areas were more affected (higher best frequencies for which the pinna is more di-rectionally selective [96]) and generally showed a decrease in spike rate with ear turn (Fac cells). More caudal units showed less effect (lower best frequencies) and often more spikes with ipsilateral (contra-lateral to the sound source) ear turn (EI cells). The space map can therefore be af-fected by pinna position.

A related problem is that of Pöppels' par-adox (115): what happens to the register be-tween the visual and auditory space maps when the eyes are moved in the orbit? An early study in the cat by Harris et al. (52)

suggested that this paradox is not resolved in the cat—the maps are not in register during a saccade and the cat circumvents this problem behaviorally: Gaze direction change is carried out by a saccade followed by a head movement that recenters the eyes in their orbits. On the other hand, Jay and Sparks (61,62) showed that SC auditory receptive fields do change with eye position in awake monkeys trained to make saccades to a target without moving the head. Auditory receptive fields (62) and auditory inputs to saccade-related cells (62) were based on retinal and not head coordinates. Electrical stimulation of the SC in cats evokes eye and pinna movements in roughly the same direction (139), and auditory and visual facilitation is shown by many cells in the deep motor layers of SC (71,93,94,112). It may therefore be possible that Pöppels paradox can be compensated for by synchronous pinna and eye movements in the cat and that it only becomes acute for an animal with immobile pinnae and mobile eyes such as monkeys.

CONCLUSIONS

I have tried to give a general overview of what is known about the coding of auditory information in the colliculi. The review is perhaps rather biased toward binaural effects and the representation of auditory space, but this represents the degree of our present state of knowledge of collicular function. Even such a simple task as the coding of sound source direction has been proved to be full of unexpected surprises: The role of high-frequency binaural interactions in the mapping of auditory space in the SC and the lack of representation of the IPD system. It might be helpful to regard these systems as basically independent: The SC as a reflex control center responsible for "where is it?" and the IPD system as a spatial cross-correlation more interested in exactly "what is happening there." Destruction of the auditory cortex results

in the inability to make an appropriate response to an object in the contralateral sound field in cats, dogs, and monkeys ([54,55,65,66] but not in rats [67]), but reflex directed head movements remain (54,55). Such quick reflex movements are reduced by SC lesions (147). Such effects were originally described in the visual system (the "two systems" theory [128,153]). Patients with large visual cortex lesions can make directed responses to objects in the blind areas without having a visual percept as such (18) and hamsters retain visual localization ability after visual cortex lesions but not after SC lesions (128). The first steps in correlating the reactions of the IPD cells with psychophysical data have been made (sections on IPD cells: BMLD and IPD cells: other psychophysical effects), and it is hoped that studies correlating physiological data with psychophysical effects will attract increasing attention in the future. Modern anatomical studies of IC—the revised parcellation of the subnuclei and the overlapping but separate projections to the central nucleus laminae—have also raised new and interesting problems of collicular function. The study of the processing of complex signals with known psychophysical properties and the correlation with anatomical substrates in the colliculi will provide interesting problems for experimental study for a long time to come.

ACKNOWLEDGMENTS

The work carried out in our laboratory was supported by the Deutsche Forschungsgemeinschaft (SFB 45). The cat BMLD experiments were carried out in conjunction with Frank Pillman, and the gerbil 2DG data are from a joint research project with Prof. H. Scheich of the Technical University in Darmstadt. The guinea pig IC recordings were performed with Alan Palmer and Adrian Rees of the Institute for Hearing Research, Nottingham, England, and were partially supported by a twinning grant from the European Training Programme in Brain and Behaviour Research. I thank my head of department, Prof. R. Klinke, for his help and encouragement during the writing of this review. Alan Palmer, Adrian Rees, and Elaine Caird made helpful comments on the manuscript. I thank Gerald Langner for helpful discussions and access to unpublished data.

REFERENCES

1. Adams JC. Ascending projections to the inferior colliculus. *J Comp Neurol* 1979;183:519–538.
2. Aitkin LM, Blake DW, Fryman S, Bock GR. Responses of neurones in the rabbit inferior colliculus. II. Influence of binaural tonal stimulation. *Brain Res* 1972;47:91–101.
3. Aitkin LM. *The auditory midbrain: structure and function in the central auditory pathway.* Clifton, NJ: Humana, 1986.
4. Aitkin LM, Bush BMH, Gates GR. The auditory midbrain of a marsupial. The brush-tailed possum (Trichosorus vulpeculus). *Brain Res* 1978;150:29–44.
5. Aitkin LM, Dickhaus H, Schult W, Zimmermann M. External nucleus of inferior colliculus: auditory and spinal somatosensory afferents and their interactions. *J Neurophysiol* 1978;41:837–847.
6. Aitkin LM, Fryman S, Blake DW, Webster WR. Responses of neurones in the rabbit inferior colliculus. I. Frequency specificity and topographic arrangement. *Brain Res* 1972;47:77–90.
7. Aitkin LM, Gates GR, Phillips SC. Responses of neurons in inferior colliculus to variations in sound-source azimuth. *J Neurophysiol* 1984;52:1–17.
8. Aitkin LM, Kenyon CE, Philpott P. The representation of the auditory and somatosensory systems in the external nucleus of the cat inferior colliculus. *J Comp Neurol* 1981;196:25–40.
9. Aitkin LM, Martin RL. The representation of stimulus azimuth by high best-frequency azimuth-selective neurons in the central nucleus of the inferior colliculus of the cat. *J Neurophysiol* 1987;57:1185–1200.
10. Aitkin LM, Pettigrew JD, Calford MB, Philips SC, Wise LZ. Representation of stimulus azimuth by low-frequency neurons in inferior colliculus of the cat. *J Neurophysiol* 1985;53:43–59.
11. Aitkin LM, Philips SC. Is the inferior colliculus an obligatory relay in the cat auditory system? *Neurosci Lett* 1984;44:259–264.
12. Aitkin LM, Schuck DM. Low frequency neurons in the lateral central nucleus of the cat inferior colliculus receive their input predominantly from the medial superior olive. *Hear Res* 1985;17:87–93.
13. Aitkin LM, Webster WR, Veale JL, Crosby DC. Inferior colliculus. I. Comparison of response properties of neurons in the central, pericentral, and external nuclei of adult cat. *J Neurophysiol* 1975;38:1196–1207.
14. Andersen RA, Roth GL, Aitkin LM, Merzenich MM. The efferent projections of the central nucleus and the pericentral nucleus of the inferior colliculus of the cat. *J Comp Neurol* 1980;194:649–662.
15. Batra R, Kuwada S, Stanford TR. Temporal coding of envelopes and their delays in the inferior colliculus of the unanesthetized rabbit. *J Neurophysiol* 1989;61:257–268.
16. Bilsen FA, Goldstein JL. Pitch of dichotically delayed noise and its possible spectral basis. *J Acoust Soc Am* 1974;55:292–296.
17. Blauert J, Lindemann W. Spatial mapping of auditory events for various degrees of internal coherence. *J Acoust Soc Am* 1986;79:806–813.
18. Blythe IM, Bromley JM, Kennard C, Ruddock KH. Visual discrimination of target displacement remains after damage to striate cortex in humans. *Nature* 1986;320:619–621.
19. Bock GR, Webster WR. Spontaneous activity of single units in the inferior colliculus of anesthetized and unanesthetized cats. *Brain Res* 1974;76:150–154.
20. Boudreau JC, Tsuchitani C. Binaural interaction in the cat superior olive S segment. *J Neurophysiol* 1968;31:442–454.
21. Brunso-Bechtold JK, Thompson GC, Masterton RB. HRP study of the organization of auditory afferents ascending to central nucleus of inferior colliculus in cat. *J Comp Neurol* 1981;197:705–722.
22. Caird DM, Klinke R. Processing of binaural stimuli by cat superior olivary complex neurons. *Exp Brain Res* 1983;52:385–399.
23. Caird DM, Klinke R. Processing of interaural time and intensity differences in the cat inferior colliculus. *Exp Brain Res* 1987;68:379–392.
24. Caird D, Pillmann F, Klinke R. Responses of single cells in the cat inferior colliculus to binaural masking level difference signals. *Hear Res* 1989;43:1–24.
25. Caird D, Scheich H, Klinke R. Functional organization of auditory cortical fields in the Mongolian gerbil (Meriones unguiculatus): binaural 2-deoxyglucose patterns.*J Comp Physiol* 1991;168:13–26.
26. Calford MB, Moore DR, Hutchings ME. Central and peripheral contributions to the coding of acoustic space by neurons in the inferior colliculus of the cat. *J Neurophysiol* 1986;55:587–603.
27. Calford MB, Pettigrew JD. Frequency dependence of directional amplification at the cat's pinna. *Hear Res* 1984;14:13–19.
28. Carlile S, Pettigrew AG. Directional properties of the auditory periphery in the guinea pig. *Hear Res* 1987;31:111–122.

29. Carlile S, Pettigrew AG. Distribution of frequency sensitivity in the superior colliculus of the guinea pig. *Hear Res* 1987;31:123–136.

30. Carney LH, Yin TCT. Responses of low-frequency cells in the inferior colliculus to interaural time differences of clicks: excitatory and inhibitory components. *J Neurophysiol* 1989; 62:144–161.

31. Chan JCK, Musicant AD, Hind JE. Directional properties of the cat external ear. In: *IUPS Satellite Symposium on Hearing*. San Francisco: University of California Press, 1986;67.

32. Chan JCK, Yin TCT, Musicant AD. Effects of interaural time delays of noise stimuli on low-frequency cells in the cat's inferior colliculus. II. Responses to band-pass filtered noises. *J Neurophysiol* 1987;58:543–561.

33. Clopton BM, Winfield JA. Tonotopic organization in the inferior colliculus of the rat. *Brain Res* 1973;56:355–358.

34. Coleman JR, Clerici WJ. Sources of projections to subdivisions of the inferior colliculus in the rat. *J Comp Neurol* 1987;262:215–226.

35. Coles RB, Guppy A. Biophysical aspects of directional hearing in the tammar wallaby (Macropus Eugenii). *J Exp Biol* 1986;121:371–394.

36. Cranford JL. Auditory masking-level differences in the cat. *J Comp Physiol Psychol* 1975;89:219–223.

37. Crow G, Langford TL, Moushegian G. Coding of interaural time differences by some high frequency neurons of the inferior colliculus: responses to noise bands and two-tone complexes. *Hear Res* 1980;3:147–153.

38. Dräger UC, Hubel DH. Responses to visual stimulation and relationship between visual, auditory, and somatosensory inputs in mouse superior colliculus. *J Neurophysiol* 1975;38: 690–713.

39. Druga R, Syka J. Ascending and descending projections to the inferior colliculus of the rat. *Physiol Bohemoslov* 1984;33:31–42.

40. Druga R, Syka J. Projections from auditory structures to the superior colliculus in the rat. *Neurosci Lett* 1984;45:247–252.

41. Ehret G, Merzenich MM. Auditory midbrain responses parallel spectral integration phenomena. *Science* 1985;227:1245–1247.

42. Ehret G, Moffat AJM. Inferior colliculus of the house mouse. II. Single unit responses to tones, noise and tone-noise combinations. *J Comp Physiol [A]* 1985;156:619–635.

43. Ehret G, Moffat AJM. Inferior colliculus of the house mouse. III. Response probabilities and thresholds of single units to synthesized mouse calls compared to tone and noise bursts. *J Comp Physiol [A]* 1985;156:637–644.

44. Fitzpatrick KA. Cellular architecture and topographic organization of the inferior colliculus of the squirrel monkey. *J Comp Neurol* 1975; 164:185–208.

45. Fuzessery ZM, Pollack GD. Determinants of sound location selectivity in bat inferior colliculus: a combined dichotic and free-field stimulation study. *J Neurophysiol* 1985;54:757–781.

46. Fuzessery ZM, Wenstrup JJ, Pollack GD. A representation of horizontal sound location in the inferior colliculus of the mustache bat (Pteronotis p. parnellii). *Hear Res* 1985;20:85–89.

47. Glendenning KK, Hudson KA, Nudo RJ, Masterton RB. Acoustic chiasm. II: Anatomical basis of binaurality in lateral superior olive of cat. *J Comp Neurol* 1985;232:261–285.

48. Glendenning KK, Masterton RB. Acoustic chiasm: efferent projections of the lateral superior olive. *J Neurosci* 1983;3:1521–1537.

49. Goldberg JM, Brown PB. Response of binaural neurons of dog superior olivary complex to dichotic tonal stimuli: some physiological mechanisms of sound localization. *J Neurophysiol* 1969;32:613–636.

50. Guinan JJ Jr, Guinan SS, Norris BE. Single auditory units in the superior olivary complex. I. Response to sounds and classifications based on physiological properties. *Int J Neurosci* 1972;4:1201–1204.

51. Harnischfeger G. Single unit study in the inferior colliculus of the house mouse (Mus musculus). *Neurosci Lett* 1978;9:279–284.

52. Harris LR, Blakemore C, Donaghy M. Integration of visual and auditory space in the mammalian superior colliculus. *Nature* 1980;288: 56–59.

53. Harrison JM, Downey P. Intensity changes at the ear as a function of the azimuth of a tone source: a comparative study. *J Acoust Soc Am* 1970;47:1509–1518.

54. Heffner HE. Effects of auditory cortex ablation on localization and discrimination of brief sounds. *J Neurophysiol* 1978;41:963–976.

55. Heffner HE, Masterton RB. Contribution of auditory cortex to sound localization in the monkey (Macacca mulatta). *J Neurophysiol* 1978;38:1340–1358.

56. Henning GB. Lateralization of transient signals and types of delay. In: Klinke R, Hartmann R, eds. *Hearing—physiological bases and psychophysics*. Berlin: Springer, 1983;196–201.

57. Hirsch JA, Chan JCK, Yin TCT. Responses of neurons in the cat's superior colliculus to acoustic stimuli. I. Monaural and binaural response properties. *J Neurophysiol* 1985;53: 726–745.

58. Inbody SB, Feng AS. Binaural response characteristics of single neurons in the medial superior olivary nucleus of the albino rat. *Brain Res* 1981;210:361–366.

59. Irvine DRF. The auditory brainstem: a review of the structure and function of auditory brainstem processing mechanisms. In: Ottoson D, ed. *Sensory physiology*, vol 7. Berlin/New York: Springer, 1986.

60. Irvine DRF. Interaural intensity differences in the cat: changes in sound pressure level at the two ears associated with azimuthal displacements in the frontal horizontal plane. *Hear Res* 1987;26:267–286.

61. Jay MF, Sparks DL. Sensorimotor integration in the primate superior colliculus. I. Motor convergence. *J Neurophysiol* 1987;57:22–34.

62. Jay MF, Sparks DL. Sensorimotor integration

in the primate superior colliculus. II. Coordinates of auditory signals. *J Neurophysiol* 1987;57:35–55.

63. Jeffress LA. A place theory of sound localization. *J Comp Psychol* 1948;41:35–39.
64. Jenkins WM, Masterton RB. Sound localization: effects of unilateral lesions in central auditory system. *J Neurophysiol* 1982;47:987–1016.
65. Jenkins WM, Merzenich MM. Role of cat primary cortex for sound localization behaviour. *J Neurophysiol* 1984;52:819–847.
66. Kavanagh GL, Kelly JB. The effects of auditory cortical lesions on minimum audible angles for sound localization in the ferret. *Neuroscience* 1984;9:956.
67. Kelly JB, Kavanagh GL. Effects of auditory cortical lesions on pure-tone sound localization by the albino rat. *Behav Neurosci* 1986;100:569–575.
68. Khanna SM, Stinson MR. Specification of the acoustical input to the ear at high frequencies. *J Acoust Soc Am* 1985;77:577–589.
69. King AJ, Hutchings ME. Spatial response properties of acoustically responsive neurons in the superior colliculus of the ferret: a map of auditory space. *J Neurophysiol* 1987;57:596–624.
70. King AJ, Palmer AR. Cells responsive to free-field auditory stimuli in guinea-pig superior colliculus: distribution and response properties. *J Physiol (Lond)* 1983;342:361–381.
71. King AJ, Palmer AR. Integration of visual and auditory information in bimodal neurones in the guinea pig superior colliculus. *Exp Brain Res* 1985;60:492–500.
72. Knudsen EI. Auditory and visual maps of space in the optic tectum of the owl. *J Neurosci* 1982;2:1177–1194.
73. Knudsen EI. Subdivisions of the inferior colliculus in the barn owl (Tyto alba). *J Comp Neurol* 1983;218:174–186.
74. Knudsen EI. Auditory properties of space-tuned units in owl's optic tectum. *J Neurophysiol* 1984;52:709–723.
75. Knudsen EI, Knudsen PF. Space-mapped auditory projections from the inferior colliculus to the optic tectum in the barn owl (Tyto alba). *J Comp Neurol* 1983;218:187–196.
76. Knudsen EI, Konishi M. Space and frequency are represented separately in auditory midbrain of the owl. *J Neurophysiol* 1978;41:870–884.
77. Knudsen EI, Konishi M. Center-surround organization of auditory receptive fields in the owl. *Science* 1978;202:778–780.
78. Knudsen EI, Konishi M. Mechanisms of sound localization in the barn owl (Tyto alba). *J Comp Physiol [A]* 1979;133:13–21.
79. Kudo M, Niimi K. Ascending projections of the inferior colliculus in the cat: an autoradiographic study. *J Comp Neurol* 1980;191:545–556.
80. Kuwada S, Batra R, Stanford TR. Monaural and binaural response properties of neurons in the inferior colliculus of the rabbit: effects of sodium pentobarbital. *J Neurophysiol* 1989;61:269–282.

81. Kuwada S, Stanford TR, Batra R. Interaural phase-sensitive units in the inferior colliculus of the unanesthetized rabbit: effects of changing frequency. *J Neurophysiol* 1987;57:1338–1360.
82. Kuwada S, Yin TCT. Binaural interaction in low-frequency neurons in inferior colliculus of the cat. I. Effects of long interaural delays, intensity, and repetition rate on interaural delay function. *J Neurophysiol* 1983;50:981–999.
83. Kuwada S, Yin TCT, Syka J, Buunen TJF, Wickesberg RE. Binaural interaction in low-frequency neurons in inferior colliculus of the cat. IV. Comparison of monaural and binaural response properties. *J Neurophysiol* 1984;51:1306–1325.
84. Langner G. Neuronal mechanisms for pitch analysis in the time domain. *Exp Brain Res* 1981;44:450–454.
85. Langner G. Evidence for neuronal periodicity detection in the auditory system of the guinea fowl: implications for pitch analysis in the time domain. *Exp Brain Res* 1983;52:333–355.
86. Langner G. Time coding and periodicity pitch. In: Michelsen A, ed. *Time resolution in auditory systems.* Berlin/New York: Springer, 1984;108–121.
87. Langner G, Schreiner C, Merzenich MM. Covariation of latency and temporal resolution in the inferior colliculus of the cat. *Hear Res* 1987;31:197–201.
88. Langner G, Schreiner C. Periodicity coding in the inferior colliculus of the cat. I. Neuronal mechanisms. *J Neurophysiol* 1988;60:1799–1822.
89. Leiman AL, Hafter ER. Responses of inferior colliculus neurons to free field auditory stimuli. *Exp Neurol* 1972;35:431–449.
90. Maffi CL, Aitkin LM. Differential neural projections to regions of the inferior colliculus of the cat responsive to high frequency sounds. *Hear Res* 1987;26:211–219.
91. Martin RL, Webster WR, Servière J. The frequency organization of the inferior colliculus of the guinea pig: a ^{14}C-2-deoxyglucose study. *Hear Res* 1988;33:245–256.
92. Meininger V, Pol D, Derer P. The inferior colliculus of the mouse. A Nissl and Golgi study. *Neuroscience* 17:1159–1179.
93. Meredith MA, Nemitz JW, Stein BE. Determinants of multisensory integration in superior colliculus neurons. I. Temporal factors. *J Neurosci* 1987;7:3215–3229.
94. Meredith MA, Stein BE. Visual, auditory and somatosensory convergence on cells in superior colliculus results in multisensory integration. *J Neurophysiol* 1986;56:640–662.
95. Merzenich MM, Reid MD. Representation of the cochlea within the inferior colliculus of the cat. *Brain Res* 1974;77:397–415.
96. Middlebrooks JC. Binaural mechanisms of spatial tuning in the cat's superior colliculus distinguished using monaural occlusion. *J Neurophysiol* 1987;57:688–701.
97. Middlebrooks JC, Knudsen EI. A neural code

for auditory space in the cat's superior colliculus. *J Neurosci* 1984;4:2621–2634.

98. Middlebrooks JC, Knudsen EI. Changes in external ear position modify the spatial tuning of auditory units in the cat's superior colliculus. *J Neurophysiol* 1987;57:672–687.

99. Moiseff A, Konshi M. Neuronal and behavioural sensitivity to binaural time differences in the owl. *J Neurosci* 1981;1:40–48.

100. Moiseff A, Konishi M. Binaural characteristics of units in the owl's brainstem auditory pathway: precursors of restricted spatial receptive fields. *J Neurosci* 1983;3:2553–2562.

101. Møller AR, Rees A. Dynamic properties of the responses of single neurons in the inferior colliculus of the rat. *Hear Res* 1986;24:203–215.

102. Moore DR, Hutchings ME, Addison PD, Semple MN, Aitkin LM. Properties of spatial receptive fields in the central nucleus of the cat inferior colliculus. II. Stimulus intensity effects. *Hear Res* 1984;13:175–188.

103. Moore DR, Semple MN, Addison PD. Some acoustic properties of neurones in the ferret inferior colliculus. *Brain Res* 1983;269:69–82.

104. Moore DR, Semple MN, Addison PD, Aitkin LM. Problems of spatial receptive fields in the central nucleus of the cat inferior colliculus. I. Responses to tones of low intensity. *Hear Res* 1984;13:159–174.

105. Morest DK, Oliver DL. The neuronal architecture of the inferior colliculus in the cat: defining the functional anatomy of the auditory midbrain. *J Comp Neurol* 1984;222:209–236.

106. Nordeen KW, Killacky HP, Kitzes LM. Ascending auditory projections to the inferior colliculus in the adult gerbil, Meriones unguiculatus. *J Comp Neurol* 1983;214:131–143.

107. Nudo RL, Masterton RB. Stimulation-induced (14C)2-deoxyglucose labelling of synaptic activity in the central auditory system. *J Comp Neurol* 1986;245:553–565.

108. Oliver DL, Morest DK. The central nucleus of the inferior colliculus of the cat. *J Comp Neurol* 1984;222:237–264.

109. Osen KK. Projection of the cochlear nuclei on the inferior colliculus in the cat. *J Comp Neurol* 1972;144:355–372.

110. Palmer AR, King AJ. A monaural space map in the guinea pig superior colliculus. *Hear Res* 1985;17:267–280.

111. Palmer AR, Rees A, Caird DM. Interaural delay sensitivity to tones and broad band signals in the guinea-pig inferior colliculus. *Hear Res* 1990;50:71–86.

112. Peck CK. Visual-auditory interactions in cat superior colliculus: their role in the control of gaze. *Brain Res* 1987;420:162–166.

113. Phillips DP, Calford MB, Pettigrew JD, Aitkin LM, Semple MN. Directionality of sound pressure transformation at the cat's pinna. *Hear Res* 1982;8:13–28.

114. Popelar J, Syka J. Response properties of neurons in the inferior colliculus of the guinea pig. *Acta Neurobiol Exp (Warsz)* 1982;42:299–310.

115. Pöppel E. Comment on "Visual system's view of acoustic space". *Nature* 1973;243:231.

116. Rees A, Møller AR. Responses of neurons in the inferior colliculus of the rat to AM and FM tones. *Hear Res* 1983;10:301–330.

117. Rees A, Møller AR. Stimulus properties influencing the responses of inferior colliculus neurons to amplitude-modulated sounds. *Hear Res* 1987;27:129–143.

118. Rees A, Palmer AR. Rate intensity functions and their modification by broadband noise for neurones in the guinea-pig inferior colliculus. *J Acoust Soc Am* 1988;83:1488–1498.

119. Rockel AJ, Jones EG. The neuronal organization of the inferior colliculus of the adult cat. I. The central nucleus. *J Comp Neurol* 1973;147:11–60.

120. Rose JE, Greenwood DD, Goldberg JM, Hind JE. Some discharge characteristics of single neurons in the inferior colliculus of the cat. I. Tonotopical organisation, relation of spike counts to tone intensity and firing patterns of single elements. *J Neurophysiol* 1963;26:294–320.

121. Rose JE, Gross NB, Geisler CD, Hind JE. Some neural mechanisms in the inferior colliculus of the cat which may be relevant to localization of a sound source. *J Neurophysiol* 1966;29:288–314.

122. Roth GL, Aitkin LM, Andersen RA, Merzenich MM. Some features of the spatial organization of the central nucleus of the inferior colliculus of the cat. *J Comp Neurol* 1978;182:661–680.

123. Roth GL, Kochhar RK, Hind JE. Interaural time differences: implications regarding the neurophysiology of sound localization. *J Acoust Soc Am* 1980;68:1643–1657.

124. Ryan A, Miller J. Single unit responses in the inferior colliculus of the awake and performing rhesus monkey. *Exp Brain Res* 1978;32:389–407.

125. Ryan AF, Woolf NK, Sharp FR. Tonotopic organization in the central auditory pathway of the Mongolian gerbil: a 2-deoxyglucose study. *J Comp Neurol* 1982;207:369–380.

126. Saint-Marie RL, Ostapoff EM, Morest DK, Wenthold RJ. Glycine-immunoreactive projection of the cat lateral superior olive: possible role in midbrain ear dominance. *J Comp Neurol* 1989;279:382–396.

127. Schreiner C, Langner G. Periodicity coding in the inferior colliculus of the cat. II. Topographical organization. *J Neurophysiol* 1988;60:1823–1840.

128. Schneider GE. Two visual systems. *Science* 1969;163:895–902.

129. Schuller G. Natural ultrasonic echoes from wing beating insects are encoded by collicular neurons in the CF-FM bat, Rhinolophus ferrumequinum. *J Comp Physiol* 1984;155:121–128.

130. Semple MN, Aitkin LM. Representation of sound frequency and laterality by units in central nucleus of cat inferior colliculus. *J Neurophysiol* 1979;42:1626–1639.

131. Semple MN, Aitkin LM. Physiology of pathway from dorsal cochlear nucleus to inferior colliculus revealed by electrical and auditory stimulation. *Exp Brain Res* 1980;41:19–28.

132. Semple MN, Aitkin LM, Calford MB, Pettigrew JD, Phillips DP. Spatial receptive fields in the cat inferior colliculus. *Hear Res* 1983;10:203–215.

133. Semple MN, Kitzes LM. Single unit responses in the gerbil inferior colliculus: different consequences of contralateral and ipsilateral auditory stimulation. *J Neurophysiol* 1985;53:1467–1482.

134. Semple MN, Kitzes LM. Binaural processing of sound pressure level in the inferior colliculus. *J Neurophysiol* 1987;57:1130–1147.

135. Servière J, Webster WR, Calford MB. Isofrequency labelling revealed by a combined (^{14}C)2-deoxyglucose, electrophysiological, and horseradish peroxidase study of the inferior colliculus of the cat. *J Comp Neurol* 1984;228:463–477.

136. Schneiderman A, Henkel CK. Banding of lateral superior olivary nucleus afferents in the inferior colliculus: a possible substrate for sensory integration. *J Comp Neurol* 1987;266:519–534.

137. Schneiderman A, Oliver DL, Henkel CK. Connections of the dorsal nucleus of the lateral lemniscus: an inhibitory parallel pathway in the ascending auditory system? *J Comp Neurol* 1988;276:188–208.

138. Sokoloff L, Reivich M, Kennedy C, et al. The (^{14}C)deoxyglucose method for the measurement of local cerebral glucose utilization: theory, procedure, and normal values in the conscious and anaesthetized albino rat. *J Neurochem* 1977;28:897–916.

139. Stein BE, Clamann HP. Control of pinna movements and sensorimotor register in cat superior colliculus. *Brain Behav Evol* 1981;19:180–192.

140. Stiebler I. Tone-threshold mapping in the inferior colliculus of the house mouse. *Neurosci Lett* 1986;65:336–340.

141. Stiebler I. A distinct ultrasound-processing area in the auditory cortex of the mouse. *Naturwissenschaften* 1987;74:96.

142. Stiebler I, Ehret G. Inferior colliculus of the house mouse. I. A quantitative study of tonotopic organization, frequency representation, and tone-threshold distribution. *J Comp Neurol* 1985;238:65–76.

143. Stillman RD. Responses of high-frequency inferior colliculus neurons to interaural intensity differences. *Exp Neurol* 1972;36:118–126.

144. Sullivan WE, Konishi M. Neural map of interaural phase difference in the owl's brainstem. *Proc Natl Acad Sci USA* 1986;83:8400–8404.

145. Syka J, Radionova EA, Popelaar J. Discharge characteristics of neuronal pairs in the rabbit inferior colliculus. *Exp Brain Res* 1981;44:11–18.

146. Takahashi T, Konishi M. Selectivity for interaural time difference in the owl's midbrain. *J Neurosci* 1986;6:3413–3422.

147. Thompson GC, Masterton RB. Brain stem auditory pathways involved in reflexive head orientation to sound. *J Neurophysiol* 1978;41:1183–1202.

148. Wagner HT, Takahashi T, Konishi M. Representation of interaural time difference in the central nucleus of the barn owl's inferior colliculus. *J Neurosci* 1987;7:3105–3116.

149. Wakeford OS, Robinson DE. Lateralization of tonal stimuli by the cat. *J Acoust Soc Am* 1974;55:649–652.

150. Webster WR, Servière J, Brown M. Inhibitory contours in the inferior colliculus as revealed by the 2 deoxyglucose method. *Exp Brain Res* 1984;56:577–581.

151. Webster WR, Servière J, Crewther D, Crewther S. Isofrequency 2-DG contours in the inferior colliculus of the awake monkey. *Exp Brain Res* 1984;56:427–437.

152. Webster WR, Servière J, Martin R, Brown M. Uncrossed and crossed inhibition in the inferior colliculus of the cat: a combined 2-deoxyglucose and electrophysiological study. *J Neurosci* 1985;5:1820–1832.

153. Weiskrantz L, Warrington EK, Sanders MD, Marshall J. Visual capacity in the hemianopic field following restricted occipital ablation. *Brain* 1974;97:709–728.

154. Wenstrup JJ, Ross LS, Pollak GD. Binaural response organization within a frequency-band representation of the inferior colliculus: implications for sound localization. *J Neurosci* 1986;6:962–973.

155. Willard FH, Ryugo GP. Anatomy of the central auditory system. In: Willott JF, ed. *The auditory psychobiology of the mouse.* Springfield, IL: Charles C Thomas, 1983;210–304.

156. Willott JF. Central nervous system physiology. In: Willott JF, ed. *The auditory psychobiology of the mouse.* Springfield, IL: Charles C Thomas, 1983;305–338.

157. Wise LZ, Irvine DRF. Auditory response properties of neurons in deep layers of cat superior colliculus. *J Neurophysiol* 1983;49:674–685.

158. Wise LZ, Irvine DRF. Interaural intensity difference sensitivity based on facilitatory binaural interaction in cat superior colliculus. *Hear Res* 1984;16:181–188.

159. Wise LZ, Irvine DRF. Topographic oranization of interaural intensity difference sensitivity in deep layers of cat superior colliculus: implications for auditory spatial representation. *J Neurophysiol* 1985;54:185–211.

160. Yin TCT, Chan JCK, Carney LH. Effects of interaural time delays of noise stimuli on low-frequency cells in the cat's inferior colliculus. III. Evidence for cross-correlation. *J Neurophysiol* 1987;58:562–583.

161. Yin TCT, Chan JCK, Irvine DRF. Effects of interaural time delays of noise stimuli on low-frequency cells in the cat's inferior colliculus. I. Responses to wide-band noise. *J Neurophysiol* 1986;55:280–300.

162. Yin TCT, Chan JCK, Kuwada S. Characteristic delays and their topographical distribution in

the inferior colliculus of the cat. In: Webster WR, Aitkin LM, eds. *Mechanisms of hearing.* Clayton, Australia: Monash University Press, 1983;94–99.

163. Yin TCT, Hirsch JA, Chan JCK. Responses of neurons in the cat's superior colliculus to acoustic stimuli II. A model of interaural intensity sensitivity. *J Neurophysiol* 1985;53:746–758.

164. Yin TCT, Kuwada S. Binaural interaction in low-frequency neurons in inferior colliculus of the cat. II. Effects of changing rate and direction of interaural phase. *J Neurophysiol* 1983; 50:1000–1019.

165. Yin TCT, Kuwada S. Binaural interaction in low-frequency neurons in inferior colliculus of the cat. III. Effects of changing frequency. *J Neurophysiol* 1983;50:1020–1042.

166. Yin TCT, Kuwada S, Sujaku Y. Interaural time sensitivity of high-frequency neurons in the inferior colliculus. *J Acoust Soc Am* 1984;76: 1401–1410.

167. Zook JM, Casseday JH. Convergence of ascending pathways at the inferior colliculus of the mustache bat, Pteronotus parnellii. *J Comp Neurol* 1987;261:347–361.

168. Zook JM, Winer JA, Pollak GD, Bodenhamer BD. Topology of the central nucleus of the mustache bat's inferior colliculus: correlation of single unit properties and neuronal architecture. *J Comp Neurol* 1985;231:530–546.

Neurobiology of Hearing: The
Central Auditory System, edited by
R. A. Altschuler et al.
Raven Press, Ltd., New York © 1991.

12

Anatomy of the Medial Geniculate Body

Jeffery A. Winer

*Division of Neurobiology, Department of Molecular and Cell Biology, University of California,
Berkeley, California 94720-2097*

Since the neuron doctrine propounds the view that the primary element in the brain is the nerve cell and the circuits it forms (108), the present account considers the neurons and their arrangement in the mammalian medial geniculate body, a structure essential for normal hearing. Such patterns might help to predict the flow of information to and from the many nuclei that comprise the medial geniculate body, to clarify the distinctions between these centers, and to suggest the nature of the thalamic auditory information reaching the cerebral cortex. Since both the inferior colliculus and the auditory cortex project to the medial geniculate body, the neural circuits linking them, as well as the intrinsic organization of the auditory thalamus, probably cooperate in the genesis and control of tonotopy, binaurality, and other axes of organization. A perspective on medial geniculate body functional organization is afforded by a comparison with the cochlear nuclear complex, where the bifurcation of primary auditory axons from the VIIIth nerve immediately establishes multiple central neural representations of the map of frequency arising in the cochlear neurosensory epithelium (36,71). Within even single subdivisions of the cochlear nuclei, there are clear structural differences among the types of neurons (21,26), and variations in their pharmacological organization (42), connections (27–29), and physiology (111). Thus,

different neuronal populations probably contribute to more than one functional circuit besides that devoted to tonotopic organization. Analogous arguments can be made for the medial geniculate body, and for the nuclei of the superior olivary complex, the trapezoid body, the lateral lemniscus, the inferior colliculus, and for the subdivisions of auditory cortex.

Progress has been comparatively slower in deciphering the functional architecture of the medial geniculate body, particularly its neurochemistry, physiological organization, and behavioral role. Recent work reveals that it, like other auditory synaptic stations, is actually a complex of several nuclei, each containing a few distinct neuronal types, a particular set of connections, and a characteristic intrinsic organization. These attributes may help to identify homologous neurons, nuclei, and circuits in different species, and they form the basis for the present analysis.

This account is largely from work on adult cats, unless otherwise noted. Normal material from rats, bats (*Pteronotus p. parnellii* and *Antrozous pallidus*), squirrels (*Sciureus carolinensis*), opossums (*Didelphis virginiana*), monkeys (*Macaca fascicularis*), and humans (*Homo sapiens*) was available and included Nissl preparations, Golgi impregnations, semithin toluidine blue-stained material, and fiber stains from the Bodian, Weil, Weigert, or Gallyas methods. For many of the nonhuman species, experiments with injections of horseradish peroxidase or tritiated amino acids or other tracers in the midbrain, thalamus, or cerebral cortex were studied.

SUBDIVISIONS OF THE MEDIAL GENICULATE BODY

In transverse sections, the medial geniculate body extends from midway through the rostrocaudal extent of the superior colliculus to the posterior one-third of the ventrobasal complex. Laterally, it is bordered by the hippocampus; dorsally, by the lateral geniculate body; medially, by the midbrain reticular formation and lateral mesence-

phalic nucleus; and ventrally, by the subparafascicular and suprapeduncular nuclei.

Ventral Division

Among the three primary parts of the medial geniculate body, the ventral division is largest in size, has the most stereotyped pattern of neuronal architecture, receives a highly topographic midbrain and corticofugal input, and contains the most precise physiological representation of frequency.

Structure

Only a few different types of neurons occur in the ventral division, and these have

TABLE 1. *List of abbreviations*

AAF	anterior auditory field	LPc	lateral posterior nucleus, caudal part
AI	primary auditory cortical field	LTS	lateral tegmental system
AII	secondary auditory cortical field	M	medial division
APt	anterior pretectum	MB	mammillary bodies
Aq	cerebral aqueduct	ML	medial lemniscus
BIC	brachium of the inferior colliculus	MRF	mesencephalic reticular formation
BSC	brachium of the superior colliculus	MZ	marginal zone
BV	blood vessel	oligo.	oligodendroglial cell
CC	cerebral cortex	OT	optic tract
CG	central gray	Ov	*pars ovoidea* (ventral division)
CN	central nucleus of the inferior colliculus	PC	posterior commissure
CP	cerebral peduncle	PL	posterior limitans nucleus (dorsal
CSC	commissure of the superior colliculus		division)
D	dorsal nucleus *or* dorsal division	POl	lateral part of the posterior nuclear
DC	dorsal cortex of the inferior colliculus		complex
DD	deep dorsal nucleus (dorsal division)	Pt	pretectum
Dm	dorsomedial zone of the inferior	r	rat
	colliculus	RN	red nucleus
DS	superficial dorsal nucleus (dorsal	SC	superior colliculus
	division)	SCo	spinal cord
EE	excitatory-excitatory binaural area	SF/daz	suprasylvian fringe/dorsal auditory
EI	excitatory-inhibitory binaural area		cortical zone
Ep	posterior ectosylvian cortical field	Sg	suprageniculate nucleus (dorsal
Ex	external nucleus of the inferior colliculus		division)
GABA	gamma-aminobutyric acid	SN	substantia nigra
GAD	glutamic acid decarboxylase	SOC	superior olivary complex
Glu	glutamate	Spf	subparafasicular nucleus
Hip	hippocampus	SpN	suprapeduncular nucleus
IBIC	interstitial nucleus of the brachium of	Te	temporal cortical field
	the inferior colliculus	ts	tree shrew
Ins	insular cortical field	V	ventral nucleus *or* ventral division
Ip	interpeduncular nucleus	Vb	ventrobasal complex
LGB	lateral geniculate body	Vl	ventrolateral nucleus (dorsal division)
LMN	lateral mesencephalic nucleus	IIIn	oculomotor nerve
LP	lateral posterior nucleus	3V	third ventricle
		D,M,L,V	dorsal, medial, lateral, ventral

a relatively clear and stereotyped arrangement (Fig. 1A:*V*). Ventral division cells are present at all rostrocaudal levels except the caudal one-fifth of the medial geniculate body; they constitute the bulk of the lateral, free surface of the posterior face of the thalamus, and the ventral division extends to the rostral tip (146). It contains many large, tufted neurons with bushy dendritic arbors (Table 2) whose long axis is usually oriented from dorsal to ventral (Fig. 3). These tufted cells (Fig. 2B:*2*) are readily distinguished from dorsal division neurons (Fig. 1A:*DS, D, DD*), whose dendritic fields usually have a more stellate branching pattern (Fig. 2E:*1–3*), and from medial division cells (Fig. 2H), which are generally larger and have more diverse patterns of dendritic branching.

Most tufted cell primary dendrites are confined to zones 30 to 100 μm wide, whose long axis follows the somatic orientation (Figs. 2A, 3, 7B). Bushy dendrites may extend dorsoventrally for 200 to 300 μm, forming parallel rows of higher-order tufts. Most tufts have a common orientation, and the configuration of the dendritic arbor is highly planar. Ascending axons afferent to ventral division neurons, particularly those believed to arise from the inferior colliculus (55,88), have a characteristic preterminal arrangement, forming long rows parallel to the tufted cell dendrites (Fig. 4: *black profiles*). Together, the dendrites of tufted neurons and these axons comprise the fibrodendritic laminae (Figs. 6, 14N) that are a hallmark of ventral division organization (84) and probably subserve the orderly arrangement of best frequencies, which change along a more or less lateral (low frequency) to medial (high frequency) axis (4,49). Thus, isofrequency contours run caudorostrally. Laminae are longest and least curved in the most lateral part of the ventral division (Fig. 1A:*V*), and shorter and more coiled and irregular in the medial part, the *pars ovoidea* (Fig. 1A:*Ov*), where their planar configuration is obscured while the tufted mode of dendritic

branching is preserved. Tufted cell axons are myelinated and devoid of branches in animals more than a few days old, and they typically arise from the soma or a dendritic trunk (Fig. 3).

A second ventral division cell type is the small stellate neurons or Golgi type II cells (Fig. 14B:*1,5*), whose flask-shaped somata are some two-thirds the size of those of tufted neurons; they constitute about 40% of the cells in the cat ventral division. Analogous neurons are common constituents of both the dorsal (Fig. 5A: *stippled cell*) and medial (Fig. 14J:*1–5*) divisions in most species (although not all; see the section on comparative anatomy). Their thin, sparsely spinous, and delicate dendrites have a stellate configuration with simple, Y-shaped branches ranging from 150 μm (Fig. 5A: *stippled cell*) to 400 μm long (145). Many of their dendrites are presynaptic to those of principal neurons and contribute to local circuits (see below). Stellate cells have unmyelinated axons about half as thick as that of the tufted cell, and they have many intrinsic branches near tufted cell dendrites (Fig. 14N: *axodendritic ending*). Other axons (Fig. 4: *hollow outlines*), perhaps of cortical origin (Figs. 8B, E, H, K; 9B), also form a conspicuous element in the neuropil, as do those arising from the thalamic reticular nucleus (80).

At the ultrastructural level, the comparative simplicity of this neuronal circuitry encourages a rigorous analysis of synaptic relations. Thus, the ascending, tendril-like axons arising in the inferior colliculus terminate chiefly on the intermediate dendrites of principal neurons and the distal dendrites of Golgi type II cells (88) where they form asymmetric synapses containing predominantly round vesicles (55). In contrast, Golgi type II axons make symmetric, flat vesicle-containing synapses upon the intermediate and distal dendrites of principal neurons, as well as on the distal dendrites of other Golgi type II cells. Besides these more or less conventional synaptic arrangements, the Golgi type II cells also

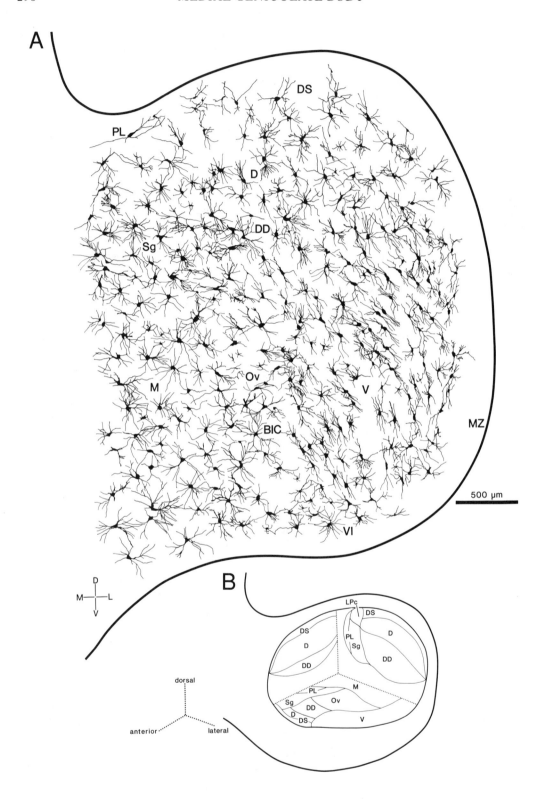

TABLE 2. *Summary of the types of neurons in the principal nuclei of the medial geniculate body*

Division	Nucleus	Type	Somatic size (μm)	Somatic shape	Dendritic branching pattern	Projection to cortex	Possible transmitter[a]
Ventral	Ventral[b]	1. Large bushy cell	15 × 18	Oval or oblate	Tufted	Yes	Glutamate (Glu)
		2. Small stellate cell	10 × 12	Flask-shaped	Radiate	No[c]	Glutamic acid decarboxylase (GAD)[d]
Dorsal	Dorsal[e]	3. Principal stellate cell	15 × 25–30	Round or oblate	Radiate	Yes	?
		4. Principal bushy cell	15 × 20–25	Triangular or flattened	Tufted	Yes	?
		5. Small stellate cell	12 × 18	Elongated and flattened	Radiate	No	GAD
		6. Large stellate cell	15 × 25–30	Elongated or flask-shaped	Radiate	No	GAD
	Suprageniculate	7. Large principal stellate cell	20 × 30	Spherical	Radiate	Yes	Glu
		8. Small stellate cell	10 × 15	Flask-shaped	Radiate	No	GAD
	Posterior limitans	9. Elongate principal cell	15 × 20–25	Flattened	Stellate	Yes	Glu
		10. Small stellate cell	≈10 × 12	Oval or elongated	Stellate	?	?
Medial	Medial	11. Medium-sized stellate cell	25 × 35	Round or oblate	Radiate	Yes	Glu
		12. Tufted cell	20 × 40	Elongated or rectangular	Tufted	Yes	Glu
		13. Elongated cell	25 × 30–35	Slightly elongated	Radiate	Yes	?
		14. Large, weakly tufted cell	35 × 40	Oval	Tufted	Yes	Glu
		15. Small stellate cell	15 × 20–25	Triangular	Radiate	No	GAD

[a]Based on immunocytochemical work in the rat for glutamate (D.T. Larue and J. A. Winer, *unpublished observations*) and on studies of GAD in the rat (64,145) and of GAD and GABA in the cat (D. T. Larue et al., *in preparation*).
[b]The *pars ovoidea* of the ventral division has a comparable set of cell types and a different pattern of neuropil architecture (84).
[c]Some neurons whose somatodendritic form resembles that of stellate cells are labeled after horseradish peroxidase injections of AI (142).
[d]GAD is the metabolic precursor of GABA; their respective patterns of immunolabeling are considered here as identical.
[e]Local differences between dorsal division nuclei are omitted here (for details, see ref. 148).

have an intrinsic role since their dendrites are often presynaptic to those of principal cells. Such arrangements, termed synaptic nests or glomeruli, occur in many different thalamic sensory nuclei (35,87,106) and entail multiple synaptic endings on dendritic spines or shafts, between which are interspersed axon terminals of midbrain origin (55) and corticofugal (88) afferents. A surrounding neuroglial sheath could spatially segregate neighboring glomeruli. There is a phylogenetic difference in the number and complexity of synaptic nests, with rats having only a few or none in the main sensory

FIG. 1. Neuronal architecture and subdivisions of the medial geniculate body in an adult cat. **A:** Principal divisions in a transverse view from two serial, 160-μm-thick sections through the caudal one-third of the auditory thalamus. Note the prevalence of bushy cells with tufted dendrites (see Table 2) in the ventral nucleus (*V*), while more medially placed neurons in *pars ovoidea* (*Ov*) have a less orderly laminar disposition. Dorsal division (*DS, D, DD, Sg, PL*) cells have predominantly radiate dendritic branching, while medial division (*M*) neurons are larger and have a weakly tufted or radiate branching pattern. Planachromat, N. A. 0.35, × 200. **B:** Axonometric reconstruction of medial geniculate subdivisions after dissection of the optic tract and lateral thalamus. For abbreviations, see Table 1. (Modified from ref. 147.)

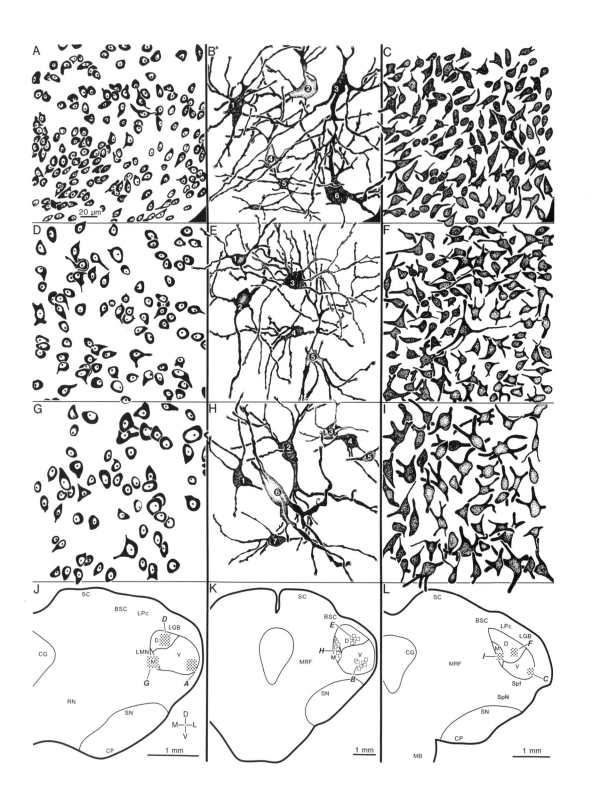

thalamic nuclei (128), cats having a large number (87,88), and primates still more (107).

Corticothalamic axons terminate mainly on the distal dendrites of principal neurons and on the somata and dendrites of Golgi type II cells. These endings typically are somewhat smaller than those of midbrain or intrinsic origin and contain round synaptic vesicles (88).

Connections

Brainstem Input

Inferior colliculus axons are the dominant (Table 3) input to the ventral division, where they terminate both in the ventral nucleus and in the *pars ovoidea* (61,81). Nearly 90% of brainstem input originates in the ipsilateral inferior colliculus (116). Topographically, this pathway appears to preserve the tonotopic pattern in the central nucleus of the inferior colliculus, where cells representing lower frequencies lie dorsal to neurons whose characteristic frequencies are higher (114). Thus, neurons situated more laterally in the ventral division receive input from more dorsal, low-frequency parts of the central nucleus. This arrangement is not unexpected since the laminar arrangement of central nucleus disc-shaped cell dendrites and the afferent axonal plexus has certain parallels with that in the ventral division, allowing for differences in laminar orientation and neuronal form between it and the auditory thalamus (89,99,149,152). Several types of central nucleus neurons may project to the ventral division (97); whether or not particular kinds of central nucleus neurons terminate in some specific pattern within monaural or binaural medial geniculate subregions, as do thalamic neurons projecting to auditory cortex (77), is uncertain. Some evidence favoring segregation is the structural diversity of horseradish peroxidase-filled axons arising in the central nucleus of the bat inferior colliculus and terminating in the ventral nucleus (136). Some axons are comparatively fine and form perisomatic terminals (Fig. 6B:*17,18*), others are much larger and probably end upon both dendrites and peri-

---

FIG. 2. Nissl-stained, Golgi-impregnated, and horseradish peroxidase-labeled neurons in the three primary divisions of the rat medial geniculate body. **A:** Ventral division, with neuronal somata oriented ventromedial-to-dorsolateral and containing medium-sized and small cells. Protocol for panels A–I: planapochromat, N.A. 0.65, × 500. Scale in panel A applies to panels A–I. **B:** Golgi-impregnated neurons, most with a tufted branching pattern (*1–6*) less developed than in the cat (see Fig. 3), and a small stellate cell (*7*). Golgi-Cox technique, 120-μm-thick section. **C:** Thalamic neurons labeled by injection of horseradish peroxidase in area 41; 60-μm-thick section, tetramethylbenzidine method. **D:** Dorsal division Nissl-stained cells without a particular somatic orientation and showing a range of sizes. Protocol as in panel A. **E:** Golgi-impregnated dorsal division cells, including large principal radiate (*2,3*) and weakly tufted (*4,5*) neurons, and a small stellate cell with sparse dendrites (*1*). Protocol as in panel B. **F:** Dorsal division cells projecting to auditory cortex include both large radiate and weakly tufted neurons. Protocol as in panel C. **G:** Medial division neurons in a Nissl preparation, showing a few large and more medium-sized neurons without obvious somatic orientation. Protocol as in panel A. **H:** Golgi-impregnated medial division cells, including large radiate (*1,3*) tufted (*2*), elongated (*4,7*), small stellate (*5*), and magnocellular (*6*) neurons. Protocol as in panel B. **I:** Medial division neurons retrogradely labeled by auditory cortex injection of horseradish peroxidase; compare these cells with neurons in Nissl material (panel G). Protocol as in panel C. **J–L:** Loci for panels A–I. Golgi-impregnated neurons appear larger than they are due to extracellular accretion of mercuric salts in the Golgi-Cox technique. Planachromat, N. A. 0.15, × 34. For abbreviations, see Table 1. (Modified from ref. 144.)

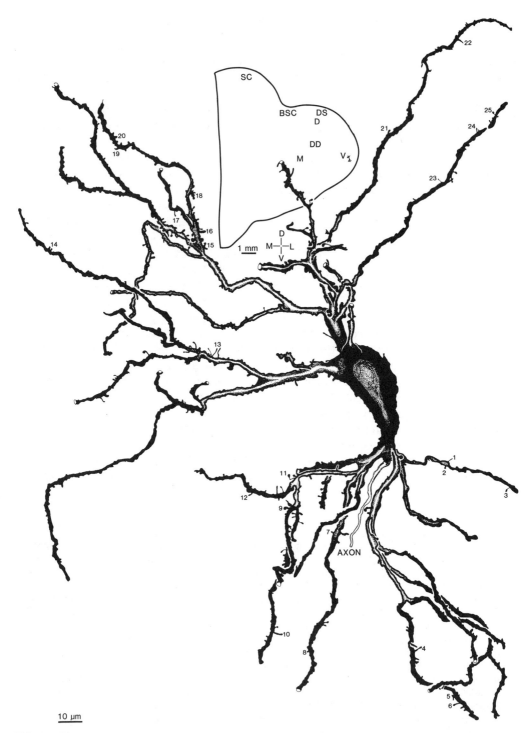

FIG. 3. Characteristic bushy principal neuron with tufted dendritic arbors from the cat ventral division. Each dendritic trunk gives rise to several tufts, some of whose distal parts recurve or form elaborate arrays limited to a small number of fibrodendritic laminae. Most of the dendritic appendages are on the intermediate segments and include short spines (*1,7,8,14,19–21,23,24*), long appendages (*4,10,13*), short, pedunculated spines (*2,3,12,17,25*), long and pedunculated appendages (*6,11*), complex spines (*5,15,18*), and thick appendages (*9,16,22*). Rapid Golgi method; 41-day-old cat. Planapochromat, N. A. 1.32, ×2,000. For abbreviations, see Table 1.

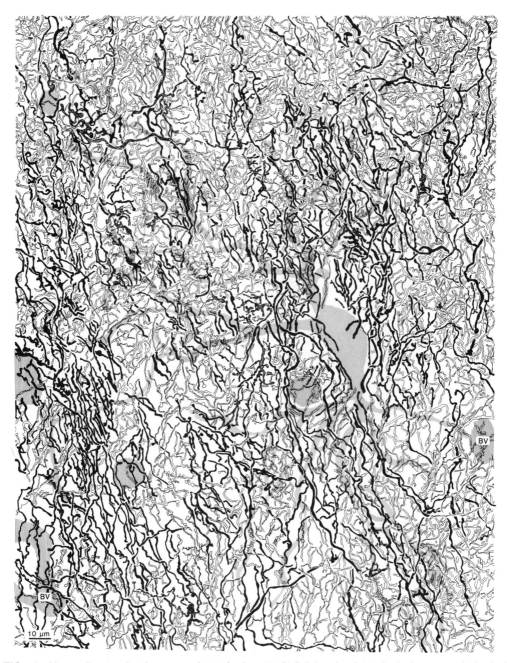

FIG. 4. Neuropil organization near the tufted ventral division bushy principal neuron (*stippled*) shown in Fig. 3. Many of the second- and higher-order dendrites lie parallel to medium-sized axons believed to be of midbrain origin (*solid black*) and terminating (see Table 3) in the ventral division of the medial geniculate body (see also Fig. 6). These axons form conspicuous fascicles oriented ventrolaterally and, with the principal cell dendrites, comprise the fibrodendritic laminae described in Golgi preparations (84,85,90,143). Other, somewhat thinner axonal profiles (*open outlines*) may be of cortical origin and are sparse near the perikaryon and more numerous near the distal dendrites. Still other axons (*hatched outlines:* center, upper left and right, lower center) have a more tortuous course, one or more collateral branches, and fine, elaborate secondary processes; these may represent Golgi type II cells. Protocol as in Fig. 3. For abbreviations, see Table 1.

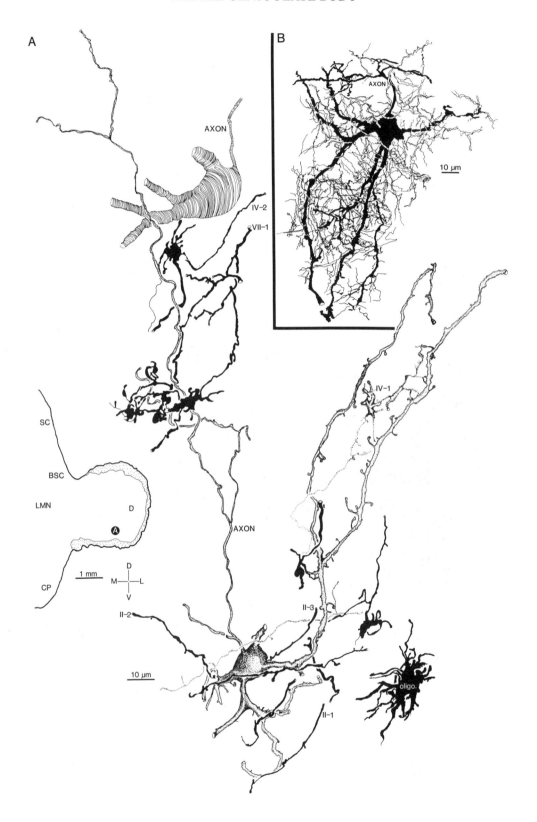

A

AXON

IV-2

VII-1

B

AXON

10 μm

SC

BSC

LMN

D

Ⓐ

CP

1 mm

D
M—L
V

AXON

IV-1

II-2

10 μm

II-3

II-1

oligo.

karya (Fig. 6B:*10*), and still others have elaborate terminal arrays in the neuropil (Fig. 6B:*33*).

A second source of afferents to the ventral division arises from neurons in the dorsal cortex of the inferior colliculus in the rat (38,65); whether this projection is topographic is unknown. Large inferior colliculus injections also label substantial regions beyond those usually considered as part of the auditory thalamus (66). In the cat, neurons and cells in the dorsomedial (nonlaminated) part of the central nucleus of the inferior colliculus and from the external nucleus of the inferior colliculus project more medially, to the *pars ovoidea*. While the dorsomedial zone receives heavy input from the auditory cortex (33), the external nucleus has both spinal cord and auditory afferents (7), suggesting that the functional arrangement within the *pars ovoidea* might differ from that prevailing at lower frequencies in the more lateral part of the ventral nucleus (83).

Axons from the thalamic reticular nucleus cells, all of which are GABAergic (46), also terminate in the rat ventral division, especially in the ventral nucleus (80), and in the ventral and dorsal divisions in the cat (117). Sparse cholinergic immunoreactive axons occur in the rat ventral division; their source is unknown (68), but may (in the cat) include immunopositive neurons whose somata lie in the peribrachial area and laterodorsal tegmental nucleus (130). A moderately dense plexus of histaminergic axons is also found in the rat medial geniculate body (50).

Thalamocortical Projection

Axons from the ventral nucleus and the *pars ovoidea* terminate in layer IIIb–IV of primary auditory cortex (AI) (93,101,127), and in an area just rostral to it, the anterior auditory field (8). Neurons in AI in anesthetized preparations are sharply tuned and tonotopically arranged (76), as are cells in the anterior auditory field (60). Thalamic input to AI (or to presumably homologous cortical field[s]) has a strongly topographic arrangement (92) consistent with the tonotopic sequences in each, and there is a comparable organization in other species (18, 63,100,110,123). While the thalamocortical neurons in the lateral part of the ventral nucleus are more or less uniformly oriented in both the rat (Fig. 8A, D, G, J) and cat (Fig. 7D), those in the *pars ovoidea* have a less clear disposition (Fig. 7B, C). They are mingled with fibers from the brachium of the inferior colliculus, thalamofugal axons, and corticothalamic fibers, which, together, obscure the relatively simple laminar arrangement of the low-frequency sector of the ventral nucleus and produce a more complex tonotopic arrangement at higher frequencies (49).

Most ventral division neurons projecting to AI (Fig. 7D:*1*) probably represent tufted cells (Fig. 3). However, some labeled neurons are far smaller and have an oval or drumstick-shaped somatodendritic profile (Fig. 7D:*2*) like that of Golgi type II neurons; such cells might function both as a local circuit and as a projection neuron (142; see also ref. 37). From 5% to 20% of the

---

FIG. 5. Two Golgi type II cells and some afferent axons in the caudal extremity of the dorsal nucleus. **A:** Typical small stellate cell, characteristic of several medial geniculate body subdivisions, with a locally branching axon near the dendrites of a bushy neuron (*hatched*). Axonal endings are of several types, including thick, sinuous fibers (*II-1–3*), grumous axons (*IV-1,2*), and large fibers with grape-like terminals (*VII-1*). Note the length and variety of the dendritic appendages. Rapid Golgi method, 41-day-old cat. Semi-apochromat, N. A. 1.25, ×1,250. **B:** Fine terminal axonal plexus near a small stellate Golgi type II cell with a locally branching axon. Several types of axons are present. Rapid Golgi method, 25-day-old cat. Planapochromat, N. A. 1.32, ×1,250. For abbreviations, see Table 1. (Modified from ref. 148.)

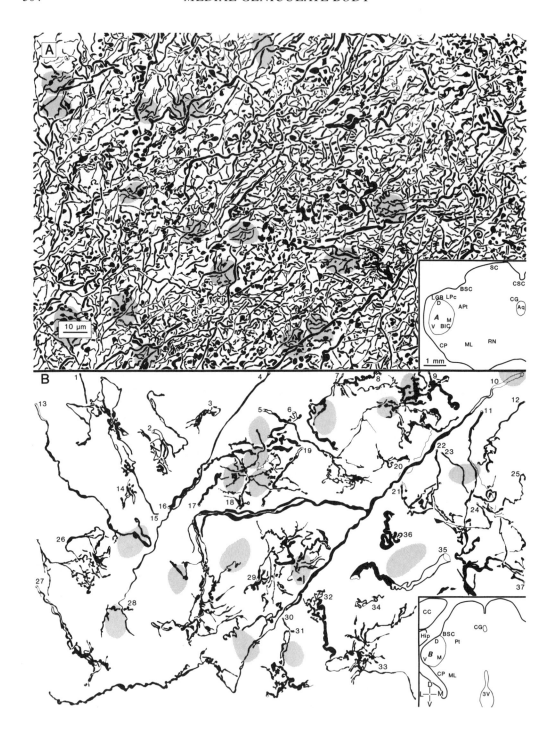

cells in the ventral division and in the lateral part of the posterior thalamic nucleus project to more than one cortical field (82), suggesting that multiple, independent, and parallel thalamocortical pathways exist.

Corticothalamic Projection

Both the ventral nucleus and the *pars ovoidea* receive a massive cortical input (Table 4) along their entire caudal-to-rostral length (Fig. 8B, E, H, K:*V*). In the rat, this projection is heavier quantitatively than the comparable corticofugal input to either the dorsal or the medial divisions. Thus, many silver grains lay in the auditory thalamic neuropil after cortical injections of [³H] leucine (Fig. 9B), which is consistent with the interpretation that corticogeniculate axons terminate preferentially upon principal cell dendrites (Fig. 14N), as they do in the cat (87,88).

All parts of the medial geniculate complex receive cortical input (Fig. 8), and there is evidence, both in the cat and the rat ventral division, that this projection is both topographic (8,33,102) and reciprocal with the cortex (8,31,144). Reciprocity between corticothalamic (Fig. 8B, E, H, K) and thalamocortical projections (Fig. 8A, D, G, J) is obvious at low power in the rat but by no means perfect. Thus, when the number of retrogradely labeled neurons (Fig. 9A: *stippled cells*) is compared with the number of silver grains in particular thalamic sectors (Fig. 9B) after combined cortical injection of horseradish peroxidase and [³H]leucine, the pattern of projections is more complex than would be predicted by a simple linear model of reciprocity (Fig. 9D). Some zones contain many labeled neurons (Fig. 9A:*1*) and have about the same number of silver grains (Fig. 9B) as those with far fewer labeled neurons (Fig. 9A:*15*), while other zones devoid of retrograde labeling receive many corticothalamic endings (compare Fig. 9A, B). Similar patterns of nonreciprocity have been reported in the cat (8); while their significance is unknown, they may be related to segregation of connections among monaural or binaural auditory thalamic subregions (77).

Neurochemistry

With the advent of methods to identify neuronal populations immunoreactive for various neurotransmitter candidates, such as gamma-aminobutyric acid (GABA) and its metabolic precursor, glutamic acid de-

---

FIG. 6. Horseradish peroxidase-filled preterminal and terminal axonal branches in the ventral nucleus of the medial geniculate body after inferior colliculus injections. **A:** In the rat after a large injection; compare with the orientation of somata in Nissl material (Fig. 2A) and dendrites in Golgi preparations (Fig. 2B), each with a dorsolateral-to-ventromedial arrangement. Many afferents form fine, tendril-like *boutons de passage,* while others have a more complex, gnarled configuration (*lower right*); see also Fig. 4. Nissl stained-somata are shown (*stippled outlines*). Heavy metal-intensified 3,3'-diaminobenzidine. Planapochromat, N. A. 1.32, ×2,000. (From K. D. Games and J. A. Winer, *unpublished observations.*) **B:** In the mustached bat (*Pteronotus p. parnellii*) following iontophoretic injections centered at the 60 kHz locus (136) of the dorsoposterior division of the central nucleus of the inferior colliculus (152); many of these axons enter from the dorsomedial aspect of the medial geniculate body and run parallel to the tufted dendrites of principal cells (149), whose somata are indicated (*stippled outlines*). Several types of terminal arrangement occur, including small endings with relatively simple *boutons* (3,4,6,7,12,14,15,18,20–25,28,30,34,37), small *boutons* with complex terminal appendages (1,2,5,26,27,31,33), large-caliber axons with simple terminal processes (8,13,16,17,19,32,35,36), and large, thick axons with complex terminal fields (9–11,29). Protocol as in panel A. For abbreviations, see Table 1. (From J. J. Wenstrup and J. A. Winer, *unpublished observations;* see also ref. 136.)

TABLE 3. *Ascending inputs to the medial geniculate body*

Medial Geniculate Body

Ascending Inputs		VENTRAL DIVISION		DORSAL DIVISION						MEDIAL DIVISION
		V	Ov	DS	D	DD	Sg	Vl	PL	M
INFERIOR COLLICULUS	CN	strong	strong	weak	weak	weak	weak	weak	unknown	moderate
	Dm	weak	strong	weak	moderate	strong	weak	weak	unknown	moderate
	DC	strong (r)	strong (r)	weak	strong	strong (ts)	moderate (r)	moderate	weak (r)	moderate (r)
	Ex	weak	strong (r)	weak	weak	weak	weak	moderate	moderate (r)	moderate
BRAIN STEM	LTS	weak	weak	weak	moderate	strong	strong	unknown	unknown	strong
	SOC	weak (r)	weak (r)	weak	weak	weak	weak	unknown	unknown	moderate
	SCo	weak (ts)	weak (ts)	weak (ts)	moderate (ts)	weak (ts)	weak (ts)	weak (ts)	weak (ts)	moderate (ts)
	other	[1][2][3] [4]	weak	weak	[4][5][6] [7]	weak	[4][8][9] [4] [10]		weak	[4][11][12] [13][14]

STRENGTH OF PROJECTION: ● strong ● moderate ● weak • absent ○ unknown

[1]From the thalamic reticular nucleus in the rat (80).
[2]From the thalamic reticular nucleus (117).
[3]Cholinergic input from an unknown source in the rat (68).
[4]From the ventrolateral medullary nucleus (56).
[5]From the nucleus sagulum in the tree shrew (98).
[6]From the nucleus sagulum (6).
[7]From the thalamic reticular nucleus (117).
[8]From the superior colliculus in the cat and the opossum (90).
[9]From the nucleus of the brachium of the inferior colliculus and the deep layers of the superior colliculus (24).
[10]From the nuclei of the lateral lemniscus in the rat (65).
[11]From the ventral nucleus of the lateral lemniscus (139).
[12]From the spinal cord in the cat and the monkey (12).
[13]From the vestibular nuclei (16,115).
[14]From the superior colliculus (43).

carboxylase (GAD), or for glutamate (Glu), it is now possible to relate the types of neurons defined in morphological and connectional studies to particular neural circuits with more precision and to compare architectonic subdivisions among species.

Only a comparatively few, perhaps 1%, of the neurons in the rat ventral division are GAD positive (GAD+). However, these include cells with intensely immunoreactive dendrites up to 400 μm long and terminating in delicate, axon-like arrays, often near the dendrites or somata of larger, GAD− neurons (64,145). There is a wide range in somatic size among the GAD+ neurons (Fig. 14B:*1–5*), and the immunoreactive axon terminals (puncta) are of moderate size (Fig. 14K), in contrast to those of the medial division (Fig. 14M), and they are more numerous than dorsal division puncta (Fig. 14L). A comparable pattern, although with many more GAD+ neurons, prevails in the cat, where the immunopositive puncta, as well as the somatic immunostaining, differentiate the subdivisions (Fig. 11). Thus, the marginal zone has sparse immunoreactivity, while only a few micrometers away, in the ventral division, the GAD+ puncta are uniformly dense (Fig. 11A). In the cat, as in the rat, the GAD+ ventral division somata vary in size (Fig. 10D:*12,13; 16,20*) and there are differences in the number of GAD+ somatic puncta (Fig. 11A:*1,2,5*). Perhaps one-third or more (112) of the neurons in the cat ventral division are GAD+ (Fig. 11A:*V,Ov*), and the largest neuronal profiles generally are GAD− (Fig. 11A:*7–13*). GAD+ neurons are also reported in the squirrel monkey medial geniculate body (126) and are comparatively rare in the mustached bat (149). While the physiological actions of iontophoretically administered GABA on single neuron responses in the medial geniculate body are unknown, in other thalamic nuclei, low-frequency rhythmic discharges are generated and modulated by thalamic reticular nucleus input (129).

In the rat, the large proportion of Glu+ neurons in the ventral division is striking (Fig. 12A:*V,Ov*) and may approximate the proportion of thalamocortical relay neurons labeled with horseradish peroxidase (Fig. 8D). In size, shape, and dendritic orientation, the Glu+ neurons resemble principal cells in Golgi preparations (Fig. 11N: *hatched neuron*).

Iontophoretic administration of acetylcholine quickly depolarizes many medial geniculate cells and is followed by a hyperpolarization, either alone or combined with a slow depolarization. In contrast, half of the guinea pig medial geniculate neurons are hyperpolarized, then slowly depolarized, by this regimen (72). In other thalamic sensory nuclei (guinea pig lateral geniculate body), intracellular studies describe single-spike and bursting action potentials with different ionic mechanisms and significant species variations in the patterns of polarization (73). Cat medial geniculate neurons exhibit a fast onset/offset response to 5-hydroxytryptamine and dopamine-mediated depression, while the norepinephrine-induced depression was more protracted. GABA is a potent depressant with a rapid time course of recovery (133), while norepinephrine (in guinea pig) causes a slow depolarization and extends the slow membrane time constant (74).

Functional Organization

Many ventral division units are narrowly tuned and part of a rigid tonotopic sequence (4) that broadens slightly in the *pars ovoidea*, and the vast majority of cells receive some type of binaural input (134). In unanesthetized preparations, both broadly and sharply tuned neurons are found in the guinea pig, of which 20% of the sample had narrower tuning that that of VIIIth nerve fibers (131). In lightly anesthetized cats, the distribution and sharpness of tuning show considerable local variation: units with

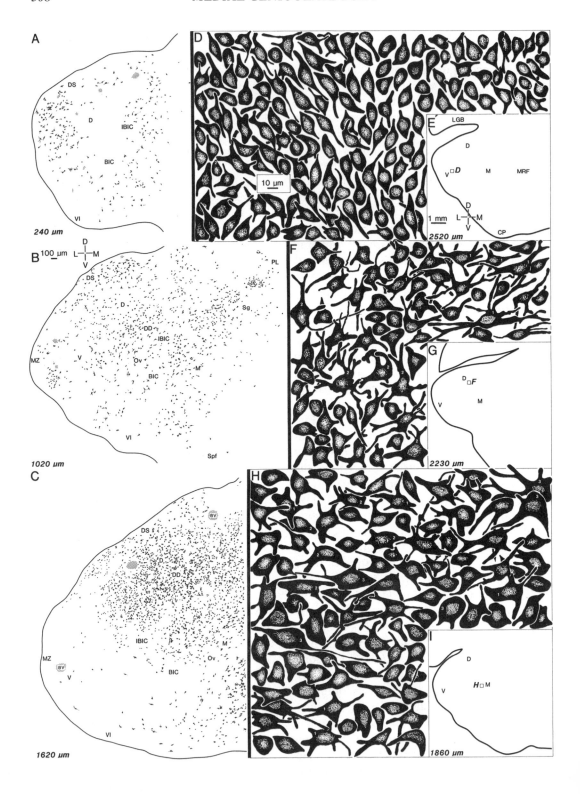

sharpest characteristic frequency are concentrated in the lateral part of the ventral division, and the most narrowly tuned units occur more rostrally (83). Their predominant response to brief tonal stimuli is transient and has a short latency (23). Some neurons respond to species-specific vocalizations at or near the unit best frequency (132). It is uncertain whether the cortical segregation of excitatory-excitatory (EE) and excitatory-inhibitory (EI) bands in AI subregions (48,77) arises in the thalamus, since the spatial arrangement of binaural ventral division cells is unclear (25). Different binaural response types do not appear to be preferentially distributed within the medial geniculate body (23). While there is a correlation between interaural phase difference sensitivity and EI response types, the change in discharge rate to various phase and intensity differences is too coarse to permit fine spatial resolution (51).

Studies of the response properties of ventral division neurons reveal several interesting changes consequent to reversible cooling of auditory cortex. Thus, click-evoked, late reverberatory discharges were affected, while tone- or click-evoked, nonreverberatory responses were unchanged. However, cooling increased the background rate of nonreverberatory units, leading to the conclusion that more than one functionally distinct corticogeniculate pathway exists (120).

Behavioral studies of carnivores find that medial geniculate lesions centered in the ventral division profoundly alter performance in the middle part of the audiogram (45), while in rodents comparable ablations have little effect (59), nor do ventral division lesions in lagomorphs alter the conditioned cardiac response to auditory stimuli (52). In view of the high level of metabolic activity within the medial geniculate complex (95), it is not surprising that toxic agents have a pronounced metabolic effect (13).

Dorsal Division

From an architectonic perspective, this division has the largest number of nuclei in the medial geniculate complex, and it is second in size only to the ventral division. In contrast, however, it has no conspicuous laminar organization, it receives midbrain axons from many auditory and nonauditory sources, it has a lighter pattern of corticofugal input than does the ventral division,

FIG. 7. Distribution of retrogradely labeled neurons in subdivisions of the cat medial geniculate body after horseradish peroxidase injections in various auditory cortical areas, and the somatodendritic form of thalamocortical relay neurons. **A–C:** Thalamic labeling from cortical injections in area AII, slightly encroaching upon the insular cortex and the caudal part of AI (see *V* in panel B). Many labeled neurons are in the posterior limitans nucleus (*PL* in panel B), and the zone of transport includes most of the dorsal division while largely sparing the ventral division except along the medial border (panel C). Lower left, distance from caudal tip of the medial geniculate body in these and in panels E, G, and I. Tetramethylbenzidine chromogen. Planapochromat, N. A. 0.32, ×200. **D:** Ventral division neurons labeled by an AI injection, most large and having polarized dendrites (*1*) with a dorsolateral-to-ventromedial arrangement (see Fig. 3), and among which a few smaller cells (*2*) are scattered. Planachromat, N. A. 0.65, ×800. Same protocol for panels F, H. **E:** Location of labeled neurons in panel D. **F:** Dorsal nucleus cells labeled by an AII injection, including neurons with varied somatodendritic profiles and sizes, many resembling large bushy (*1*) or large stellate (*2*) cells. **G:** Locus of labeled neurons in panel F. **H:** Labeled medial division neurons marked by the injection described in panel A. These neurons are comparatively larger than cells in the ventral (A) and dorsal (B) nuclei and include radiate (*1*) and elongate (*2*) neurons, and some of the largest medial geniculate perikarya (*3*), as well as some smaller neurons. **I:** Location of labeled cells in panel H. For abbreviations, see Table 1.

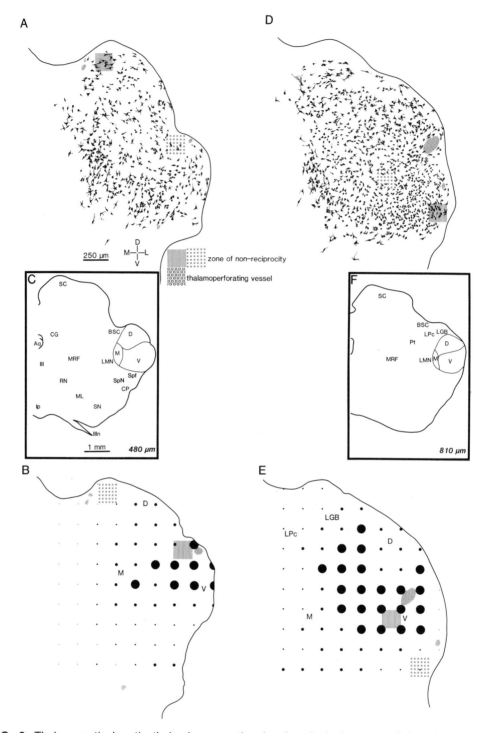

FIG. 8. Thalamocortical-corticothalamic connectional reciprocity in the rat medial geniculate complex. Retrogradely labeled thalamic neurons (**upper panels**) and anterograde autoradiographic transport (**lower panels**) from adjacent pairs of sections after auditory cortical injection of a mixture of horseradish peroxidase and [³H]leucine. **Middle panels:** Cytoarchitectonic boundaries (distance from caudal tip is at the lower right). *Vertical hatching* (upper panels): Zone with many retrogradely labeled somata; *small squares* (lower panels): corresponding locus in the matching autoradiograph that receives a disproportionately smaller anterograde projection; *small squares* (upper panels): zone of sparse retrograde labeling; *vertical hatching* (lower panels): corresponding locus in the matching autoradiograph that receives a heavier anterograde projection than predicted by the degree of retrograde transport. Blood vessels (*small open circles*) were used as fiducial marks. For panels

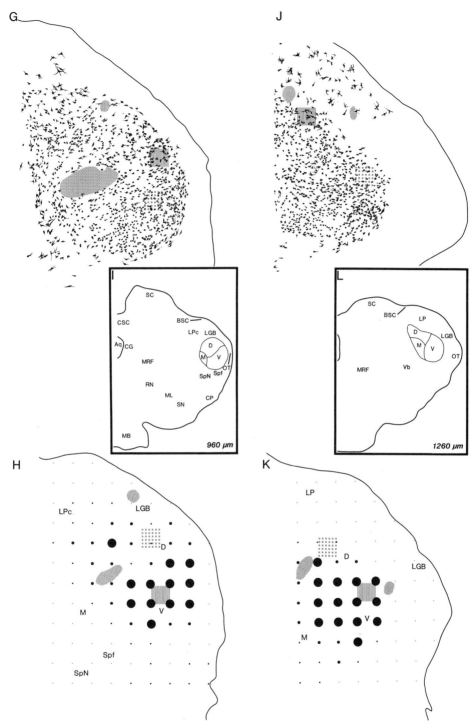

A, B, D, E, G, H, J, K: Planapochromat, N. A. 0.32, ×200; for panels **C, F, I, L:** planachromat, N. A. 0.15, ×23. Dot size in panels B, E, H, K is proportional to the strength of input; *tiny dots:* 0–100 silver grains/14,400 μm² (background; see Fig. 9C, D); *small dots:* 101–500 grains (sparse labeling); *medium-sized dots:* 501–2,000 grains (moderate labeling); *large dots:* 2,001–10,000 grains (heavy labeling). There is some extraauditory labeling in the lateral geniculate (D, E) and lateral posterior (G, H) nuclei since the injection invaded their cortical targets, but the heaviest transport is to the medial geniculate complex. Zones of nonreciprocity occur in both the ventral (J, K) and dorsal divisions (G, H), and the overall input to the ventral division is heavy, while that to the dorsal and medial divisions is moderate or light. For abbreviations, see Table 1. (Modified from ref. 144.)

TABLE 4. *Auditory thalamocortical and corticothalamic projections*

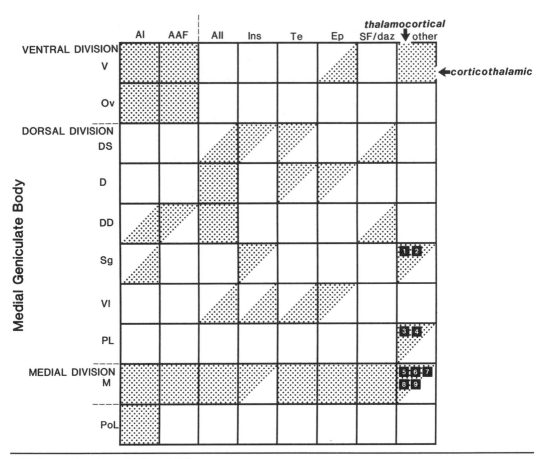

¹To the caudoputamen in the rat (65).
²To the putamen (118) and to the caudate nucleus (47).
³To the cerebral cortex (142).
⁴To the medial thalamus in the rat (65).
⁵Includes somatic sensory (54) and auditory cortex (92,150).
⁶To the caudoputamen in the rat (65) and to the amygdala and putamen in the northern native cat (62).
⁷To the amygdala in the rat (65).
⁸To the amygdala (118).
⁹To the putamen (118).

FIG. 9. Comparison of thalamocortical-corticothalamic reciprocity in adjacent, horseradish peroxidase-processed material and from [³H]leucine-labeled autoradiographs. **A:** Retrogradely labeled neurons (*stippled cells*) and unlabeled cells (*open circles*) in the ventral nucleus (see panel E for location). This section and the matching autoradiograph were aligned by their shape and blood vessels, and the number of neurons and silver grains were counted in 15 successive 120×120-μm grids (*1,15* in panel A) and plotted against each other (D). Planapochromat, N. A. 0.65, ×500. **B:** [³H]leucine anterograde transport; neural somata (*open circles*). **C:** Typical background autoradiographic labeling in the ventral nucleus of the contralateral medial geniculate body (see panel D). **D:** Direct comparisons of retrograde-anterograde labeling in the ventral nucleus, showing instances of anterograde and retrograde reciprocity and of nonreciprocity. **E:** Thalamic loci for analysis of retrograde (*left*) and anterograde (*right*) labeling. Planachromat, N. A. 0.15, ×23. For abbreviations, see Table 1. (Modified from ref. 144.)

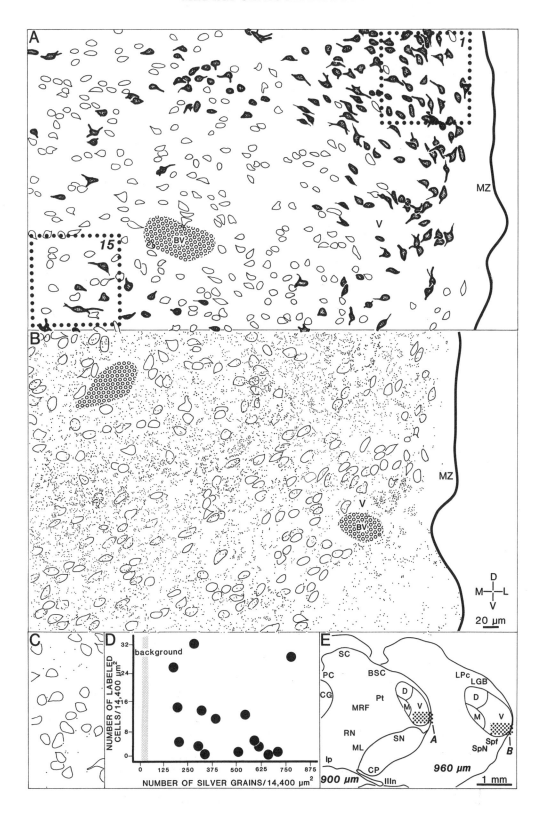

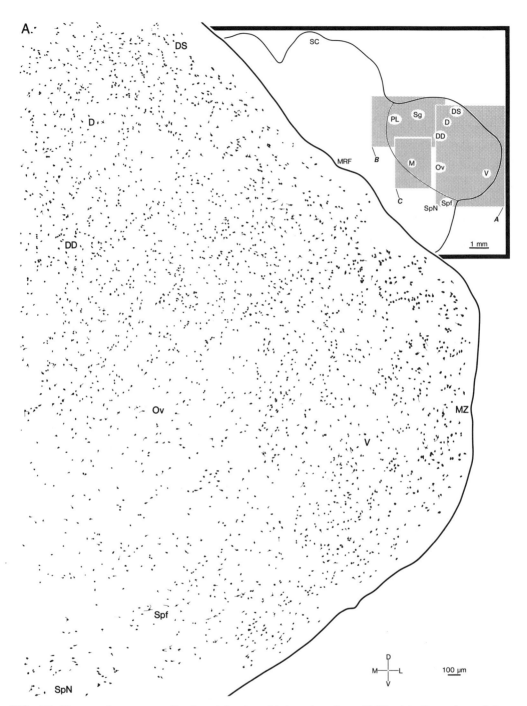

FIG. 10. Neurons immunoreactive for glutamic acid decarboxylase (GAD+) in the cat medial geniculate body. **A:** Ventral and dorsal divisions, both with many GAD+ cells, and somewhat fewer cells in the *pars ovoidea* than in the ventral nucleus (*V*), while the marginal zone has no immunopositive neuronal perikarya (see also Fig. 11A). Many zones devoid of GAD+ neurons contain either blood vessels or fibers. Protocol for panels A–C: planapochromat, N. A. 0.32, ×200. **B:** Dorsal division GAD+ neurons, noteworthy for the small size of the cells in the dorsal nuclei proper (*DS,D,DD*), and the much larger suprageniculate nucleus (*Sg*) immunoreactive cells adjoining the smaller, GAD+ posterior limitans (*PL*) neurons. **C:** Medial division (*M*) GAD+ neurons, with diverse shapes and sizes and at a somewhat lower concentration than in the ventral (A) and dorsal (B) divisions. **D–F:** GAD+ cells at higher magnification from the medial geniculate body. **D:** Ventral

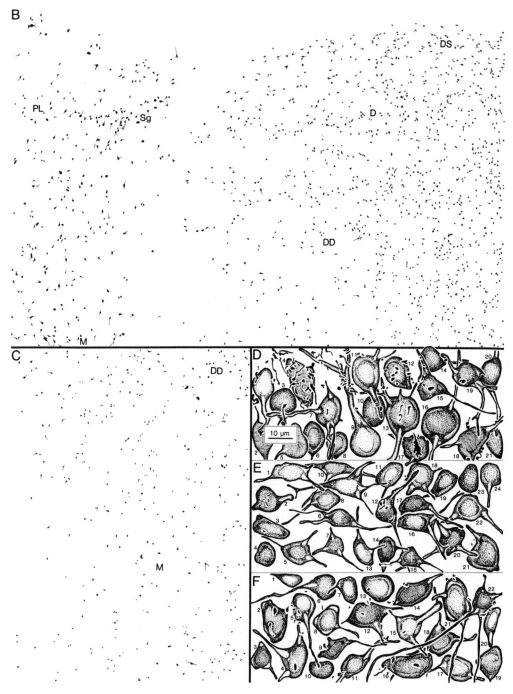

nucleus, where many cells (*9,11,15,19*) have a preferred dorsomedial-to-ventrolateral dendritic orientation, while others (*8,12,21*) show little dendritic immunostaining. Dots represent axosomatic puncta (cf. Fig. 11). Protocol for panels D–F: planapochromat, N. A. 1.32, ×2,000. **E:** Dorsal nucleus, where the GAD+ neurons range from small (*13,14*) to medium-sized (*9,22*) with occasional larger cells (*21*), and the neurons have a preferred medial-to-lateral orientation; with a few exceptions (*4,23*), they show moderate dendritic immunostaining. **F:** Medial division GAD+ cells, many of which are comparable in size to ventral nucleus neurons while others are diverse in form, show little preferential orientation, and some have extensive dendritic immunoreactivity. For abbreviations, see Table 1. For more details, see ref. 145.

315

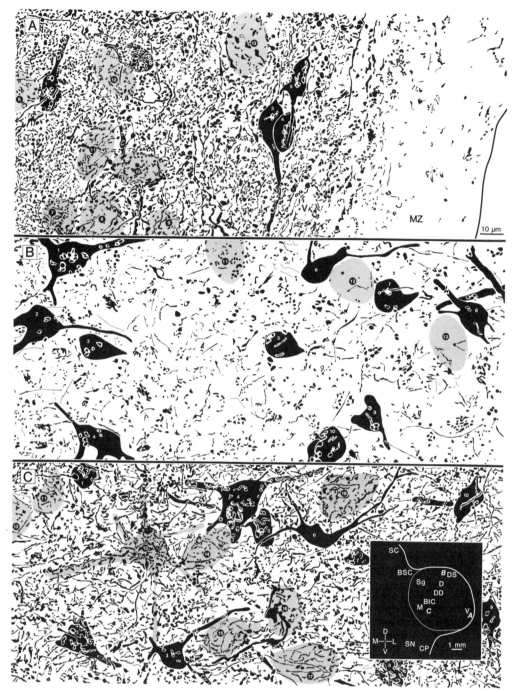

FIG. 11. GAD+ (*black*) and GAD–(*stippled*) neurons and puncta (putative axon terminals, *fine black profiles*) in the three major medial geniculate divisions (*inset*) in the cat. **A:** Ventral nucleus, where the largest silhouettes (*11,13*) are GAD– and probably correspond to tufted neurons (Fig. 3; Table 2), and the smaller, GAD+ profiles may represent Golgi type II cells (142). Note the sparse marginal zone (*MZ*) immunostaining and the rather uniform density of puncta in the ventral nucleus. Protocol for panels A–C: planapochromat, N. A. 1.32, ×2,000. **B:** Dorsal nucleus, where the biggest neurons (*11–13*) are GAD–, and most GAD+ cells are small (*5,6,9*) or medium-sized (*1,2,4*), and could correspond to the two varieties of local circuit neurons described in rapid Golgi preparations (148). There are fewer puncta than in the ventral and medial divisions. **C:** Medial division, showing small (*1,7,8*), medium-sized (*2,3,5,6*), and large (*4*) GAD+ cells among yet larger GAD– (*13–18*) neurons. Puncta density approaches that in the ventral division, but single puncta may be larger. For abbreviations, see Table 1.

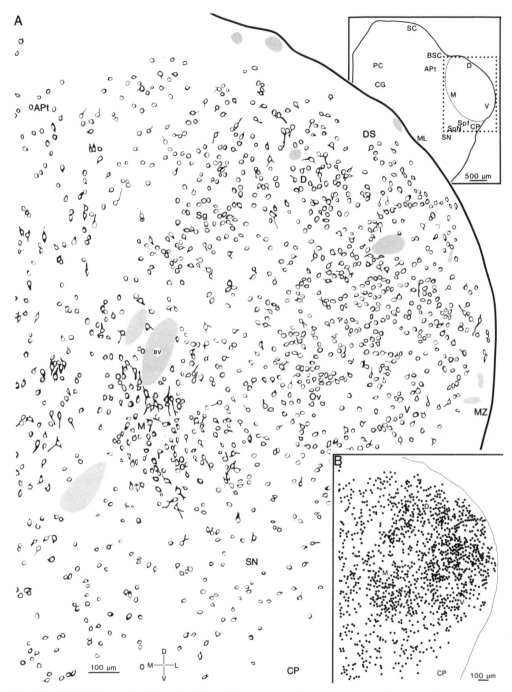

FIG. 12. Distribution of glutamate (Glu+) immunoreactive neurons in the rat medial geniculate body. **A:** Many ventral division (*V, Ov*) Glu+ cells have a dorsomedial-to-ventrolateral dendritic orientation, while superficial dorsal nucleus (*DS*) cells show less dendritic immunostaining. Medial division (*M*) neurons are conspicuously larger, have intense dendritic immunoreactivity, and are readily distinguished from the slightly smaller suprageniculate nucleus (*Sg*) Glu+ cells. Planapochromat, N. A. 0.65, ×500. **B:** Density plot of Glu+ cells, whose distribution is uniform and heavy in the three primary divisions. For abbreviations, see Table 1.

and any tonotopic arrangement is far less precise.

Structure

Diverse neuronal populations are present in the dorsal division, whose nuclei span the full anteroposterior course of the medial geniculate complex (Fig. 1B) and, in the cat, constitute most of the extreme caudal tip (90,146–148,151). These nuclei form much of the dorsal surface of the medial geniculate body and have even been considered to represent a distinct lobe (109) or as part of the ventral (principal) division in other architectonic schemes (113). However, on the basis of data from Golgi preparations (Fig. 1A), thalamocortical connections (Fig. 7F), patterns of corticothalamic input (Fig. 8B, E, H, K), and from differences in immunocytochemical organization (Fig. 11B), the dorsal division is considered here as a distinct architectonic entity.

Neurons with a stellate dendritic branching pattern and a radiating field are the prevalent type (Figs. 1A, 2E). However, regional architectonic variations in neuronal form and in connectivity, intrinsic architecture, and physiological organization all confirm that further subdivisions occur, although there is a basic continuity in neuronal morphology and the arrangement of neuropil throughout.

In the dorsal nuclei, which lie above the ventral division and dorsolateral to the medial division, four types of neuron occur, including the large stellate neurons noted above (Fig. 2E:2) and the cells with a more tufted dendritic arrangement (Fig. 2E:5). Still larger stellate cells with radiating dendrites are common in the suprageniculate nucleus of the dorsal division (Fig. 1A:Sg) and, although far fewer in number, are found in the medial division as well (Fig. 1A:M).

Large stellate neurons dominate the dorsal nuclei and are recognized by their oval soma and dichotomous dendritic branch-

ing. They have thick dendrites that arise from any part of the soma and radiate irregularly to fill a spherical field. These dendritic fields often overlap with one another or with those of the bushy neurons, among which they mingle. There is only a weak laminar pattern of dendritic organization in the dorsal nuclei except in the most superficial part (Fig. 1A:DS), where cells with more tufted dendrites are prominent, whereas in the deep dorsal nucleus radiate cells are the prevailing type (Fig. 1A:DD).

Bushy cells have somata more oblate than those of radiate neurons, and their dendrites form tufts, some quite elaborate (147) but devoid of systematic orientation except as noted above. Both stellate and bushy neurons have dendritic fields comparable in size to those of ventral division bushy neurons, and their large, unmyelinated axon has few or no local branches. In mature animals, each type of large neuron has moderate numbers of short appendages on their intermediate dendrites.

Two classes of neuron with an intrinsic axon are recognized in the superficial dorsal, dorsal, and deep dorsal nuclei. Small stellate cells have three to five thin, sparsely branched dendrites, smooth or with a few long spines on their intermediate parts, and a slender unmyelinated axon (Fig. 5A: *stippled cell*) with many local collaterals. A larger and rarer variety of interneuron has fewer axonal branches and a more heterogeneous neuronal architecture (147,148).

These many delicate interneuronal axons contribute to the fine, lacy texture of the dorsal division neuropil in rapid Golgi preparations (Fig. 5B), and they are complemented by eight other types of axon likely to be of extrinsic origin (143,148). While the correlation between a particular type of axon, its origin, and thalamic termination cannot always be made, for some varieties, such as the type I axon, a plausible correspondence exists. Thus, these axons probably arise from the posterior cortex of the inferior colliculus (61) and travel in the brachium of the inferior colliculus before terminating in broad, diffuse arrays through much of the dorsal division (148). Others, such as the type VI axons, may be of cortical origin, and they enter the medial geniculate body extrabrachially, from its rostral pole, before terminating as fine, beaded profiles. Still others, such as the type IV axons, are brachial in origin but from an unknown source and have complex shapes and a primarily peridendritic distribution (Fig. 5A:*IV-1,IV-2*). While some axons form fascicles, the overall texture of the plexus is devoid of the systematic laminar pattern seen in the ventral division (Figs. 1A, 4, 6A).

Suprageniculate nucleus principal cells are larger than those in other parts of the dorsal division (Table 2), have somewhat fewer primary dendritic branches (Fig. 1A:*Sg*), and possess a thick, myelinated axon without local collaterals. Their regular pattern of stellate branching and radiate dendritic fields distinguish them from medial division neurons, which are much more diverse in size and shape and dendritic configuration. A second, much smaller stellate cell has a local, unmyelinated axon that contributes to the neuropil, whose irregular texture and ventromedial-to-dorsolateral arrangement (148) is dominated by axons probably arising in the lateral tegmental system (86). Many of the same types of axons identified in the dorsal nuclei also occur here, although in somewhat simpler form.

Posterior limitans nucleus principal cells occupy a small, elongated wedge between the brachium of the superior colliculus and the suprageniculate nucleus, where their long, thin dendrites ramify (Fig. 1A:*PL*). A second, much smaller stellate neuron with a local, unmyelinated axon occurs (Table 2). However, the neuropil is coarser than in other dorsal division nuclei and irregularly arranged axonal fascicles criss-cross the nucleus either vertically or horizontally (148); the sources of these afferents are unknown, although in the rat some arise in the inferior colliculus (65).

Connections

Brainstem Input

Dorsal division nuclei receive significant projections from many parts of the inferior colliculus with the exception of the central nucleus (Table 3). A second ascending pathway arises from the lateral tegmental system of the midbrain (86). Both of these sources include nuclei that lie outside the classical lemniscal pathway that is represented by the anteroventral cochlear nucleus, related nuclei near the trapezoid body, the central nucleus of the inferior colliculus, the ventral nucleus of the medial geniculate body, and the primary auditory cortex (2). Most of these secondary or lemniscal adjunct auditory pathways are dominated by neurons with radiating dendrites without an obvious laminar organization, and which are broadly tuned and respond to nonauditory as well as auditory stimuli (146).

Both the dorsomedial zone (61) and the dorsal cortex (9) of the inferior colliculus project to the dorsal nucleus of the medial geniculate body, as does the lateral tegmental system (86). Many of these axons ascend through the brachium of the inferior colliculus to form endings mainly in the thalamic neuropil (148). Both the dorsomedial zone and the dorsal cortex receive a massive projection from the primary auditory cortex (33), providing a common source of descending feedback between what might otherwise be regarded as parallel pathways. Input to the deep dorsal nucleus arises mainly from the medial aspect of the central nucleus of the inferior colliculus and from the pericentral nucleus (116).

Lateral tegmental projections arise chiefly from the vicinity of the nuclei lying medial and ventral to the brachium of the inferior colliculus, and they form fine and widely or sparsely ramified preterminal axonal segments in the dorsal nucleus (86). Similar patterns occur in the deep dorsal nucleus, except that the projections from the dorsomedial zone in the tree shrew (98) and the lateral tegmental system in the cat (86) are slightly heavier, and the preterminal axons have more diverse forms, including medium-sized fibers with cup-like endings that might correspond to a type of axon forming peridendritic baskets through much of the dorsal division in rapid Golgi preparations (148).

In the suprageniculate nucleus, the axons from the dorsal cortex are still present beside those of lateral tegmental origin. Lesions in the area between the brachium of the inferior colliculus and the spinothalamic tract or just medial to the brachium itself cause heavy preterminal degeneration, consisting of diffuse axonal arrays (as in the dorsal nucleus) and including medium-sized, sparsely ramified endings (86) resembling the grumous axons in Golgi material (148). Horseradish peroxidase injections in the suprageniculate nucleus label neurons in the nucleus of the brachium of the inferior colliculus and in the deep layers of the superior colliculus (24).

Ventrolateral nucleus neurons lie within the confines of the ventral division, from whose cells they are distinguished by their more radiate branching pattern (Fig. 1A). As in other dorsal division nuclei, their midbrain input arises largely from the dorsal cortex and the external nucleus of the inferior colliculus (24). These same sources also project to the posterior limitans nucleus.

Thalamocortical Projection

Dorsal division neurons project exclusively to cortical targets outside AI (8,92), where their axons terminate mainly in layer IV (127). These nonprimary areas, which include the second auditory cortex (AII), and insular, temporal, posterior ectosylvian, and suprasylvian fringe fields (Table 4), share several physiological traits, including broadly tuned neurons without an apparent tonotopic organization (76) and a lack of clear segregation into monaural and binaural subregions (124), in contrast to AI (48).

Neurons in the superficial dorsal nucleus project to both the insular and temporal cortex; however, few if any of these cells project by multiple axonal branches to more than one cortical field (10). Dorsal nucleus neurons project to AII (8) and to temporal and posterior ectosylvian cortex, without obvious topographic organization (105). Both of the large varieties of dorsal nucleus neurons, the bushy and stellate cells (Figs. 2F; 7F:1,2), probably project to the cerebral cortex (Table 2). Cells in the deep dorsal nucleus appear to project to only one cortical area, AII (8,10), also without any clear topography (150).

Suprageniculate nucleus neurons send their axons to insular cortex (10). Only the large neurons are retrogradely labeled after cortical injections (Fig. 7B:Sg), and it is unknown if their projection has a systematic pattern with respect to frequency.

Ventrolateral nucleus cells are labeled by injections in the posterior ectosylvian gyrus along its dorsoventral axis (19,150). Because of their midbrain and cortical affiliations and their structure, these neurons are considered as part of the dorsal division despite their physical location within the ventral division (143).

Corticothalamic Projection

Patterns of cortical input to the dorsal division in the rat are distinguished from those to the ventral division in two ways: first, the projection to the latter is always lighter (Fig. 8B, E, H, K:D), quantitatively about half of the ventral division value (145); second, several nuclei in the cat dorsal division either project to a cortical field without receiving a reciprocal corticothalamic projection (Table 4,DS→Ins) or the converse (DD→Ep), in contrast to the more consistently reciprocal ventral and medial division patterns. Thus, every dorsal division nucleus contains at least one example of such nonreciprocity with respect to cortical connectivity (Table 4). It is unclear what physiological significance either pattern might have.

Neurochemistry

In the rat, the dorsal division is remarkable for the small number of GAD+ cells (145) and the sparse, exceedingly fine immunoreactive puncta (Fig. 14L), which number about one-fourth the value in the ventral (Fig. 14K) and medial (Fig. 14M) divisions. Despite their comparatively low density, the GAD+ neurons are diverse in somatodendritic form (Fig. 14E:*1–5*), receive only a few somatic puncta, and have little dendritic immunoreactivity beyond their initial 100 μm.

In the cat, many more dorsal division neurons are GAD+, and such cells are common in all subdivisions (Fig. 10A, B) and, as in the rat (145), they are variable in size and shape, ranging from tiny cells less than 10 μm in diameter and devoid of dendritic immunostaining (Fig. 10E:*4,23*) to much larger cells (Fig. 10E:*21*), some immunoreactive as far as their initial dendritic branch points (Fig. 10E:*6*). Immunopositive puncta (Fig. 11B) are similar in relative size and shape to those in the rat (Fig. 14L), and dorsal division GAD+ neurons typically receive only a few (Fig. 11B:*3,5,7,8*) or no (Fig. 11B:*6*) such endings, as do GAD– cells (Fig. 11B:*11–13*). Some neurons, especially larger ones, receive more puncta (Fig. 11B:*1,6*), although never as many as some ventral division neurons (Fig. 11A:*1,2*). Neurons immunoreactive for enkephalin occur in the dorsal and medial divisions (32).

Many Glu+ neurons occur throughout the rat dorsal division. Their disposition is consistent with both thalamic connectional (Fig. 11D, E) and cytoarchitectonic boundaries (30), the relative number of GABAergic neurons (145), and with the hypothe-

sis that many glutamatergic cells could project to the cerebral cortex.

Functional Organization

As might be expected on the basis of their midbrain (Table 3) and cortical (Table 4) connections, dorsal division neurons have different, and more diverse, physiological response patterns than do ventral and medial division neurons. Thus, no systemic tonotopic organization has been found in these nuclei, the discharge patterns of single cells to tonal stimuli are more heterogeneous than those in the ventral division, and minimum discharge latencies are about 1.5 to 4 times longer. Ventrolateral nucleus neurons display characteristic dorsal division response profiles (23; see also ref. 83). Despite the absence of a clear tonotopic representation, some bat dorsal division cells may convey information to particular cortical fields concerned with the construction of temporal delay lines (125).

In some dorsal division cells, the discharges to tonal stimuli are often more varied and complex than those in the ventral division, including mixed or prolonged excitatory-inhibitory patterns (3,23, 138) and cells with bursting, irregular spike trains (1). These neurons thus appear well adapted to encode the complex, rapidly modulated acoustic signals relevant to biological communication. Other dorsal division cells respond to somatic sensory as well as auditory input (69,70), and many have little spontaneous activity and low thresholds.

Medial Division

While it is the smallest of the main divisions of the auditory thalamus, the medial division has the most diverse types of neurons, receives input from many different sources, including nonauditory afferents, has the widest distribution of thalamocor-

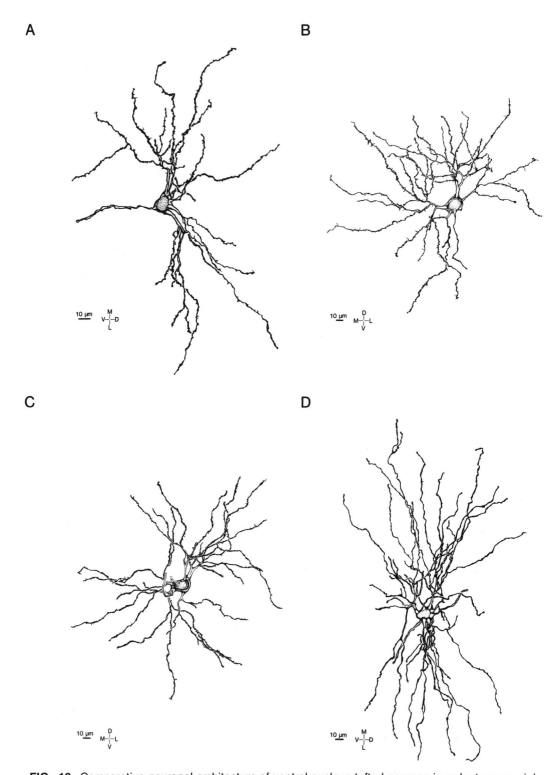

FIG. 13. Comparative neuronal architecture of ventral nucleus tufted neurons in rodent, marsupial, chiropteran, and primate species. **A:** From the rat (*Rattus norvegicus*) in the ventral and lateral part of the ventral nucleus, showing moderately well-developed dendritic tufts. Protocol for panels A–D: planapochromat, N. A. 1.32, ×2,000. **B:** From the opossum (*Didelphis virginiana*), in which dendritic tufts overlap at their tips and the shape of the dendritic field is nearly spherical. **C:** From the pallid bat (*Antrozous pallidus*), which resembles the opossum in size and orientation. **D:** From the human (*Homo sapiens*), where the long, laminar axis runs from lateral-to-medial, the dendritic field is relatively much larger, and the dendrites are strongly tufted.

tical and subcortical projections, and contains broadly tuned neurons responsive to several modalities other than audition.

Structure

In spite of the structural variability among medial division neurons, no further regional subdivision is warranted on architectonic grounds since both the medial division and each type of cell is represented in all but the most caudal parts of the auditory thalamus. With the exception of the magnocellular neurons, these cells approximate in somatic size those in other medial geniculate subdivisions (84), but they have no preferred somatodendritic orientation (Fig. 1A:*M*), and their packing density is lower (Fig. 2G).

Most medial division neurons have a stellate dendritic configuration and a simple, dichotomous branching pattern. When cells with tufted dendrites occur, this trait is not as strongly expressed as in the ventral and dorsal divisions (Fig. 2B, E, H), nor are the bushy dendrites oriented preferentially.

Medium-sized stellate cell dendrites may span the width of the medial division (146), and their arbors overlap one another (143). Their long, sparsely branched dendrites are gnarled and irregular and have occasional appendages. This neuron and each of the following types (with the exception of the small stellate cell) have a comparatively thick, myelinated axon without local branches.

Tufted cells are nearly as large and have a few stout dendrites that project irregularly (Fig. 2H:*2*); they may have a considerable number of appendages. Some dendrites run parallel to the brachial axons, while others cross them.

Elongated cells have a few irregularly stellate branches with a preferred medial-to-lateral orientation. Their branching pattern ranges from comparatively simple and dichotomous (Fig. 2H:*4*) to weakly tufted and slightly more elaborate (Fig. 2H:*7*); these dendrites have a few or a moderate number of appendages (146).

Magnocellular neurons are the largest medial geniculate cells (Fig. 2H:*6*), and their many long and thick dendrites form wavy tufts that radiate irregularly among the brachial axons; their size and weakly tufted arbors distinguish them from the adjoining suprageniculate nucleus principal cells, which have a stellate branching pattern and a more spherical dendritic field (Fig. 1A:*M,Sg*). These large medial division cells are more numerous in the caudal one-half of the medial geniculate body.

A tiny Golgi type II cell with a simple stellate dendritic configuration and a locally projecting axon also occurs (Figs. 2H:*5*, 14J:*5*). While the dendrites usually are short, they often have many complex appendages, some up to 5 μm long, and the axonal branches are exceedingly fine and typically sparser than those of Golgi type II cells in other divisions (146).

In semithin, 1- to 2-μm thick, plastic-embedded and toluidine blue-stained sections, the complexity of medial division neuropil readily distinguishes it from the ventral and dorsal divisions. Large, heavily myelinated brachial axons run from medial to lateral and form terminal branches studded with *boutons de passage*. Many axons are destined for the *pars ovoidea,* while others pass to the lateral part of the ventral nucleus. A second type of axon, the serpentine endings, are much thicker and form elaborate terminal arrays up to 100 μm wide along the medial-to-lateral axis. Crossing the beaded fibers and the serpentine axons at right angles are small fascicles containing thin or medium-sized axons, perhaps of cortical origin; other axonal types also occur. None of these axonal varieties has been traced to a particular origin, nor is there any knowledge of medial division ultrastructure.

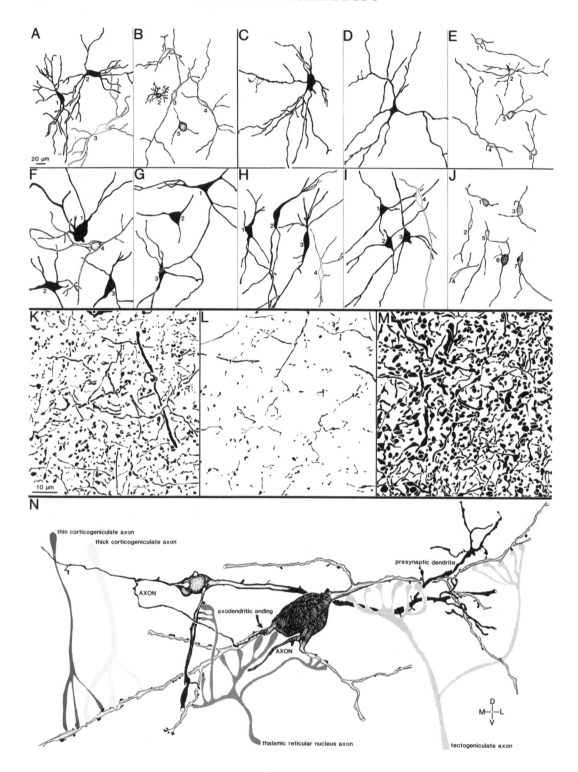

Connections

Brainstem Input

At least 11 separate ascending sources project to the medial division (Table 3). These include axons from nuclei such as the central nucleus of the inferior colliculus (9,61,81), whose functional contributions are clearly auditory (2), in contrast to axons from the external nucleus of the inferior colliculus (24), many of whose cells have receptive fields broadly tuned to auditory input, while other neurons respond to somatic stimuli (7). Besides the diversity of brainstem afferents to the medial division, the strength of these projections (except in the case of input from the lateral tegmental system of the midbrain, where the preterminal degeneration is considerable [86]) is usually sparse to moderate, resembling the pattern in the dorsal division more closely than that in the ventral division (Table 3).

In the medial division, as in the dorsal division, it is unknown whether the afferent input is topographically organized. Since there is a clearly arranged tonotopic sequence of best frequencies in the central nucleus of the inferior colliculus (75), in the superior olivary complex and related nuclei (135), and in the nuclei of the lateral lemniscus (5), some input from narrowly tuned auditory neurons may reach medial division neurons, perhaps to be degraded by convergence for some other purpose.

Thalamocortical Projection

Medial division neurons project to all of the auditory cortical fields (Table 4), and more rostrally, to the somatic sensory cortex (10). These projections terminate primarily in layers I and VI in auditory cortex in both cat (78,94) and rat (119), in contrast to those from the ventral division, which end chiefly in layer IV (93,127) and are larger in caliber and probably form a denser terminal plexus than those to layer I. After horseradish peroxidase injections within layer IV, only about 10% of the labeled thalamic neurons were in the medial division, while after layer I injections nearly 50% of these cells lay in the medial division (79), and the overall layer IV:layer I ratio is 82%:18% (78). Thus, the medial division

---

FIG. 14. Primary features of rat medial geniculate organization with emphasis on neuronal structure, intrinsic organization, and patterns of connectivity. **A–J:** Main types of neurons identified in Golgi preparations (30,144). Key: *black,* likely to be Glu+ and GAD− and to project to the auditory cortex; *stippled,* probably GAD+; *open,* some may be GAD+, others Glu+ or have unknown affiliations. **A** and **B:** Ventral division. **A:** Tufted cells with bushy dendrites (*1–3*). **B:** Small cells, including stellate neurons (*1,3–5*) and tiny, possibly neurogliaform, cell (*2*). **C–E:** Dorsal division. **C:** Tufted principal cell. **D:** Radiate principal cell. **E:** Small stellate cells (*1–5*). **F–J:** Medial division neurons. **F:** Magnocellular principal neurons (*1–4*). **G:** Large radiate cells (*1–3*). **H:** Medium-sized tufted cells (*1–4*). **I:** Smooth multipolar cells (*1–4*). **J:** Small stellate cells (*1–7*). **K–M:** Patterns of GAD+ puncta in medial geniculate divisions. Planachromat, N. A. 0.45, ×312. Same scale for all panels. **K:** Ventral division, with medium-sized and moderately dense puncta. **L:** Dorsal division, containing small puncta sparsely distributed. **M:** Medial division, with large, coarse puncta that are moderately dense. Planapochromat, N. A. 1.32, ×2,000. **N:** Some possible circuit arrangements in the ventral division based on a synthesis of work in the rat (30,144), bat (136,149), cat (84–88,146–148), human (141), and other species. In this model, dendrites of Golgi type II cells (*dark stippling*) are presynaptic to those of principal neurons (*hatched*), while axons of midbrain origin (*tectogeniculate axon*) contact the tufted cell proximal and distal dendrites. Cortical inputs, which may comprise more than one class (*thin* and *thick corticogeniculate axon*) end along distal dendrites, while GAD+ afferents (*thalamic reticular nucleus axon*) synapse upon intermediate dendrites and somata. Thus, tufted principal neurons could receive at least two independent varieties of GABAergic input, and two types of excitatory endings. (From ref. 144, with permission.)

projection can be described as moderate, bilaminar, and widespread. At least three types of medial division neurons project to the cortex, including large stellate, elongate, and magnocellular varieties (Fig. 7H:1–3, respectively). A comparable laminar distribution of anterogradely labeled axon terminals occurs in primate auditory cortex, except that layer III is more heavily labeled (22,53). Other, subcortical projections give the medial division access to telencephalic limbic centers (Table 4).

Corticothalamic Projection

Descending cortical axons essentially recapitulate the pattern of thalamocortical inputs, at least on a global scale (8), with the possible exception of insular cortex (102; see also ref. 33). Corticofugal axons to the medial division stained by the reduced silver method are reported to be medium sized or thick (102), but far finer than subcortical afferents, and to extend the rostrocaudal length of the medial division, but not through its mediolateral dimension, after AI lesions (33). Quantitatively, the cortical input in the rat is much lighter than that to the ventral division (Fig. 8B, E, H, K) and approximates that to the dorsal division (144).

Neurochemistry

GAD-immunoreactive neurons are comparatively common in the rat medial division, considering its modest size. These neurons constitute a diverse population ranging in size from less than 10 μm to more than 20 μm in diameter and are about 25% larger than GAD+ ventral and dorsal division cells (145). Many of these perikarya, as well as those of GAD− neurons, receive an assortment of somatic puncta. As in the dorsal division, there were few GAD+ neurons whose dendritic immunoreactivity extended beyond 80 to 100 μm.

Puncta (Fig. 14M) were just as numerous as those in the ventral division (Fig. 14K) but are much larger and coarser. Their spatial distribution conforms to and confirms the architectonically and connectionally defined borders of the medial division.

In the cat medial division, the proportion of GAD+ neurons is substantial (Fig. 10C) and might include several types of neuron, ranging from the smallest medial division cells (Fig. 10F:1,20) to medium-sized (Fig. 10F:13,19) and larger cells (Fig. 10F:12,21), including some almost as large as the tufted neurons (Fig. 11C:4) and resembling them in shape and size (Table 2). As in the rat, the concentration of puncta is uniformly heavy (Fig. 11C), but the absolute value may be lower than in the ventral division (Fig. 11A). However, there are some striking differences in the density of axosomatic puncta onto single neurons, some GAD+ cells receiving moderate numbers (Fig. 11C:2) and others few (Fig. 11C:6), while certain GAD− neurons have many (Fig. 11C:13).

There is a conspicuous concentration of Glu+ multipolar neurons in the rat medial division (Fig. 12A). While the proportion of such cells may be similar to that in the ventral division (Fig. 12B), it suggests that the number of presumptively excitatory medial division neurons is substantial and, in view of the diverse medial division neuronal arhitecture, perhaps correspondingly varied.

Functional Organization

Medial division cells have broad tuning curves and, while the full frequency range represented along the basilar membrane is conserved, there is little in the way of any systematic arrangement (1,23). Many cells are driven by auditory and nonauditory stimuli, the latter including somatic sensory, vestibular, and visual inputs (11, 16,69,70,137), and some of these neurons project to areas as remote as the anterior suprasylvian cortex (17). Response latencies were ≈1.5 times longer than those in the ventral division, and ≈1–3 times those of the dorsal division. However, about one-third of medial division cells discharged in a sustained pattern, twice the number of such units in other subdivisions (23). Some medial division cells show long-term potentiation in the cat (41), while others form associative responses to appetitive or aversive stimuli in, respectively, the cat (121), rat (15,34), and rabbit (40). Subcortical projections from the medial division to the limbic forebrain play a crucial enabling role in the formation of acoustically conditioned autonomic or behavioral responses (67).

COMPARATIVE ANATOMY AND PHYSIOLOGY

There may be trends in medial geniculate organization common to distantly related species and, perhaps more importantly, some interspecific differences with functional significance. Most medial geniculate nuclei recognized in the cat can also be identified in the opossum, despite differences in shape or size, and such subdivisions are comparable on the basis of their cytoarchitecture, neuronal architecture, connectivity, neurochemistry, and, in certain respects, intrinsic organization (90,151). Thus, the tufted cell in the opossum ventral nucleus (Fig. 13B) is readily compared to its proscriptive homologue in the cat (Fig. 3), although the tufted pattern of branching is less well developed. This neuron projects to the primary auditory cortex in both species. While midbrain inputs are similar in the two species, there are important differences in neurochemical and intrinsic organization (see below). A broad range of neuronal variation is represented by the rubric, tufted, and an analogous argument could be made for other denominators. By the same token, a laminar organization of the ventral division is apparent in all species studied, despite differences in laminar dimensions, orientation, and neuronal configuration

(30,96,151). Even relatively minute thalamic subdivisions are readily identified in parallel studies of architectonic, connectional, and immunocytochemical organization (149,151).

Among the most striking species differences is the degree of neuropil development. In rodents, marsupials, avians, and insectivores, for example, the neuropil is comparatively sparse and the neurons closely packed, while in carnivores and primates packing density is much lower, the proportion of Golgi type II neurons is larger, and the neuropil is correspondingly more developed. In human material, single medial geniculate neurons may be separated by neuropil zones up to 500 μm or more wide, while in rats the typical distance is less than 50 μm. This trend is correlated with the number and relative complexity of Golgi type II neurons, which are reported to be nonexistent in some rat thalamic nuclei (122,140) and numerous in humans (109,141). This is consistent with the differences relative to the numbers of GAD+ neurons in the rat (145) and cat (Fig. 10). Thus, while tufted neurons in both species might have a comparable neuronal architecture (Fig. 13A, D), the synaptic arrangements, particularly the pattern of intrinsic organization, may differ between them.

A thalamic auditory representation has also been described in leopard frogs on the basis of evoked potentials (91) and in a single unit analysis (39). Tract-tracing experiments show that two subdivisions of the auditory thalamus have different patterns of ascending input, one (the central nucleus) chiefly from brainstem acoustic nuclei, while the other (the posterior nucleus) is dominated by reticular, tegmental, and ventral thalamic projections. Posterior nucleus cells show nonlinear summation to tones at different frequencies, while central nucleus cells do not (44).

In reptiles, a pathway from the central nucleus of the torus semicircularis in the midbrain has been traced to the central part of the nucleus reuniens (posterior part) in the thalamus (103), and from the thalamus to the telencephalic dorsal ventricular ridge (104). A comparable midbrain auditory relay in birds, the lateral mesencephalic nucleus, projects to the thalamic nucleus ovoidalis (57), which then sends fibers to the dorsal ventricular ridge (58). A topographic projection between nucleus ovoidalis and its telencephalic target in field "L" is reported (20), and there is evidence of a tonotopic arrangement in some parts of the avian auditory thalamus (14).

ACKNOWLEDGMENTS

This work was supported by U.S. Public Health Service grant R01 NS16832-11, a Deafness Research Foundation grant, and University of California Faculty Research grants. Antiserum to GAD and generous technical guidance were given by Drs. D. E. Schmechel and E. Mugnaini. Antisera to glutamate and helpful advice were contributed by Dr. R. J. Wenthold, and by Drs. J. E. Madl and A. J. Beitz. J. G. Van de Vere conscientiously typed the manuscript, and D. T. Larue and J. M. Popowits provided essential help. I am grateful to my colleagues, particularly to Drs. K. D. Games and J. J. Wenstrup, for sharing their data and ideas with me. Citations of the relevant literature were completed in 1989.

REFERENCES

1. Aitkin LM. Medial geniculate body of the cat: responses to tonal stimuli of neurons in medial division. *J Neurophysiol* 1973;36:275–283.
2. Aitkin LM. *The auditory midbrain. Structure and function in the central auditory pathway.* Clifton, NJ: Humana Press, 1986.
3. Aitkin LM, Prain SM. Medial geniculate body: unit responses in the awake cat. *J Neurophysiol* 1974;37:512–521.
4. Aitkin LM, Webster WR. Medial geniculate body of the cat: organization and responses to tonal stimuli of neurons in ventral division. *J Neurophysiol* 1972;35:365–380.
5. Aitkin LM, Anderson DJ, Brugge JF. Tono-topic organization and discharge characteristics of single neurons in nuclei of the lateral lemniscus of the cat. *J Neurophysiol* 1970;33: 421–440.
6. Aitkin LM, Calford MB, Kenyon CE, Webster WR. Some facets of the organization of the principal division of the cat medial geniculate body. In: Syka J, Aitkin LM, eds. *Neuronal mechanisms of hearing.* London: Plenum, 1981;163–181.
7. Aitkin LM, Dickhaus H, Schult W, Zimmermann M. External nucleus of inferior colliculus: auditory and spinal somatosensory afferents and their interactions. *J Neurophysiol* 1978;41:837–847.
8. Andersen RA, Knight PL, Merzenich MM. The thalamocortical and corticothalamic connections of AI, AII, and the anterior auditory field (AAF) in the cat: evidence for two largely segregated systems of connections. *J Comp Neurol* 1980;194:663–701.
9. Andersen RA, Roth GL, Aitkin LM, Merzenich MM. The efferent projections of the central nucleus of the inferior colliculus in the cat. *J Comp Neurol* 1980;194:649–662.
10. Bentivoglio M, Molinari M, Minciacchi M, Macchi G. Organization of cortical projections of the posterior complex and intralaminar nuclei of the thalamus as studied by means of retrograde tracers. In: Macchi G, Rustioni A, Spreafico, eds. *Somatosensory integration in the thalamus.* Amsterdam: Elsevier, 1983;337–363.
11. Berkley KJ. Response properties of cells in ventrobasal and posterior group nuclei of the cat. *J Neurophysiol* 1973;36:940–952.
12. Berkley KJ. Spatial relationships between the terminations of somatic sensory and motor pathways in the rostral brainstem of cats and monkeys I. Ascending somatic sensory inputs to lateral diencephalon. *J Comp Neurol* 1980; 193:283–317.
13. Bertoni JM, Sprenkle PM. Lead acutely reduces glucose utilization in the rat brain especially in higher auditory centers. *Neurotoxicology* 1988;9:235–242.
14. Bigalke-Kunz B, Rübsamen R, Dörrscheidt GJ. Tonotopic organization and functional characterization of the auditory thalamus in a songbird, the European starling. *J Comp Physiol* 1987;161:255–265.
15. Birt D, Nienhuis R, Olds M. Separation of associative from non-associative short latency changes in medial geniculate and inferior colliculus during differential conditioning and reversal in rats. *Brain Res* 1979;167:129–138.
16. Blum PS, Abraham LD, Gilman S. Vestibular, auditory, and somatic input to the posterior thalamus of the cat. *Exp Brain Res* 1979;34:1–9.
17. Blum PS, Day MJ, Carpenter MB, Gilman S. Thalamic components of the ascending vestibular system. *Exp Neurol* 1979;64:587–603.
18. Bonke BA, Bonke D, Scheich H. Connectivity

of the auditory forebrain in the guinea fowl (*Numida meleagris*). *Cell Tissue Res* 1979;200: 101–121.

19. Bowman EM, Olson CR. Visual and auditory association areas of the cat's posterior ectosylvian gyrus: thalamic afferents. *J Comp Neurol* 1988;272:15–29.

20. Brauth SE, McHale CM, Brasher CA, Dooling RJ. Auditory pathways in the budgerigar. I. Thalamo-telencephalic projections. *Brain Behav Evol* 1987;30:174–199.

21. Brawer JR, Morest DK, Kane EC. The neuronal architecture of the cochlear nucleus of the cat. *J Comp Neurol* 1974;155:251–300.

22. Burton H, Jones EG. The posterior thalamic region and its cortical projection in new world and old world monkeys. *J Comp Neurol* 1976;168:249–302.

23. Calford MB. The parcellation of the medial geniculate body of the cat defined by the auditory response properties of single units. *J Neurosci* 1983;3:2350–2364.

24. Calford MB, Aitkin LM. Ascending projections to the medial geniculate body of the cat: evidence for multiple, parallel auditory pathways through the thalamus. *J Neurosci* 1983;3:2365–2380.

25. Calford MB, Webster WR. Auditory representation within principal division of cat medial geniculate body: an electrophysiological study. *J Neurophysiol* 1981;45:1013–1028.

26. Cant NB. The fine structure of two types of stellate cells in the anterior division of the anteroventral cochlear nucleus of the cat. *Neuroscience* 1981;12:2643–2655.

27. Cant NB. Identification of cell types in the anteroventral cochlear nucleus that project to the inferior colliculus. *Neurosci Lett* 1982;32:241–246.

28. Cant NB, Casseday JH. Projections from the anteroventral cochlear nucleus to the lateral and medial superior olivary nuclei. *J Comp Neurol* 1986;247:457–476.

29. Cant NB, Gaston KC. Pathways connecting the right and left cochlear nuclei. *J Comp Neurol* 1982;212:313–326.

30. Cheff SJ, Larue DT, Winer JA. The rat medial geniculate complex: nuclear architecture, neuronal organization, and neocortical connections. *Proc Soc Neurosci* 1987;13:548.

31. Colwell SA. Thalamocortical-corticothalamic reciprocity: a combined anterograde-retrograde tracer technique. *Brain Res* 1975;92:443–449.

32. Covenas R, Romo R, Cheramy A, Cesselin F, Conrath M. Immunoctyochemical study of enkephalin-like cell bodies in the thalamus of the cat. *Brain Res* 1986;377:355–361.

33. Diamond IT, Jones EG, Powell TPS. The projection of the auditory cortex upon the diencephalon and brain stem in the cat. *Brain Res* 1969;15:305–340.

34. Edeline J-M, Dutrieux G, Neuenschwander-El Massioui N. Multiunit changes in hippocampus and medial geniculate body in free-behaving rats during acquisition and retention of a conditioned response to a tone. *Behav Neural Biol* 1988;50:61–79.

35. Famiglietti EV. Dendro-dendritic synapses in the lateral geniculate nucleus of the cat. *Brain Res* 1970;20:181–191.

36. Fekete DM, Rouiller EM, Liberman MC, Ryugo DK. The central projections of intracellularly labeled auditory nerve fibers in cats. *J Comp Neurol* 1984;229:432–450.

37. Friedlander MJ, Lin C-S, Stanford LR, Sherman SM. Morphology of functionally identified neurons in lateral geniculate nucleus of the cat. *J Neurophysiol* 1981;46:80–129.

38. Fullerton BC. Morphological studies of the inferior colliculus and the medial geniculate body in the rhesus monkey and the albino rat. Doctoral dissertation, Northeastern University, Boston, MA, 1978.

39. Fuzessery ZM, Feng AS. Mating cell selectivity in the thalamus and midbrain of the leopard frog (*Rana p. pipiens*): single and multiunit analysis. *J Comp Physiol* 1983;150:333–344.

40. Gabriel M, Miller JD, Saltwick SE. Multiple-unit activity of the rabbit medial geniculate nucleus in conditioning, extinction, and reversal. *Physiol Psychol* 1976;4:124–134.

41. Gerren RA, Weinberger NM. Long term potentiation in the magnocellular medial geniculate nucleus of the anesthetized cat. *Brain Res* 1983;265:138–142.

42. Godfrey DA, Carter JA, Lowry OH, Matschinsky FM. Distribution of gamma-aminobutyric acid, glycine, glutamate and aspartate in the cochlear nucleus of the rat. *J Histochem Cytochem* 1978;26:118–126.

43. Graham J. An autoradiographic study of the efferent connections of the superior colliculus in the cat. *J Comp Neurol* 1977;173:629–654.

44. Hall JC, Feng AS. Evidence for parallel processing in the frog's auditory thalamus. *J Comp Neurol* 1987;258:407–419.

45. Heffner RS, Heffner HE. Hearing loss in dogs after lesions of the brachium of the inferior colliculus and medial geniculate. *J Comp Neurol* 1984;230:207–217.

46. Houser CR, Vaughn JE, Barber RP, Roberts E. GABA neurons are the major cell type of the nucleus reticularis thalami. *Brain Res* 1980;200:341–354.

47. Hu H, Jayarman A. The projection pattern of the suprageniculate nucleus to the caudate nucleus in cats. *Brain Res* 1986;368:201–203.

48. Imig TJ, Adrián HO. Binaural columns in the primary auditory field (A1) of cat auditory cortex. *Brain Res* 1977;138:241–257.

49. Imig TJ, Morel A. Topographic and cytoarchitectonic organization of thalamic neurons related to their targets in low-, middle-, and high-frequency representations in cat auditory cortex. *J Comp Neurol* 1984;227:511–539.

50. Inagaki N, Yamatodani A, Ando-Yamamoto M, Tohyama M, Watanabe T, Wada H. Organiza-

tion of histaminergic fibers in the rat brain. *J Comp Neurol* 1988;273:283–300.

51. Ivarsson C, de Ribaupierre Y, de Ribaupierre F. Influence of auditory localization cues on neuronal activity in the auditory thalamus of the cat. *J Neurophysiol* 1988;59:586–606.

52. Jarrell TW, Gentile CG, Romanski LM, McCabe PM, Schneiderman N. Involvement of cortical and thalamic auditory regions in retention of differential bradycardiac conditioning to acoustic conditioned stimuli in rabbits. *Brain Res* 1987;412:285–294.

53. Jones EG, Burton H. Areal differences in the laminar distribution of thalamic afferents in cortical fields of the insular, parietal, and temporal regions of primates. *J Comp Neurol* 1976;168:197–248.

54. Jones EG, Powell TPS. Anatomical organization of the somatosensory cortex. In: Iggo A, ed. *Handbook of sensory physiology, volume 2: somatosensory system.* Berlin: Springer-Verlag, 1973;579–620.

55. Jones EG, Rockel AJ. The synaptic organization in the medial geniculate body of afferent fibres ascending from the inferior colliculus. *Z Zellforsch* 1971;113:44–66.

56. Kamiya H, Itoh K, Yasui Y, Ino T, Mizuno N. Somatosensory and auditory relay nucleus in the rostral part of the ventrolateral medulla: a morphological study in the cat. *J Comp Neurol* 1988;273:421–435.

57. Karten HJ. The organization of the ascending auditory pathway in the pigeon (*Columba livia*). I. Diencephalic projections of the inferior colliculus (nucleus mesencephalicus lateralis, pars dorsalis). *Brain Res* 1967;6:409–427.

58. Karten HJ. The ascending auditory pathway in the pigeon (*Columba livia*). II. Telencephalic projections of the nucleus ovoidalis thalami. *Brain Res* 1968;11:134–153.

59. Kelly JB, Judge PW. Effects of medial geniculate lesions on sound localization by the rat. *J Neurophysiol* 1985;53:361–372.

60. Knight PL. Representation of the cochlea within the anterior auditory field (AAF) of the cat. *Brain Res* 1977;130:447–467.

61. Kudo M, Niimi K. Ascending projections of the inferior colliculus in the cat: an autoradiographic study. *J Comp Neurol* 1980;191:545–556.

62. Kudo M, Aitkin LM, Nelson JE. Auditory forebrain organization of an Australian marsupial, the northern native cat (*Dasyurus hallucatus*). *J Comp Neurol* 1989;279:28–42.

63. Kudo M, Glendenning KK, Frost SB, Masterton RB. Origin of mammalian thalamocortical projections. I. Telencephalic projections of the medial geniculate body in the opossum (*Didelphis virginiana*). *J Comp Neurol* 1986;245:176–197.

64. Larue DT, Winer JA. Architecture of GAD-immunoreactive dendrites in rat medial geniculate complex: a possible substrate for dendrodendritic relations. *Proc Soc Neurosci* 1987;13:549.

65. LeDoux JE, Ruggiero DA, Reis DJ. Projections to the subcortical forebrain from anatomically defined regions of the medial geniculate body in the rat. *J Comp Neurol* 1985;242:182–213.

66. LeDoux JE, Ruggiero DA, Forest R, Stornetta R, Reis DJ. Topographic organization of convergent projections to the thalamus from the inferior colliculus and spinal cord in the rat. *J Comp Neurol* 1987;264:123–146.

67. LeDoux JE, Sakaguchi A, Reis DJ. Subcortical efferent projections of the medial geniculate nucleus mediate emotional responses conditioned to acoustic stimuli. *J Neurosci* 1984;4:683–698.

68. Levey AI, Hallanger AE, Wainer BH. Choline acetyltransferase immunoreactivity in the rat thalamus. *J Comp Neurol* 1987;257:317–332.

69. Lippe WR, Weinberger NM. The distribution of click evoked activity within the medial geniculate body of the anesthetized cat. *Exp Neurol* 1973;39:507–523.

70. Lippe WR, Weinberger NM. The distribution of sensory evoked activity within the medial geniculate body of the anesthetized cat. *Exp Neurol* 1973;40:431–444.

71. Lorente de Nó R. *The primary acoustic nuclei.* New York: Raven Press, 1981.

72. McCormick DA, Prince DA. Actions of acetylcholine in the guinea-pig and cat medial and lateral geniculate nuclei, *in vitro. J Physiol (Lond)* 1987;392:147–165.

73. McCormick DA, Prince DA. Neurotransmitter modulation of thalamic neuronal firing pattern. *J Mind Behav* 1987;8:573–590.

74. McCormick DA, Prince DA. Noradrenergic modulation of firing pattern in guinea pig and cat thalamic neurons, *in vitro. J Neurophysiol* 1988;59:978–996.

75. Merzenich MM, Reid MD. Representation of the cochlea within the inferior colliculus of the cat. *Brain Res* 1974;77:397–415.

76. Merzenich MM, Knight PL, Roth GL. Representation of the cochlea within primary auditory cortex of the cat. *J Neurophysiol* 1975;38:231–249.

77. Middlebrooks JC, Zook JM. Intrinsic organization of the cat's medial geniculate body identified by projections to binaural response-specific bands in the primary auditory cortex. *J Neurosci* 1983;3:203–225.

78. Mitani A, Itoh K, Mizuno N. Distribution and size of thalamic neurons projecting to layer I of the auditory cortical fields of the cat compared to those projecting to layer IV. *J Comp Neurol* 1987;257:105–121.

79. Mitani A, Itoh K, Nomura S, Kudo M, Kaneko T, Mizuno N. Thalamocortical projections to layer I of the primary auditory cortex in the cat: a horseradish peroxidase study. *Brain Res* 1984;310:347–350.

80. Montero VM. Ultrastructural identification of axon terminals from the thalamic reticular nucleus in the medial geniculate body in the rat: an EM autoradiographic study. *Exp Brain Res* 1983;51:338–342.

81. Moore RY, Goldberg JM. Ascending projections of the inferior colliculus in the cat. *J Comp Neurol* 1963;121:109–135.

82. Morel A, Imig TJ. Thalamic projections to fields A, AI, P and VP in the cat auditory cortex. *J Comp Neurol* 1987;265:119–144.

83. Morel A, Rouiller E, de Ribaupierre Y, de Ribaupierre F. Tonotopic organization in the medial geniculate body (MGB) of lightly anesthetized cats. *Exp Brain Res* 1987;69:24–42.

84. Morest DK. The neuronal architecture of the medial geniculate body of the cat. *J Anat* 1964;98:611–630.

85. Morest DK. The laminar structure of the medial geniculate body of the cat. *J Anat* 1965; 99:143–160.

86. Morest DK. The lateral tegmental system of the midbrain and the medial geniculate body: study with Golgi and Nauta methods in cat. *J Anat* 1965;99:611–634.

87. Morest DK. Dendrodendritic synapses of cells that have axons: the fine structure of the Golgi type II cell in the medial geniculate body of the cat. *Z Anat Entwickl-Gesch* 1971;133:216–246.

88. Morest DK. Synaptic relationships of Golgi type II cells in the medial geniculate body of the cat. *J Comp Neurol* 1975;162:157–194.

89. Morest DK, Oliver DL. The neuronal architecture of the inferior colliculus in the cat: defining the functional anatomy of the auditory midbrain. *J Comp Neurol* 1984;222:209–236.

90. Morest DK, Winer JA. The comparative anatomy of neurons: homologous neurons in the medial geniculate body of the opossum and the cat. *Adv Anat Embryol Cell Biol* 1986;97:1–96.

91. Mudry KM, Constantine-Paton M, Capranica RR. Auditory sensitivity of the diencephalon of the leopard frog (*Rana p. pipiens*). *J Comp Physiol [A]* 1977;114:1–13.

92. Niimi K, Matsuoka H. Thalamocortical organization of the auditory system in the cat studied by retrograde axonal transport of horseradish peroxidase. *Adv Anat Embryol Cell Biol* 1979;57:1–56.

93. Niimi K, Naito F. Cortical projections of the medial geniculate body in the cat. *Exp Brain Res* 1974;19:326–342.

94. Niimi K, Ono K, Kusunose M. Projections of the medial geniculate nucleus to layer 1 of the auditory cortex in the cat traced with horseradish peroxidase. *Neurosci Lett* 1984;45:223–228.

95. Nudo RJ, Masterton RB. Stimulation-induced [^{14}C]2-deoxyglucose labeling of synaptic activity in the central auditory system. *J Comp Neurol* 1986;245:553–565.

96. Oliver DL. A Golgi study of the medial geniculate body in the tree shrew, *Tupaia glis*. *J Comp Neurol* 1982;209:1–16.

97. Oliver DL. Neuron types in the central nucleus of the inferior colliculus that project to the medial geniculate body. *Neuroscience* 1984;11:409–424.

98. Oliver DL, Hall WC. The medial geniculate body of the tree shrew, *Tupaia glis*. I. Cytoarchitecture and midbrain connections. *J Comp Neurol* 1978;182:423–458.

99. Oliver DL, Morest DK. The central nucleus of the inferior colliculus in the cat. *J Comp Neurol* 1984;222:237–264.

100. Olsen JF. Processing of biosonar information by the medial geniculate body of the mustached bat. Doctoral dissertation, Washington University, St. Louis, MO, 1986.

101. Peterson BA, Winer JA. Projections of the cat medial geniculate body to the primary auditory cortex (AI). *Proc Soc Neurosci* 1988;14:492.

102. Pontes C, Reis FF, Sousa-Pinto A. The auditory cortical projections onto the medial geniculate body in the cat. An experimental anatomical study with silver and autoradiographic methods. *Brain Res* 1975;91:43–63.

103. Pritz MB. Ascending connections of a midbrain auditory area in a crocodile, *Caiman crocodilus*. *J Comp Neurol* 1974;153:179–198.

104. Pritz MB. Ascending connections of a thalamic auditory area in a crocodile, *Caiman crocodilus*. *J Comp Neurol* 1974;153:199–214.

105. Raczkowski D, Diamond IT, Winer J. Organization of thalamocortical auditory system in the cat studied with horseradish peroxidase. *Brain Res* 1976;101:345–354.

106. Ralston HJ. Evidence for presynaptic dendrites and a proposal for their mechanism of action. *Nature* 1971;230:585–587.

107. Ralston III HJ. The synaptic organization of the ventrobasal thalamus in the rat, cat and monkey. In: Macchi G, Rustioni A, Spreafico R, eds. *Somatosensory integration in the thalamus*. Amsterdam: Elsevier, 1983;241–250.

108. Ramón y Cajal S. The structure and connexions of neurons. Nobel Lecture, 1906. Reprinted in: *The Nobel lectures in physiology or medicine*. Amsterdam: Elsevier, 19XX;220–256.

109. Ramón y Cajal S. *Histologie du système nerveux de l'homme et des vertébrés* (Azoulay L, transl.) Paris: Maloine, 1911. (Reprinted by Consejo Superior de Investigaciones Çientificas, Madrid, 1972.)

110. Redies H, Brandner S, Creutzfeldt OD. Anatomy of the auditory thalamocortical system of the guinea pig. *J Comp Neurol* 1989;282:489–511.

111. Rhode WS, Smith PH. Encoding timing and intensity in the ventral cochlear nucleus of the cat. *J Neurophysiol* 1986;56:261–286.

112. Rinvik E, Ottersen OP, Storm-Mathisen J. Gamma-aminobutyrate-like immunoreactivity in the thalamus of the cat. *Neuroscience* 1987; 21:781–805.

113. Rose JE, Woolsey CN. The relations of thalamic connections, cellular structure and evocable electrical activity in the auditory region of the cat. *J Comp Neurol* 1949;91:441–466.

114. Rose JE, Greenwood DD, Goldberg JM, Hind JE. Some discharge characteristics of single neurons in the inferior colliculus of the cat. I. Tonotopical organization, relation of spike-counts to tone intensity, and firing patterns of

single elements. *J Neurophysiol* 1963;36:294–320.

115. Roucoux-Hanus M, Boisacq-Schepens N. Ascending vestibular projections: further results at cortical and thalamic levels in the cat. *Exp Brain Res* 1977;29:283–292.

116. Rouiller EM, de Ribaupierre F. Origin of afferents to physiologically defined regions of the medial geniculate body of the cat: ventral and dorsal divisions. *Hear Res* 1985;19:97–114.

117. Rouiller EM, Colomb E, Capt M, de Ribaupierre F. Projections of the reticular complex of the thalamus onto physiologically characterized regions of the medial geniculate body. *Neurosci Lett* 1985;53:227–232.

118. Russchen FT. Amygdalopetal projections in the cat. II. Subcortical afferent connections. A study with retrograde tracing techniques. *J Comp Neurol* 1982;207:157–176.

119. Ryugo DK, Killackey HP. Differential telencephalic projection of the medial and ventral divisions of the medial geniculate body of the rat. *Brain Res* 1974;82:173–177.

120. Ryugo DK, Weinberger NM. Corticofugal modulation of the medial geniculate body. *Exp Neurol* 1976;51:377–391.

121. Ryugo DK, Weinberger NM. Differential plasticity of morphologically distinct neuron populations in the medial geniculate body of the cat during classical conditioning. *Behav Biol* 1978;22:275–301.

122. Saporta S, Kruger L. The organization of thalamocortical relay neurons in the rat ventrobasal complex studied by the retrograde transport of horseradish peroxidase. *J Comp Neurol* 1977;174:187–208.

123. Scheel M. Isofrequency laminae in the medial geniculate body of the rat as shown by injections of WGA-HRP into the auditory cortex. *Neurosci Lett Suppl* 1984;18:S245.

124. Schreiner CE, Cynader MS. Basic functional organization of second auditory cortical field (AII) of the cat. *J Neurophysiol* 1984;51:1284–1305.

125. Shannon SL, Wong D. Interconnections between the medial geniculate body and the auditory cortex in an FM bat. *Proc Soc Neurosci* 1987;13:1469.

126. Smith Y, Séguéla P, Parent A. Distribution of GABA-immunoreactive neurons in the thalamus of the squirrel monkey (*Saimiri sciureus*). *Neuroscience* 1987;22:579–591.

127. Sousa-Pinto A. Cortical projections of the medial geniculate body in the cat. *Adv Anat Embryol Cell Biol* 1973;48:1–42.

128. Špaček J, Lieberman AR. Ultrastructural and three-dimensional organization of synaptic glomeruli in rat somatosensory thalamus. *J Anat (Lond)* 1974;117:487–516.

129. Steriade M, Deschênes M, Domich L, Mulle C. Abolition of spindle oscillations in thalamic neurons disconnected from nucleus reticularis thalami. *J Neurophysiol* 1985;54:1473–1497.

130. Steriade M, Paré D, Parent A, Smith Y. Projec-

tion of cholinergic and non-cholinergic neurons of the brainstem core to relay and associational thalamic nuclei in the cat and macaque monkey. *Neuroscience* 1988;25:47–67.

131. Tanaka H, Taniguchi I. Tuning characteristics of neurons in the medial geniculate body of unanesthetized guinea pigs. *Proc Jpn Acad* 1986;62:352–354.

132. Tanaka H, Taniguchi I. Response properties of neurons in the medial geniculate body of unanesthetized guinea pigs to the species-specific vocalized sound. *Proc Jpn Acad* 1987;63:348–351.

133. Tebēcis AK. Effects of monoamines and amino acids on medial geniculate neurones of the cat. *Neuropharmacology* 1970;9:381–390.

134. Toros A, Rouiller E, de Ribaupierre Y, Ivarsson C, Molden H, de Ribaupierre F. Changes of functional properties of medial geniculate body neurons along the rostro-caudal axis. *Neurosci Lett Suppl* 1979;3:S5.

135. Tsuchitani C. Lower auditory brain stem structures of the cat. In: Naunton RF, Fernández C, eds. *Evoked electrical activity in the auditory nervous system*. New York: Academic Press, 1978;373–401.

136. Wenstrup JJ, Winer JA. Projections to the medial geniculate body from physiologically defined frequency representations of the mustached bat's inferior colliculus. *Proc Soc Neurosci* 1987;13:324.

137. Wepsic JG. Multimodal sensory activation of cells in magnocellular medial geniculate nucleus. *Exp Neurol* 1966;15:299–318.

138. Whitfield IC, Purser D. Microelectrode study of the medial geniculate body in unanesthetized free-moving cats. *Brain Behav Evol* 1972;6:311–322.

139. Whitley JM, Henkel CK. Topographical organization of the inferior collicular projection and other connections of the ventral nucleus of the lateral lemniscus in the cat. *J Comp Neurol* 1984;229:257–270.

140. Williams MN, Faull RLM. The disribution and morphology of identified thalamocortical projection neurons and glial cells with reference to the question of interneurons in the ventrolateral nucleus of the rat thalamus. *Neuroscience* 1987;21:767–780.

141. Winer JA. The human medial geniculate body. *Hear Res* 1984;15:225–247.

142. Winer JA. Identification and structure of neurons in the medial geniculate body projecting to primary auditory cortex (AI) in the cat. *Neuroscience* 1984;13:395–413.

143. Winer JA. The medial geniculate body of the cat. *Adv Anat Embryol Cell Biol* 1985;86:1–98.

144. Winer JA, Larue DT. Patterns of reciprocity in auditory thalamocortical and corticothalamic connections: study with horseradish peroxidase and autoradiographic methods in the rat medial geniculate body. *J Comp Neurol* 1987;257:282–315.

145. Winer JA, Larue DT. Anatomy of glutamic acid

decarboxylase immunoreactive neurons and axons in the rat medial geniculate body. *J Comp Neurol* 1988;274:47–68.

146. Winer JA, Morest DK. The medial division of the medial geniculate body of the cat: implications for thalamic organization. *J Neurosci* 1983;3:2629–2651.

147. Winer JA, Morest DK. The neuronal architecture of the dorsal division of the medial geniculate body of the cat. A study with the rapid Golgi method. *J Comp Neurol* 1983;221:1–30.

148. Winer JA, Morest DK. Axons of the dorsal division of the medial geniculate body of the cat: a study with the rapid Golgi method. *J Comp Neurol* 1984;224:344–370.

149. Winer JA, Wenstrup JJ. Anatomy of the mustached bat's medial geniculate body: cytoarchitectonics, neuronal architecture, and GAD-immunoreactivity. *Proc Soc Neurosci* 1987;13:324.

150. Winer JA, Diamond IT, Raczkowski D. Subdivisions of the auditory cortex of the cat: the retrograde transport of horseradish peroxidase to the medial geniculate body and posterior thalamic nuclei. *J Comp Neurol* 1977;176:387–418.

151. Winer JA, Morest DK, Diamond IT. A cytoarchitectonic atlas of the medial geniculate body of the opossum, *Didelphys virginiana,* with a comment on the posterior intralaminar nuclei of the thalamus. *J Comp Neurol* 1988;274:422–448.

152. Zook JM, Winer JA, Pollak GD, Bodenhamer RD. Topology of the central nucleus of the mustache bat's inferior colliculus: correlation of single unit response properties and neuronal architecture. *J Comp Neurol* 1985;231:530–546.

Neurobiology of Hearing: The
Central Auditory System, edited by
R. A. Altschuler et al.
Raven Press, Ltd., New York © 1991.

13

Stimulus Processing in the Auditory Cortex

*Dennis P. Phillips, †Richard A. Reale, and †John F. Brugge

*Department of Psychology, Dalhousie University, Halifax, Nova Scotia, Canada B3H 4J1;
†Department of Neurophysiology and Waisman Center on Mental Retardation and Human
Development, University of Wisconsin-Madison, Madison, Wisconsin 53706

The auditory areas of cerebral cortex are targets of a remarkable complex family of ascending pathways that originate from the two ears (for review, see refs. 1,2). Auditory cortex, in turn, sends projections to thalamic and midbrain targets, an arrangement that lends itself to cortical modulation of ascending activity. It is, therefore, not surprising to find that auditory cortical neurons can respond to acoustic events within the animal's environment in ways quite different from the initial representation of that sound encoded by cochlear nerve fibers. In this chapter, we describe some of the dominant aspects of the physiology of auditory cortical neurons, and we do so with two emphases that reflect the foci of much of the more recent research in this area. The first is an exploration of the mechanisms that shape the selectivity of cortical neurons for particular stimuli or stimulus configurations. The second is an examination of the extent to which those mechanisms may be emergent properties of the auditory forebrain rather than preserved properties that derive from mechanisms developed in the auditory periphery and brainstem.

It is beyond the scope of this chapter to examine all of the recent developments in our knowledge of the structure and function of acoustic sensory cortex. The reader is referred to other authors for historical backgrounds to the more recent studies (3–

6), for reviews of the functions and functional architecture of the auditory cortex in cats and monkeys (7–11), and for detailed accounts of the organization of auditory cortex of the bat (12–16), where knowledge of behaviorally relevant stimulus parameters has guided both empirical studies and modeling of central auditory processing. Our attention here is directed primarily to studies in cats and primates in which the "stimulus-response" themes have generally employed as stimuli relatively simple signals that are not typically heard in isolation but that are components of naturally occurring sound. This has been a powerful approach that often permits a straightforward correlation between neural events and selected stimulus parameters.

Most of auditory cortical research still concerns the physiology of the primary auditory cortical field (AI), although the presence of multiple auditory cortical areas has been known for more than four decades (17). Therefore, unless stated to the contrary, most of our discussion is applied to field AI. Area AI is distinguishable from surrounding auditory areas in both cats and primates by a number of structural and functional features including cytoarchitecture (18–20), tonotopic organization (20–24), and the patterns of thalamocortical innervation (11,19,25,26). In those studies in which two or more of these features were examined together, there is rather good agreement regarding the boundaries and organization of this field. The more fundamental issue of whether field AI, or any other cortical area, can be intimately related to its functional role in acoustically guided behavior has mainly been addressed in the bat (for review, see refs. 12,15,16), although relevant new data in the cat have appeared in recent years (27).

We begin by providing a description of the static spectral selectivity of cortical neurons determined with a pure-tone stimulus delivered either monaurally or binaurally. This acoustic probe is of unchanging frequency and is presented in isolation. We then proceed to a discussion of the binaural sensitivity of AI neurons followed by an examination of the effects of broadband noise masking on the tonal sensitivity of these cells. Next we turn to examine the cortical coding of more complex time-varying tonal stimuli, including amplitude (AM) and frequency (FM) modulations, and from there to the coding of animal vocalizations and the effects of imposing behavioral relevance on the stimulus probes.

In contrast to the output of a single auditory nerve fiber, the response of a single AI neuron to a pure-tone stimulus is frequently transient in nature, consisting of one spike or a burst of but a few action potentials having, on the average, an onset latent period of about 10 to 12 msec. Sustained responses may also be recorded, and occasionally a neuron exhibits an "off" response. Thus, between the auditory nerve and cortex we recognize in the majority of AI neurons a transformation in the time structure of the sound-evoked discharge, and these temporal response patterns are sensitive to general anesthesia, to a state of arousal, and to the behavioral context within which a stimulus tone is delivered, as we discuss in later sections. These more dynamic characteristics of AI neurons are superimposed on the cells' more static properties, which are determined by anatomical constraints imposed at the periphery or lower auditory brainstem. Thus, for example, regardless of the temporal properties of the evoked response of a given AI neuron, that cell's output is restricted to a limited range of frequency and intensity imposed by the mechanical tuning properties of the basilar membrane, the afferent innervation pattern of the organ of Corti, and the degree of convergence of frequency-selective neurons at various levels of the auditory central neuroaxis.

PURE-TONE RESPONSE AREA

Frequency selectivity is commonly illustrated by a threshold tuning curve, which plots the threshold intensity as a function of stimulus frequency. The shapes of the curves can vary considerably among central auditory neurons. The majority of reported AI tuning curves are narrow and V-shaped (28) and reminiscent of those derived from primary auditory nerve fibers (29). The tip of such a tuning curve defines the neuron's characteristic (or best) frequency (CF), and, like primary afferent fibers, one interprets the CF as corresponding to a small region of the cochlear partition to which the neuron is ultimately connected. For both the nerve (29–31) and cortex (28), the range of CFs derived from such tuning curves spans most of the audible frequencies for the species under study, with the greatest sensitivity at frequencies to which the animal is also behaviorally most sensitive.

Figure 1A depicts a typical response area (i.e., the domain of frequency-intensity pairings that affect the cell's discharge) of a cochlear nerve fiber determined with pure-tone stimuli. The accompanying inset plots the V-shaped threshold tuning curve as well as tuning curves for suprathreshold discharge rates. Within this response area, it is possible to describe quantitatively the neural response strength and the temporal discharge pattern, both of which change with changes in sound frequency and level.

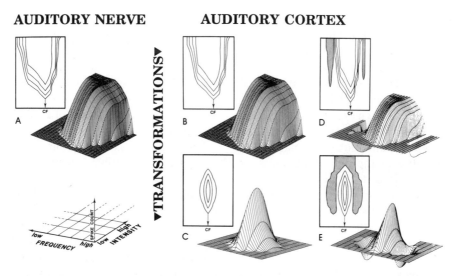

FIG. 1. Idealized response areas obtained with pure-tone stimuli for an auditory nerve fiber (**A**) and auditory cortex neurons (**B–E**). In the auditory nerve, spike count is always greater (net excitation) than the baseline within the effective frequency-intensity domain. In the auditory cortex, spike count may be greater or less than (net inhibition) the baseline at appropriate frequency-intensity pairings. Insets show threshold (just detectable change in spike count from baseline) and suprathreshold tuning curves for each response area. Inhibitory domains are shaded. See text for additional details.

For auditory cortical neurons, the curve plotting spike count as a function of stimulus strength at various stimulus frequencies usually takes one of two forms (32–35). For most AI neurons, these curves are sigmoidal in shape with spike count rising in a monotonic fashion over a typical range of some 10 to 30 dB, although some have a dynamic range of 70 dB; beyond this range the counts remain at or near their maximal value. The general form of this function is usually constant across the effective frequency range, as illustrated in Fig. 1B, although thresholds become progressively higher as the frequency departs further from CF. Neurons with these properties have the V-shaped threshold tuning curves mentioned previously. All cochlear nerve fibers so far recorded display monotonic rate-level functions (29,36,37). So too do many neurons in the anteroventral and posteroventral cochlear nuclei (38,39), lateral superior olivary nucleus (40,41), inferior colliculus (42), and medial geniculate body

(43), which together comprise one route linking the cochlea with the cortex. It might be reasonably argued, therefore, that despite some evidence that the dynamic ranges of cortical neurons might be slightly narrower than those of cochlear nerve fibers (compare, e.g., refs. 44,45), the primary-like forms of the spike-count-versus-sound pressure level (SPL) function and tuning curve reflect a preservation by certain cortical cells of coding properties seen at the level of cochlear output.

For a second class of AI neurons (Fig. 1C), spike count is a nonmonotonic function of stimulus intensity: as tone intensity is raised, the count rises to a maximum and then declines, in some cases to zero. The functions and response area are, thus, somewhat bell shaped, and the tone level evoking the maximal discharge has been termed the "most effective SPL" (33) or "best SPL" (46). Whereas these cells maintain their general form across the breadth of their effective frequency ranges (32,35), the best SPL is not necessarily constant across this same range (35,47). Thus, the notion of "best SPL" is for many neurons germane only for tones at or near the cell's CF. For cells with similar CFs in any given animal, the best SPLs vary relatively widely, covering much of the dynamic range of hearing (33,47). This raises the possibility that one cortical code for stimulus level might reside in the identity of the neural elements excited by the relevant stimulus (33,48). This idea that the intensity level of a sound may be coded by a "place" mechanism raises the question of whether there exists an orderly and continuous physiological map of stimulus intensity in the transformation from cochlea to cortex. The most compelling evidence for this latter idea comes from the work on the bat (46). Similar evidence has not appeared in other mammals, although within AI of the cat there appears to be a partial segregation of neurons having monotonic and nonmonotonic spike-count functions (35).

There are a few instances in which inhibitory responses to tonal stimuli have been observed directly in auditory cortical neurons, if one includes fields outside of AI (33,49,50). More commonly, the existence and/or disposition of inhibitory regions within a response area has been inferred from studies using stimuli consisting of two-tone probes (34,51,52) or tones and noise (35). These studies suggest that in addition to the two forms of AI neuron response areas described above there may be other forms distinguished by the shape of their spike-count-versus-intensity functions and by the presence of inhibitory regions. One simple variation, shown in Fig. 1D, exhibits a monotonic spike-count-versus-intensity function to tones, but the use of noise as an acoustic stimulus suggests that inhibitory domains flank the excitatory region of the response area. For these cells, the spike-count function is monotonic in shape when tones are employed and nonmonotonic when broadband noise is the stimulus (35). AI cells that show a nonmonotonic re-

sponse to increasing levels of a CF tone and either fail to be excited by noise or do so only at low SPLs suggest other variants of response area, like the one illustrated in Fig. 1E. This response area is composed of not only a highly sensitive excitatory frequency-intensity domain but equally sensitive domains producing inhibition.

These conclusions are unremarkable in the sense that similar neuronal types have been described for the cochlear nuclear complex (38,53–55). Since all cochlear nerve fibers so far studied exhibit monotonically increasing rate-level functions for tones, it has been argued that the high-intensity descending limb of the nonmonotonic functions seen for central neurons must be produced by inhibitory inputs at CF (42,53,54). In the dorsal cochlear nucleus (DCN), there is little doubt that this is the case; inhibitory response areas flanking the excitatory one at CF have been directly observed (38,53), and some of the underlying circuitry has been worked out (56). Although, as mentioned previously, there are quantitative differences between these cortical and subcortical responses, there is still a formal similarity between the excitatory and inhibitory domains observed in cochlear nuclei and AI, suggesting that certain pathways from the cochlear nuclei to the cortex may act to preserve this form of response area organization. These pathways may be separate from, but parallel to, those carrying primary-like information from the auditory periphery.

Within AI (and presumably other fields as well) neurons of similar CF are arrayed parallel to radial cell columns. The volume of tissue containing neurons of similar CF resembles a strip-like structure that runs roughly orthogonal to the high-to-low frequency tonotopic axis (22,24,33). This represents still another transformation, a spatial one, from the linear tonotopic map (Fig. 2A) on the basilar membrane to a three-dimensional frequency map within central auditory synaptic stations, including auditory cortex (Fig. 2B).

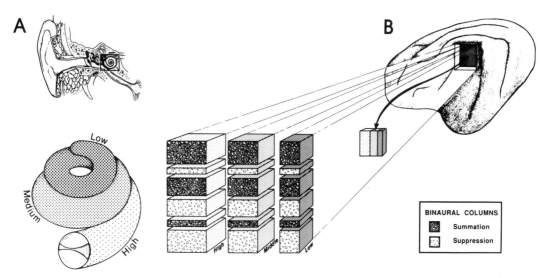

FIG. 2. Schematized transformation of the one-dimensional spatial frequency representation recognized within the cochlea of the inner ear (**A**) to the three-dimensional spatial organization in the primary auditory cortex (**B**). Isofrequency contours (low, middle, high) extend across the field AI in a sheet-like fashion. In addition to a tonotopic representation, AI is also shown to possess a binaural organization in which binaural columns (summation and suppression; terms from ref. 58) are elongated in a direction perpendicular to isofrequency sheets. See text for additional details.

BINAURAL INTERACTIONS

Almost all neurons recorded in AI of the cat receive input from both ears (57–61). Much, if not all, of the initial convergence of information from the two cochlear nuclei occurs in the auditory brainstem, notably in neurons of the superior olivary complex (SOC) (1,2,62–65). A comparison of the responses of cortical and brainstem neurons to variations in the interaural temporal and intensive parameters of static tonal stimuli leaves little doubt that the cortex preserves many of the binaural interaction patterns developed in the brainstem (28,32,33,63, 66–70).

SENSITIVITY TO INTERAURAL INTENSITY DIFFERENCES

Most AI neurons receive a short-latency excitatory input from the contralateral ear. The input from the ipsilateral ear may be excitatory, inhibitory, or mixed, and is pre-

sumed to have a CF close to that of the contralateral input (67). For neurons receiving an excitatory input from the contralateral ear and an inhibitory input from the ipsilateral ear (EI cells), the strength of the neural response evoked by a binaural CF tone pulse depends on the relative amplitudes of the signals at the two ears (32,33,66,71). For these neurons, sensitivity to interaural intensity differences (IIDs) is manifested as a sigmoidal relation of spike count to IID. Spike count tends to be maximal for IIDs favoring the excitatory ear, and minimal for IIDs favoring the ipsilateral ear; it is most sensitive to IIDs ranging close to 0 dB or slightly favoring the contralateral ear. The contribution of neural timing to these functions is seen clearly in experiments in which time-intensity trading is examined; the response latency advantage of the inhibitory input, deriving from a higher tone level at the ipsilateral ear, is offset by a stimulus timing difference favoring the excitatory ear (32,72).

To the extent that it is possible to extrapolate from IIDs to the free-field loci of sound sources that might generate those IIDs, these data have interesting implications for spatial representation in the cortex (64,71,73,74). Both the most effective IIDs and those associated with the steeply graded portion of the IID response function are those that might be generated by sound sources mainly in the acoustic hemifield contralateral to the neuron in question. This suggests that following the binaural comparison occurring in the brainstem, higher auditory nuclei encode spatial information mainly for contralateral sound sources. Moreover, once the relevant interaural comparison has been made at the level of the SOC nuclei, then the more rostral auditory centers on each side of the brain have sufficient information to be independently capable of localizing sound sources in the contralateral auditory hemifield. We shall return to these issues in the paragraphs that follow.

Cells sensitive to IIDs are by no means restricted to those in the EI group. Some cortical neurons (PB cells) receive (apparently) subthreshold excitatory inputs from each ear that are able to sum and to evoke vigorous spike discharges, if the stimuli at the two ears are synchronous in time and equivalent in amplitude (71,75,76). Other cortical neurons derive a supra(spike) threshold excitatory input from each ear (EE cells). For some of these cells, it is likely that binaural stimuli of near-zero intensity disparity evoke spike counts that are greater than those that would be predicted from a linear summation of the monaural responses. Such neurons are likely involved selectively in the processing of acoustic information derived from sources in the frontal sound field (77,78). In other cases, these neurons are insensitive to IIDs over the physiologically relevant range of IIDs (71).

Most of the cells sensitive to IIDs and, therefore, to one binaural intensity cue for sound localization, have CFs greater than about 2.5 kHz. A number of recent studies have mapped this high CF region of AI with respect to the spatial distribution of neuron types distinguished by the binaural interactions (58,59,61). These studies revealed a partial segregation of binaural cell types within AI that overlays the continuous representation of tonal frequency. Both single-unit studies and the mapping experiments suggest that most or all binaural cell types are represented across this entire high-frequency representation of AI.

The areal segregation of binaural cell types has been alternately termed a "binaural column" or a "binaural band." The geometric description of a column or band translates into a three-dimensional volume of cortical tissue that is elongated orthogonal to isofrequency contours in AI (58, 59,79–81). Figure 2B presents one simple organizational scheme, in which AI is composed of only two classes of binaural columns (i.e., summative and suppressive) that are arrayed in an alternating fashion across the field.

More recent studies of binaural interactions have focused on the invariance of functional cell types along a radial column of single neurons and on the transformations of column boundaries, particularly with regard to variations in stimulus intensity (60,61,71). The diversity of intensity effects on cells sensitive to IIDs suggests that the topography of cell types is more accurately described as a mosaic in which the various recognized components can form several distinct patterns. The invariance of cortical maps has been of continuing interest (82) and is broadly related to the issue of stimulus context, which we shall discuss more fully in later sections.

Particularly interesting evidence has been presented on the afferent and efferent connections of binaural columns. First, these bands in AI appear to derive their input from largely nonoverlapping populations of thalamic neurons (81). This suggests that the binaural columns in AI are manifestations of a tightly ordered thalamocortical projection system. Second, callosal connectivity among AI neurons appears to be restricted to those elements with "summative" binaural interactions (80). If, as one might reasonably assume, "summative" refers to EE and PB cell types, then this finding suggests that *inter*hemispheric information transfer is restricted to those neural elements whose spatial selectivity is constrained to the frontal sound field or is otherwise minimal. Third, the AI neurons participating most densely in ipsilateral, corticocortical connections appear to be those with "suppressive" (presumably EI) patterns of binaural interaction (83). These data suggest that *intra*hemispheric information transfer is limited to those neural elements whose spike output is restricted to responses to sound sources in the contralateral hemifield. Within AI, local connections are constrained by the CFs but not apparently by the binaural interactions of the participating elements (84,85).

These findings may be significant for several reasons. They suggest that each cerebral hemisphere derives spatial information mainly, if not only, from sound sources in the contralateral hemifield (64,71,86,87). They tend to lay to rest the notion that it is a comparison of activity in the two cerebral hemispheres that is the basis of sound localization ability, for each hemisphere is independently capable of localizing sound sources in the contralateral acoustic hemifield; the neurons that communicate interhemispherically are precisely those that convey little or no information about sound source location within a hemifield. These data also provide a neurophysiological basis for the related finding that in animals, unilateral lesion of AI results in sound localization deficits only for responses to sound sources in the hemifield contralateral to the lesion (27,74,88,89). Finally, since the more removed multimodal regions of the cerebral cortex likely derive their acoustic input at least in part from the auditory cortex and since such connectivity might be constrained to neurons that are ultimately EI elements, these data may pro-

vide a partial basis for the observation that acoustic attentional deficits in humans following unilateral parietal cortical lesions are largely limited to sound sources in the hemifield contralateral to the cerebral damage (86).

SENSITIVITY TO INTERAURAL PHASE DIFFERENCES

It has long been known that certain cat and monkey auditory cortical neurons are exquisitely sensitive to small shifts in the interaural phase of binaurally presented low-frequency tones (32,33,76,90). This sensitivity is believed to be imparted to cortical neurons by binaural mechanisms operating at brainstem levels and has been taken to underlie a listener's ability to localize the source of a low-frequency tone using interaural phase cues (70,91). Yin and colleagues (65) in particular characterized in great detail the phase sensitivity of neurons in the SOC and the inferior colliculus (ICC) using both static and dynamic stimuli including low-frequency tones of slightly different frequencies at each ear, which simulates some elements of a sound moving around the head along the horizontal plane and results in the perception of "binaural beats" (for review, see ref. 65). It has been recently shown that AI neurons in the cat preserve these same encoding properties (90). It is also recognized that lateralization is possible when interaural time differences are constructed from the waveform envelopes of dichotically presented high-frequency carrier signals (e.g., transients, noise, and tones) whose amplitudes are modulated at relatively low rates (92–96). Indeed, the ability to lateralize sinusoidal AM has been known for some time (97–100). Yin et al. (65) and Crow et al. (101) have reported what may be, in part, the physiological basis for this: neurons in the ICC of the cat are very sensitive to the interaural time differences between modulation envelopes when a high-frequency carrier is modulated by a low-frequency sinusoid. Apparently, timing information that is carried by the phase disparity between the two AM waveforms is encoded within the central nervous system (CNS).

There is no demonstrable degradation in the sensitivity to static binaural listening cues in the transmission of the information from brainstem to cortex. Low-frequency interaural delay sensitivity is recorded equally well at comparable frequencies at thalamic (43) and cortical levels (90) as it is in the brainstem. Few phase-sensitive cells of the ICC phase-lock to the individual cycles of a low-frequency tone, and such timing behavior is even rarer in the auditory thalamus (102,103) and has never been reported in auditory cortex. Thus, in the transformation from phase-locking in monaural channels to interaural phase sensitivity a period-time code has apparently been traded for one based on rate and/or place. The situation may be analogous to that previously described for AM sounds, namely, from the periphery to the cortex there is a transformation from a mechanism that is dominated by temporal processing of information to one in which time or phase information is conveyed by spike rate or by a particular neuron or pool of neurons. The analogy suggests a possible common mechanism for encoding low-frequency tones and AM high-frequency carriers, which is especially interesting considering the fact that the information pertaining to the two signal types originates from very disparate parts of the basilar membrane and may be conveyed to the cortex over quite different ascending parallel pathways (104). In the inferior colliculus (105) and auditory cortex, AM phase-sensitive cells are also sensitive to IIDs of the carrier signal, which means that certain central auditory neurons are capable of encoding interaural level differences and, if the signal is temporally modulated, interaural phase differences (IPD) as well.

ROLE OF CORTEX IN SOUND LOCALIZATION

We mentioned above that animals in which AI has been unilaterally lesioned show marked deficits in their ability to localize sound sources in the acoustic hemifield contralateral to the lesion. Since the initial binaural comparison of basilar membrane phase or amplitude takes place in the caudal brainstem, the specific contribution(s) of the cortex to sound localization is of interest.

One line of evidence on this issue has come from studies of animals with bilateral cortical ablations (106–108). These experiments indicated that the deficits revealed in tests of such animals might be task dependent. The experiments in each case required the animal only to perform a left-versus-right free-field discrimination, but performance varied from chance to near-normal levels according to the nature of the response required. This suggests that the bilaterally lesioned animal may retain the sensory ability to discriminate sound source laterality but may be unable to use that sensory information in the performance of some motor tasks.

Whatever their precise nature, the contralaterality of the deficits resulting from unilateral lesions is most clearly revealed in tasks requiring the animal to discriminate sound source location within an acoustic hemifield (27,74,88). These animals retain the ability to make discriminations of sound source laterality but perform at chance levels on tasks requiring discrimination of source location within the hemifield contralateral to the lesion. Jenkins and Merzenich (27) provided a new insight into the cortical processing of sound localization information, using a refinement of the free-field task. They made unilateral lesions of AI in cats but confined the damage to relatively restricted CF sectors as revealed in prior electrophysiological mapping of that area. In subsequent sound localization tasks using pure tones, the behavioral deficits were evident only for contralateral sources and largely for signals whose frequencies were deprived of cortical representation because of the lesion. This has the important implication that whatever the nature of AI's contribution to the performance on localization tasks, an essential component of the cortical processing is performed within frequency-specific channels. This conclusion is entirely consistent with the knowledge that the brainstem coding of interaural disparities is performed within a tonotopic framework and that the organization of afferent input to the cortex is tonotopically constrained.

SENSITIVITY TO WIDEBAND NOISE MASKING

The spike-count function of an AI neuron determined with pure-tone probes can be shifted along the intensity axis by acoustically combining the tones with a background of continuous noise (45,109). Once the noise level is above threshold for bringing about this sensitivity shift, then further increments in the noise level are matched by adjustments in the cell's sensitivity to tones (34,48). A similar shift in the latency-versus-intensity curve is observed under these conditions, indicating that the noise exerts a threshold elevation on the response to tones. There is an approximately linear relationship between the shift (expressed in dB) measured at the mid-point of the spike-count functions and the intensity of the continuous noise background. There is no systematic change in the detailed shape of the shifted function when the shift and dynamic range are less than 15 dB (45). However, for neurons with a wider dynamic range, continuous noise backgrounds that produce shifts greater than 15 dB also have the consequence of compressing the dynamic range. In general, these noise backgrounds do not produce a background rate

of discharge nor do they restrict the maximal spike count elicited by pure tones.

A comparison of the effects of continuous noise masking in the auditory nerve (36,110,111) with those seen in the cortex provides evidence on the factors shaping the cortical responses. Figure 3 provides, schematically, families of CF-tone intensity functions for tone pulses delivered in the presence of continuous wideband noise of increasing intensity level (shown by dashed curves a,b,c). All auditory nerve fibers are excited by wideband noise and show only modest adaptation of their firing rates when the signal is maintained. A noise background, therefore, foreshortens the range of spike rates available to encode the intensity of a tone presented against that background. As a result, only that portion of a spike-count function that survives this baseline elevation appears shifted along the intensity axis. This effect may reflect constraints on tone-evoked basilar membrane motion at the locus innervated by that fiber, imposed by a more widespread mechanical response to the noise (36). It is interesting to note that both the psychophysical data and the neural data show that the slope of the function relating sensitivity shift to noise level is close to unity. Thus, these sensitivity shifts may be the neural correlates of the perceptual tone threshold elevations seen under similar listening conditions (112,113).

The magnitude of the shift in dynamic range of a cortical cell may reflect to a large degree peripheral transduction mechanisms. Unlike auditory nerve fibers (111), however, threshold elevations for cortical cells are typically greatest for CF tones and decline for frequencies more distant from CF (45). This differential susceptibility to noise across the cortical cell's response area implies that the cortical neuron receives partially independent inputs across its effective tone frequency range and, therefore, that the frequency-intensity response domain of a cortical cell might ac-

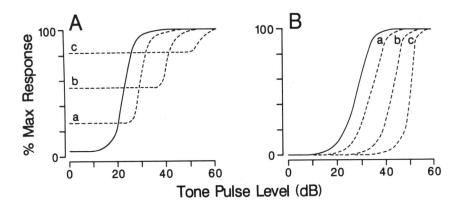

FIG. 3. Schematic spike-count-versus-intensity functions that might be obtained from an auditory nerve fiber (**A**) and an auditory cortical neuron (**B**), for characteristic frequency (CF) tones alone (*solid lines*) and for CF tones presented with continuous wideband noise backgrounds of increasing intensity level (*dashed lines* marked a,b,c). Each family of curves has been normalized to its maximum. In A, note that increasing the level of the background noise raises the baseline of response and displaces the function toward higher tone SPLs. The slope of the functions retains its unmasked value. In B, continuous noise does not elevate the baseline but shifts the tone intensity function toward higher SPLs and, in some cases, steepens its slope. See text for details.

tually represent the envelope of a multiplicity of inputs, unlike an auditory nerve fiber, which represents the output of but a single inner hair cell.

Comparison of parts A and B of Fig. 3 also suggests that, unlike the case for auditory nerve fibers (36), background noise of sufficient level to shift the tone-pulse spike-count function of a cortical neuron (e.g., more than about 10–15 dB) may also steepen the ascending slope of that function (45). Furthermore cortical cells, unlike eighth nerve fibers, receive multiple convergent inputs at CF, and these need not have identical thresholds. Thus, masking noise is likely to shift the sensitivity of only those inputs whose thresholds are exceeded by the noise level. As a result, those inputs will have their thresholds in closer register than would be found in the unmasked state. Even modestly suprathreshold signals would then be able to activate more of those inputs than would an unmasked signal of the same suprathreshold level. On the assumption that the cortical cell's spike output reflects the summation of the mag-

nitude of its input, it follows that the masking may result in a steepened spike-count function.

These observations may be relevant to the neural basis of perceived loudness (for discussion, see ref. 48). We have already seen that the shift of the spike-count function in the presence of background noise may be a neural correlate of the perceptual sensitivity shifts seen under similar stimulus conditions. The steepening of the function may equally be related to the increased rate of loudness growth for signals masked by noise (113). In this respect, cochlear pathology sometimes results in elevated thresholds and steepened rate-level functions in primary afferent fibers, and these responses, in turn, have been implicated in the neural basis of loudness recruitment (114–116). The recent data on noise masking in cortical neurons provide a striking parallel. If perceived loudness is, in fact, related to the firing level of the relevant neurons, then this parallel may have a noteworthy ramification, namely, that the mechanisms underlying loudness recruitment in cochlear pathology are peripheral in locus, while those underlying that in noise masking are central.

It should be noted that cortical neurons exhibiting nonmonotonic spike-count functions are no less affected by background noise than are cells showing monotonic behavior (45,109). Since in the former case the most effective SPL varies with noise level, it is perhaps reasonable that such neurons also possess a "best signal-to-noise ratio." This notion is tantamount to a definition of acoustic contrast and is a concept that may be worthy of further examination.

SENSITIVITY TO MODULATIONS OF AMPLITUDE OR FREQUENCY

There is widespread occurrence in nature of temporal variations in the frequency and amplitude of sounds. These modulations are richly represented in vocalizations produced by most animals, including cats and kittens (117–119), as well as in a variety of other biologically important sounds that fill the ambient environment. There is now considerable evidence that certain of these temporal variations in a sound wave serve as information-bearing elements that are of particular importance to the animal and, moreover, that the auditory nervous system may have, in some species at least, evolved mechanisms for their detection and transmission (120–122). Hence, it is not surprising that interest in the sensitivity of individual auditory cortical elements to complex sounds has a history almost as long as that of single-unit studies of the cortex per se (52,123). Among mammals, the bat auditory system is the one that has been studied most extensively as regards processing of complex sounds. The bat's auditory cortex in particular possesses an apparent division of labor in which neurons encoding different information-bearing elements related to echolocation are highly organized and spatially segregated in different cortical fields (12–14).

An individual mammalian auditory nerve fiber faithfully transmits spectral and temporal information about those components of a complex acoustic waveform that activate the narrow region of the basilar membrane innervated by that fiber. Accordingly, ensembles of auditory nerve fibers innervating collectively a wide region of the cochlear partition transmit the full array of spectral and temporal information contained in that sound (124,125) to multiple tonotopically organized nuclei of the cochlear complex of the brainstem. However, information pertaining to elements of a complex sound need not be restricted within the auditory CNS to parallel pathways isolated from one another, as is the situation with auditory nerve fibers by virtue of their afferent innervation patterns in the cochlea. Rather, at successively higher auditory centers of the brain incoming information is directed over converging and diverging paths (82,126), an arrangement that may provide mechanisms for combining, integrating, and detecting biologically relevant, information-bearing elements of a sound. Watanabe and Katsuki (127) arrived at such a conclusion in their study of neuronal responses to tape-recorded cat vocalizations at several levels of the auditory pathway. One may interpret in the same way the results of the studies in monkey of cortical neurons responding to species-specific vocalizations (128–131). Suga (12–14) refers to this arrangement as "parallel and hierarchical" signal processing and has evidence that such mechanisms are operating in the bat central auditory system. Considering the divergent and convergent anatomical projections found in the central auditory pathways it is not likely that such mechanisms will be fully revealed at cortical levels through the sole use of spectrally simple, temporally static, pure tones or, at the other extreme, with particular complex stimuli such as conspecific vocalizations. Rather, some of the underlying mechanisms might be better understood at this time by the application of complex signals that are a vital part of the animals' natural acoustic world and whose parameters can be systematically varied.

Vertebrate auditory systems process acoustic signals both in the frequency (spectral) and temporal domains. Extensive studies of threshold tuning curves and their spatial (tonotopic or cochleotopic) representations provide evidence for spectral analyses operating at all levels of the auditory pathway including the cortex, as mentioned earlier. Many natural sounds, and those used in communication especially, are characterized not only by a rich spectrum but by a wide range of temporal fluctuations in frequency and intensity. Moreover, a complex sound that is either stationary or moving creates a continuing fluctuation in the rate and timing of the inputs to the two ears that is reflected, in turn, in the fluctuations in spike output of central auditory neurons receiving and transmitting binaural input. While there is a great deal of evidence for the processing of this kind of acoustic information at the level of the auditory nerve and brainstem, with the possible exception of the bat, little is known about the mechanisms for coding of temporal fluctuations in sounds at higher forebrain levels, and almost nothing as regards binaural processing of such signals.

Analyzing responses to such temporal fluctuations may be accomplished, in part, by using well-controlled AM or FM sounds. AM of pure-tone or other carrier signals can generate a variety of sounds that differ markedly in their spectral and temporal properties and therefore in the range of neural mechanisms that they are likely to activate. Two of the most convenient forms of AM employ a high-frequency, pure-tone carrier whose amplitude varies with time in either a sinusoidal or linear manner.

A steady-state sinusoidal AM signal produces a simple line spectrum with three components, corresponding to the carrier frequency and to two symmetrically located side bands that represent the sum and difference of the carrier and modulation frequencies. In mammals (132–134), fish (135), and frogs (136), the waveform periodicity of a sinusoidal AM signal is faithfully reproduced in the temporal rhythm of spikes in single auditory nerve fibers. Furthermore, the low-pass filter characteristics exhibited by auditory nerve fibers in response to such a signal are, for the most part, consistent with those of a model derived from human psychophysics that behaves roughly as a linear envelope detector (137,138). The periodicity of the modulation envelope in sinusoidal AM signals is the hallmark that suggests that this form of AM may be particularly useful in the study of the neural basis of the perception of the pitch of complex sounds (139,140) in which pseudorandom noise is used as the carrier signal (141).

In contrast, a linear AM signal may be a more analytic stimulus because the three consequential stimulus parameters (rate of amplitude change, depth of amplitude change, and repetition rate of the modulation envelope) may be independently varied (142). Recently, Phillips and colleagues (143,144) have used this attribute of linearly modulated signals to infer some of the essential components in a modulated signal's spectrum for which single cortical neurons appear to possess particular sensitivities. The observations of the responsiveness of AI neurons to linear AM signals have a number of implications, only some of which are dealt with here. Primarily, they emphasize the sensitivity of cortical neurons to transient stimulus events and to the short-term spectra of those events. This point takes on special significance from the point of view of modern psychoacoustics in which behavioral sensitivity to AM and short-term spectral processes has been shown to be involved in the perception of complex signals, including speech (145–149).

Band-pass characteristics of central auditory neurons responding to AM signals may differ considerably from those exhibited in the auditory nerve, indicating that temporal selectivity arises from neural mechanisms in the central auditory system (136,141,150). Within the auditory brainstem different AM-sensitive neurons may be tuned to different modulation frequencies, a situation that constitutes an array of temporal filters within the central auditory pathways. Schreiner and Langner (151) have inferred from mapping studies that the central nucleus of the ICC of the cat contains a systematic topographic representation of the best modulation frequency for AM tones. They also argue that a combined spectrotemporal filtering of an input signal by an ICC neuron provides a good approximation to the unit's response to a complex sound.

The responses of cat AI single neurons to linear AM tones have shown that rapid versus slow modulation rates will differentially affect a unit's response depending on the intensity level of the carrier tone (144). When the intensity level of the carrier was close to a unit's absolute threshold and the depth of amplitude change was small (6 dB), rapid AM was typically more effective than slow AM in evoking spike discharges. This finding likely follows from the fact that near threshold levels of stimulation, rapid amplitude increments are most able to synchronize afferent neural inputs (152). Furthermore, since the depth of modulation was small, only the most sensitive of a cortical cell's inputs would have been available to be activated by the AM contribution to the sound's spectrum. At high intensity levels of the carrier, slow AM usually became increasingly effective, while rapid AM decreased in effectiveness for most neurons. This superior effectiveness of the spectral contribution from the slow AM was attributed to the wider range of inputs impinging on the cell at suprathreshold intensity levels and the concomitant adaptation of the most sensitive of these inputs by the maintained carrier tone (45,144). On the other hand, the broader spectrum of the rapid AM may contain sufficient energy, at suprathreshold carrier levels, to activate inhibitory re-

sponse areas of cortical cells (35,143). This argument is strengthened by the finding that these behaviors were most marked in cells with a nonmonotonic rate response for tone pulses, i.e., in those neurons previously believed to be most likely to have inhibitory response areas.

In the central auditory pathways of frogs (136), bats (153), rats (154), and cats (151) the most sharply AM-tuned neurons need not exhibit significant synchronization of the spikes to a particular phase of the modulation envelope, which implies that the coding and representation of AM rate is accomplished at successively higher levels in the auditory CNS without the need to preserve the fine structure of the stimulus waveform. In a qualitative study of AM sensitivity of auditory cortical neuron clusters in the cat (155–157), it was reported that neurons in the major auditory cortical areas are sensitive to AM, that such neurons are tuned to a best modulation frequency, that fields A (anterior) and AI had predominantly higher temporal resolution than fields AII, P, and VP (second, posterior and ventroposterior, respectively), that within field A, best modulation frequency is correlated with CF, and that with the possible exception of field A, the overall temporal resolution was far below that recorded at brainstem levels. The optimal modulation frequencies for cortical neurons appear to be low, in the range of 1 to 50 Hz, regardless of the field. These optimal temporal frequencies are lower than those seen in brainstem neurons (141,150,158–160), which are, in turn, lower than those seen in cochlear nerve fibers (150). Thus, all evidence points to a general reduction in temporal resolution as information ascends the auditory system (151,155,156,159,161–163). The trend toward lower frequency tuning to periodic temporal stimulus variations at rostral levels of the auditory pathway is paralleled by a similar one in the ability to lock spike responses to transients at high repetition rates (164–167). The reasons for the lower temporal tuning of cells in the cortex is not known. Interestingly, however, there may be reason to believe that some of the temporal modulation frequencies that are important in speech discriminations might be quite low and in the range that is optimal for cortical neurons (168,169).

Much of the work of Schreiner and colleagues was aimed at broadly surveying AM sensitivity and mapping the distribution of best modulation frequencies of neuron clusters located for the most part in the middle cortical layers receiving direct thalamic input. While multiunit recording of this kind is useful in mapping the summed, net response of the neuronal cluster, it reveals little about the individual constituent elements that may have very divergent stimulus-response properties, as Phillips and Irvine (170), among others, have pointed out. Thus, the processing of temporal information appears to involve, first, a transformation in the lower auditory brainstem from a periodicity code in the auditory nerve to a central temporal-filter mechanism and, second, a general decrease in temporal resolution from brainstem to cortex.

FM, like AM, is an important information-bearing element of ambient sounds, especially vocalizations of both cats and humans (117–119,171–175). Sinex and Geisler (176) reported that auditory nerve fibers were uniformly sensitive to FM tones that swept through the response area and that there was no significant sensitivity to the direction of the sweep. By the first synapse in the cochlear nuclei, there are already substantial transformations in this eighth nerve input (142,150,167,177–179) and this is further elaborated at midbrain levels (141,159,180).

Even though there have been reports over the years regarding auditory cortical responses to sweep tones (52,123,181–183), the first to make systematic use of FM tones as acoustic stimuli were Whitfield and Evans (123). Their work in a free sound field on what was described as AI in the cat clearly shows that there are some neurons whose steady-state (pure tone) response area properties predict accurately the cell's response to linear or sinusoidal FM sounds. It also shows, however, that for a substantial number of cells there is no such relationship and that the essential stimulus parameter is direction of frequency excursion. Some cells responded to FM tones completely outside the boundaries of the steady-state response area.

Phillips et al. (184) found that AI cells required at least part of a linear excursion to be within the neuron's excitatory response area and that the direction of FM be toward CF. The more recent quantitative studies of these neurons revealed that direction preference to such FMs is close to perfect; further, the strength of response for modulations in that direction was closely correlated with the slope of the spike-count-versus-frequency function measured over the FM excursion (these functions may be thought of as horizontal slices through the response area; they typically have a maximum at, or close to, CF). For linear FMs of ongoing signals, then, neural directional preference is mirror symmetric about CF. Most of the results of Phillips et al. (184) were obtained with short (2 kHz) ramps. In those few cases in which broad FM ramps were also employed (e.g., 50 kHz), it was shown that the mechanisms for directional selectivity for broad and narrow ramps were clearly quite different.

One interpretation of these findings draws on the notion of adaptation to the effective level of the carrier tone that precedes the FM (109,144). Viewed in this framework, the ability of an FM signal to evoke spike discharges would, in part, reflect the extent to which the FM transient improves the stimulus effectiveness beyond the adapted threshold. It follows from this account that neural preference for the direction of frequency change would always favor FMs toward CF and that the strength of responses for that direction of FM would follow the slope of the frequency-response function. This line of argument suggests that the range of effective FM excursions would vary with carrier amplitude, since the width of cortical cell response areas also varies with tone level. To date there is no evidence on this question.

Apparently, when sinusoidal FM is employed, a cortical neuron may respond within a more-or-less restricted range of modulation rates between 0.5 and 15 Hz (185), which overlaps the range of human detection thresholds as determined by Kay and Matthews (186). If this sensitivity is found to be widespread in the cortex, it would suggest that the upper limit of effective sinusoidal modulation is determined largely by the repetition rate of the modulation envelope.

Whitfield and Evans (123) described two other forms of sensitivity to FM direction. In some neurons, they found that the preferred direction of FM was fixed and independent of the locus of the FM excursion within the excitatory response area. In other neurons, FM stimuli were effective in evoking spikes discharges, while static tone pulses were not (see also ref. 52). These observations were among the first to indicate clearly that knowledge of a cortical neuron's excitatory frequency tuning curve is an insufficient basis with which to explain responsiveness to complex sounds. The circuitry that shapes these responses in cortical neurons is largely unknown. Excitatory responses to wideband complex sounds in neurons inhibited by tone pulses is, however, not without precedent in the auditory system. In the DCN, such neurons have been studied in some detail, as has the neural connectivity responsible for these properties (53,56,187).

Suga (52,171) has provided detailed accounts of the sensitivity of bat cortical neurons to linear FMs presented in the form of brief tone pulses. In addition to determining the shape of a neuron's excitatory re-

sponse area, Suga mapped inhibitory response areas using tone-on-tone methods. In some neurons, these were asymmetric (i.e., located on only one side of the excitatory response area) and in others they were found on both sides of CF. Suga found that FM pulses initiated within the excitatory response area and in which the direction of frequency change was away from CF were effective in evoking spike discharges. In contrast, FM pulses initiated in inhibitory response areas were ineffective in evoking spikes, even if they subsequently passed through CF. These data suggested that the effectiveness of FM pulses was related to the temporal sequence with which the stimulus activated the excitatory and inhibitory response areas. This notion has received some confirmation in intracellular studies of cochlear nucleus neurons (177) and in cortical neurons by studies that showed that responses to successive tones of different frequencies mimicked those to FM pulses with the same direction of frequency change (52).

Since these properties were revealed using brief, high-frequency stimuli, it is arguable whether the cortical neurons were continuously tracking the waveform of the stimulus (176). It is probable that responses to FM pulses are dominated by the afferent events evoked by pulse onset. In the case of FMs initiated in the inhibitory response area, it is possible that the inhibitory response outlasts the triggering stimulus and thus suppresses the response to the later stimulus elements within the excitatory response area. In contrast, FMs beginning close to CF may have already triggered the afferent events leading to spike discharges by the time the stimulus has invaded any inhibitory response area. These are precisely the opposite patterns of behavior seen with comparable FMs embedded in continuous carrier tones (184). The contrast between the two sets of observations points to the importance of the acoustic setting in which the relevant stimulus component occurs: that the response to one stimulus element may be significantly altered by the presence of preceding stimulus components.

RESPONSES TO VOCALIZATIONS

Wollberg and Newman (130) were the first to describe the responses of cortical neurons in the monkey to conspecific vocalizations. They found that cortical cells varied widely in their selectivity for vocalizations. Some cells responded to only a single member of the repertoire of vocalizations with which they were tested, while other cells were much less selective. Subsequent work on this topic sought to relate the selectivity of cortical neurons for one or another vocalization to that neuron's static response area. These studies confirmed the variability in the selectivity of cortical cells for the conspecific and other vocalizations but were in disagreement about the extent to which there existed a relationship between neural response areas and effective vocalizations. One study found negligible correspondence (131), whereas others revealed that a significant relationship was present in 60% to 75% of cases examined (188–190). For the most part, these analyses were qualitative, both in the sense that complete response-area data were rarely obtained and in the sense that relationships were typically sought as to whether the relevant vocalizations evoked an excitatory or inhibitory response per se. Nevertheless, there has been agreement among these researchers that cortical neurons should not be thought of as passive acoustic filters, a conclusion confirmed in the most recent studies using AM and FM stimuli (see above).

Two other related findings also have led to an important line of research (130,131). First, it was observed that the spike discharges evoked in auditory cortical neurons by a vocalization typically were locked to particular components of the complex sound. Second, the time structure of the

discharge for a given vocalization varied among cortical neurons responsive to that vocalization (190,191). These data indicate that rather than responding to any long-term average of the spectral properties of the vocalizations, cortical cells follow the time structure of the stimulus, component by component, and the fashion in which they do so is neuron specific. This specificity may follow from the overlap of the spectra of the transients in the stimulus with a neuron's highly individual neural excitatory-inhibitory response area.

These observations raised the further question of the conditions under which a given vocalization component was effective in evoking spike discharges. Wollberg and Newman (130) found that if elements of a vocalization were deleted and replaced by silence, then responses to a later component were often significantly enhanced. Newman and Symmes (129) reported that primate cortical responses to isolated vocalization fragments were typically greater in strength than responses to the same fragment embedded in the complete vocalization from which it was drawn. Similarly, Steinschneider et al. (192) showed that the responses of monkey cortical neurons to a synthetic human vowel sound were significantly modified by the preceding consonant. These observations confirm that the responses to one element of a complex sound may considerably modify the strength (or presence) of an excitatory response to a subsequent stimulus element.

Further evidence on the sensitivity of auditory cortical neurons to the temporal ordering of elements in a complex sound was provided in two studies by Glass and Wollberg (193,194). In one study (193), they examined the effects of reversing conspecific vocalizations, a strategy that preserves the frequency content of the stimulus but reverses the temporal order of the elements. The manipulation had diverse effects on cortical cells. In some instances, reversal of the vocalization eliminated spike responses to that stimulus. In other cases, the stimulus reversal resulted in a broadly comparable reversal in the cadence of spike discharges. In still other neurons, the temporal ordering of spike responses was altered in an unpredictable fashion. In the same year, Glass and Wollberg (194) described the responses of cortical neurons in awake monkeys to sequences of normal and reversed vocalizations and made comparable findings. Responses to a given vocalization were typically stronger when that vocalization was presented in isolation rather than as an element of a continuous sequence. Reversal of the sequence produced findings on spike-train cadences comparable to those seen with single vocalizations.

To what extent these properties are unique to cortical neurons is unclear. The cortical data indicated that the short-term temporal ordering of stimulus elements within a complex sound has a powerful effect on responsiveness to a given acoustic element, and comparable findings have been made in at least some brainstem neurons for human speech sound sequences (195,196). At a somewhat more mechanistic level, there is evidence that stimulus energy falling in side-band inhibitory domains modifies the response to energy falling simultaneously within the excitatory response area of cochlear nuclear cells (197). Whether these effects are as general among neurons of the auditory brainstem as they appear to be among cortical cells is unknown.

It should be clear from the foregoing paragraphs that while some of the stimulus factors that shape cortical responses to vocalizations have been identified, there is still much to learn before a quantitative model of the neural mechanisms configuring those responses can be fully developed. One of the promising features of the research to date, however, is that the responses to sounds as complex as naturally occurring vocalizations appear to be shaped by response factors that are similar in form to those described more quantitatively in parametric studies of responses to complex tonal stimuli. Although this does not mean that the excitatory, inhibitory, and adaptive properties of cortical cells revealed in the tone or tone-noise studies are necessarily the same mechanisms that configure responses to complex vocalizations, the correspondence opens up a potentially fruitful line of further research.

We have already commented on the fact that cortical neurons may be sensitive to the gross form of the short-term spectra of brief stimulus events and that this kind of sensitivity is compatible with the requirements of a recent model of human speech perception. It is noteworthy that this correspondence extends at least one level further. Another continuing line of research has focused on the effects of cortical lesions on complex sound perception. There is some agreement that discrimination between sounds differing in a single stimulus dimension (e.g., frequency, intensity, direction of frequency change) is relatively unaffected by AI ablations (198–201). In addition, deficits in the discrimination of longer term tonal patterns appear to result more from damage to insular-temporal cortical regions than from damage to AI (202–204). On the other hand, primates with bilateral lesions of AI show marked impairments in discrimination of conspecific vocalizations (205), a faculty that, in primates, might be more dependent on the integrity of the left auditory cortex than the right (206,207). Humans with (presumed) bilateral AI lesions often show a neurological syndrome termed "pure word deafness" (208), again possibly somewhat lateralized to the left hemisphere (209). In any event, the term "pure word deafness" may be a misnomer, since there is some evidence that the speech discrimination deficits in these patients might be only the most obvious manifestation of a more general deficit in the processing of temporally complex sounds (210–215). It is likely, then, that the contribution of AI to speech discrimination is a strictly sensory-analytic one.

A more ethologically driven approach to the coding of vocalizations may be found in a series of studies from Suga's laboratory (12–16,216). For the bat, it is a comparison of the emitted sonar pulse and the returning echos that provides biologically important information to the individual. In the mustached bat, the emitted pulse is highly stereotyped, consisting of a 15-msec duration constant-frequency (cf) component followed by a descending, roughly linear frequency sweep about 6 to 10 kHz wide and 3 msec in duration. The first harmonic of the cf portion of the pulse is roughly 30 kHz; the biologically relevant signal includes the second, third, and fourth harmonics of both the pulse and the echo. The total duration of the pulses, and their repetition rate, varies during the approach phase of the behavior.

The cf portion of the signal is suitable for the detection of the velocity of the target relative to the bat. This follows from the fact that any radial motion between the bat and the source of the echo will result in a Doppler-shifted echo; the frequency difference between the cf portion of the pulse and the echo may be as great as 2 kHz and is well within the spatial resolving power of the bat's auditory nervous system. Suga et al. (217) provided detailed descriptions of the region of the mustached bat's cortex in which a majority of neurons were tuned to combinations of cf components that could reasonably be expected to occur in a comparison of harmonically related pulses and echos. In these neurons, responses to either element of the combination were relatively poor but were dramatically facilitated by the combination. In particular, many of these neurons showed narrow tuning to the frequency of the echo cf component and therefore to the frequency disparity between the pulse and the echo and thus of the relative velocity of the target. Moreover, within the cf/cf combination processing areas of the cortex, neurons are spatially arrayed according to their target velocity tuning.

By contrast with the cf/cf (i.e., pulse/echo) comparison, the comparison between the FM pulse/echo elements (FM/FM) may provide the bat with information on target distance. The FM portions of the signal have broad, short-term spectra, and the neurons in the bat's FM/FM processing area are themselves more broadly tuned than those of the cf/cf area. This broad tuning largely precludes sensitivity to target velocity information. On the other hand, the FM/FM combination neurons are very sensitive to the delay between the pulse and the echo FM components, while the cf/cf combination-sensitive neurons show poorer delay sensitivity (217). Within the cortical area containing high concentrations of FM/FM neurons, these cells are often finely tuned to echo delay and therefore to target distance. In at least some cases, these neurons were also tuned to the amplitude of the pulse FM component, which is a second acoustic parameter that might provide information on target distance (following from the inverse-square law). The factors shaping the amplitude tuning are likely similar to those shaping the nonmonotonic spike-count-versus-level functions in other bat cortical regions (46) and in cortical areas of other mammals (see above). As in the cf/cf cortical area, neurons in the FM/FM area were found to be topographically arrayed according to their preferred delays, at least over the behaviorally relevant range.

CORTICAL REPRESENTATION OF SOUND-TIME STRUCTURE

The preceding section raises the question of the temporal grain with which the time structure of a sound is represented in the spike activity of cortical neurons. This issue is only beginning to be studied explicitly. One useful distinction to emerge has been that between the steady-state and transient responses of cortical neurons (218,219). The steady-state temporal response of a neuron underlies the ability of that cell to time-lock spikes to stimulus periodicities. Studies using pure tones (220), modulated signals (156,158), and other sounds (166,220) are in broad agreement that the steady-state temporal response of cortical neurons is competent only for periodicities less than about 100 Hz. This is more than an order of magnitude poorer than that seen in the auditory brainstem and cochlear nerve (103,132,134,150,154,167, 221). It has the important consequence that, whereas the cochlear nerve has the ability to represent many speech and other sounds on a temporal basis (125,176,222, 223), the cortex has no temporal representation of the fine time structure (time waveform) of those sounds. In this respect, the strictly temporal representation of steady-state vowels is, by comparison with that in the cochlear nerve, already significantly degraded in the cochlear nucleus neurons thought to receive the most temporally faithful auditory nerve input (224). This suggests that the poor steady-state response seen in the cortex might reflect a cumulative degradation of the signal at each synaptic station in the afferent path to it.

The further ramification of these observations is that if the behavioral discrimination of two sounds relies solely on discrimination of steady-state periodicities, then the cortex is unlikely to be directly involved in mediating that behavior. It is perhaps for this reason that cats deprived of the auditory cortex bilaterally retain the ability to discriminate interaural phase differences as small as 15 µsec (225). Similarly, if we accept that the human discrimination of spoken vowels is based on temporal (c.f. spectral) representations of the signals, then it is noteworthy that vowel discrimination survives bilateral lesion of the auditory cortex in humans (for review, see ref. 226). The discrimination of sounds whose identities reside in their fine periodic time structure may rely more on brainstem processing in which the temporal structure of the sounds is better represented.

In contrast to the poverty of the cortex's steady-state temporal response, the precision with which the transient responses of cortical neurons can encode stimulus event times is comparable to that seen in the cochlear nerve (219). The "jitter" in the first-spike times of transient responses can be smaller than a few hundred microseconds in many cortical cells, and this degree of timing precision could possibly support a neural temporal resolution of about a millisecond. Interestingly, in humans, behavioral temporal resolution is of the same order and is grossly worse after bilateral cortical lesions (219,226). The same degree of transient response precision is demonstrably capable of supporting a representation of the timing of phonetically relevant components of speech sounds (e.g., voice onset times [192]), and it is often the discrimination of speech sounds with this temporal grain that is most severely impaired in patients with bilateral cortical lesions (210, 212,226).

These observations mesh well with our foregoing description of the responses to vocalizations. Recall that studies in awake monkeys typically showed that the timing of spikes in responses to primate conspecific vocalizations is nonrandom and appears to follow the transient content of the sound. This presumably reflects both the sensitivity of cortical neurons to brief stimulus events and the temporal precision of those cells' transient responses. The spectral composition of each transient event is thought to be represented by those neurons of the tonotopic array that are activated. Note that it is this precision of transient response timing that, in bats, makes possible the neural representation of pulse/echo delays used in target distance estimation.

The reasons for the relative preservation of transient response timing in cortical neurons are not known with certainty. As Rhode and Smith (221) have pointed out, one means of enhancing the precision of transient response timing is by an averaging process applied to convergent, nearly synchronous inputs (the jitter theoretically could decline with the square root of the number of inputs). Since the input to cortical neurons is indeed derived from a highly convergent afferent pathway, a neural substrate for such an averaging process exists. The impoverished steady-state temporal response of cortical cells reflects at least two factors. One is that cortical cells, at least in anesthetized animals, are rapidly adapting (109). The second is that convergence of inputs, while enhancing the transient response, might result in a more even distribution of subsequent spike times.

PLASTICITY OF AUDITORY CORTICAL NEURONAL RESPONSES

Hubel and colleagues (227) were the first to report that, in the awake cat, the responsiveness of cortical auditory neurons might depend on factors other than any inherent effectiveness of the stimulus. Specifically, they showed that responses to acoustic stimuli were exhibited by some neurons only if the cat "attended" to the sound, typically by orienting its head to the source. Whether the apparent benefits of appropriate head orientation actually reflected "attentional" processes rather than peripheral acoustic advantages conferred by pinna directionality (228,229) is not known in this case. Later work showed that, in unanesthetized monkeys, the overall responsiveness of single auditory cortical neurons to acoustic stimuli may fluctuate over time. This nonstationarity may sometimes be stimulus specific (128,230), whereas some of these variations may be associated with the arousal state (33). These data indicate that some cortical neurons may be labile in their responsiveness and raise the possibility that this plasticity might be the medium through which attentional processes may shape cortical responses. This, along with a desire to visualize cortical auditory processing uncontaminated by general anesthetic effects, led to interest in the con-

tribution of attentional processes and behavioral relevance to the stimulus-response properties of cortical cells.

There have been a host of experiments that have used subtle, and often insightful, variations on paradigms that introduce behavioral relevance to the stimuli with which cortical neurons are studied. This includes requiring the experimental animals to indicate detection of the stimulus by means of an operant response (231,232) or by using the sound as a conditioned stimulus (for review, see ref. 233).

Both simple attention to the stimulus and the requirement of a behavioral response may significantly modify cortical neuron responses to an acoustic signal. Most commonly, authors have described stronger responses in the attending than in the nonattending animal (232,234–239). In some neurons in which there is a suppressed background spontaneous rate, a particularly salient evoked response results (240, 241). There is increasing evidence that attention may suppress stimulus-evoked spike discharges in a significant proportion of cortical cells (233,242–244) and that the effects may extend to spontaneous discharges (241,243).

The question of whether behavioral arousal, attention, or performance may be able to impose a response specificity that is not present in the unattending or anesthetized animal is more complex (233,238,239). It appears, however, to be the general conclusion that differences in the attentiveness to a stimulus in a behavioral paradigm exert rather little effect on the basic response properties of cortical neurons, including frequency tuning, input-output functions, and spatial selectivity (236,238,243), although there is now evidence that even some of these basic measures are influenced by the presence of anesthetics (245). This conclusion extends to the effects of direct electrical stimulation of the reticular formation on a cortical neuron's selectivity for vocalizations (246).

It is likely that some neurons in subcortical auditory nuclei are also influenced by behavioral state (247–252). The wealth of data on this issue is too detailed to be reviewed comprehensively here, but some features of it do warrant brief mention. First, at levels as caudal as the ICC, attentional effects are sometimes seen in the shortest latency evoked discharges (248, 251). Although there is evidence that brainstem neural discharges are directly affected by cooling auditory cortex (240), the latency data suggest that descending corticofugal influences are not the sole contributors to attentional effects on brainstem neurons. Second, at thalamic levels, plasticity of evoked response is more common among neurons of the magnocellular division of the medial geniculate body than among those of the ventral division (252). This point may be of specific significance since the magnocellular division is a component of what has been called the "lemniscal adjunct system" that parallels the "lemniscal line system" in the ascending auditory pathways (253,254). In this terminology, the lemniscal line system is viewed as being composed of narrowly tuned neurons connected by highly ordered convergent and divergent pathways that are tonotopically constrained and that confer these properties to certain auditory cortical fields. In contrast, neurons in the lemniscal adjunct system are thought to receive highly convergent, often multimodal, sensory input that is ultimately reflected in the more nonspecific sound-evoked responses of certain other cortical fields. This contrast, which has perhaps been most demonstrable at midbrain and thalamic levels, might extend to the cortex (233,255) both in terms of the connectivity patterns of those regions and the susceptibility to behavioral state of neural responses. In this regard, some of the most compelling and robust effects of behavioral state are exhibited by neurons in cortical fields outside the tonotopically organized ones (128,230,237,256, 257). Weinberger and Diamond (233) studied the frequency-response functions of neurons in cortical fields ventral to AI. These cells are often broadly tuned to tonal frequency (24,258). These authors showed that if a tone, but not specifically its frequency, was behaviorally relevant, the effects of attention/arousal were global across a neuron's response area, whether those effects were facilitatory or inhibitory. In contrast, if the frequency of the tone was a parameter determining the stimulus' relevance, then the effects, suppressive or facilitative, were selective, and most were marked for frequencies at or close to the behaviorally relevant one(s). These data suggest that observations of the stimulus selectivity of some cortical neurons in the untrained animal might show the *potential range* of effective inputs received by a neuron, but that the expression of this range might be narrowed by the imposition of behavioral relevance on a subset of those inputs.

Finally, Ryan and Miller (251) made some interesting observations on the spike discharge patterns of collicular neurons. They reported that in the nonperforming monkey, some neurons discharged transiently at the onset and offset of a tonal stimulus. When the monkey was required to respond operantly to the onset of a stimulus, they observed that the same neurons continued to respond to stimulus onset but ceased to respond to its offset. These data necessarily indicate that the neural circuitry-shaping responses to individual components of a complex response must be relatively independent, a conclusion that extends to cortical neurons (144,234).

CONCLUSIONS: INFORMATION PROCESSING IN THE AUDITORY CORTEX

In this chapter, we have tried to review some recent advances in our understanding of auditory cortical physiology. We have paid particular attention to neural mechanisms that shape cortical unit physiology to gain insight into the extent to which these mechanisms might be elaborations on, rather than preservations of, processes developed in the auditory brainstem.

An often repeated question of the auditory system is the extent to which elaboration of cochlear nerve input is serial and hierarchical rather than parallel in organization (259). In the auditory as well as other sensory modalities, it now appears to be the general consensus that both principles operate (260,261). On the one hand, it is perfectly clear that some AI neurons have acquired properties that are developed in spatially segregated brainstem nuclei. Thus, a cortical neuron may have a response area organization reminiscent of that in the DCN, but the binaural interaction exhibited by a lateral superior olivary cell. In this sense, the afferent pathways to the cortex are necessarily hierarchical and convergent in organization. On the other hand, it is equally clear that the convergence of input on the AI cells, even those of the same CF and binaural interaction type, is markedly incomplete. This results in discontinuous territories within AI that preserve response properties reflecting one or the other dominant afferent input. In this sense, the input to AI is at least partially parallel in form, and a similar argument may be made for the various fields that lie outside AI (11,260,262).

The specifically transient nature of the responses of many cortical neurons is by no means unique to cells at this locus. There is, however, some evidence that transient responses become progressively more common at successive nuclei along the ascending auditory pathway (28), and this transformation may be an emergent property of central auditory processing. It may be that this metamorphosis confers on cortical cells sensitivity and salient responses to transient and dynamic stimulus events that fill the ambient acoustic environment. A cortical cell's sensitivity to rise-time, for instance, is usually manifested as the presence or absence of spike responses, whereas a cochlear nerve fiber may show only a slight modulation of its discharge rate (263). Even complex vocalizations in awake animals appear to evoke cortical responses for which the time structure of spike discharges tends to follow that of the transient elements in the stimulus. The circuits that shape such responses may be partially independent since individual response components may be differentially susceptible to the effects of behavior state. The total response, however, may not be a simple summation of independent responses since the time course of the response to one component may significantly alter the response to the next.

It is probable that we do not appreciate most of the advantages that the complexity and intricacy of this so-called hierarchical-parallel processing mechanism has provided to the neocortex. It seems clear that the stringently topographic afferent pathway from the cochleas to the cortex imposes a tonotopic and functional framework within which processing of acoustic information other than static pure tones takes place. A well-studied case is that of sound localization. The neurophysiological data indicate that in the afferent auditory pathways, including field AI, the neural coding of binaural localization cues for sources of a particular tonal frequency is performed, for the most part, by neurons with CFs at, or close to, that frequency. There are examples, however, of neurons capable of encoding both IIDs and IPDs when pure tones are employed as stimuli (264). There is even more evidence to show that high CF neurons are capable of encoding monaural and binaural temporal information provided the high-frequency carrier is modulated at relatively low frequency (65,265). By the same token, animals with cortical lesions limited to a restricted iso-frequency plane show deficits in sound localization ability primarily for those contra-laterally located signals with dominant spectral content deprived of cortical representation (27).

A final question concerns the existence in the auditory cortex of "grandmother cells," i.e., neurons whose stimulus requirements are so strict that they could be satisfied only by a signal of extraordinary spectral and temporal complexity, which would presumably be coded by discharges after the conclusion of a precisely ordered temporal concatenation of stimulus components. On this issue we concur with Symmes (266) in that the data available to date provide little support for this notion, at least in AI. Moreover, the preceding arguments we have made about the nature of cortical physiology render it unlikely that AI might even be a viable site for the presence of any such neurons. First, the existence of stringent tonotopic constraints on the afferent connectivity of AI neurons suggests that these cells do not receive a sufficiently convergent input (across the frequency domain) to encompass such sensitivity. Second, cortical neurons typically show responses that are dominated by short-term stimulus events and are highly idiosyncratic in their sensitivity to the temporal ordering of events. It seems much more likely that the grandmother acoustic stimulus will be coded in the spatial and temporal distribution of evoked discharges across the mosaic of cortical neurons, rather than in the identity of a few specific elements.

ACKNOWLEDGMENTS

We thank Carol Dizack and Yvonne Slusser for their artful illustrations, Shirley Hunsaker for photography, and S. E. Hall for comments on previous versions of this manuscript. Research described here was supported by grants U0442 and E2745 from the Natural Sciences and Engineering Research Council of Canada (DPP), a Dalhousie University Research Development Award (DPP), NSF grant BNS-8215777 (JFB and RAR) and NIH grants NS24559, HD03352, NS12732 (JFB and RAR).

REFERENCES

1. Aitkin LM, Irvine DRF, Webster WR. Central neural mechanisms of hearing. In: Darian-Smith I, ed. *Handbook of physiology—the nervous system III*. Washington, DC: American Physiological Society, 1984;675–737.
2. Phillips DP. Introduction to anatomy and physiology of the central auditory nervous system. In: Jahn AF, Santos-Sacchi JR, eds. *Physiology of the ear*. New York: Raven Press, 1988;407–429.
3. Brugge JF. Progress in neuroanatomy and neurophysiology of auditory cortex. In: Tower DB, ed. *The nervous system, volume 3*. New York: Raven Press, 1975;97–111.
4. Brugge JF. Auditory cortical areas in primates. In: Woolsey CN, ed. *Cortical sensory organization, volume 3, multiple auditory areas*. Clifton, NJ: Humana Press, 1982;59–70.
5. Evans EF. Cortical representation. In: de Reuck AVS, Knight J, eds. *Hearing mechanisms in vertebrates*. Boston: Little, Brown, 1968;272–295.
6. Goldstein MH Jr, Abeles M. Note on tonotopic organization of primary auditory cortex in the cat. *Brain Res* 1975;100:188–191.
7. Brugge JF. Patterns of organization in auditory cortex. *J Acoust Soc Am* 1985;78:353–359.
8. Fitzpatrick KA, Imig TJ. Organization of auditory connections. The primate auditory cortex. In: Woolsey CN, ed. *Cortical sensory organization, volume 3, multiple auditory areas*. Clifton, NJ: Humana Press, 1982;71–109.
9. Brugge JF, Reale RA. Auditory cortex. In: Peters A, Jones EG, eds. *Cerebral cortex, volume 4*. New York: Plenum, 1985;229–271.
10. Imig TJ, Reale RA, Brugge JF. Patterns of cortico-cortical projections related to physiological maps of the cat's auditory cortex. In: Woolsey CN, ed. *Cortical sensory organization, volume 3, multiple auditory areas*. Clifton, NJ: Humana Press, 1982;1–41.
11. Imig TJ, Morel A. Organization of the thalamocortical auditory system in the cat. *Annu Rev Neurosci* 1983;6:95–120.
12. Suga N. Functional organization of the auditory cortex. Representation beyond tonotopy in the bat. In: Woolsey CN, ed. *Cortical sensory organization, volume 3, multiple auditory areas*. Clifton, NJ: Humana Press, 1982;157–218.
13. Suga N. The extent to which biosonar information is represented in the bat auditory cortex. In: Edelman GM, Gall WE, Cowan WM, eds. *Dynamic aspects of neocortical function*. New York: Wiley, 1984;315–373.
14. Suga N. Parallel-hierarchical processing of complex sound in the bat auditory system. In: Gall WE, Cowan WM, Edelman GM, eds. *Functions of the auditory system*. New York: Academic Press, 1986.
15. Suga N, Kuzirai K, O'Neill WE. How biosonar information is processed in the bat cerebral

cortex. In: Syka J, Aitkin LM, eds. *Neuronal mechanisms of hearing.* New York: Plenum Press, 1981;197–219.

16. Suga N, Niwa H, Taniguchi I. Representation of biosonar information in the auditory cortex of the mustached bat, with emphasis on target velocity information. In: Ewert J-P, Capranica RR, Ingle DJ, eds. *Advances in vertebrate neuroethology.* New York: Plenum Press, 1983; 829–867.

17. Woolsey CN, Walzl EM. Topical projection of nerve fibers from local regions of the cochlea to the cerebral cortex of the cat. *Bull Johns Hopkins Hosp* 1942;71:315–344.

18. Imig TJ, Ruggero MA, Kitzes LM, Javel E, Brugge JF. Organization of auditory cortex in the owl monkey (Aotus trivirgatus). *J Comp Neurol* 1977;171:111–128.

19. Rose JE, Woolsey CN. The relations of thalamic connections, cellular structure and evocable electrical activity in the auditory region of the cat. *J Comp Neurol* 1949;91:441–466.

20. Merzenich MM, Brugge JF. Representation of the cochlear partition of the superior temporal plane of the macaque monkey. *Brain Res* 1973;50:275–296.

21. Aitkin LM, Merzenich MM, Irvine DR, Clarey JC, Nelson JE. Frequency representation in auditory cortex of the common marmoset (Callithrix jacchus jacchus). *J Comp Neurol* 1986; 252:175–185.

22. Merzenich MM, Knight PL, Roth GL. Representation of cochlea within primary auditory cortex in the cat. *J Neurophysiol* 1975;38:231–249.

23. Phillips DP, Judge PW, Kelly JB. Primary auditory cortex in the ferret (Mustela putorius): neural response properties and topographic organization. *Brain Res* 1988;443:281–294.

24. Reale RA, Imig TJ. Tonotopic organization in auditory cortex of the cat. *J Comp Neurol* 1980;192:265–291.

25. Imig TJ, Morel A. Topographic and cytoarchitectonic organization of thalamic neurons related to their targets in low-, middle-, and high-frequency representations in cat auditory cortex. *J Comp Neurol* 1984;227:511–539.

26. Morel A, Imig TJ. Thalamic projections to fields A, AI, P, and VP in the cat auditory cortex. *J Comp Neurol* 1987;265:119–144.

27. Jenkins WM, Merzenich MM. Role of cat primary auditory cortex for sound-localization behavior. *J Neurophysiol* 1984;52:819–847.

28. Phillips DP, Irvine DR. Responses of single neurons in physiologically defined primary auditory cortex (AI) of the cat: frequency tuning and responses to intensity. *J Neurophysiol* 1981;45:48–58.

29. Kiang NYS, Watanabe T, Thomas EC, Clark LF. Discharge patterns of single fibers in the cat's auditory nerve. In: *MIT research monograph no. 35.* Cambridge, MA: MIT Press, 1965.

30. Liberman MC. Auditory nerve responses from cats raised in a low-noise chamber. *J Acoust Soc Am* 1978;63:442–455.

31. Liberman MC. The cochlear frequency map for the cat: labeling auditory nerve fibers of known characteristic frequency. *J Acoust Soc Am* 1982;72:1441–1449.

32. Brugge JF, Dubrovsky NA, Aitkin LM, Anderson DJ. Sensitivity of single neurons in auditory cortex of cat to binaural tonal stimulation; effects of varying interaural time and intensity. *J Neurophysiol* 1969;32:1005–1024.

33. Brugge JF, Merzenich MM. Responses of neurons in auditory cortex of the macaque monkey to monaural and binaural stimulation. *J Neurophysiol* 1973;36:1138–1158.

34. Phillips DP, Cynader MS. Some neural mechanisms in the cat's auditory cortex underlying sensitivity to combined tone and wide-spectrum noise stimuli. *Hear Res* 1985;18:87–102.

35. Phillips DP, Orman SS, Musicant AD, Wilson GF. Neurons in the cat's primary auditory cortex distinguished by their responses to tones and wide-spectrum noise. *Hear Res* 1985;18:73–86.

36. Costalupes JA, Young ED, Gibson DJ. Effects of continuous noise backgrounds on rate response of auditory nerve fibers in cats. *J Neurophysiol* 1984;51:1326–1344.

37. Sachs MB, Abbas PJ. Rate versus level functions for auditory-nerve fibers in cats: tone burst stimuli. *J Acoust Soc Am* 1974;56:1835–1847.

38. Evans EF, Nelson PG. The responses of single neurons in the cochlear nucleus of the cat as a function of their location and anesthetic state. *Exp Brain Res* 1973;17:402–427.

39. Goldberg JM, Brownell WE. Discharge characteristics of neurons in anteroventral and dorsal cochlear nuclei of cat. *Brain Res* 1973; 64:35–54.

40. Tsuchitani C, Boudreau JC. Encoding of stimulus frequency and intensity by cat superior olive S-segment cells. *J Acoust Soc Am* 1967; 42:794–805.

41. Tsuchitani C. Functional organization of lateral cell groups of cat superior olivary complex. *J Neurophysiol* 1977;40:296–318.

42. Rose JE, Greenwood DD, Goldberg JM, Hind JE. Some discharge characteristics of single neurons in the inferior colliculus of the cat. I. Tonotopical organization, relation of spike counts to tone intensity, and firing patterns of single elements. *J Neurophysiol* 1963;26:294–320.

43. Aitkin LM, Webster WR. Medial geniculate body of the cat: organization and responses to tonal stimuli of neurons in ventral division. *J Neurophysiol* 1972;35:365–380.

44. Palmer AR, Evans EF. Cochlear fiber rate-intensity functions: no evidence for basilar membrane nonlinearities. *Hear Res* 1980;2:319–326.

45. Phillips DP, Hall SE. Spike-rate intensity functions of cat cortical neurons studied with com-

bined tone-noise stimuli. *J Acoust Soc Am* 1986;80:177–187.

46. Suga N, Manabe T. Neural basis of amplitude-spectrum representation in auditory cortex of the mustached bat. *J Neurophysiol* 1982;47:225–255.

47. Phillips DP, Orman SS. Responses of single neurons in posterior field of cat auditory cortex to tonal stimulation. *J Neurophysiol* 1984;51:147–163.

48. Phillips DP. Stimulus intensity and loudness recruitment: neural correlates. *J Acoust Soc Am* 1987;82:1–12.

49. Evans EF, Whitfield IC. Classification of unit responses in the auditory cortex of the unanesthetized and unrestrained cat. *J Neurophysiol* 1964;171:476–492.

50. Goldstein MH Jr, Hall JL, Butterfield BO. Single-unit activity in the primary auditory cortex of unanesthetized cats. *J Acoust Soc Am* 1968;43:444–455.

51. Shamma SA, Symmes D. Patterns of inhibition in auditory cortical cells in awake squirrel monkeys. *Hear Res* 1985;19:1–13.

52. Suga N. Functional properties of auditory neurones in the cortex of echo-locating bats. *J Physiol (Lond)* 1965;181:671–700.

53. Young ED, Brownell WE. Responses to tones and noise of single cells in dorsal cochlear nucleus of unanesthetized cats. *J Neurophysiol* 1976;39:282–300.

54. Greenwood DD, Maruyama N. Excitatory and inhibitory response areas of auditory neurons in the cochlear nucleus. *J Neurophysiol* 1965;28:863–892.

55. Shofner WP, Young ED. Excitatory/inhibitory response types in the cochlear nucleus: relationship to discharge patterns and responses to electrical stimulation of the auditory nerve. *J Neurophysiol* 1985;54:917–940.

56. Voight HF, Young ED. Evidence of inhibitory interactions between neurons in dorsal cochlear nucleus. *J Neurophysiol* 1980;44:76–96.

57. Hall JL, Goldstein MH Jr. Representation of binaural stimuli by single units in primary auditory cortex of unanesthetized cats. *J Acoust Soc Am* 1968;43:456–461.

58. Imig TJ, Adrian HO. Binaural columns in the primary field (A1) of cat auditory cortex. *Brain Res* 1977;138:241–257.

59. Middlebrooks JC, Dykes RW, Merzenich MM. Binaural response-specific bands in primary auditory cortex (AI) of the cat: topographical organization orthogonal to isofrequency contours. *Brain Res* 1980;181:31–48.

60. Phillips DP, Irvine DR. Some features of binaural input to single neurons in physiologically defined area AI of cat cerebral cortex. *J Neurophysiol* 1983;49:383–395.

61. Reale RA, Kettner RE. Topography of binaural organization in primary auditory cortex of the cat: effects of changing interaural intensity. *J Neurophysiol* 1986;56:663–682.

62. Brugge JF, Geisler CD. Auditory mechanisms of the lower brainstem. *Annu Rev Neurosci* 1978;1:363–394.

63. Caird D, Klinke R. Processing of binaural stimuli by cat superior olivary complex neurons. *Exp Brain Res* 1983;52:385–399.

64. Phillips DP, Brugge JF. Progress in neurophysiology of sound localization. *Annu Rev Psychol* 1985;36:245–274.

65. Yin TCT, Kuwada S. Neuronal mechanisms of binaural interactional. In: Edelman GM, Gall WE, Cowan WM, eds. *Dynamic aspects of neocortical function.* New York: Wiley, 1984;263–313.

66. Benson DA, Teas DC. Single unit study of binaural interaction in the auditory cortex of the chinchilla. *Brain Res* 1976;103:313–338.

67. Boudreau JC, Tsuchitani C. Binaural interaction in the cat superior olive S-segment. *J Neurophysiol* 1968;31:442–454.

68. Guinan JJ, Guinan SS, Norris BE. Single auditory units in the superior olivary complex. I. Responses to sounds and classification based on physiological properties. *Int J Neurosci* 1972;4:101–120.

69. Kuwada S, Yin TC. Binaural interaction in low-frequency neurons in inferior colliculus of the cat. I. Effects of long interaural delays, intensity, and repetition rate on interaural delay function. *J Neurophysiol* 1983;50:981–999.

70. Rose JE, Gross NB, Geisler CD, Hind JE. Some neural mechanisms in the inferior colliculus of the cat which may be relevant to localization of a sound source. *J Neurophysiol* 1966;29:288–314.

71. Phillips DP, Irvine DR. Responses of single neurons in physiologically defined area AI of cat cerebral cortex: sensitivity to interaural intensity differences. *Hear Res* 1981;4:299–307.

72. Durlach NI, Colburn HS. Binaural phenomena. In: Carterette EC, Friedman MP, eds. *Handbook of perception, volume 4, hearing.* New York: Academic Press, 1978;365–466.

73. Irvine DR. Interaural intensity differences in the cat: changes in sound pressure level at the two ears associated with azimuthal displacements in the frontal horizontal plane. *Hear Res* 1987;26:267–286.

74. Jenkins WM, Masterton RB. Sound localization: effects of unilateral lesions in central auditory system. *J Neurophysiol* 1982;47:987–1016.

75. Kitzes LM, Wrege KS, Cassady JM. Patterns of responses of cortical cells to binaural stimulation. *J Comp Neurol* 1980;192:455–472.

76. Orman SS, Phillips DP. Binaural interactions of single neurons in posterior field of cat auditory cortex. *J Neurophysiol* 1984;51:1028–1039.

77. Aitkin LM, Rawson JA. Frontal sound source location is represented in the cat cerebellum. *Brain Res* 1983;265:317–321.

78. Aitkin LM, Boyd J. Responses of single units in cerebellar vermis of the cat to monaural and binaural stimuli. *J Neurophysiol* 1975;38:418–429.

79. Brugge JF, Imig TJ. Some relationships of bin-aural response patterns of single neurons to cortical columns and interhemispheric connec-tions of auditory area AI of cat cerebral cortex. In: Naunton RF, Fernandez C, eds. *Evoked electrical activity in the auditory nervous sys-tem.* New York: Academic Press, 1978;487–503.

80. Imig TJ, Brugge JF. Sources and terminations of callosal axons related to binaural and fre-quency maps in primary auditory cortex of the cat. *J Comp Neurol* 1978;182:637–660.

81. Middlebrooks JC, Zook JM. Intrinsic organi-zation of the cat's medial geniculate body iden-tified by projections to binaural response-spe-cific bands in the primary auditory cortex. *J Neurosci* 1983;3:203–224.

82. Merzenich MM, Colwell SA, Andersen RA. Auditory forebrain organization: thalamocorti-cal and corticothalamic connections in the cat. In: Woolsey CN, ed. *Cortical sensory organi-zation, volume 3, multiple auditory areas.* Clif-ton, NJ: Humana Press, 1982;43–57.

83. Imig TJ, Reale RA. Ipsilateral corticocortical projections related to binaural columns in cat primary auditory cortex. *J Comp Neurol* 1981; 203:1–14.

84. Matsubara JA, Phillips DP. Intracortical con-nections and their physiological correlates in the primary auditory cortex (AI) of the cat. *J Comp Neurol* 1988;268:38–48.

85. Reale RA, Brugge JF, Feng JZ. Geometry and orientation of neuronal processes in cat pri-mary auditory cortex (AI) related to character-istic-frequency maps. *Proc Natl Acad Sci USA* 1983;80:5449–5453.

86. Phillips DP, Gates GR. Representation of the two ears in the auditory cortex: a reexamina-tion. *Int J Neurosci* 1982;16:41–46.

87. Masterton RB, Imig TJ. Neural mechanisms for sound localization. *Annu Rev Physiol* 1984;46: 275–287.

88. Kavanagh GL, Kelly JB. Contribution of audi-tory cortex to sound localization by the ferret (Mustela putorius). *J Neurophysiol* 1987;57: 1746–1766.

89. Strominger NL. Localization of sound after unilateral and bilateral ablation of auditory cor-tex. *Exp Neurol* 1969;25:521–533.

90. Reale RA, Brugge JF. Auditory cortical neu-rons are sensitive to static and continuously changing interaural phase cues. *J Neurophysiol* 1990;64:1247–1260.

91. Goldberg JM, Brown PB. Response of binaural neurons of dog superior olivary complex to di-chotic tonal stimuli: some physiological mech-anisms of sound localization. *J Neurophysiol* 1969;32:613–636.

92. Hafter ER, Dye RH, Neutzel JM. Lateraliza-tion of high-frequency stimuli on the basis of time and intensity. In: Klinke R, Hartman R, eds. *Hearing-physiological basis and psycho-physics,* Berlin: Springer-Verlag, 1980;202–208.

93. Harris CG. Binaural interactions of impulsive stimuli and pure tones. *J Acoust Soc Am* 1960;32:685–692.

94. Klumpp RG, Eady HR. Some measurements of interaural time difference thresholds. *J Acoust Soc Am* 1956;28:859–860.

95. Yost WA. Lateralization of filtered transients. *J Acoust Soc Am* 1976;60:178–181.

96. McFadden D, Pasanen E. Lateralization at high frequencies based on interaural time differ-ences. *J Acoust Soc Am* 1976;59:634–639.

97. Henning GB. Detectability of interaural de-lay in high-frequency complex waveforms. *J Acoust Soc Am* 1974;55:84–90.

98. Leakey DM, Sayers BMA, Cherry C. Binaural fusion of low- and high-frequency sounds. *J Acoust Soc Am* 1958;30:222–223.

99. Nuetzel JM, Hafter ER. Lateralization of com-plex waveforms: effects of fine structure, am-plitude, and duration. *J Acoust Soc Am* 1976; 60:1339–1346.

100. Neutzel JM, Hafter ER. Lateralization of com-plex waveforms: spectral effects. *J Acoust Soc Am* 1981;69:1112–1118.

101. Crow G, Langford TL, Moushegian G. Coding of interaural time differences by some high-fre-quency neurons of the inferior colliculus: re-sponses to noise bands and two-tone com-plexes. *Hear Res* 1980;3:147–153.

102. De Ribaupierre F, Rouiller E, Toros A, De Ri-baupierre Y. Transmission delay of phase-locked cells in the medial geniculate body. *Hear Res* 1980;3:65–77.

103. Rouiller E, De Ribaupierre Y, De Ribaupierre F. Phase-locked responses to low frequency tones in the medial geniculate body. *Hear Res* 1979;1:213–226.

104. Roth GL, Aitkin LM, Anderson RA, Merzen-ich MM. Some features of the spatial organi-zation of the central nucleus of the inferior col-liculus of the cat. *J Comp Neurol* 1978;182: 661–680.

105. Blatchley BJ, Brugge JF. Sensitivity to binaural intensity and phase difference cues in kitten in-ferior colliculus. *J Neurophysiol* 1990;64:582–597.

106. Heffner H. Effect of auditory cortex ablation on localization and discrimination of brief sounds. *J Neurophysiol* 1978;41:963–976.

107. Ravizza RJ, Masterton RB. Contribution of neocortex to sound localization in opossum (Didelphis virginiana). *J Neurophysiol* 1972;35: 344–356.

108. Heffner HE, Masterton RB. Contribution of auditory cortex to sound localization in the monkey (Macaca mulatta). *J Neurophysiol* 1975;38:1340–1358.

109. Phillips DP. Temporal response features of cat auditory cortex neurons contributing to sensi-tivity to tones delivered in the presence of con-tinuous noise. *Hear Res* 1985;19:253–268.

110. Gibson DJ, Young ED, Costalupes JA. Similar-ity of dynamic range adjustment in auditory nerve and cochlear nuclei. *J Neurophysiol* 1985;53:940–958.

111. Kiang NYS, Moxon EC. Tails of tuning curves

of auditory nerve fibers. *J Acoust Soc Am* 1974;55:620–630.

112. Hawkins JE Jr, Stevens SS. The masking of pure tones and of speech by white noise. *J Acoust Soc Am* 1950;22:6–13.

113. Stevens SS, Guirao M. Loudness functions under inhibition. *Percept Psychophys* 1967;2:459–466.

114. Harrison RV. Rate-vs-intensity functions and related AP responses in normal and pathological guinea pig and human cochleas. *J Acoust Soc Am* 1981;70:1036–1044.

115. Harrison RV. The physiology of the normal and pathological cochlear neurones—some recent advances. *J Otolaryngol* 1985;14:345–356.

116. Harrison RV, Prijs VF. Single cochlear fiber responses in guinea pigs with longterm endolymphatic hydrops. *Hearing Res* 1984;14:79–84.

117. Brown KA, Buchwald JS, Johnson JR, Mikolich DJ. Vocalization in the cat and kitten. *Dev Psychobiol* 1978;11:559–570.

118. Kay RH. Hearing modulations in sound. *Physiol Rev* 1980;62:894–969.

119. Buchwald JS. Development of vocal communication in an experimental model. In: Friedman SL, Sigman M, eds. *Preterm birth and psychological development*. New York: Academic Press, 1981;107–126.

120. Margoliash D. Acoustic parameters underlying the response of song-specific neurons in the white-crowned sparrow. *J Neurosci* 1983;3:1029–1057.

121. Fuzessary ZM, Feng AS. Mating call selectivity in the thalamus and midbrain of the leopard frog (Rana p. pipiens): single and multiunit analyses. *J Comp Physiol* 1983;150:333–344.

122. Margoliash D, Konishi M. Auditory representation of autogenous song in the song-system of white-crowned sparrows. *Proc Natl Acad Sci USA* 1985;82:5997–6000.

123. Whitfield IC, Evans EF. Responses of auditory cortical neurons to stimuli of changing frequency. *J Neurophysiol* 1965;28:655–672.

124. Kim DO, Molnar CE. A population study of cochlear nerve fibers: comparison of spatial distributions of average rate and phase-locking measures of responses to single tones. *J Neurophysiol* 1979;42:16–30.

125. Young ED, Sachs MB. Representation of steady-state vowels in the temporal aspects of the discharge patterns of populations of auditory-nerve fibers. *J Acoust Soc Am* 1979;66:1381–1403.

126. Merzenich MM, Roth GL, Andersen RL, Knight PL, Colwell SA. Some basic features of organization of the central auditory nervous system. In: Evans EF, Wilson JP, eds. *Psychophysics and physiology of hearing*. New York: Academic Press, 1977;485–497.

127. Watanabe T, Katsuki Y. Response patterns of single auditory neurons of the cat to species-specific vocalizations. *Jpn J Physiol* 1974;24:135–155.

128. Manley JA, Muller-Preuss P. Response variability of auditory cortex cells in the squirrel

monkey to constant acoustic stimuli. *Exp Brain Res* 1978;32:171–180.

129. Newman JD, Symmes D. Feature detection by single units in squirrel monkey auditory cortex. *Exp Brain Res Suppl* 1979;2:140–145.

130. Wollberg Z, Newman JD. Auditory cortex of squirrel monkey: response patterns of single cells to species specific vocalizations. *Science* 1972;175:212–214.

131. Newman JD, Wollberg Z. Multiple coding of species-specific vocalizations in the auditory cortex of squirrel monkeys. *Brain Res* 1973;54:287–304.

132. Javel E. Coding of amplitude modulated tones in the chinchilla auditory nerve: implications for the pitch of complex tones. *J Acoust Soc Am* 1980;68:133–146.

133. Smith RL, Brachman ML. Adaptation in auditory nerve fibers: a revised model. *Biol Cybern* 1980;44:107–120.

134. Palmer AR. Encoding of rapid amplitude fluctuations by cochlear-nerve fibres in the guinea pig. *Arch Otolaryngol* 1982;236:197–202.

135. Fay RR. Psychophysics and neurophysiology of temporal factors in hearing by the goldfish: amplitude modulation detection. *J Neurophysiol* 1980;4:312–332.

136. Rose GJ, Capranica RR. Sensitivity to amplitude modulated sounds in the anuran auditory nervous system. *J Neurophysiol* 1985;53:446–465.

137. Rodenberg M. Investigations of temporal effects with amplitude modulated signals. In: Evans EF, Wilson JP, eds. *Psychophysics and physiology of hearing*. New York: Academic Press, 1977;429–439.

138. Viemeister NF. Temporal factors in audition: a system analysis approach. In: Evans EF, Wilson PJ, eds. *Psychophysics and physiology of hearing*. New York: Academic Press, 1977;419–428.

139. Small AM. Periodicity pitch. In: Tobias JV, ed. *Foundations of modern auditory theory, volume I*. New York: Academic Press, 1970;3–54.

140. Ritsma RJ. Frequencies dominant in the perception of the pitch of complex sounds. *J Acoust Soc Am* 1967;42:191–198.

141. Møller AR, Rees A. Dynamic properties of the responses of single neurons in the inferior colliculus of the rat. *Hear Res* 1986;24:203–215.

142. Erulkar SD, Butler RA, Gerstein GL. Excitation and inhibition in cochlear nucleus. II. Frequency modulated tones. *J Neurophysiol* 1968;31:537–548.

143. Phillips DP. Effect of tone-pulse rise time on rate-level functions of cat auditory cortex neurons: excitatory and inhibitory processes shaping responses to tone onset. *J Neurophysiol* 1988;59:1524–1539.

144. Phillips DP, Hall SE. Responses of single neurons in cat auditory cortex to time-varying stimuli: linear amplitude modulations. *Exp Brain Res* 1987;67:479–492.

145. Cutting JE, Rosner BS. Categories and bound-

aries in speech and music. *Percept Psychophys* 1974;16:564–570.

146. Blumstein SE, Stevens KN. Acoustic invariance in speech production: evidence from measurements of the spectral characteristics of stop consonants. *J Acoust Soc Am* 1979;66: 1001–1017.

147. Blumstein SE, Stevens KN. Perceptual invariance and onset spectra for stop consonants in different vowel environments. *J Acoust Soc Am* 1980;67:648–662.

148. Stevens KN. Acoustic correlates of some phonetic categories. *J Acoust Soc Am* 1980;68: 836–842.

149. Stevens KN, Blumstein SE. Invariant cues for place of articulation in stop consonants. *J Acoust Soc Am* 1978;64:1358–1368.

150. Møller AR. Dynamic properties of primary auditory fibers compared with cells in the cochlear nucleus. *Acta Physiol Scand* 1976;98: 157–167.

151. Schreiner CE, Langner G. Coding of temporal patterns in the central auditory nervous system. In: Edelman GM, Hassler S, Gall WM, eds. *Functions of the auditory system.* New York: Wiley, 1986.

152. Goldstein MH Jr, Kiang N-YS. Synchrony of neural activity in electric responses evoked by transient acoustic stimuli. *J Acoust Soc Am* 1958;30:107–114.

153. Schuller G. Coding of small sinusoidal frequency and amplitude modulations in the inferior colliculus of the "CF-FM" bat, Rhinolophus ferrumequinum. *Exp Brain Res* 1979;34: 117–132.

154. Møller AR. Responses of units in the cochlear nucleus to sinusoidally amplitude-modulated tones. *Exp Neurol* 1974;45:105–117.

155. Schreiner CE, Urbas JV. Representation of amplitude modulation in the auditory cortex of the cat. I. The anterior auditory field (AAF). *Hear Res* 1986;21:227–241.

156. Schreiner CE, Urbas JV. Representation of amplitude modulation in the auditory cortex of the cat. II. Comparison between cortical fields. *Hear Res* 1988;32:49–63.

157. Schreiner CE, Urbas JV, Mehrgardt S. Temporal resolution of amplitude modulation and complex signals in the auditory cortex of the cat. In: Klinke R, Hartman R, eds. *Hearing—physiological bases and psychophysics.* New York: Springer-Verlag, 1983;169–174.

158. Muller-Preuss P. On the mechanisms of call coding through auditory neurons in the squirrel monkey. *Eur Arch Psychiatry Neurol Sci* 1986; 236:50–55.

159. Rees A, Møller AR. Responses of neurons in the inferior colliculus of the rat to AM and FM tones. *Hear Res* 1983;10:301–330.

160. Rees A, Møller AR. Stimulus properties influencing the responses of inferior colliculus neurons to amplitude-modulated sounds. *Hear Res* 1987;27:129–143.

161. Nelson PG, Erulkar SD, Bryan JS. Responses of units of the inferior colliculus to time varying acoustic stimuli. *J Neurophysiol* 1966;29: 834–860.

162. Vartanyan IA. Impulse activity of neurons of rat's inferior colliculus in response to amplitude modulated sound signals. In: Gersuni GV, Rose J, eds. *Sensory processes at the neuronal and behavioral levels.* New York: Academic Press, 1971;210–219.

163. Gersuni GV, Vartanyan IA. Time-dependent features of adequate sound stimuli and the functional organization of central auditory neurons. In: Møller AR, ed. *Basic mechanisms in hearing.* New York: Academic Press, 1973; 623–673.

164. Rouiller E, De Ribaupierre F. Neurons sensitive to narrow ranges of repetitive acoustic transients in the medial geniculate body of the cat. *Exp Brain Res* 1982;48:323–326.

165. Godfrey DA, Kiang NYS, Norris BE. Single unit activity in the dorsal cochlear nucleus of the cat. *J Comp Neurol* 1975;162:269–284.

166. De Ribaupierre F, Goldstein MH Jr. Cortical coding of repetitive acoustic pulses. *Brain Res* 1972;48:205–225.

167. Møller AR. Unite responses in the rat cochlear nucleus to repetitive, transient sounds. *Acta Physiol Scand* 1969;75:542–551.

168. Bregman AS, Abramson J, Doehring P, Darwin CJ. Spectral integration based on common amplitude modulation. *Percept Psychophys* 1985; 37:483–493.

169. Plomp R. The role of modulation in hearing. In: Klinke R, Hartmann R, eds. *Hearing—physiological bases and psychophysics.* Berlin: Springer-Verlag, 1983;270–276.

170. Phillips DP, Irvine DR. Methodological considerations in mapping auditory cortex: binaural columnns in AI of cat. *Brain Res* 1979;161:342–346.

171. Suga N. Analysis of frequency-modulated and complex sounds by single auditory neurones of bats. *J Physiol (Lond)* 1968;198:51–80.

172. Watanabe T. Fundamental study of the neural mechanism in cats subserving the feature extraction process of complex sounds. *Jpn J Physiol* 1972;22:569–583.

173. Winter P, Ploog D, Latta J. Vocal repertoire of the squirrel monkey (Saimiri sciureus). *Exp Brain Res* 1966;1:359–384.

174. Watanabe T, Ohgushi K. FM sensitive auditory neuron. *Proc Jpn Acad* 1968;44:968–973.

175. Newman JD. Perception of sounds used in species-specific communication: the auditory cortex and beyond. *J Med Primatol* 1978;7:98–105.

176. Sinex DG, Geisler CD. Auditory-nerve fiber responses to frequency-modulated tones. *Hear Res* 1981;4:127–148.

177. Britt R, Starr A. Synaptic events and discharged patterns of cochlear nucleus cells. II. Frequency modulated tones. *J Neurophysiol* 1976;31:179–193.

178. Møller AR. Coding of amplitude and frequency modulated sounds in the cochlear nucleus of the rat. *Acta Physiol Scand* 1972;86:223–238.

179. Møller AR. Unit responses in the rat cochlear

nucleus to tones of rapidly varying frequency and amplitude. *Acta Physiol Scand* 1971;81: 540–556.

180. Nelson PG, Erulkar SD, Bryan BJS. Responses of units of the inferior colliculus to time-varying acoustic stimuli. *J Neurophysiol* 1966;29:834–860.

181. Bogdanski DF, Galambos R. Studies of the auditory system with implanted electrodes. In: Rasmussen GL, Windle WF, eds. *Neural mechanisms of the auditory and vestibular systems.* Springfield, IL: Charles C. Thomas, 1960;137–151.

182. Suga N. Recovery cycles and responses to frequency-modulated tone pulses in auditory neurones of echolocating bats. *J Physiol (Lond)* 1964;175:50–80.

183. Whitfield IC. The electrical responses of the unanesthetized auditory cortex in the intact cat. *Electroencephalogr Clin Neurophysiol* 1957;9:35–42.

184. Phillips DP, Mendelson JR, Cynader MS, Douglas RM. Responses of single neurones in cat auditory cortex to time-varying stimuli: frequency-modulated tones of narrow excursion. *Exp Brain Res* 1985;58:443–454.

185. Evans EF. Neural processes for the detection of acoustic pattern and for sound localization. In: Schmitt FO, Worden FG, eds. *Neurosciences. Third study program.* Cambridge, MA: MIT Press, 1974;131–145.

186. Kay RH, Matthews DR. On the existence in human auditory pathways of channels selectively tuned to the modulation present in frequency-modulated tones. *J Physiol (Lond)* 1972;225:657–678.

187. Young ED, Voight HF. Response properties of type II and type III units in the dorsal cochlear nucleus. *Hear Res* 1982;6:153–169.

188. Newman JD, Wollberg Z. Responses of single neurons in the auditory cortex of squirrel monkeys to variants of a single call type. *Exp Neurol* 1973;40:821–824.

189. Sovijarvi ARA. Detection of natural complex sounds by cells in the primary auditory cortex of the cat. *Acta Physiol Scand* 1975;93:318–335.

190. Winter P, Funkenstein HH. The effect of species-specific vocalization on the discharge of auditory cortical cells in the awake squirrel monkey (Saimiri sciureus). *Exp Brain Res* 1973;18:489–504.

191. Miller JM, Beaton RD, O'Connor T, Pfingst BE. Response pattern complexity of auditory cells in the cortex of unanesthetized monkeys. *Brain Res* 1974;69:101–113.

192. Steinschneider M, Arezzo J, Vaughan HG Jr. Speech evoked activity in the auditory radiations and cortex of the awake monkey. *Brain Res* 1982;252:353–365.

193. Glass I, Wollberg Z. Responses of cells in the auditory cortex of awake squirrel monkeys to normal and reversed species-specific vocalizations. *Hear Res* 1983;9:27–33.

194. Glass I, Wollberg Z. Auditory cortex responses to sequences of normal and reversed squirrel monkey vocalizations. *Brain Behav Evol* 1983; 22:13–21.

195. Rupert AL, Caspary DM, Moushegian G. Response characteristics of cochlear nucleus neurons to vowel sounds. *Ann Otol Rhinol Laryngol* 1977;86:37–48.

196. Watanabe T, Sakai H. Responses of the cat's collicular auditory neuron to human speech. *J Acoust Soc Am* 1978;64:333–337.

197. Moore TJ, Cashin JL Jr. Response patterns of cochlear nucleus neurons to excerpts from sustained vowels. *J Acoust Soc Am* 1974;56:1565–1576.

198. Butler RA, Diamond IT, Neff WD. Role of auditory cortex in discrimination of changes in frequency. *J Neurophysiol* 1957;20:108–120.

199. Kelly JB, Whitfield IC. Effects of auditory cortical lesions on discriminations of rising and falling frequency-modulated tones. *J Neurophysiol* 1971;34:802–816.

200. Thompson RF. Function of auditory cortex in frequency discrimination. *J Neurophysiol* 1960; 23:321–334.

201. Swisher L. Auditory intensity discrimination in patients with temporal-lobe damage. *Cortex* 1967;3:179–193.

202. Colavita FB, Szeligo FV, Zimmer SD. Temporal pattern discrimination in cats with insular-temporal lesions. *Brain Res* 1974;79:153–156.

203. Kaas J, Axelrod S, Diamond IT. An ablation study of the auditory cortex in the cat using binaural tonal patterns. *J Neurophysiol* 1967; 30:710–724.

204. Kelly JB. The effects of insular and temporal lesions in cats on two types of auditory pattern discrimination. *Brain Res* 1973;62:71–87.

205. Hupfer K, Jurgens U, Ploog D. The effect of superior temporal lesions on the recognition of species-specific calls in the squirrel monkey. *Exp Brain Res* 1977;30:75–87.

206. Hefner HE, Heffner RS. Effect of unilateral and bilateral auditory cortex lesions on the discrimination of vocalizations by Japanese macaques. *J Neurophysiol* 1986;56:683–701.

207. Heffner HE, Heffner RS. Temporal lobe lesions and perception of species-specific vocalizations by macaques. *Science* 1984;226:75–76.

208. Goldstein MN. Auditory agnosia for speech ("pure word deafness"). *Brain Lang* 1974;1: 195–204.

209. Metz-Lutz M-N, Dahl E. Analysis of word comprehension in a case of pure word deafness. *Brain Lang* 1984;23:13–25.

210. Albert ML, Bear D. Time to understand. A case study of word deafness with reference to the role of time in auditory comprehension. *Brain* 1974;97:373–384.

211. Miceli G. The processing of speech sounds in a patient with cortical auditory disorder. *Neuropsychologia* 1982;20:5–20.

212. Auerbach SH, Allard T, Naeser N, Alexander MP, Albert ML. Pure word deafness. Analysis of a case with bilateral lesions and a defect at

the prephonemic level. *Brain* 1982;105:271–300.

213. Rosati G, De Bastiani P, Paolina E, Prosser S, Arslan E, Artioli M. Clinical and audiological findings in a case of auditory agnosia. *J Neurol Neurosurg Psychiatry* 1982;227:21–27.

214. Saffran EM, Marin SM, Yeni-Komshian GH. An analysis of speech perception in word deafness. *Brain Lang* 1976;3:209–228.

215. von Stockert TR. On the structure of word deafness and mechanisms underlying the fluctuation of disturbances of higher cortical functions. *Brain Lang* 1982;16:133–146.

216. Suga N, Niwa H, Taniguchi I, Margoliash D. The personalized auditory cortex of the mustached bat: adaptation for echolocation. *J Neurophysiol* 1987;58:643–654.

217. Suga N, O'Neill WE, Kujirai K, Manabe T. Specificity of combination-sensitive neurons for processing of complex biosonar signals in auditory cortex of the mustached bat. *J Neurophysiol* 1983;49:1573–1626.

218. Phillips DP. Timing of spike discharges in cat auditory cortex neurons: implications for encoding of stimulus periodicity. *Hear Res* 1989; 40:137–146.

219. Phillips DP, Hall SE. Response timing constraints on the cortical representation of sound time structure. *J Acoust Soc Am* 1990;88:1403–1411.

220. Steinschneider M, Arezzo J, Vaughan HG Jr. Phase-locked cortical responses to a human speech sound and low-frequency tones in the monkey. *Brain Res* 1980;198:75–84.

221. Rhode WS, Smith PH. Encoding timing and intensity in the ventral cochlear nucleus of the cat. *J Neurophysiol* 1986;56:261–286.

222. Delgutte B. Representation of speech-like sounds in the discharge patterns of auditory-nerve fibers. *J Acoust Soc Am* 1980;68:843–857.

223. Carney LH, Geisler CD. A temporal analysis of auditory-nerve fiber responses to spoken stop consonant-vowel syllables. *J Acoust Soc Am* 1986;79:1896–1914.

224. Palmer AR, Winter IM, Darwin CJ. The representation of steady-state vowel sounds in the temporal discharge patterns of the guinea pig cochlear nerve and primarylike cochlear nucleus neurons. *J Acoust Soc Am* 1986;79:100–113.

225. Cranford JL. Auditory cortex lesions and interaural intensity and phase-angle discrimination in cats. *J Neurophysiol* 1979;42:1518–1526.

226. Phillips DP, Farmer ME. Acquired word deafness, and the temporal grain of sound representation in the primary auditory cortex. *Behav Brain Res* 1990;40:85–94.

227. Hubel DH, Henson CO, Rupert A, Galambos R. "Attention" units in the auditory cortex. *Science* 1959;129:1279–1280.

228. Phillips DP, Calford MB, Pettigrew JD, Aitkin LM, Semple MN. Directionality of sound pressure transformation at the cat's pinna. *Hear Res* 1982;8:13–28.

229. Musicant AD, Chan JCK, Hind JE. Direction-dependent spectral properties of cat external ear: new data and cross-species comparisons. *J Acoust Soc Am* 1990;87:757–781.

230. Glass I, Wollberg Z. Lability in the responses of cells in the auditory cortex of squirrel monkeys to species-specific vocalizations. *Exp Brain Res* 1979;34:489–498.

231. Pfingst BE, O'Connor TA. Characteristics of neurons in auditory cortex of monkeys performing a simple auditory task. *J Neurophysiol* 1981;45:16–34.

232. Miller JM, Dobie RA, Pfingst BE, Hienz RD. Electrophysiologic studies of the auditory cortex in the awake monkey. *Am J Otolaryngol* 1980;1:119–130.

233. Weinberger NM, Diamond DM. Physiological plasticity in auditory cortex: rapid induction by learning. *Prog Neurobiol* 1987;29:1–55.

234. Beaton R, Miller JF. Single cell activity in the auditory cortex of the unanesthetized, behaving monkey: correlation with stimulus controlled behavior. *Brain Res* 1975;100:543–562.

235. Benson DA, Hienz RD. Single-unit activity in the auditory cortex of monkeys selectively attending left vs. right ear stimuli. *Brain Res* 1978;159:307–320.

236. Pfingst BE, O'Connor TA, Miller JM. Response plasticity of neurons in auditory cortex of the rhesus monkey. *Exp Brain Res* 1977; 29:393–404.

237. Kraus N, Disterhoft JF. Response plasticity of single neurons in rabbit auditory association cortex during tone-signalled learning. *Brain Res* 1982;246:205–215.

238. Miller JM, Sutton D, Pfingst B, Ryan A, Beaton R, Gourevitch G. Single cell activity in the auditory cortex of rhesus monkeys: behavioral dependency. *Science* 1972;177:449–451.

239. Benson DA, Hienz RD, Goldstein MH Jr. Single-unit activity in the auditory cortex of monkeys actively localizing sound sources: spatial tuning and behavioral dependency. *Brain Res* 1981;219:249–267.

240. Orman SS, Humphrey GL. Effects of changes in cortical arousal and of auditory cortex cooling on neuronal activity in the medial geniculate body. *Exp Brain Res* 1981;42:475–482.

241. Weinberger NM, Hopkins W, Diamond DM. Physiological plasticity of single neurons in auditory cortex of the cat during acquisition of the pupillary conditioned response: I. Primary field (AI). *Behav Neurosci* 1984;98:171–188.

242. Hocherman S, Benson DA, Goldstein MH Jr, Heffner HE, Hienz RD. Evoked unit activity in auditory cortex of monkeys performing a selective attention task. *Brain Res* 1976;117:51–68.

243. Kitzes LM, Farley GR, Starr A. Modulation of auditory cortex unit activity during the performance of a conditioned response. *Exp Neurol* 1978;62:678–697.

244. Hocherman S, Itzhaki A, Gilat E. The response of single units in the auditory cortex of rhesus monkeys to predicted and to unpredicted sound stimuli. *Brain Res* 1981;230:65–86.

245. Kuwada S, Stanford TR, Batra R. Interaural phase-sensitive units in the inferior colliculus of the unanesthetized rabbit: effects of changing frequency. *J Neurophysiol* 1987;57:1338–1360.

246. Newman JD, Symmes D. Arousal effects on unit responsiveness in squirrel monkey auditory cortex. *Brain Res* 1974;78:125–138.

247. Imig TJ, Weinberger NM, Westenberg IS. Relationships among unit discharge rate, pattern, and phasic arousal in the medial geniculate nucleus of the waking cat. *Exp Neurol* 1972; 35:337–357.

248. Gabriel M, Saltwick SE, Miller JD. Conditioning and reversal of short-latency multiple-unit responses in the rabbit medial geniculate nucleus. *Science* 1975;189:1108–1109.

249. Humphrey GL, Orman SS. Activity of the auditory system related to cortical arousal. *Exp Neurol* 1977;55:520–537.

250. Oleson TD, Ashe JH, Weinberger NM. Modification of auditory and somatosensory system activity during pupillary conditioning in the paralyzed cat. *J Neurophysiol* 1975;38:1114–1139.

251. Ryan A, Miller J. Effects of behavioral performance on single-unit firing patterns in inferior colliculus of the rhesus monkey. *J Neurophysiol* 1977;40:943–956.

252. Ryugo DK, Weinberger NM. Differential plasticity of morphologically distinct neuron populations in the medial geniculate body of the cat during classical conditioning. *Behav Neural Biol* 1978;22:275–301.

253. Graybiel AM. Some fiber pathways related to the posterior thalamic region in the cat. *Brain Behav Evol* 1972;6:363–393.

254. Graybiel AM. The thalamocortical projection of the so-called posterior nuclear group: a study with anterograde degeneration methods in the cat. *Brain Res* 1973;49:229–244.

255. Andersen RA, Roth GL, Aitkin LM, Merzenich MM. The efferent projections of the central nucleus and the pericentral nucleus of the inferior colliculus in the cat. *J Comp Neurol* 1980;194:649–662.

256. Diamond DM, Weinberger NM. Physiological plasticity of single neurons in auditory cortex of the cat during acquisition of the pupillary conditioned response: II. Secondary field (AII). *Behav Neurosci* 1984;98:189–210.

257. Vaadia E, Benson DA, Hienz RD, Goldstein MH Jr. Unit study of monkey frontal cortex: active localization of auditory and of visual stimuli. *J Neurophysiol* 1986;56:934–952.

258. Schreiner CE, Cynader MS. Basic functional organization of second auditory cortical field (AII) of the cat. *J Neurophysiol* 1984;51:1284–1305.

259. Webster WR, Aitkin LM. Central auditory processing. In: Gazzaniga M, Blakemore C, eds. *Handbook of psychobiology*. New York: Academic Press, 1975;325–364.

260. Merzenich MM, Kaas JH. Principles of organization of sensory-perceptual systems in mammals. In: Sprague JM, Epstein AN, eds. *Progress in psychobiology and physiological psychology, volume 9*. New York: Academic Press, 1980;1–42.

261. Stone J, Dreher B, Leventhal A. Hierarchical and parallel mechanisms in the organization of visual cortex. *Brain Res Rev* 1979;1:345–394.

262. Andersen RA, Knight PL, Merzenich MM. The thalamocortical and corticothalamic connections of AI, AII, and the anterior auditory field (AAF) in the cat: evidence for two largely segregated systems of connections. *J Comp Neurol* 1980;194:663–701.

263. Delgutte B, Kiang NYS. Speech coding in the auditory nerve. IV. Sounds with consonant-like dynamic characteristics. *J Acoust Soc Am* 1984;75:897–907.

264. Brugge JF, Anderson DJ, Aitkin LM. Responses of neurons in the dorsal nucleus of the lateral lemniscus of cat to binaural tonal stimulation. *J Neurophysiol* 1970;33:441–458.

265. Brugge JF, Blatchley B. Encoding of amplitude-modulated tones by neurons of the inferior colliculus of kitten (abstract). *Association for Research in Otolaryngology*, 12th annual meeting, 1989.

266. Symmes D. On the use of natural stimuli in neurophysiological studies of audition. *Hear Res* 1981;4:203–214.

Neurobiology of Hearing: The Central Auditory System, edited by R. A. Altschuler et al.
Raven Press, Ltd., New York © 1991.

14

Cellular Organization of the Cat's Auditory Cortex

Donald Wong

Departments of Anatomy and of Otolaryngology and Head-Neck Surgery, Indiana University School of Medicine, Indianapolis, Indiana 46202-5120

A precise identification of areas in the cerebral cortex that subserve specific functions typically requires a combination of experimental approaches. Like other sensory cortices, the auditory cortex has been defined according to such anatomical criteria as cytoarchitecture, topographical organization, and connectivity and such neurophysiological criteria as evoked potentials and single-unit mapping studies. The historical background leading to the development of our current definition of the auditory cortex is not recapitulated in this chapter, since such coverage is already found in a number of reviews (6,17,87). Over the past decade more detailed single-unit mapping of the auditory cortex has revealed numerous functional subregions with varying degrees of tonotopic order (58). Co-extensive with a part of this tonotopic organization is a functional organization according to ear dominance and binaural interaction (23,44). To delineate the connectional patterns of these functional maps, neuroanatomical tracing methods were further incorporated into electrophysiological mapping experiments (24,27,28).

This review focuses on the cellular organization of the cat's auditory cortex since the cytoarchitecture, laminar organization, and synaptic connections of the auditory cortex have not to date received the atten-tion appropriate to their importance. A cellular perspective on the auditory cortex provides a basis for comparing the organizational schemes among the sensory cortices. The interconnections between specific functional subregions of auditory cortex may also provide insights into the possible stages of cortical processing important for generating auditory perception.

First, this chapter presents a brief description of the anatomical location of the parts of the cat's auditory cortex that have been known for several decades. The functional organization as determined by tonotopy is then introduced (the previous chapter by Phillips et al. covers sound processing as it relates to functional organization) since these functional subregions and their borders currently provide the clearest and most precise location of the different auditory cortical subregions. The thalamocortical connections are not discussed here since excellent reviews already exist (e.g., see ref. 25 for review), and the cortical connections as they relate to the neuronal architecture of the medial geniculate body are described in another chapter (see chapter by Winer). The laminar organization and connections of the auditory cortex are related to both frequency analysis and binaural processing. Hence, this chapter reviews the cellular organization, corticocortical connectivity, and related functions of the auditory cortex.

LOCATION OF THE AUDITORY CORTEX

The location of the primary auditory cortex (AI) and its surrounding belt of auditory subregions was defined in the cat by a number of anatomical and physiological criteria: cytoarchitecture (60), thalamic connections (61), and evoked potentials (see ref. 87 for review). The auditory cortex is located on the lateral surface of the brain and is generally described with respect to the ectosylvian gyri and associated sulci (Fig. 1). About half of the auditory cortex is exposed on the ectosylvian gyri with the remaining part extending into the banks of the suprasylvian, anterior ectosylvian and posterior ectosylvian sulci. AI lies across the middle ectosylvian gyrus, extending caudally into the banks of the dorsal tip of the posterior ectosylvian sulcus and into a small part of the posterior ectosylvian gyrus. In the rostral part of AI, the ventral border extends to the tip of the anterior ectosylvian sulcus. Ventral to AI lies the secondary auditory cortex (AII) and posterior to both AI and AII on the posterior ectosylvian gyrus is another auditory zone, originally termed Ep by Ades (2).

The first functional maps in which the auditory cortex was parceled into individual subregions were derived from a number of evoked-potential studies (19,61,87). These electrophysiological studies provided the foundation for all subsequent single-unit mapping studies. Evoked-potential studies revealed a cochleotopic representation in AI: high sound frequencies processed by the more basal part of the cochlea are represented in the more rostral part of AI and low sound frequencies by the more apical part of the cochlea are represented in the more caudal part of AI (88). In cortical regions adjoining the primary area, a separate cochleotopic representation, and hence fre-

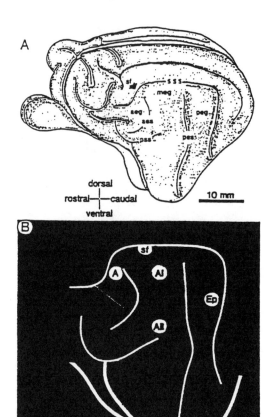

FIG. 1. A and **B:** General location of the cat's auditory cortex with respect to the gyral and sulcal pattern on the lateral surface of the cerebral cortex. The primary auditory cortex (AI) is located in the middle ectosylvian gyrus (meg). The AII subregion lies ventral to AI and occupies part of the meg between the anterior ectosylvian sulcus (aes), posterior ectosylvian sulcus (pes), and pseudosylvian sulcus (pss). The anterior (A) subregion occupies part of the anterior ectosylvian gyrus (aeg) and the Ep subregion occupies part of the posterior ectosylvian gyrus (peg). The suprasylvian fringe (sf) is deep in the banks of the suprasylvian sulcus (sss). (Modified from ref. 74, with permission.)

quency axis, was also deduced by Woolsey (87) on the basis of evoked-potential maps of other investigators.

Although zones mapped by evoked potentials were consistent with cytoarchitectonically defined fields (60), precise tonotopic organization was definitively demonstrated first by Merzenich et al. (43) in mapping characteristic frequencies of single and multiple units. More importantly, these cellular mapping experiments revealed the functional borders and, hence, the areal extent of AI. The definition of the different subregions with reference to the visible sulcal pattern, which served in the past as a principal guide for subdividing the auditory cortex, was found to be unreliable due to wide variation of these anatomical landmarks from animal to animal.

The comprehensive frequency-mapping study by Reale and Imig (58) is the basis for our current knowledge of the multiple tonotopic subregions constituting much of the auditory cortex. Four distinct regions of the auditory cortex are known to be tonotopically organized with complete representation of best frequency: primary (AI), anterior (A) (originally defined as AAF [anterior auditory field] by Knight [39]), posterior (P), and ventroposterior (VP) fields (Fig. 2). P and VP are caudal and ventral to AI, mostly in the banks of the posterior ectosylvian sulcus (both forming part of Ep as originally mapped by Woolsey [87]). The anterior field adjoins AI at its rostral border, occupying the anterior ectosylvian gyrus, the rostral part of the middle ectosylvian gyrus, and extending into the adjoining part of the suprasylvian sulcus. AI occupies mainly the middle ectosylvian gyrus, a central location with respect to the surrounding auditory cortical region. The highest best frequency of both A and AI are represented at the A/AI border. Progressively lower best frequencies in A are represented more rostroventrally along the anterior ectosylvian gyrus, and in AI are represented more caudally along the middle ectosylvian gyrus. Dorsoventrally oriented isofrequency contours, first detailed in AI by Merzenich et al. (43), traverse an expanse of 4 to 7 mm of the middle ectosylvian gyrus. The lowest best frequencies of AI and P are contiguously represented at the AI/P border. Moreover, AII is not simply defined as the

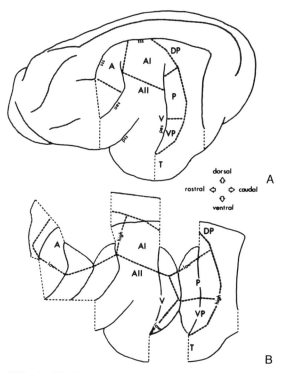

FIG. 2. Fields comprising the cat's auditory cortex as defined by electrophysiological mapping of single neurons according to their best frequency. The auditory fields and their physiological borders are shown on the cortical surface (**A**) and on an unfolded cortex exposing the sulcal banks (**B**). *Heavy dotted lines* show the borders of tonotopic fields where the high and low frequencies are represented. Dorsoposterior (DP), posterior (P), ventroposterior (VP), and temporal (T) auditory fields. (From ref. 27, with permission.)

region immediately ventral to AI and between the anterior and posterior ectosylvian sulci as originally described by Woolsey (87). Reale and Imig (58) further subdivided this ventral region into two parts: AII located in the rostral part of the middle ectosylvian gyrus and a ventral auditory area (V) along the caudal part of the middle ectosylvian gyrus and extending into the rostral bank of the posterior ectosylvian sulcus. Since AII neurons exhibit broad frequency tuning and multiple best frequencies, the determination of a precise tonotopy was not possible in AII. AII extends at least 4 mm ventrally from the AI/ AII border. Area V is tonotopically organized, but its frequency representation often shows no fixed relationship with respect to the representation of other tonotopic fields (A, AI, P, VP). The auditory belt surrounding AI also contains two areas not well mapped: a dorsoposterior (DP) area, named by its relative location to AI, and the temporal area (T) located in the most ventral part of Ep.

The multiple tonotopic regions of the auditory cortex form a crescent-shaped region in the ectosylvian cortex ventral to the suprasylvian sulcus. Surrounding these multiple tonotopic zones is a belt of auditory cortex consisting of AII, DP, V, and T subregions. These belt regions are identifiable from physiological mapping studies and, with the possible exception of V, have no clear tonotopy. A region along the dorsal margin of AI, referred to as the dorsal zone (DZ) by Middlebrooks and Zook (47), is distinguishable from AI by its frequency specificity and binaural responses. The DZ region may refer to the same region that Reale and Imig (58) mapped as the DP field (see previously).

LAMINAR ORGANIZATION OF THE PRIMARY AUDITORY CORTEX

The neocortex is a laminated structure and functionally distinct regions often exhibit clear anatomical differences in their cytoarchitecture (56). A sharp cytoarchitectonic border demarcating areas 17–18 in the primate visual cortex is one of the most striking examples in the cerebral cortex (21,22). In a classic Nissl study of the cat's auditory cortex, Rose (60) distinguished the AI area from the suprasylvian-fringe (SF) area, AII, and Ep, subregions all forming a belt around AI. A characteristic cytoarchitectonic feature of AI is that layers II–IV are indistinguishable in Nissl-stained coronal sections, since the cellular population in these layers appear fairly uniform in den-

sity (60). In the Nissl-stained coronal sections, the relatively cell-sparse layer V appears as a lightly stained band. These features distinguish AI from other primary sensory cortices. Delineating the cytoarchitectonic borders of AI from the surrounding auditory belt is often difficult, since lamination and the relative contribution of different cell-types often change gradually across the borders of contiguous regions.

Winer (74–77) has provided an extensive analysis of the laminar organization of the cat's AI based on architectonic studies in Nissl, Golgi, and fiber preparations. Distinguishing the individual layers of AI is greatly facilitated when preparations stained from several techniques are compared. In AI of the cat, the six layers make up a thickness of about 2 mm (Fig. 3). Each layer can be divided into an inner and an outer half. Layer I is cell sparse, consisting mainly of neuropil. On the basis of its fiber architecture, this layer can be further subdivided into a superficial (Ia) and a deeper (Ib) stratum. Layer Ia contains many myelinated axons and few ascending dendritic branches, whereas layer Ib contains many unmyelinated axons along with more extensive apical dendrites from the deeper layers (66,68).

Winer delineated several of the layers according to the cytoarchitectonic criteria originally used by Rose (60) and described in more detail the laminar distribution of distinctive cell-types. These morphological cell-types and laminar location were further confirmed in an electrophysiological study in which intracellular injections of horseradish peroxidase (HRP) were made into AI cells after electrical stimulation from a number of brain regions (49). In general, the border between layers II and III in AI is characterized by a difference in the number of pyramidal cells. In Nissl-stained preparations, layer II contains a large population of small nonpyramidal cells with round or flask-shaped somata. The few pyramidal cells in layer II are smaller and have less elaborate dendritic arbors than

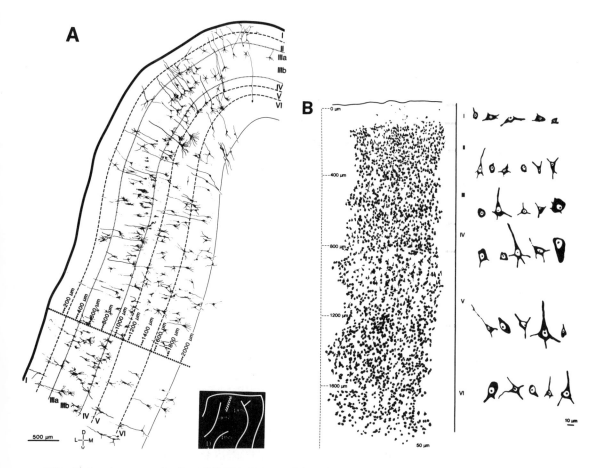

FIG. 3. Laminar organization of the six layers of the primary auditory cortex (AI). **A:** The representative cell-types of each layer are drawn from the Nissl-stained tissue. Inset shows the location where the coronal section was cut in AI. (From ref. 75, with permission.) **B:** The packing density and representative cell-types are drawn from Golgi-impregnated tissue. (From ref. 74, with permission.)

those in layer III. The medium-sized pyramidal cells mark the border between layers II and III. Layer III, about 400 μm in thickness, is the thickest layer of AI. Numerous pyramidal cells of various sizes are found in this layer along with a sizable proportion of morphologically diverse nonpyramidal cells. The nonpyramidal cells in layer III include tufted cells, bipolar cells, multipolar cells, and several kinds of stellate cells. Layer III can be subdivided further into two tiers (IIIa, IIIb) of about equal thickness. Small cells with oval-shaped somata and numerous small pyramidal cells prevail in layer IIIa, while medium-sized

and large pyramidal cells are more common in layer IIIb, where their laterally directed basal dendrites often demarcate the layer IIIb/IV border. Most layer-III pyramidal cells have tangentially directed basal dendrites aligned along the dorsoventrally oriented isofrequency contours, whereas the nonpyramidal cells have dendritic fields that are spheroidal and less polarized vertically than those found in layer IV.

Layer IV is a thin lamina (200–250 μm thick) consisting mainly of small, densely packed nonpyramidal neurons that are often aligned in vertical columns. Although pyramidal cells encroach onto layer IV from both above and below, few pyramidal cells actually reside in layer IV.

A feature of AI, particularly in layer IV, is the *pronounced* vertical disposition of the dendritic and axonal fields of most cells (74). This columnar arrangement, long known to exist throughout the cerebral cortex (e.g., see ref. 73), appears more highly developed in Golgi preparations of the auditory cortex than of other cortical areas. The morphological polarization of neurons has been observed in newborn cats as young as 1 month where the somata in layers III to VI are arranged in slender rows, whereas alternating columns of somata and neuropil 50 to 75 μm wide are found in the adult.

A dominant feature of layer V, much like layer III, is the presence of numerous pyramidal cells, some of which are the largest neurons in AI; a significant number of these also have an inverted orientation. An outer, cell-sparse but fiber-rich zone (Va) is distinct from the inner, more densely packed half (Vb). Layer VI contains large cell-free zones filled with myelinated axons that are accentuated by clusters of pyramidal, modified pyramidal, and horizontally oriented nonpyramidal cells.

The laminar cytoarchitecture is complemented by a myeloarchitecture where axonal profiles become increasingly dense from layer II to III. There are few myelinated fibers in layer II in toluidine-blue stained or reduced-silver preparations. The myeloarchitecture of IIIa is dominated by radial bundles of medium-sized axons that are interspersed among columns of apical dendrites arising from deeper lying pyramidal cells. A denser texture is found in the fiber architecture of IIIb with more lateral-running profiles. Hence, a radial organization is evident in layer-III fibers in silver preparations, with the large vertical fascicles prevailing over the finer fibers of the horizontally oriented plexus (Fig. 4). Still deeper across the IIIb/IV border, the number of small axons traversing obliquely is diminished and replaced with a dramatic increase of a plexus consisting of laterally directed fibers.

A population of relatively large ascending axons, often Golgi-impregnated in layers IIIb and IVa, may be of thalamic origin. Layers III and IV of the cat AI are known to be the principal thalamic-recipient layers (54,67,84). Layer I also receives a sparse geniculocortical projection. Autoradiographic studies involving injections of tritiated amino acids into the ventral medial geniculate body (MGB) have revealed labeling of thalamocortical terminals and preterminals in bands as broad as 675 μm thick in layers III and IV (84). The specific morphological cell-types receiving direct MGB projections were identified by Mitani and co-workers (48,49) in intracellular recordings and labeling of AI neurons after subcortical electrical stimulation. Fast-conducting MGB-fibers were found to project monosynaptically to stellate, tufted, and fusiform cells in layer IV and slow-conducting MGB-fibers to project to horizontal cells in layer I.

PATTERNS OF CORTICOTHALAMIC AND CORTICOTECTAL PROJECTIONS

The pattern of subcortical connections provides another important basis for the parcellation of the auditory cortex into distinct subregions. A distinctive pattern of connections exists between each subregion of auditory cortex and the cytoarchitectonic subdivisions of the MGB. The specific MGB subdivisions (as defined by Morest [51,52]) that give rise to thalamocortical projections or receive corticothalamic projections were determined by tract-tracing studies, in which anterograde and retrograde labels were injected into individual subregions defined by cytoarchitecture (37,79) or physiological mapping (3,50). In anterograde tracing of corticothalamic projections from frequency-mapped cortical zones, Andersen et al. (3) found that both AI and A project to the vertical division of

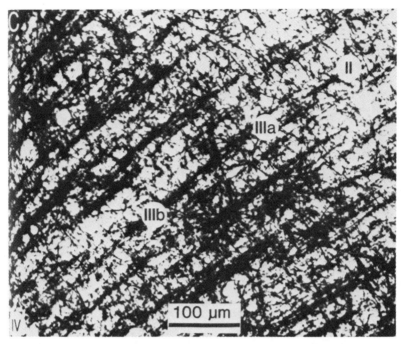

FIG. 4. Myeloarchitecture of layer III in the primary auditory cortex. A radial organization is apparent in the vertically oriented fascicles of fibers in layer III against a fine plexus of laterally directed fibers. Liesegang stain of 30-μm-thick coronal section. (From ref. 75, with permission.)

the MGB (connections with ventral MGB more extensive with AI than with A), with smaller projections to the deep dorsal nucleus (Dd), medial division (M), and lateral division of the posterior thalamic group (POl). Corticothalamic projections of AII terminate in the caudal dorsal nucleus (Dc), the ventral lateral nucleus (VL), and the medial division (M). Morel and Imig (50) revealed from tracing thalamocortical projections that each of the four tonotopic fields, A, AI, P, VP, has its distinctive set of connections with both tonotopic and nontonotopic thalamic subnuclei. Segregated regions of both tonotopically organized ventral nucleus of the MGB and POl provide a major projection to one cortical field and minor projections to one or more other fields. This pattern of thalamocortical projections is likely matched by a similar pattern of corticothalamic projections as Andersen et al. (3) demonstrated.

Andersen et al. (3) proposed two func-tionally distinct and segregated systems of connections between the auditory thalamus and cortex: a *cochleotopic system* consisting of neurons sharply tuned to sound frequency, and a *diffuse system* consisting of broadly tuned neurons. The cochleotopic system includes the connections between more rostral subdivisions of the MGB (e.g., laminated part of ventral division, deep dorsal and medial divisions) and tonotopically organized AI, A, P, and VP cortical areas. In contrast, the diffuse system is characterized by a pattern of connections between more caudal parts of the MGB (e.g., Dc, VL, and M) and such cortical areas as AII and T.

Several subregions of the auditory cortex also are distinguishable on the basis of their differential pattern of corticotectal projections. In anterograde tracing studies with tracer injections made into physiologically identified cortical loci, terminal labeling of fibers from areas AI, A, and AII to the in-

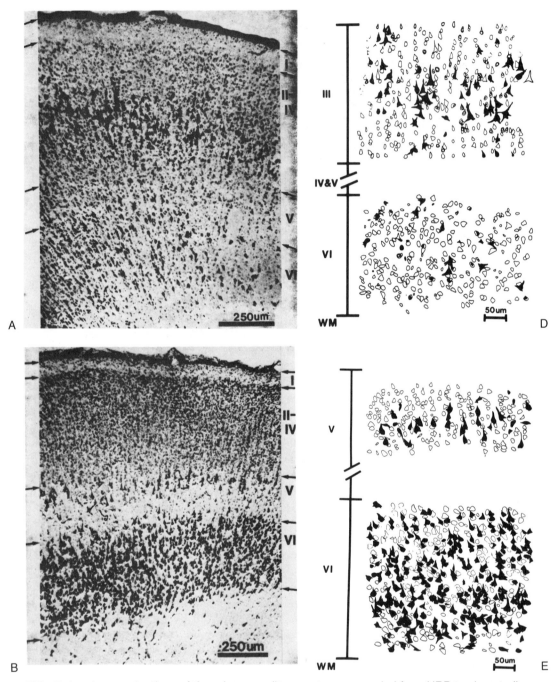

FIG. 5. Laminar connections of the primary auditory cortex as revealed from HRP-tracing studies. Callosal cells (**A,D**) connecting the primary auditory cortex of both cerebral hemisphere, cortico-thalamic cells (**B,E**) projecting to the ipsilateral medial geniculate body, and cortico-collicular cells (**C,F**) projecting to the ipsilateral inferior colliculus are shown. Camera-lucida drawings of the layers with HRP-labeled cells (*darkened*) are shown on the right. Length of rectangle in C is 750 μm. Coronally cut frozen sections reacted with tetramethylbenzidine and counterstained with thionin. (From ref. 37, with permission.) (*Figure continues.*)

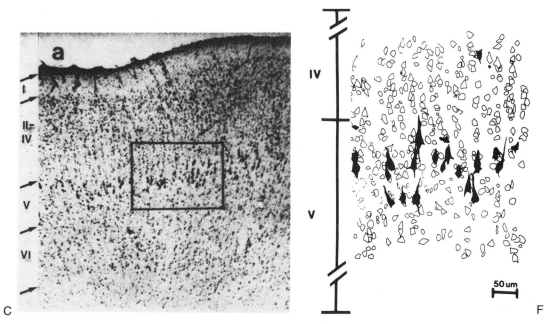

FIG. 5. *Continued.*

ferior colliculus was determined (4). AI sends fibers that terminate in the caudal part of the inferior colliculus: the dorso-medial division of the central nucleus bilaterally and the pericentral nucleus ipsilaterally. Area A exhibits a similar, but weaker, cortico-collicular projection than AI. These corticotectal projections are topographically organized with respect to the orderly frequency maps in A and AI. AII projections to the inferior colliculus terminate ipsilaterally in the lateral part of, and bilaterally in the medial part of, the pericentral nucleus. While the corticotectal projections from AI are systematically arranged according to sound frequency, the AII projections to the colliculus are more diffuse. Hence, the subcortical projections, to both the MGB and inferior colliculus, reflect the frequency organization of cortical fields where these fibers arise.

Laminar Origin of Subcortical Projections

The laminar origin in AI of corticofugal cells was first described on the basis of ret-rograde cell-labeling with HRP (37). Corti-cothalamic cells originate from both layers V and VI (Fig. 5B, E). A distinct population of cells, including relatively large pyramidal cells in the outer rim of layer V, project from AI to the ventral MGB. In contrast, the inner rim of layer V (Vb as described by Winer [74]) is almost free of corticogeniculate cells (cf. ref. 49). Most of the corticogeniculate projections from AI, however, arise from layer VI, where about 50% of the cells project to the ventral MGB. These corticofugal cells are small pyramidal or fusiform in morphology (37).

The large pyramidal cells (about 20 μm in diameter) located in the outer rim of layer V also project to the central nucleus of the inferior colliculus (Fig. 5C, F). Although this population of cortico-collicular cells is co-extensive with the population of corticogeniculate cells, no pyramidal cells in the outer rim of layer V were double labeled in studies using HRP and fluorescent dyes to determine whether dually projecting cells exist in a single layer (85). The ratio of corticogeniculate to cortico-collicular cells in layer V is about 1:1.

The double-labeling studies also did not reveal dually projecting cells among the corticogeniculate and callosal cells (see below) in layer VI (85). A relatively large number of corticogeniculate cells are distributed homogeneously along the horizontal axis of layer VI, while a much smaller number of callosal cells are scattered among them. The corticogeniculate cells in layer VI are relatively uniform in size, consisting mainly of small pyramidal cells (10–15 μm in diameter), each with several basal dendrites and a single apical dendrite. A small number of corticogeniculate cells have round somata and several radiating processes. The callosal cells are generally located more superficial than the corticogeniculate cells. The ratio of corticogeniculate to callosal cells in layer VI is about 5.5:1. Thus, individual layers in the cat's auditory cortex may project to more than one site. In layer V or VI of AI, dual projections arise from separate populations of neurons that overlap topographically but have distinctive patterns of projections.

CORTICO-CORTICAL CONNECTIONS

Associational and Callosal Connections of Tonotopic Regions

The efferent cortico-cortical connections of tonotopically organized subregions of the auditory cortex, both associational and callosal, have been traced anatomically after injections of anterograde tracers within electrophysiologically defined tonotopic zones (27). Fields A, AI, P, and VP all receive inputs converging from other auditory fields in the same hemisphere. These tonotopically organized areas provide callosal projections to one or more tonotopic areas of the contralateral hemisphere so that regions representing similar best frequencies are interconnected. When a single cortical injection is placed within a tonotopic area, multiple patches of anterograde labeling are often found in several functionally defined

fields both ipsilaterally and contralaterally. Such a pattern of labeled terminals suggests that cortico-cortical neurons give rise to divergent projections even within a single target area, typically distributed in a cortical band along an isofrequency contour. The association connections of A, AI, P, and VP are reciprocal, with adjacent fields more strongly connected than more distant fields (e.g., ipsilateral connections between A and VP are sparse). Callosal connections are stronger between homotypic than heterotypic regions. The tonotopically organized regions also project to several areas of the surrounding auditory belt. For example, AII is reciprocally interconnected with these multiple tonotopic zones. The complex network of interconnections suggests that a greater functional cooperation exists between adjoining regions than between more widely separated regions.

Laminar Pattern of Cortico-Cortical Connections

The laminar distribution of callosal cells has been examined with retrograde cell-labeling after HRP injection into the auditory cortex (Fig. 5A, D). Imig and Brugge (24) initially reported callosal cells in AI that originate from two tiers, mainly from layers III and IV with relatively few callosal cells from layers V–VI. Kelly and Wong (37) attributed over three-quarters of the callosal cells to layer III and the remaining population of callosal cells to layer VI. On the basis of connectional studies of AI, Code and Winer (8,9) argued that few if any callosal cells originate from layer IV since the pyramidal cells labeled in the more superficial tier are likely to be almost exclusively in layer IIIb, a layer dominated by pyramidal cells of varying sizes. The pyramidal neurons at the III/IV border are likely to have processes encroaching into layer IV but somata actually located in layer IIIb. Morphologically diverse callosal cells originate from layer III of AI and include both pyramidal and nonpyramidal cells (8,37,49). When correlated with Golgi material, about two-thirds of the callosal cells are pyramidal (8). A much smaller percentage of callosal cells of varying morphology is found in layers V and VI. Even though combined electrophysiological-neuroanatomical tracing studies have mapped functionally distinct binaural bands and have correlated their location with reference to zones containing callosal cells and terminals (24), the morphological cell-types and laminar position of cortical neurons exhibiting a particular aural dominance are still not well understood.

The callosal cells are not homogeneously distributed in these layers but rather form clusters between zones relatively free of these cells (24,37). These clusters are more evident in layer III, spanning up to 1,100 μm along the horizontal extent of the layer, with areas some 500 μm wide between the clusters of far fewer callosal cells (Fig. 6a). The clustered pattern in layer III is not as distinctive in layer VI, where the callosal-cell population is relatively small.

Autoradiographic studies have revealed that callosal axons also terminate in irregular patches within AI after contralateral AI injections of tritiated amino acids (9, 24,29,37). Patches of labeled terminals form a complex topography on the cortical surface when examined in tangentially cut sections (24). A laminar analysis of coronal sections showed that these terminal fields form radial patches oriented orthogonally to the pial surface (9,37). In contrast to the two-tier origin of callosal-cell clusters, callosal axons project to all cortical layers of AI and, hence, to layers without callosal cells. Although it is not possible to distinguish preterminals from terminals in light microscopic autoradiography, many callosal axons appear to terminate in layers I, II, and III. Some callosal terminals, however, also may be found in layers V and VI among the *en passant* fibers ascending to more superficial layers (37). The patches of callosal terminals are variable in width,

varying from about 400 to 800 μm. The spaces separating the densely labeled terminals range in width from 250 to 800 μm. These interpatch areas are not entirely devoid of labeled terminals, especially in the superficial layers (Fig. 6b). Density measurements revealed that the heaviest anterograde labeling is found in layer III, the layer also containing most of the callosal cells. Layer IV, the thalamic-recipient layer, contains the least anterograde labeling.

The possibility exists that some regions of AI give rise to callosal connections but do not receive them. This lack of complete reciprocity (Fig. 6b) was suggested by the histologic observation that autoradiographically labeled patches of callosal terminals were considerably narrower in width (on the average) than HRP-labeled clusters of callosal cells (9,37). Direct evidence that callosal-cell clusters and terminal patches are not co-extensive is clearly demonstrated by simultaneous retrograde and anterograde labeling in HRP-reacted sections cut in the coronal plane (Fig. 6b). However, complete overlap of callosal-cell clusters and callosal-terminal patches is found at least in the high-frequency-represented (rostral) part of AI in histologic sections cut tangentially along layer III (Fig. 6c, d) (26). Patterns of complete reciprocity and nonreciprocity are known to exist in other sensory cortices (62,63,81) and in the motor cortex (55). Electron-microscopic studies will be necessary to show conclusively if some callosal cells in the cat's auditory cortex actually lack reciprocal innervation. Callosal cells may share the same binaural properties as the associational cells in the interpatch regions (28; see Phillips et al., previous chapter).

The callosal connection between AI of both hemispheres, although discontinuous, is nevertheless extensive throughout the entire AI. This pattern of connection contrasts with the restricted callosal interconnections found in both the primary visual and primary somatosensory cortices of the

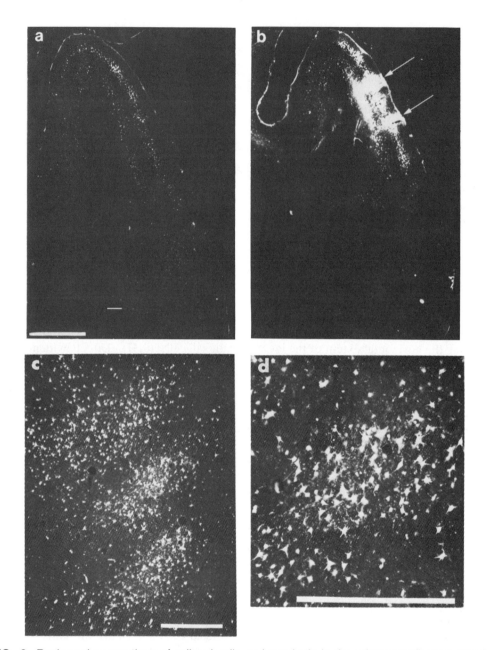

FIG. 6. Reciprocal connections of callosal cells and terminals in the primary auditory cortex (AI) from anterograde and retrograde HRP-labeling experiments. **a:** Clusters of callosal-cell labeling are seen from anterograde and retrograde labeling (2-mm calibration bar for a and b). **b:** Incomplete reciprocity of callosal-cell clusters and callosal-terminal bands is seen in transverse section. (From ref. 37, with permission.) **c** and **d** (both calibration bars represent 500 μm): Complete reciprocity in three labeled patches is seen in a tangential section of AI where high frequencies are represented. Calibration bar is 2 mm for a and b. (From ref. 26, with permission.)

cat and monkey. In the primary visual cortex (area 17) of the cat, callosal cells originate and terminate only at the 17/18 cytoarchitectonic border, an area representing the vertical meridian of the visual field (62–64). The rest of area 17 does not establish callosal connections (7,12,13,20). Similarly, in the primary somatosensory cortex of the monkey, callosal cells originate from and terminate in only regions representing more axial parts of the body, such as the face, trunk, and proximal limbs (12,33,35,36). The callosal connection is reciprocal with an exact correspondence between zones of callosal cells and terminals (34). The parts of the primary somatosensory cortices representing distal limbs are not connected by the corpus callosum. The widespread callosal connection between the primary auditory cortices provides a bilateral link of sound frequencies and ear dominance. However, the exact role of this interhemispheric connectivity in cortical sound processing is not known. Callosal innervation does not appear to be essential in shaping the binaural properties observed at AI (5). AI preserves many of the binaural interactions already generated at the brainstem levels. Moreover, regions in AI, which are callosally connected, contain binaural neurons exhibiting summation responses (24). Since it is likely that summation neurons are location insensitive (or minimally spatially selective), it appears that the ability of the auditory cortex to localize sound (53) is *not* mediated by *inter*hemispheric comparison of auditory information (see Phillips et al., previous chapter).

Neurons in all six layers of AI give rise to associational projections to other ipsilateral auditory cortical areas. After injection of HRP into AII, cells labeled in AI were mainly in layers III (40%) and V (25%) with the remaining cells about equally distributed in layers II, IV, and VI (80). Only a few scattered cells in layer I were labeled. Labeled AI cells were clustered in small aggregates between zones of little cell labeling. Although the loci of tracer injections were not mapped physiologically, a general topographic pattern of AI-to-AII projection was nevertheless found, with areas of presumably similar frequency being most heavily interconnected. HRP-labeled AI cells in layers II and III were pyramidal and nonpyramidal cells. Furthermore, when HRP-reacted tissue was compared to Golgi-impregnated tissue, the ipsilaterally projecting cortico-cortical cells in layer II were identified as medium-sized pyramidal, bipolar, and multipolar cells, and those in layer III included small and large pyramidal cells. In addition to this diverse morphological population of AI, other subregions of auditory cortex also send convergent cortico-cortical inputs to AII. Functional segregation may exist at the laminar level, since layer II is the source of intrahemispheric projections while layer III is the source of both intrahemispheric (associational) and interhemispheric (callosal) projections. In contrast to the widespread laminar origin of associational fibers from the cat AI, the associational fibers from both the primary visual and somatosensory cortices appear to be species dependent, with a laminar segregation confined mainly to layer III and possibly layer V.

INTERCONNECTIONS OF CORTICAL BINAURAL COLUMNS

Topographical Distribution of Binaural Columns in the Primary Auditory Cortex

Functional columns with similar sensitivity to binaural stimuli were found to be coextensive with the tonotopic map in AI. In examining the functional organization of the cat's auditory cortex, Abeles and Goldstein (1) found that neurons exhibiting similar binaural interactions were clustered in a columnar fashion. Using a classification scheme according to binaural interaction and aural dominance, two main types of binaural columns, summation and suppression, were mapped in the higher frequency representation of AI (23,44). In the higher frequency domain of AI, summation columns occupy about two-thirds of the total area and suppression columns one-third. These columns extend from layers III–VI. Neurons in suppression columns are termed excitatory/inhibitory (EI): monaural stimulation of the dominant (usually contralateral) ear results in an excitatory response, whereas binaural stimulation results in a neural response smaller than that of the dominant ear (inhibition by the nondominant ear). Neurons in summation columns are termed excitatory/excitatory (EE): monaural stimulation of either ear results in an excitatory response, while binaural stimulation results in a facilitated response greater than the neural response to stimulation of either ear alone. Hence, binaural stimulation is more effective in driving summation neurons than suppression neurons.

When the topographical distribution of these binaural interaction columns are correlated with the tonotopic map, the columns are found to vary greatly in shape and size. Some suppression columns are relatively large, elongated bands spanning up to 4 mm rostrocaudally and representing over two octaves in AI. Summation and suppression bands alternate along the dorsoventral direction of AI (Fig. 7).

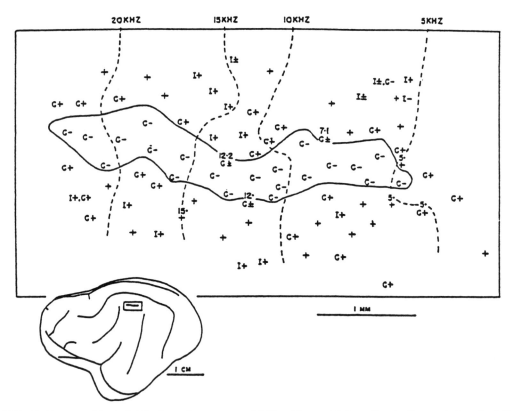

FIG. 7. Topographical distribution of neurons exhibiting binaural interaction in the rostral part of AI where high frequencies are represented. A large contralateral dominant suppression column (C−) extends orthogonally across isofrequency contours of over two octaves in the physiologically mapped primary auditory cortex (AI). Summation columns either ipsilateral dominant (I+) or contralateral dominant (C+) alternate with suppression columns along the dorsoventral direction. Inset shows the location of the binaural columns in AI. (Modified from ref. 23, with permission.)

The functional organizations according to binaural columns and best frequency exist in an overlapping fashion in AI. Binaural information, such as interaural time difference (ITD) and interaural intensity difference (IID), provides spatial cues important for sound localization. Yet, it remains unclear how the topographical distribution of binaural columns is specifically related to sound localization, a role long attributed to the auditory cortex (e.g., see ref. 53). The localization of sound sources by freely moving animals is processed along frequency channels in AI, since unilateral lesions at specific isofrequency contours result in frequency-specific contralateral deficits (30). While sound-localizing mechanisms involving binaural processing may operate over the tonotopically organized AI, the auditory cortex may actually play no main sensory role (10), at least in an auditory-motor task such as moving toward a sound source. Thus, it is not surprising that a neural map of auditory space is not found in AI (46), but one does exist in a sensorimotor integration center: the superior colliculus of the cat (45), barn owl (40), guinea pig (38), the bat (82). Sound location in the cerebral cortex may require higher order computational maps (see ref. 41) based on binaural interactions and tonotopy.

Cortico-Cortical Connectivity of Binaural Columns

In an elegant experiment combining neuroanatomical tracing with physiological mapping, Imig and Brugge (24) demonstrated that summation columns (+) in the high-frequency representation receive more dense callosal innervation than columns exhibiting contralateral dominant suppression (C−). Injections of tritiated amino acids were made into AI prior to neurophysiological mapping experiments in the contralateral AI according to unit binaural properties. In tangential penetrations along layer IV, electrolytic lesions were made at borders between two sequences of neurons differing in binaural responses. These marking lesions between binaural columns corresponded to the borders of callosal columns in subsequent autoradiographic processing for anterograde labeling of callosal terminals. In fact, the topography of callosal columns, as observed in histologic sections cut parallel to the cortical surface, appeared to correspond to the map reconstructed from physiological mapping of binaural responses. The configuration of these callosal columns is elongated along the frequency axis of AI and spans several octaves of frequency representation. Besides clustering of callosal terminals in columns, callosal cells in AI also are clustered in specific layers of AI, with many in layers III and IV, and the remainder in layers V and VI. Conversely, sectors containing summation (EE) neurons or ipsilateral dominant suppression (IE) neurons are located in zones containing more callosal cells than sectors containing contralateral dominant suppression (EI) or monaural contralateral neurons.

Association inputs to AI from adjacent auditory zones also were examined with respect to the binaural organization of AI (28). A pattern is observed in the projection from A to AI and the distribution of binaural response class in the high-frequency part of AI. Contralateral dominant suppression (EI) columns receive more association projections than the adjacent summation (EE) columns of AI. This difference between the associational connections of binaural columns in AI is more evident with the ipsilateral projections provided by field A than by field P. Furthermore, this difference is observed only in a limited portion of AI, with other parts of AI showing no obvious relation between innervation density of association fibers and specific type of binaural neurons. For example, neurons exhibiting contralateral dominant suppression (EI) are physiologically mapped at loci devoid of labeling.

Thus, the cortico-cortical inputs arising from the contralateral and ipsilateral auditory cortex each preferentially project to a different class of binaural columns. Summation (EE) columns in AI are more densely innervated by callosal fibers than by associational fibers originating from the ipsilateral A and P fields. Conversely, contralateral dominant suppression (EI) columns are preferentially innervated by associational than callosal projections.

INTRINSIC CORTICAL CIRCUITRY

Complex-sound processing in the auditory cortex involves contributions of thalamic, associational, and callosal inputs. Little is known, however, of the interneuronal network that modulates the multiple interlaminar inputs terminating within an auditory subregion. Many different classes of neurons throughout the six layers of AI have been shown to accumulate tritiated gamma-aminobutyric acid ([³H]GABA), and hence, these identified neurons possibly utilize this putative transmitter in mediating intracortical inhibition (78). Many local inhibitory interactions in the visual cortex have been attributed to GABAergic neurons that play a role in shaping specific visual properties of cortical cells (11,65). The bulk of the GABAergic neurons that are found within the supragranular layers of AI also are likely to participate in local circuits, although one class of distant-projecting GABAergic neurons may be associated with a subpopulation of callosal cells (78).

A variety of horizontally running axons in AI originate from layers III and IV (74,76). Pyramidal cells in layer III provide a major contribution to these intrinsic fibers, projecting laterally for as much as 1 mm mainly into layer IV. Most nonpyramidal cells project locally to targets within the immediate vicinity of the cells themselves, whereas pyramidal cells have axons that divide and project to targets remote from their laminar origin. Such intracortical patterns of axonal ramification resemble those observed in the primary visual cortex of the

cat (14,15) and the primary somatosensory cortex (see ref. 32 for review). Layer II provides an interlaminar projection to the superficial part of layer III.

In Golgi-stained preparations of the cat's auditory cortex cut parallel to the pial surface, neuronal processes and dendritic fields are oriented preferentially along the flattened middle ectosylvian gyrus (83). Golgi-impregnated stellate and pyramidal cells in layers IV and V are oriented preferentially in the dorsal to ventral direction (16). Many of the processes labeled from focal microinjections of HRP into AI radiate from the injection site and run mainly dorsoventrally along electrophysiologically mapped isofrequency contours (57). Multiple patches of transported label also are distributed ventral, dorsal, and anterior to small injections confined to AI, although the foci of labeling are asymmetrical and irregularly distributed (42). Both pyramidal and nonpyramidal cells in the patches are retrogradely labeled, mainly in layers III and IV. The characteristic frequency (CF) recorded from each of these labeled patches is similar to, or slightly higher (up to 6 kHz) than, the CF of the injected zone. No relation, however, is found between the binaural properties in injected sites and those of labeled patches. Thus, while the local interconnections within AI can span horizontal distances up to 3 mm, the function of this intrinsic cortical connectivity appears to differ significantly from the associational and callosal connections of tonotopically and binaurally related subregions.

CONCLUSION: FUTURE STUDIES

The organization of the cat's auditory cortex into multiple subregions appears to be a common feature of sensory cortex. Of the multiple visual areas mapped in the primate cerebral cortex, each cortical area analyzes primarily a specific aspect of the visual image (see ref. 72 for review). However, in the auditory cortex, little is known about the specific roles or stages of cortical processing that each subregion plays in generating perception. A notable exception is the auditory cortex of the echolocating bat, currently the only animal model in which the processing of specific aspects of sound can be attributed to identified functional subregions (see ref. 69 for review). Although the functional organization of the bat's auditory cortex is specialized for the processing of the animal's own emitted sounds and echoes, these studies will continue to unravel possible organizational schemes and computational maps important for cortical sound analysis (70,71,86). Thus, comparative studies in animals with highly developed auditory systems can provide fresh insights into shared mechanisms of spectral and temporal processing.

With the rapid emergence of powerful immunocytochemical and molecular techniques (e.g., see ref. 18), further advances are possible in relating the functional organization of a cortical subregion with its intrinsic pattern of connections. For example, the different classes of binaural columns mapped in AI are topographically distributed in a seemingly random fashion. Tracing the pattern of intracortical connections of binaural columns in AI may clarify how such a binaural organization is related to the sound analysis of this primary area. When modern and more sensitive probes are used in conjunction with neurophysiological studies, the functional properties and synaptic inputs of identified cell-types can be further established.

The ability of sensory maps to reorganize throughout life appears to be an inherent property among sensory systems (31). For example, the auditory cortex of the guinea pig has the capacity to reorganize its frequency map after partial deafness (59). To determine how malleable this functional organization is and the extent to which it is dependent on experience will require detecting the subtle connectional or synaptic changes that underlie damage-induced plasticity over time. Future studies with par-

tially deafened animals can examine how the functional properties of single cells, maps of binaural interaction and best frequency, and, hence, auditory processing are modified by reorganization in the subregions of auditory cortex.

SUMMARY

1. The cat's auditory cortex is located on the lateral surface of the cerebral cortex, occupying the ectosylvian gyri and associated sulci. The tonotopically organized AI is surrounded by a belt of auditory subregions that include (a) A, P, and VP auditory fields with tonotopic order and (b) AII, DP, and V auditory fields with no clear or consistent tonotopy.

2. The six layers of AI are distinguishable architectonically by comparing Golgi, Nissl, and fiber preparations. The characteristic columnar arrangement of cells throughout the cerebral cortex appears more highly developed in AI, especially in layer IV, where most cells exhibit a *pronounced* vertical disposition of their dendritic and axonal fields.

3. Subregions of auditory cortex can be defined by their connectivity pattern with the different nuclei comprising the MGB and the inferior colliculus.

4. Layer VI of AI gives rise to an extensive ipsilateral corticothalamic projection and layer V to a much smaller bilateral cortico-collicular projection.

5. Regions of tonotopically organized fields representing the same best frequency are reciprocally connected *intra*hemispherically by association fibers and *inter*hemispherically by callosal fibers.

6. The laminar origin of callosal cells in AI is from two tiers, with most of these cells from layer III and relatively few from layers V and VI. Association cells originate from all six layers of AI, with most of these cells from layers III and

V. Callosal and associational cells are both distributed in their layers as distinct clusters.

7. The functional organizations according to binaural interaction columns and best frequency exist in an overlapping fashion in AI.

8. Summation columns, which contain neurons with EE responses to binaural stimulation, are more densely innervated by callosal than associational fibers; conversely, contralateral dominant suppression columns, which contain neurons with EI responses to binaural stimulation, are more densely innervated by associational than callosal fibers.

9. Pyramidal and nonpyramidal cells, mainly in layers III and IV of AI, send intracortical fibers tangentially and preferentially along isofrequency contours, possibly to provide local processing of regions with similar, or slightly higher, best frequencies.

10. Studies in animals with such highly developed auditory systems as that of the bat have identified different roles in sound processing for each of the functional regions of auditory cortex. These animal models continue to provide insights into basic mechanisms underlying cortical sound processing, and hence, the functional significance of the connections linking the multiple subregions of auditory cortex.

ACKNOWLEDGMENTS

I am grateful to T. J. Imig, J. P. Kelly, and J. A. Winer for their suggestions on the organization of this chapter. The comments of M. J. Osberger were also helpful. This research was supported by NIDCD grant R01-DC00600 and a Project Development Program grant from Indiana University School of Medicine at Indianapolis.

REFERENCES

1. Abeles M, Goldstein MH. Functional architecture in cat primary auditory cortex: columnar organization and organization according to depth. *J Neurophysiol* 1970;33:172–187.
2. Ades HW. A secondary acoustic area in the cerebral cortex of the cat. *J Neurophysiol* 1943;6:59–63.
3. Andersen RA, Knight PL, Merzenich MM. The thalamocortical and corticothalamic connections of AI, AII, and the anterior auditory field (AAF) in the cat: evidence for two largely segregated systems of connections. *J Comp Neurol* 1980;194:663–701.
4. Andersen RA, Snyder RL, Merzenich MM. The topographic organization of corticocollicular projections from physiologically identified loci in the AI, AII, and anterior auditory cortical fields of the cat. *J Comp Neurol* 1980;191:479–494.
5. Brugge JF, Imig TJ. Some relationships of binaural response properties of single neurons to cortical columns and interhemispheric connections of auditory area AI of cat cerebral cortex. In: Naunton RF, Fernandez C, eds. *Evoked electrical activity in the auditory nervous system*. New York: Academic Press, 1978;487–503.
6. Brugge JF, Reale RA. Auditory cortex. In: Peters A, Jones EG, eds. *Cerebral cortex, volume 4, association and auditory cortices*. New York: Plenum Press, 1985;229–271.
7. Choudhury BP, Whitteridge D, Wilson ME. The function of the callosal connections of the visual cortex. *QJ Exp Physiol* 1965;50:214–219.
8. Code RA, Winer JA. Commissural neurons in layer III of cat primary auditory cortex (AI): pyramidal and non-pyramidal cell input. *J Comp Neurol* 1985;212:485–510.
9. Code RA, Winer JA. Columnar organization and reciprocity of commissural connections in cat primary auditory cortex (AI). *Hear Res* 1986;23:205–222.
10. Cranford JL. Auditory cortex lesion and interaural intensity and phase-angle discrimination in cats. *J Neurophysiol* 1979;42:1518–1526.
11. Daniels JD, Pettigrew JD. A study of inhibitory antagonism in cat visual cortex. *Brain Res* 1977;93:41–62.
12. Ebner EF, Myers RE. Distribution of corpus callosum and anterior commissure in cat and raccoon. *J Comp Neurol* 1965;124:353–366.
13. Fisken RA, Garey LJ, Powell TPS. The intrinsic, association, and commissural connections of area 17 of the visual cortex. *Philos Trans Soc Lond [Biol]* 1975;272:487–536.
14. Gilbert CD, Wiesel TN. Morphology and intracortical projections of functionally identified neurons in cat visual cortex. *Nature* 1979;280:120–125.
15. Gilbert CD, Wiesel TN. Laminar specialization and intracortical connections in cat primary auditory cortex. In: Schmidt FO, Worden FG,

Adelman G, Dennis SG, eds. *The organization of the cerebral cortex.* Cambridge, MA: MIT Press, 1981;163–191.

16. Glaser EM, Van der Loos H, Gissler M. Tangential orientation and spatial order in dendrites of cat auditory cortex: a computer microscope study of Golgi-impregnated material. *Exp Brain Res* 1979;36:411–431.

17. Goldstein MH, Knight PL. Comparative organization of mammalian auditory cortex. In: Popper AN, Fay RR, eds. *Comparative studies of hearing in vertebrates.* New York: Springer-Verlag, 1980;375–398.

18. Heimer L, Záborszky L, eds. *Neuroanatomical tract-tracing methods, 2: recent progress.* New York: Plenum Press. 1989.

19. Hind JE. An electrophysiological determination of tonotopic organization in auditory cortex of the cat. *J Neurophysiol* 1953;16:475–489.

20. Hubel DH, Wiesel TN. Cortical and callosal connections concerned with the vertical meridian of visual fields in the cat. *J Neurophysiol* 1967;30:1561–1573.

21. Hubel DH, Wiesel TN. Receptive fields and functional architecture of monkey striate cortex. *J Physiol (Lond)* 1968;195:215–243.

22. Hubel DH, Wiesel TN. Cells sensitive to binocular depth in area 18 of the macaque monkey cortex. *Nature* 1970;225:41–42.

23. Imig TJ, Adrián HO. Binaural columns in the primary auditory field (AI) of cat auditory cortex. *Brain Res* 1977;138:241–257.

24. Imig TJ, Brugge JF. Sources and termination of callosal axons related to binaural and frequency maps in primary auditory cortex of the cat. *J Comp Neurol* 1978;182:637–660.

25. Imig TJ, Morel A. Organization of the thalamocortical auditory system in the cat. *Annu Rev Neurosci* 1983;6:95–120.

26. Imig TJ, Morel A, Kauer CD. Covariation and distribution of callosal cell bodies and callosal axon terminals in layer III of cat primary auditory cortex. *Brain Res* 1982;251:157–159.

27. Imig TJ, Reale RA. Patterns of cortico-cortical connections related to tonotopic maps in cat auditory cortex. *J Comp Neurol* 1980;192:293–332.

28. Imig TJ, Reale RA. Ipsilateral corticocortical projections related to binaural columns in the cat primary auditory cortex. *J Comp Neurol* 1981;203:1–14.

29. Jacobson S, Trojanowski JQ. The cells of origin of the corpus callosum in the rat, cat, and rhesus monkey. *Brain Res* 1974;74:149–155.

30. Jenkins WM, Merzenich MM. Role of cat primary auditory cortex for sound localization behavior. *J Neurophysiol* 1984;52:819–847.

31. Jenkins WM, Merzenich MM. Reorganization of neocortical representations after brain injury: a neurophysiological model of the bases of recovery from stroke. *Prog Brain Res* 1987;71:249–266.

32. Jones EG. Identification and classification of intrinsic circuit elements in the neocortex. In:

Edelman GM, Gall WE, Cowan WM, eds. *Dynamic aspect of neocortical function.* New York: Wiley, 1984;7–40.

33. Jones EG, Burton H, Porter R. Commissural and cortico-cortical "columns" in the somatic sensory cortex of primates. *Science* 1975;190: 572–574.

34. Jones EG, Coulter JD, Wise SP. Commissural columns in the sensory-motor cortex of monkeys. *J Comp Neurol* 1979;188:113–136.

35. Jones EG, Powell TPS. The commissural connexions of the somatic sensory cortex in the cat. *J Anat* 1968;103:433–455.

36. Jones EG, Powell TPS. Connexions of the somatic sensory cortex of the rhesus monkey. II. Contralateral cortial connexions. *Brain* 1969; 92:717–730.

37. Kelly JP, Wong D. Laminar connections of the cat's auditory cortex. *Brain Res* 1981;212:1–15.

38. King AJ, Palmer AR. Cells responsive to free field auditory stimuli in guinea pig superior colliculus: distribution and response properties. *J Physiol (Lond)* 1983;342:361–381.

39. Knight PL. Representation of the cochlea within the anterior auditory field (AAF) of the cat. *Brain Res* 1977;130:447–467.

40. Knudsen EI. Auditory and visual maps of space in the optic tectum of the owl. *J Neurosci* 1982;2:1177–94.

41. Knudsen EI, du Lac S, Esterly SD. Computational maps in the brain. *Annu Rev Neurosci* 1987;10:41–65.

42. Matsubara JA, Phillips DP. Intracortical connections and their physiological correlates in the primary auditory cortex of the cat. *J Comp Neurol* 1988;268:38–48.

43. Merzenich MM, Knight PL, Roth GL. Representation of cochlea within primary auditory cortex in the cat. *J Neurophysiol* 1975;28:231–49.

44. Middlebrooks JC, Dykes RW, Merzenich MM. Binaural response-specific bands in primary auditory cortex (AI) of the cat: topographic organization orthogonal to isofrequency contours. *Brain Res* 1980;181:31–48.

45. Middlebrooks JC, Knudsen EI. A neural code for auditory space in the cat's superior colliculus. *J Neurosci* 1984;4:2621–2634.

46. Middlebrooks JC, Pettigrew JD. Functional classes of neurons in primary auditory cortex of the cat distinguished by sensitivity to sound location. *J Neurosci* 1981;1:107–120.

47. Middlebrooks JC, Zook JM. Intrinsic organization of the cat's medial geniculate body identified by projections to binaural response-specific bands in the primary auditory cortex. *J Neurosci* 1983;3:203–224.

48. Mitani 'A, Shimokouchi M. Neuronal connections in the primary auditory cortex: an electrophysiological study in the cat. *J Comp Neurol* 1985;235:417–429.

49. Mitani A, Shimokouchi M, Itoh K, Nomura S, Kudo M, Mizuno N. Morphology and laminar organization of electrophysiologically identified

neurons in the primary auditory cortex in the cat. *J Comp Neurol* 1985;235:430–447.

50. Morel A, Imig TJ. Thalamic projections to fields A, AI, P, and VP in the cat auditory cortex. *J Comp Neurol* 1987;265:119–144.

51. Morest DK. The neuronal architecture of the medial geniculate body of the cat. *J Anat* 1964;98:611–630.

52. Morest DK. The laminar structure of the medial geniculate body of the cat. *J Anat* 1965;99:143–160.

53. Neff WD, Fisher JF, Diamond IT, Yela M. Role of auditory cortex in discrimination requiring localization of sound in space. *J Neurophysiol* 1956;19:500–512.

54. Niimi K, Naito F. Cortical projections of the medial geniculate body in the cat. *Exp Brain Res* 1974;19:326–342.

55. Porter LL, White EL. Afferent and efferent pathways of the vibrissal region of primary motor cortex in the mouse. *J Comp Neurol* 1983;214:279–289.

56. Powell TPS, Mountcastle VB. Some aspects of the functional organization of the postcentral gyrus of the monkey: a correlation of findings obtained in a single unit analysis with architecture. *Bull Johns Hopkins Hosp* 1959;105:133–162.

57. Reale RA, Brugge JF, Feng JZ. Geometry and orientation of neuronal processes in cat primary auditory cortex (AI) related to characteristic-frequency maps. *Proc Natl Acad Sci USA* 1983;80:5449–5453.

58. Reale RA, Imig TJ. Tonotopic organization of auditory cortex in the cat. *J Comp Neurol* 1980;192:265–291.

59. Robertson D, Irvine DRF. Plasticity of frequency organization in auditory cortex of guinea pigs with partial unilateral deafness. *J Comp Neurol* 1989;282:456–471.

60. Rose JE. The cellular structure of the auditory region of the cat. *J Comp Neurol* 1949;91:409–440.

61. Rose JE, Woolsey CN. The relations of thalamic connections, cellular structure and evocable electrical activity in the auditory region of the cat. *J Comp Neurol* 1949;91:441–466.

62. Segraves MA, Rosenquist AC. The distribution of the cells of origin of callosal projections in cat visual cortex. *J Neurosci* 1982;2:1079–1089.

63. Segraves MA, Rosenquist AC. The afferent and efferent callosal connections of retinotopically defined areas in cat cortex. *J Neurosci* 1982;2:1090–1107.

64. Shatz C. Anatomy of interhemispheric connections in the visual system of Boston Siamese and ordinary cats. *J Comp Neurol* 1977;173:497–518.

65. Sillito AM. The contribution of inhibitory mechanisms to the receptive field properties of neurones in the striate cortex of the cat. *J Physiol (Lond)* 1975;250:305–329.

66. Sousa-Pinto A. The structure of the first auditory cortex (AI) of the cat. I. Light microscopic observations on its structure. *Arch Ital Biol* 1973;111:112–137.

67. Sousa-Pinto A. Cortical projections of the medial geniculate body of the cat. *Adv Anat Embryol Cell Biol* 1973;48:1–42.

68. Sousa-Pinto A, Paula-Barbosa M, Matos MDC. A Golgi and electron microscopic study of nerve cells in layer I of the cat auditory cortex. *Brain Res* 1975;95:443–458.

69. Suga N. The extent to which biosonar information is represented in the bat auditory cortex. In: Edelman GM, Gall WE, Cowan WM, eds. *Dynamic aspects of neocortical function.* New York: Wiley, 1984;315–373.

70. Suga N. Auditory neuroethology and speech processing: complex-sound processing by combination-sensitive neurons. In: Edelman GM, Gall WE, Cowan WM, eds. *Auditory function. Neurobiological bases of hearing.* New York: Wiley, 1989;679–720.

71. Suga N. Cortical computational maps for auditory imaging. *Neural Networks* 1990;3:3–21.

72. Van Essen DC, Maunsell JHR. Hierarchical organization and functional streams in the visual cortex. *Trends Neurosci* 1983;6:370–375.

73. von Economo C. *The cytoarchitectonics of the human cerebral cortex.* London: Oxford, 1929.

74. Winer JA. Anatomy of layer IV in cat primary auditory cortex (AI). *J Comp Neurol* 1984;224:535–567.

75. Winer JA. The pyramidal cells in layer III of cat primary auditory cortex (AI). *J Comp Neurol* 1984;229:476–496.

76. Winer JA. The non-pyramidal cells in layer III of cat primary auditory cortex (AI). *J Comp Neurol* 1984;229:512–530.

77. Winer JA. Structure of layer II in cat primary auditory cortex (AI). *J Comp Neurol* 1985;238:10–37.

78. Winer JA. Neurons accumulating [³H]gamma-aminobutyric acid (GABA) in supragranular layers of cat primary auditory cortex (AI). *Neuroscience* 1986;19:771–793.

79. Winer JA, Diamond IT, Raczkowski D. Subdivisions of the auditory cortex of the cat: the retrograde transport of horseradish peroxidase to the medial geniculate body and posterior thalamic nuclei. *J Comp Neurol* 1977;176:387–418.

80. Winguth SD, Winer JA. Corticocortical connections of cat primary auditory cortex (AI): laminar organization and identification of supragranular neurons projecting to AII. *J Comp Neurol* 1986;248:36–56.

81. Wise SP, Jones EG. The organization and postnatal development of the commissural system of the somatic sensory cortex in the rat. *J Comp Neurol* 1976;168:313–344.

82. Wong D. Spatial tuning of auditory neurons in the superior colliculus of the echolocating bat, *Myotis lucifugus. Hear Res* 1984;16:261–270.

83. Wong WC. The tangential organization of dendrites and axons in three auditory areas of the cat's cerebral cortex. *J Anat* 1967;101:419–433.

84. Wong D, Kelly JP. Laminar connections in the auditory cortex of the cat. *Anat Rec* 1979;193:725–726.

85. Wong D, Kelly JP. Differentially projecting cells in individual layers of the auditory cortex: a

double-labeling study. *Brain Res* 1981;230:
362–366.

86. Wong D, Shannon SL. Functional zones in the
auditory cortex of the echolocating bat, *Myotis
lucifugus. Brain Res* 1988;453:349–352.

87. Woolsey CN. Organization of cortical auditory
system: a review and a synthesis. In: Rasmussen
G, Windle W, eds. *Neural mechanisms of the
auditory and vestibular systems.* Springfield,
IL: Charles C. Thomas, 1960; 165–180.

88. Woolsey CN, Walzl EM. Topical projection of
nerve fibers from local regions of the cochlea to
the cerebral cortex of the cat. *Bull Johns Hopkins Hosp* 1942;71:315–344.

Neurobiology of Hearing: The Central Auditory System, edited by R. A. Altschuler et al.
Raven Press, Ltd., New York © 1991.

15

Properties of Sound Localization by Humans

William A. Yost and Raymond H. Dye

The Parmly Hearing Institute, Loyola University of Chicago, Chicago Illinois 60626

Almost all animals localize sound sources in their immediate environment. For most mammals, a comparison of the inputs to the two ears by the central nervous system is the basis for determining sound source location. As such, studies of binaural processing not only provide information about sound localization but often reveal fundamental characteristics of central nervous system processing.

This chapter reviews human psychophysical data and theories of binaural processing. Other chapters in this volume cover additional information about binaural processing. In addition to this review, there have been a number of reviews and books on binaural hearing published over the past two decades (4,9,12,16,19,20,33,40,79).

DUPLEX THEORY OF LOCALIZATION

From the early work of Rayleigh (55), to the classical study of Stevens and Newman (62), and up through the 1960s, the Duplex Theory of Localization was the cornerstone of binaural theories. The Duplex Theory of Localization is based on the relationship between the physics of a sound arriving at the ears and the geometry of the head. Sound reaches the ear closer to the source first, producing an interaural time or phase difference that results from the difference in path length to the two ears. Due to the presence of the head between the two ears, a sound shadow is cast that creates an interaural difference of level (IDL), with the sound at the ear farthest from the source being less intense than the sound at the ear closest to the source (see Fig. 1). Stevens and Newman (62) formalized the duplex theory of localization by suggesting that interaural differences of time (IDTs) provide a usable cue for localization at low frequencies (where IDLs are minimal) and IDLs provide the cue at high frequencies (Fig. 1), since the sound shadow cast by the head would be substantial (but interaural timing information is ambiguous at high frequencies, see ref. 73). The IDT becomes an ambiguous cue at high frequencies for periods shorter than the maximum time it takes sound to travel from one ear to the other. Thus, according to the Duplex Theory of Localization interaural time and level, each operating best over a particular frequency range, provide the basic cues for localization.

Starting in the early 1970s, a number of experiments indicated that the Duplex Theory of Localization was an oversimplification of human sound localization. The newer developments are derived from: (a) careful measurements of the IDTs and IDLs around the head and torso, (b) a greater appreciation for the fact that sounds can be localized monaurally, (c) the recognition of the importance of low-frequency envelopes for stimuli containing only high-frequency spectral components, (d) considerations of

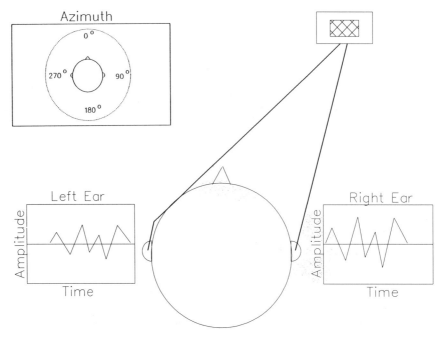

FIG. 1. A sound from a sound source arrives at the near ear (right ear) first and with a greater intensity, producing an interaural temporal and intensive difference. The interaural intensive difference is due largely to the head producing a sound shadow. As the sound source is located further toward one side of the head, the magnitude of the both interaural differences increases. The inset in the upper left shows the referent system used to describe azimuth location.

the importance of the first acoustic wave to reach the ears, and (e) observations suggesting that the shape of a sound's spectrum at the middle ear (especially in the high frequencies) contained useful information for localization. Before reviewing these findings, it will be useful to define some terms.

DEFINITION OF TERMS

When stimuli are delivered to two ears, the listening condition is *binaural* as opposed to when sound is delivered to only one ear, as in *monaural* or *monotic* conditions. In binaural conditions the stimuli can be presented *diotically,* in which case the two ears receive exactly the same stimulus, or the presentation can be *dichotic,* in which case the stimulus delivered to one ear differs from that delivered to the other

ear. Binaural tasks are often referred to as *localization, lateralization, binaural masking,* or *dichotic listening* tasks.

"Localization" usually refers to conditions involving the location of sound sources in the environment surrounding the subject. Oftentimes the environment is *anechoic,* in which case reflections are minimized as sound travels from its source to the listener. "Lateralization" refers to conditions in which sounds are presented to subjects over headphones. The term "lateralization" is derived from the fact that headphone-delivered stimuli are generally perceived to be inside the listener's head, with the sound image lying along the axis between the ears. In a lateralization task, the listeners are assumed to be using some characteristic of the intracranial images, usually their lateral positions, as the basis for response.

"Binaural masking" refers to procedures

TABLE 1. *The stimulus configurations for the maskers (N) and signals (S) used in many MLD conditions*

Binaural condition	Description	MLD
NmSm (monotic)	Masker (N) at only one ear (m); signal (S) at only one ear (m)	Referent
NoSo (diotic)	Masker (N) the same at both ears (o); signal (S) the same at both ears (o)	0 dB
NπSm	Masker (N) out of phase between ears (π); signal (S) at only one (m)	2 dB
NuSo	Masker (N) uncorrelated between ears (u); signal (S) the same at both ears (o)	6 dB
NuSπ	Masker (N) uncorrelated between ears (u); signal (S) out of phase between ears (π)	6 dB
NoSm	Masker (N) the same at both ears (o); signal (S) at only one ear (m)	10 dB
NπSo	Masker (N) out of phase between ears (π); signal (S) the same at both ears (o)	12 dB
NoSπ	Masker (N) the same at both ears (o); signal (S) out of phase between ears (π)	15 dB

MLD, masking-level difference.
The typical size of the MLD (in dB) relative to the NmSm condition is shown. The size of the MLD depends on many stimulus variables. The size of the MLDs shown represent those that might be obtained when the masker is a moderately intense continuous noise and the signal a 500-Hz tone on for 500 msec.

in which listeners are asked to detect a signal in the presence of a background masker delivered over headphones. A certain nomenclature has been developed to distinguish the different binaural (diotic and dichotic) conditions that may exist for the signal and for the masker (see Table 1). The listener's task is to detect the signal in the presence of the masking background.

"Dichotic listening" tasks are used to investigate presumed differences in the type of information processed by the two cortical hemispheres. The dichotic listening conditions involve presenting competing messages simultaneously (or nearly simultaneously) to both ears and asking listeners to indicate which of the two messages was heard. If messages delivered to one ear are reported more often than those delivered to the other ear, then the results are interpreted as indicating that the hemisphere contralateral to the ear receiving the reported message plays a dominant role in processing the information in that message set.

Localization and lateralization procedures have been used to study the binaural processes required to locate sounds. While studies of binaural masking may tap aspects of sound localization, they often are aimed at understanding the extraction of information in noisy environments due to the spatial separation of the sound sources. As explained above, dichotic listening procedures are usually not designed to study sound source localization, and therefore, they are not covered in this review.

CUES USED TO LOCATE A SOUND SOURCE

The Physical Stimulus

Over the years a number of investigators (4,13,37,43,45,60,70,71) have measured the level and phase characteristics at the ears for sounds of different spectral content arriving from different spatial locations. In general, the pattern of level variation over frequency and spatial location is quite complex, while the patterns for phase or time are less complex (but far from simple). The measurements differ greatly depending on where they are made (e.g., on a mannequin or on a live human, at the entrance to external meatus, in the concha, or in the outer ear canal, etc.).

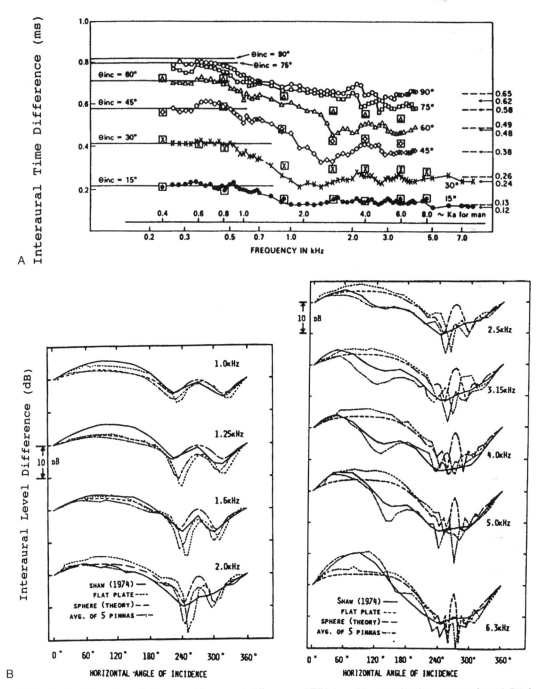

FIG. 2. A: The value of interaural temporal difference (ITD) in milliseconds shown as a function of tonal frequency (in kHz) and angle of incidence (θinc) between the loudspeaker and the acoustic mannequin, KEMAR (Knowles Electronics Mannequin for Acoustic Research). Measurements were made from microphones placed in the ear canals of KEMAR and are representative of the IDTs that exist at the ears of a normal male. As can be seen, the value of the IDTs is not constant with frequency, being somewhat larger for frequencies below approximately 800 Hz. The values at the right of the figure are the calculations of ITD based on different calculation schemes as explained by Kuhn (37). **B:** IDL is shown as a function of angle of incidence between the loudspeaker and the head and as a function of the frequency of the sound (each panel). Data from spheres and from theoretical calculations are compared to those from the KEMAR mannequin. The pattern of interaural differences is complex, especially for high-frequency stimuli. At 6.3 kHz the interaural level differences can be as large as 20 dB, whereas at 1 kHz the maximum is approximately 5 dB. (Data from ref. 37.)

Figure 2A describes the IDTs for different frequencies measured under a variety of conditions as explained in the figure caption. These data show that even for a simple stimulus originating from one point in space, the value of the IDT is frequency dependent. Therefore, interaural time per se cannot provide an unambiguous cue for localization even at low frequencies, as assumed by the Duplex Theory of Localization. At the very least, different maps of spatial position from interaural time delay must exist for different frequency channels (41).

The pattern of level differences is more complex as the spectral content of the stimulus extends to high frequencies (see Fig. 2B). Thus, there is not a simple mapping of spatial location from interaural level, especially at high frequencies where the Duplex Theory assumed that interaural level was the dominant cue for localization. The IDTs and IDLs depend not only on the location of the sound relative to the head but also on frequency and the exact path the sound takes to the ears (37).

The measurements shown in Fig. 2 can be used to describe the transfer functions of the head, torso, and pinna. That is, the sound undergoes filtering (changes in level

and phase) as it travels from its source to the ears. The filtering provided by the pinna can have a pronounced effect on localization accuracy, as we describe later in this review. No well-established description of these transfer functions has yet emerged, but if such transfer functions can be established they would provide a better description of the physical stimulus available to the nervous system than that provided by the Duplex Theory of Localization (71,72).

Localization

The early work on localization (24,46,62) established some of the basic characteristics of pure-tone localization:

1. Errors in the accuracy of localizing pure tones were less in a region below 1,500 Hz and above 2,500 Hz. The region below 1,500 Hz was assumed to be the region in which interaural time was operating as the major cue for localization, while in the region above 2,500 Hz interaural level dominated. The poorer performance in the region between 1,500 and 2,500 Hz was assumed to be due to neither cue providing its highest degree of localization information (see Fig. 3).

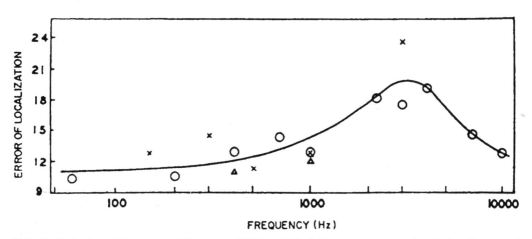

FIG. 3. Data from Stevens and Newman (62) in which listeners were asked to judge the actual location of a loudspeaker. Sinusoids covering the range of 50 to 10,000 Hz were played over the loudspeaker. The data are the mean errors in degrees of visual angle made by three blindfolded listeners in indicating the location of the loudspeaker for the various frequencies used.

2. Errors of localization were greatest for spatial areas within the geometric "cones of confusion" (see Fig. 4).

3. The accuracy for discriminating between two locations was best when the sound sources were directly in front of the listeners (the minimum audible angle [MAA] for discriminating two separated sources can be as small as 3° of visual angle) and performance deteriorated as the sources were located toward one ear (the MAA increased as much as sevenfold) (see Fig. 5).

4. The MAA was found to be frequency dependent, with frequencies below 2,000 Hz and between 4,000 and 8,000 Hz providing the smallest MAAs. As is the case for localization accuracy, the spectral region around 2,000 Hz was found to be the least useful for discriminating the separation between two pure-tone sound sources (the MAA is largest in the mid-frequency region; see Fig. 5).

5. Localization accuracy was poorer when the listener was prevented from moving his/her head.

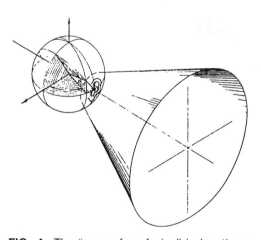

FIG. 4. The "cone of confusion" in locating a sound source. All sources on the surface of the cone produce the same interaural values of time and intensity. For sources located directly in front of the listener, the same interaural differences are also produced by a source directly behind the listener. The "confusion" can be overcome by moving the head slightly. (From ref. 46.)

Although these earlier results were consistent with the major assumptions of the Duplex Theory of Localization, more recent studies (4,5,27,39,72) using complex stimuli indicated that cues in addition to interaural time and level can be used to localize complex sounds. The information in the high-frequency portion of the spectrum can be used by listeners to localize sound sources when they are using only one ear (i.e., the other ear is blocked) (47). Localization of complex sounds in the vertical direction (up-down) and perhaps the determination of range of a complex sound source (4,50) appear to depend greatly on the distribution of energy across the spectrum, especially in the high frequencies for vertical localization (29). Localization accuracy can be altered by filtering a complex noise stimulus (5), even when source location is not changed. Thus, the spectrum of sound appears to provide usable information for determining a sound's source.

Precedence

In real world environments a sound often encounters many reflective surfaces before it reaches the ears. These reflected sound waves could produce binaural cues that would indicate the sound source was coming from the reflected surface rather than from the sound's source. Such false localizations are rarely made, even in conditions in which the reflections are intense. As long as the sound from the source reaches the ears before the reflected sound (because a reflected sound must travel a longer path than the unreflected sound), then the sound is almost always localized as coming from the source (4). It is as if the sound reaching the ears first takes precedence over the later arriving echoes in determining sound source location (see Fig. 6). Thus, the suppression of echoes in their contribution to sound localization has been called the "precedence effect" (sometimes the "law of the first wavefront" or the "Haas ef-

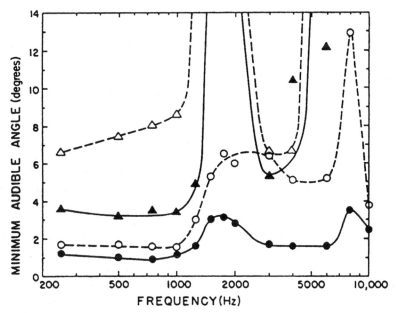

FIG. 5. The minimum audible angle (MAA) required to discriminate between two sound sources as a function of the frequency of the sinusoidal source and the initial location of the source. The *filled circles* are for sources directly in front of the listener, *open circles* are for locations 30° to one side, *filled triangles* 60° to one side, and *open triangles* 75° to one side. Notice that the MAA is smallest when the source is directly in front and when the frequencies are low or high. (From ref. 46.)

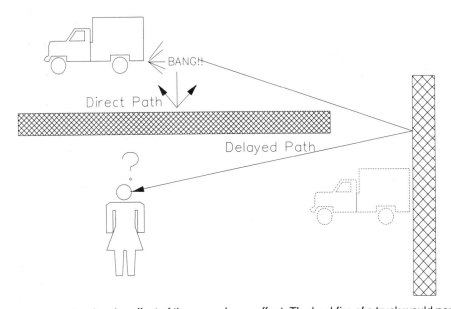

FIG. 6. A cartoon showing the effect of the precedence effect. The backfire of a truck would normally be located as coming from the rear of the truck. However, if the direct path of the sound is blocked, as shown in the cartoon, and the sound takes a delayed path to reach the ears, then the source may be misperceived as coming from the reflected surface (to the listener's right) because the most intense sound to reach the ears first comes from that direction. Thus, the first intense sound that reaches the ears dominates in determining the location of a sound source.

fect"; Gardner [15] explains the differences among the use of these terms; also see refs. 4,27,84 for reviews). The importance of the precedence effect has not been incorporated into the Duplex Theory of Localization (see refs. 52,56).

Lateralization

When simple stimuli are presented over headphones, increases in the IDT (for phase delays less then 180°) move the internalized, lateral image toward the ear receiving the stimulus leading in time, and increases in the IDL move the lateral image toward the ear receiving the more intense stimulus (7,64,76,80) (see Fig. 7).

The thresholds for discriminating between different values of interaural level, interaural time, and combinations of interaural time and level have been measured in a wide variety of conditions (see refs. 12,80 for reviews). Figure 8 is a depiction of some of the major results. Notice that signals with IDTs as small as 10 μsec and IDLs as small as 0.3 dB can be discriminated from diotic signals. Interaural time discrimination for *pure tones* is limited to frequencies below 2,000 Hz, while IDLs appear to be discriminable over a wide range of pure-tone frequencies.

In a number of experiments the interaural differences were arranged such that the ear receiving the louder stimulus also received the stimulus lagging in time. For a single source, this IDT would indicate a sound coming from one side of the head, while the IDL would indicate a sound coming from the opposite side of the head. Thus, the two interaural differences are in opposition. These experiments are often referred to as *"trading ratio"* experiments because they were designed to determine if interaural time and level were equated in some manner (see refs. 19,80 for reviews). The results from trading ratio experiments became difficult to interpret when Hafter and Jeffress (23) demonstrated that listeners were capable of hearing two images, a time image and a time-intensity traded image, rather than one generated from the trade of interaural time for interaural level (there are other difficulties in interpreting the results from many of the trading ratio studies, see ref. 67).

A number of *binaural models* have been developed to account for the data described above, especially those involving pure-tone stimuli (4,7,8,31,58,59,61). These models assume that the information from the two ears is processed via a cross-correlation mechanism. Figure 9 describes one of these models (61) and is illustrative of the major components that are included in the variations of cross-correlation proposed as models for pure-tone lateralization. Jeffress (31) originally proposed that a coincidence network (see Fig. 10) could serve as a neural cross-correlator. Cross-correlation and coincidence networks have made an appealing model for both psychoacousticians and physiologists.

In the early 1970s data from a series of experiments undermined one of the major assumptions of the Duplex Theory of Localization: that interaural time was a cue only for low frequencies (see ref. 80 for a review of this literature). Numerous studies established that complex stimuli with energy restricted to high frequencies could be lateralized on the basis of IDTs (often as well as low-frequency pure tones), *if* the high-frequency stimuli had a low-frequency temporal envelope. Figure 11 shows the data from one such study involving high-frequency pure tones that were amplitude modulated at a slow rate (28). Stimuli consisting of two tones separated by a few hundred hertz (beating stimuli), sinusoidally amplitude-modulated (SAM) tones with low-modulation frequencies, narrow bands of noise, and filtered trains of impulses could all be lateralized on the basis of IDTs of a few tens of microseconds, even when the spectral components in the stimuli are all above 2,000 Hz. Thus, binaural processing of interaural time is not limited

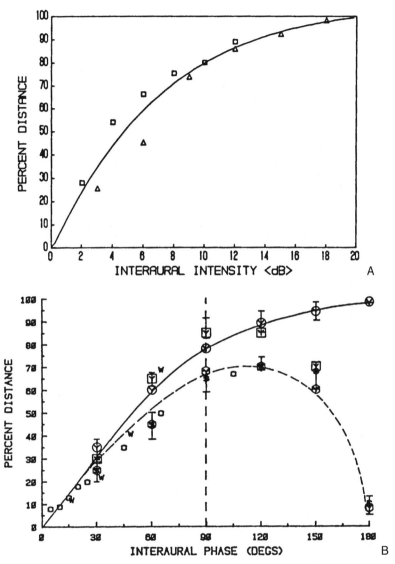

FIG. 7. The relative lateral position (0 is at midline and 100 all the way toward one ear) within the head is shown as a function of interaural level (**A**) and interaural phase (**B**) differences for pure tones. The image is located more and more toward the ear receiving the louder stimulus up to at least a 15-dB interaural level difference (data from different studies as described in ref. 80). In B, the image appears toward the ear leading in phase, up to one-half period of the stimulating tone. As the phase shift increases beyond 180°, the image appears on the other side of the head. At or near 180° the stimulus has an ambiguous location. (Data are from different studies as described in ref. 80.)

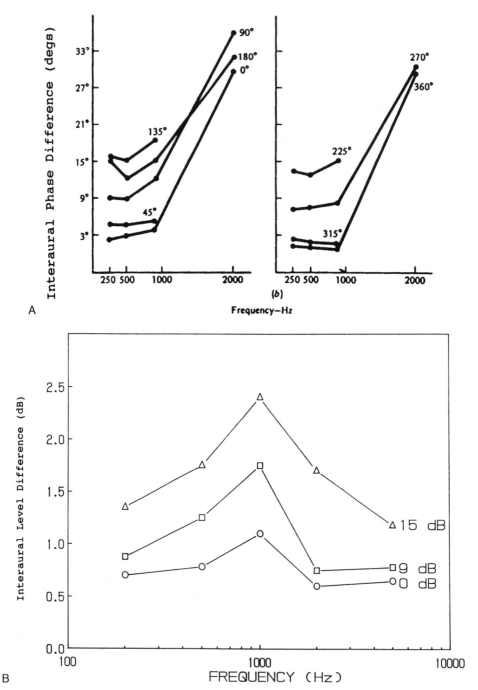

FIG. 8. The smallest amount of interaural phase difference (**A**) or level difference (**B**) required to discriminate between two stimuli are shown as a function of pure-tone frequency and the amount of interaural phase or level introduced for the referent stimulus. The just discriminable interaural level difference (IDL) is approximately 0.5 to 1.0 dB (except in the region of 1,000 Hz), when the standard stimulus has no IDL. As the IDL of the standard is increased (as the standard occupies a spatial location away from the midline toward one ear), there is a slight increase in the thresholds. A similar situation exists for discriminations of interaural phase except that interaural phase shifts can only be detected for low-frequency pure tones and the thresholds are lowest for very low frequencies. As for discriminations and interaural phase, the thresholds increase as the image is moved toward one ear by increasing the phase shift of the standard stimulus toward half of a period. (Data in A from ref. 75; B from ref. 78.)

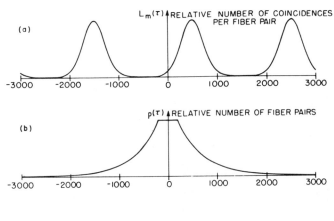

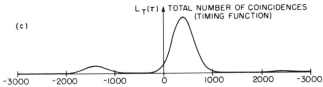

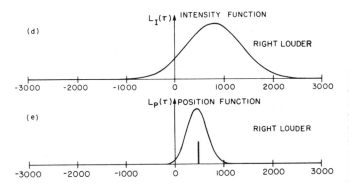

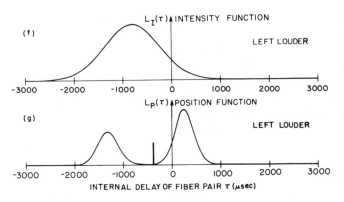

FIG. 9. The outline of the cross-correlation model of Stern and Colburn (61). In **a** the cross-correlation or coincidences for a 500-Hz tone presented with a 500-μsec interaural temporal difference favoring the right ear is shown. Information coming from the center of the network (near 0) receives the most weight (**b**), resulting in the weighted coincidences shown in **c**. If the right ear also received a more intense sound, as sound in **d**, then the intensity weighting function results in the coincidence shown in **e**. **f** and **g** show the effect of making the sound to the left ear more intense. The center of the coincidence distribution indicates the perceived location of the sound, while the discriminability between two coincidence distributions is used to account for interaural time or intensity discrimination.

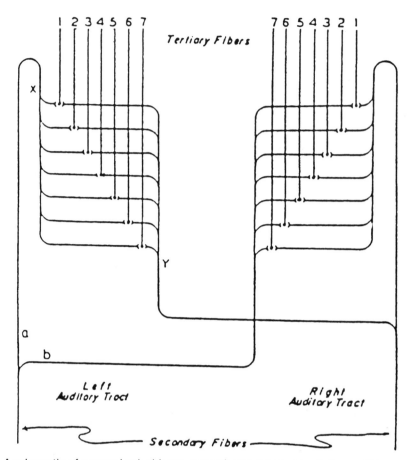

FIG. 10. A schematic of a neural coincidence network as proposed by Jeffress. If the sound arrives at both ears at the same time (sound source is directly in front of the listener), then tertiary fiber 4 would be excited, because the pulses coming from both ears would reach this fiber at the same time. If the sound came from the right side, then fibers 1, 2, or 3 would be excited depending on how far toward one ear (how large the interaural time difference) the sound source was located.

to low frequencies as assumed by the Duplex Theory of Localization.

The precedence effect (68,81,83,84) and phenomena similar to precedence (1,21) have been studied with stimuli presented over headphones. The work of Hafter and colleagues (21) has demonstrated the importance of the early arriving information contained in a train of impulsive stimuli (see Fig. 12). They model their lateralization data with a compressive time function that weighs the interaural information in the first impulses more than that in later occurring impulses. Zurek (83) suggested some form of inhibition following early arriving

information makes the system less sensitive to later arriving copies of the stimulus. Abel and Kunov (1) showed that for pure tones, IDTs at stimulus onset dominate lateralization unless long rise times are used, in which case the salience of the interaural differences at onset is reduced. Thus, in lateralization, as in localization, early arriving information often carries more weight in determining binaural performance than later arriving stimulation.

As explained above, in most listening conditions involving headphones, the sound source appears to be inside the head (internalized) and not externalized as it is

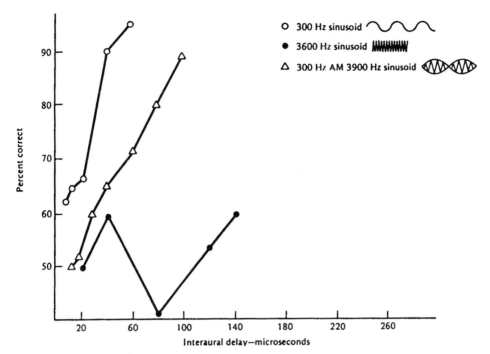

FIG. 11. Psychometric functions showing percent correct for discriminating a change in interaural temporal difference (IDT) as a function of the amount of interaural time. Data are shown for a 300-Hz sinusoid (*open circles*), a 3,600 Hz sinusoid (*filled circles*), and a 3,600-Hz sinusoid amplitude modulated at 300 Hz (*triangles*). Listeners can detect a 30- to 50-μsec interaural difference for a 300-Hz tone but cannot discriminate interaural time for the high-frequency, 3,600-Hz tone; but they can discriminate IDTs if the 3,600-Hz tone has a 300-Hz envelope provided by amplitude modulation. An example from Henning (28) showing that high frequencies can be discriminated on the basis of interaural time if the stimulus has a low-frequency temporal envelope.

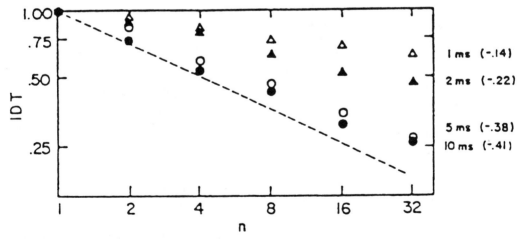

FIG. 12. Data from Hafter (21) showing the interaural difference in time (IDT) required to discriminate an interaural temporal difference for clicks IDT (expressed as normalized value; all IDTs were divided by that required to discriminate an IDT for a single click) is shown as a function of the number of clicks in the train of clicks. Each set of data represents a different click rate. That is, the frequency of the click train is increasing from the *filled circles* to the *open triangles*. The *dotted line* represents the prediction for IDT assuming that each click in the train contributes the same amount of information. The fact that the slopes of the data are less than that of the dotted lines suggests that the first clicks in the click train carry more binaural information than the later arriving clicks. This is especially true for fast click rates.

for sounds in the real world. The internalization is especially strong for spectrally simple stimuli, such as pure tones (66). However, complex sounds (speech, music, and noise bands) can be heard externalized over headphones if they are recorded with microphones placed in the ear canals of humans or mannequins and then played back over headphones (4,11,34,70,72). The filtering of the sound by the pinna appears to be the crucial transform in producing natural reproductions and accurate localizations (72). To date, the exact nature of the transform responsible for externalization and localization is not known. However, as suggested above, the transforms that sound undergoes as it travels from the source to the ears appear to provide crucial cues for localization.

OTHER PHENOMENA RELATED TO LOCALIZATION

Moving Sound Sources

Most of the work on localization has involved stationary sound sources, yet many of our experiences with real life sounds involve moving sound sources. Localization and lateralization studies have measured human sensitivity to sound source movement and to simulations of sound source movement. Threshold displacements have been obtained for moving sound sources (42) and for conditions in movement is simulated (17), and it is generally found that thresholds increase as the velocity of movement exceeds about 100°/sec (51). The binaural system also appears to be slow to respond to dynamic changes in interaural differences as assessed in other paradigms (18,35).

Auditory Space

Clearly the ability to locate the source of sounds is a necessary condition for defining auditory space. However, the subjective attribute of auditory space (that is, the ability to recreate the subjective experience of being in a real sound field when stimuli are presented over headphones) also appears to depend on aspects of early reflections and reverberation (2,4,34,63). If one listens to a recording of sound made from microphones placed in the ear canals when the sound is generated in an anechoic room, one can localize the sounds, but the subjective impression is unlike that of listening in a real-world environment. If the same recording is made in a reverberant space, a more real-world subjective impression of auditory space is obtained. A particularly important aspect of creating the subjective experience of space is the provision of early echoes of the original sounds (34).

SUMMARY

There are a variety of interaural and spectral cues that provide information about the source of a sound. It is probably time to take the Duplex Theory of Localization out of circulation as a theory of binaural processing. No general theory has emerged to take its place, probably because we have just begun to learn about many recently discovered variables that contribute to localization. The list of potential cues includes at least the following: IDTs, IDLs, interaural differences at stimulus onset, interaural delays between low-frequency envelopes of high-frequency complex sounds, the distribution of energy within the spectra of complex sounds, and the spectral transformation sounds undergo due to the filtering of the head, torso, and pinna. The information arriving at the central nervous system regarding the location of a sound source is certainly richer than proposed by the Duplex Theory of Sound Localization.

Sound source localization appears to be based on computations made by the auditory system on the incoming information. The auditory system does not have a spatial array of receptors, as exists in the eye or along the skin, which provides a direct map of space onto neural place. The receptor array in the cochlea transforms sound frequency to neural place (the ear is tonotopically, not spatiotopically organized). Thus, additional processing is required to transform aspects of the peripheral neural code into a central code indicating sound source location. The psychophysical data reviewed above provide some strong hints as to the physical variables that are coded by the auditory system in order for the computation of spatial location to take place. Some of the modeling work suggests ways in which the nervous system might make the necessary computations (e.g., coincidence networks). Clearly additional work at both the psychophysical and neural levels are required before we can develop a comprehensive theory of sound localization.

BINAURAL MASKING AND OTHER PHENOMENA RELATED TO BINAURAL ANALYSIS

Binaural Masking

In two separate experiments in 1948, Hirsh (30) and Licklider (38) discovered that thresholds for detecting masked signals could be substantially lowered if the interaural configuration of the signal was different from that of the masker. The difference in masked thresholds between a diotic and a monotic masking arrangement is usually zero, while the difference in masked thresholds between a diotic and dichotic masking arrangement can be as large as 20 or more dB, with the dichotic conditions always producing the smaller thresholds. The difference in masked thresholds between a

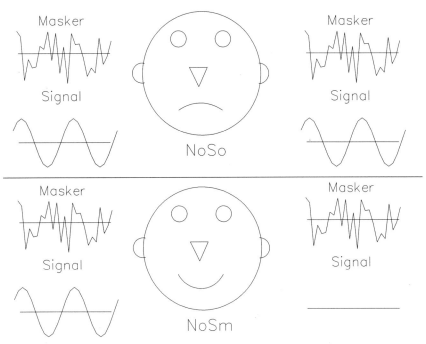

FIG. 13. If listeners are presented the same masker to both ears and the same signal to both ears (**top**), then the signal is more difficult to detect than if the masker is the same at both ears and the signal is presented to only one ear (**bottom**). The top panel represents the NoSo configuration and the bottom panel the NoSm configuration. For low-frequency pure tones and continuous broadband maskers, the signal threshold is approximately 10 dB less for the NoSm configuration than it is for the NoSo configuration.

diotic (or monotic) condition and a dichotic condition is called the "masking-level difference" (MLD) or "binaural masking-level difference" (BMLD).

Table 1 depicts some of the dichotic conditions and the typical values of the MLD as compared to the monotic case of (NmSm). The cartoon shown in Fig. 13 indicates that the NoSm condition produces approximately a 10-dB MLD. A large number of studies have been devoted to the MLD (see refs. 12,20,40 for reviews). In addition to the hierarchy of MLDs summarized in Table 1, Figs. 14 and 15 show two other relationships concerning the NoSπ conditions. Figure 15 indicates the change in the MLD with the frequency of a tonal signal and Fig. 14 shows the change in the

MLD at different frequencies as a function of a change in noise-masker level.

A similar improvement in signal detection occurs when the signal source has a different location in real space than that for the masker sound. Plomp and Mimpin (53) showed that a speech signal can be as much as 10 dB more detectable when it comes from a loudspeaker that is located at a 90° angle from a loudspeaker presenting a masking stimulus than when the signal and masker occupy the same spatial location.

A number of models have been proposed to account for the MLD. The models tend to be variations of three themes: vector models (22,33,69,74), equalization-cancellation (E-C) models (48), and neural based cross-correlation models (8). Colburn and

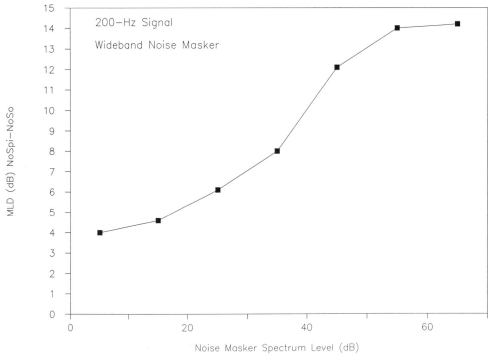

FIG. 14. The masking-level difference (MLD) for the NoSπ condition as compared to the NoSo condition is shown as a function of the frequency of the tonal signal. Data from many studies are shown (from ref. 12). The curve is a fit of the Durlach equalization-cancellation model. The MLD decreases but does not go to zero as the frequency of the tone increases. The reduction in the MLD with increasing frequency has been used to suggest that the MLD is largely due to interaural temporal differences in the signal-plus-masker waveforms.

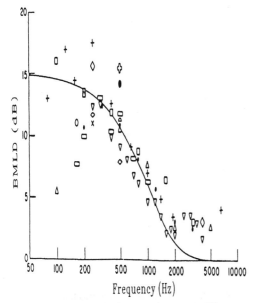

FIG. 15. The binaural masking-level difference (BMLD) for the NoSπ condition as compared to the NoSo condition is shown for a 200-Hz tonal signal and a broadband noise masker presented at different spectrum levels. The decrease in the MLD with decreases in masker level may be due to the presence of physiological noise in the outer occuled ear (From ref. 77.)

The vector models consider the addition of the signal to the masker as vector addition, as indicated in Fig. 16. The size of the MLD is assumed to be proportional to the size of the interaural phase shift ($\Delta\theta$) and/or interaural level difference (ΔR). The E-C model is described in Fig. 17, and the size of the MLD is assumed to be proportional to the signal-to-noise ratio at the output of the E-C device. A version of the cross-correlation approach was described in Fig. 9. In this model the size of the MLD is assumed to be proportional to the magnitude of the cross-correlation or the strength of coincidence along a coincidence network. Each model has its strengths and weaknesses in accounting for MLD data, and all are still used as theories for the MLD (9).

Durlach (9) pointed out that even though the three types of models are analytically different, they are all based on comparing IDTs and IDLs. As such, cross-correlation (coincidence counting) is a convenient method for modeling binaural masking, as it is for modeling lateralization and localization.

Dichotic Pitch

There is a variation of the dichotic signal-plus-noise stimulus used in the MLD procedures. In these stimulus configurations a narrow-band section of a broad-band noise delivered to one ear is different than that presented to the other ear (3,10,14,25, 36,54,82). An example of such a stimulus is shown in Fig. 18. Cramer and Huggins (10) were the first to use this type of stimulus, and they showed that listeners hear a pitch corresponding to that which would be heard if the interaurally altered section of noise were presented by itself. That is, if an interaural phase shift were produced in a nar-

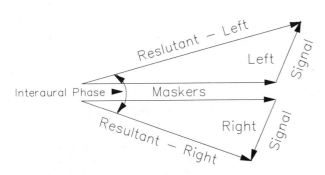

FIG. 16. An explanation for the vector models of the masking-level difference (MLD). The vector addition of the signal plus masker at each ear produces an interaural time (phase) difference and an interaural level difference. The magnitude of MLD is assumed to be proportional to the size of these two interaural differences.

Input   Output

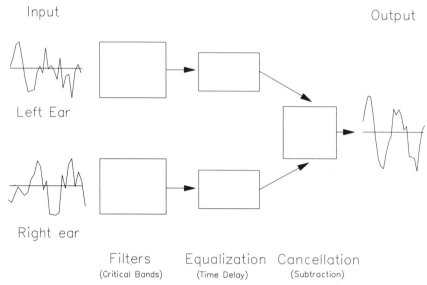

Left Ear

Right ear

Filters   Equalization   Cancellation
(Critical Bands)   (Time Delay)   (Subtraction)

FIG. 17. The block diagram of the equalization-cancellation (E-C) model of the masking-level difference (MLD). The signal and masker are filtered at each ear by internal filters, fed to an equalization stage (which produces internal noise and may involve time shifting the information at one ear), and then to the cancellation stage (where the power of the difference between the two waveforms is computed). The signal-to-noise ratio at the output of the cancellation stage determines the relative size of the MLD. Two cycles of a tone are added to a noise at the left ear and added out of phase to the same noise at the right ear (NoSπ condition). The two sinusoidal cycles are more easily identified at the output than at either of the two inputs, indicating that the E-C network makes it easier to detect a signal in the NoSπ condition than in the NmSm condition.

row band centered at 500 Hz, a noisy pitch of 500 Hz would be perceived from this dichotic stimulus. The pitch and background noise are often perceived as having different intracranial positions. No pitch can be heard while listening to the stimulus delivered to either ear alone, and the pitch does not result from any addition of energy to the stimulus. Both cross-correlation (54) and equalization-cancellation (3) models have been used to explain these dichotic pitches.

Cocktail-Party Effect

Cherry (6) observed that the ability to attend to one voice at a cocktail party, where many voices and sounds exist, may partially depend on the auditory system's ability to spatially separate sound sources. The voice of interest has a different spatial location than the other sounds, and as a con-

sequence one is able to attend to it. According to this form of the "cocktail-party effect," spatial separation and our ability to localize provide a means for extracting signals from noisy backgrounds. The MLD conditions and those leading to dichotic pitches are seen as ones that share some of the dimensions that are present in the cocktail party example. However, the literature (20) suggests that some caution may be required in assuming that the studies of the MLD relate *directly* to studies of the cocktail-party effect.

Binaural Beats

If a low-frequency tone is presented to one ear and a tone of a slightly different frequency is presented to the other ear, the sensation of a beating stimulus that moves

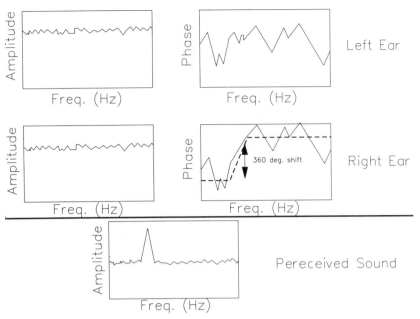

FIG. 18. An example of the amplitude and phase spectrum of a sound that yields a Cramer-Huggins pitch. A broadband stimulus with the same amplitude spectrum is delivered to both ears, but a 360° phase shift over a limited spectral region is added to the spectrum at the right ear. The phase shift produces an interaural phase difference in the spectral region of the phase shift, and listeners perceive a pitch associated with the region of the phase shift (spectral region of the interaural phase difference) in the background of noise. The lateral position of the pitch is different (toward one ear) than that of the background noise (located at or near the middle of the head).

within the head is often reported (see ref. 65; and 45). This sensation is called "binaural beats," and the internal movement of the sound is presumably caused by the slight frequency difference being interpreted by the binaural system as a changing interaural phase difference, resulting in a moving lateral image. McFadden and Pasanen (42) used binaural beats to demonstrate the ability of the binaural system to use IDTs for high-frequency stimuli having low-frequency envelopes (see the discussion earlier in this chapter). They presented a complex of two tones, 3,000 and 3,100 Hz, to one ear and a complex of 3,000 and 3,101 Hz to the other ear. The listener reported hearing a 1-Hz binaural beat, presumably because the 100-Hz envelope (3,100–3,000) at one ear interacted binaur-ally with the 101-Hz envelope (3,101–3,000) at the other ear. The 1-Hz interaural difference in the envelopes produced a 1-Hz binaural beat, that is, an image that moves back and forth across the head at a rate of once per second. A 1-Hz binaural beat was also reported when the tones presented to one ear were 2,000 and 2,050 Hz and those presented to the other ear were 3,000 and 3,051 Hz. The fact that binaural beats are reported for tone pairs presented in different frequency regions but having the same envelopes demonstrates that it is the envelopes that are important for generating the binaural interaction. These data also show that interaural timing can provide binaural information at high frequencies as long as there is a low-frequency temporal envelope.

CONCLUSIONS

This review has been based largely on the stimulus conditions that have been used to study binaural processing, especially those aspects of binaural processing that involve localization. This approach is characteristic of the stimulus-orientated approach so common in psychoacoustics (32), and it will, it is hoped, stimulate exploration of binaural processing at the neural level using similar stimuli. The list of potential physical cues for localization has grown considerably since the development of the Duplex Theory of Localization. These cues have also been used to study aspects of binaural analysis in procedures that do not directly address questions of localization. Thus, phenomena like binaural masking, dichotic pitch, and binaural beats, which may not relate directly to localization, have revealed some important aspects of binaural analysis and have contributed greatly to our understanding of the algorithms used in binaural processing.

REFERENCES

1. Abel SM, Kunov H. Lateralization based on interaural phase differences: effects of frequency, amplitude, duration, and shape of rise/decay. *J Acoust Soc Am* 1983;73:955–960.
2. Berkeley DA. Hearing in rooms. In: Yost WA, Gourevitch G, eds. *Directional hearing.* New York: Springer-Verlag, 1987.
3. Bilsen FA, Goldstein JD. Pitch of dichotically delayed noise and its possible spectral basis. *J Acoust Soc Am* 1974;55:291.
4. Blauert J. *Spatial hearing.* Cambridge, MA: MIT Press, 1983.
5. Butler RA, Planert N. The influence of stimulus band-width on localization of sound in space. *Percept Psychophys* 1976;19:103–108.
6. Cherry EC. Some experiments on the recognition of speech, with one and two ears. *J Acoust Soc Am* 1953;25:975.
7. Cherry EC, Sayers B. On the mechanism of binaural fusion. *J Acoust Soc Am* 1959;31:535.
8. Colburn HS. Theory of binaural interaction based on auditory nerve data II: detection of tones in noise. *J Acoust Soc Am* 1977;61:525–537.
9. Colburn HS, Durlach NI. Models of binaural interaction. In: Carterette EC, Friedman MP, eds.

Handbook of perception (hearing). New York: Academic Press, 1978.
10. Cramer EM, Huggins WH. Creation of pitch through binaural interaction. *J Acoust Soc Am* 1958;30:412–417.
11. Damaske P. Head-related two-channel stereophony with loudspeaker reproduction. *J Acoust Soc Am* 1971;50:1109–1111.
12. Durlach NI, Colburn HS. Binaural phenomena. In: Carterette EC, Friedman MP, eds. *Handbook of perception (hearing).* New York: Academic Press, 1978.
13. Feddersen WE, Sandel TT, Teas DC, Jeffress LA. Measurements of interaural time and intensity difference. *J Acoust Soc Am* 1955;27:1008.
14. Fourcin AJ. Binaural pitch phenomena. *J Acoust Soc Am* 1962;34:1995.
15. Gardner MB. Historical background of the Haas and/or precedence effect. *J Acoust Soc Am* 1968;43:1243–1248.
16. Gatehouse G. *Localization of sound theory and application.* Groton, CT: The Empora Press, 1982.
17. Grantham DW. Detection and discrimination of simulated motion of auditory targets in the horizontal plane. *J Acoust Soc Am* 1986;79:1939–1949.
18. Grantham DW, Luethke P. Detectability of tonal signals with changing interaural phase differences in noise. *J Acoust Soc Am* 1988;83:1117–1123.
19. Green DM, Henning GW. Audition. In: *Annual review of psychology,* vol 20. Palo Alto, CA: Annual Reviews, Inc., 1969.
20. Green DM, Yost WA. Binaural analysis. In: Keidel W, Neff DW, eds. *Handbook of sensory physiology.* Netherlands: Springer-Verlag, 1975.
21. Hafter ER. Spatial hearing and the duplex theory. How viable? In: Edelman GM, Gall WE, Cowan WM, eds. *Dynamic aspects of neocortical function.* New York: Wiley, 1984.
22. Hafter ER, Carrier SC. Masking-level differences obtained with a pulsed tonal masker. *J Acoust Soc Am* 1970;47:1041–1045.
23. Hafter ER, Jeffress LA. Two-image lateralization of tones and clicks. *J Acoust Soc Am* 1968;44:563–569.
24. Harris JD. A florilegium of experiments on directional hearing. *Acta Otolaryngol Suppl (Stockh)* 1972;S298.
25. Hartmann WM. Localization of sound in rooms. *J Acoust Soc Am* 1983;74:1380–1391.
26. Hartmann WM, Rakerd B. On the minimum audible angle—a decision theory approach. *J Acoust Soc Am* 1989;85:2031–2041.
27. Hartmann WM, Rakerd B. Localization of sounds in rooms. IV: the Franssen effect. *J Acoust Soc Am* 1989;86:1366–1373.
28. Henning GB. Detectability of interaural delay in high-frequency complex waveforms. *J Acoust Soc Am* 1974;55:84–90.
29. Herbank J, Wright D. Spectral cues used in localization of sound sources in the median plane. *J Acoust Soc Am* 1974;56:1829–1834.

30. Hirsh IJ. Binaural summation and interaural inhibition as a function of the level of masking noise. *Am J Psychol* 1948;56:205–213.

31. Jeffress LA. A place theory of sound localization. *J Comp Physiol Psychol* 1948;41:35–39.

32. Jeffress LA. Stimulus-oriented approach to detection theory. *J Acoust Soc Am* 1964;36:760–774.

33. Jeffress LA. Binaural signal detection: vector theory. In: Tobias JV, ed. *Foundations of modern auditory theory*. New York: Academic Press, 1972.

34. Kendall GS, Martens WL. Simulating the cues of spatial hearing in natural environments. Proceedings of the 1984 International Computer Music conference, Paris, 1984.

35. Kollmeier B, Gilkey RH. Binaural forward and backward masking: evidence for sluggishness in binaural detection. *J Acoust Soc Am* 1990;87:1709–1719.

36. Kubovy M, Cutting JE, McGuire RM. Hearing with the third ear dichotic perception of a melody without monaural familiarity cues. *Science* 1974;186:272–274.

37. Kuhn GF. Physical acoustics and measurements pertaining to directional hearing. In: Yost WA, Gourevitch G, eds. *Directional hearing*. New York: Springer-Verlag, 1987.

38. Licklider JCR. Influence of interaural phase relations upon the masking of speech by white noise. *J Acoust Soc Am* 1948;20:150–159.

39. Makous JC, Middlebrooks JC. Two-dimensional sound localization by human listeners. *J Acoust Soc Am* 1990;87:2188–2200.

40. McFadden DM. Masking and the binaural system. In: Eagles EL, ed. *The nervous system,* vol 3. New York: Raven Press, 1975.

41. McFadden DM. The problem of different interaural time differences at different frequencies. *J Acoust Soc Am* 1981;69:1836–1837.

42. McFadden D, Pasanen EG. Binaural beats at high frequencies. *Science* 1975;190:394–397.

43. Middlebrooks JC, Green DM. Directional dependence of interaural envelope delays. *J Acoust Soc Am* 1990;87:2149–2162.

44. Middlebrooks JC, Makous JC, Green DM. Directional sensitivity of sound pressure levels in the human ear canal. Abstracts of Midwinter Meeting, Association for Research in Otolaryngology, 1988.

45. Middlebrooks JC, Makous JC, Green DM. Directional sensitivity of sound-pressure levels in the human ear canal. *J Acoust Soc Am* 1989; 86:89–108.

46. Mills AW. Auditory localization. In: Tobias JV, ed. *Foundations of modern auditory theory,* vol II. New York: Academic Press, 1972.

47. Musicant AD, Butler RA. Influence of monaural spectral cues on binaural localization. *J Acoust Soc Am* 1985;77:202–208.

48. Osman E. A correlation model of binaural masking level differences. *J Acoust Soc Am* 1971;50:1414–1511.

49. Perrott D. Dynamic factors in sound localization. In: Gatehouse G, ed. *Localization of sound*

50. Perrott D, Saberi K. Minimum audible angle thresholds for sources varying in both elevation and azimuth. *J Acoust Soc Am* 1990;87:1728–1731.

51. Perrott DR, Tucker J. Minimum audible movement angle as a function of signal frequency and the velocity of the source. *J Acoust Soc Am* 1988;83:1522–1527.

52. Perrott D, Marlborough K, Merrill P, Strybel TZ. Minimum angle thresholds obtained under conditions in which the precedence effect is assumed to operate. *J Acoust Soc Am* 1989;85:282–288.

53. Plomp R, Mimpin AM. Effect of orientation of the speaker's head and the azimuth of a noise source and the speech-reception threshold for sentences. *Acustica* 1981;48:325–328.

54. Raatgever J, Bilsen FA. A central spectrum theory of binaural processing. Evidence from dichotic pitch. *J Acoust Soc Am* 1986;80:429–441.

55. Raleigh Lord. On our perception of sound direction. *Philos Mag* 1907;13:214–232.

56. Saberi K, Perrott DR. Lateralization thresholds obtained under conditions in which the precedence effect is assumed to operate. *J Acoust Soc Am* 1990;87:1732–1737.

57. Sayers B, Cherry EC. Mechanism of binaural fusion in the hearing of speech. *J Acoust Soc Am* 1957;29:973–986.

58. Searle CL, Braida LP, Davis MF, Colburn HS. Model for auditory localization. *J Acoust Soc Am* 1970;60:1169–1176.

59. Shamma SA, Shen N, Gopalaswamy P. Stereausis: binaural processing without neural delays. *J Acoust Soc Am* 1989;86:989–1006.

60. Shaw EAG. Transformation of sound pressure level from the free field to the eardrum in the horizontal plane. *J Acoust Soc Am* 1974;56:1848–1861.

61. Stern RM, Colburn HS. Theory of binaural interaction based on auditory-nerve data. IV. A model for subjective lateral position. *J Acoust Soc Am* 1978;64:127–140.

62. Stevens SS, Newman EB. The localization of actual sources of sound. *Am J Psychol* 1936;48:297–306.

63. Tannaka Y, Koshikawa T. Correlations between sound field characteristics and subjective ratings on reproduced music sound quality. *J Acoust Soc Am* 1989;86:603–620.

64. Teas DC. Lateralization of acoustic transients. *J Acoust Soc Am* 1962;34:1460–1465.

65. Tobias JV. Curious binaural phenomena. In: Tobias JV, ed. *Foundations of modern auditory theory,* vol II. New York: Academic Press, 1972.

66. Toole FE. In-head localization of acoustic images. *J Acoust Soc Am* 1967;41:1592.

67. Trahiotis C, Kappauf WE. Regression interpretation of differences in time-intensity trading ratios obtained in studies of laterality using the method of adjustment. *J Acoust Soc Am* 1978; 64:1041–1047.

68. Wallach H, Newman EB, Rosenzweig MR. The

theory and application. Groton, CT: Empora Press, 1982.

precedence effect in sound localization. *Am J Psychol* 1949;62:315–336.

69. Webster FA. The influence of interaural phase on masked thresholds. I. The role of interaural time deviation. *J Acoust Soc Am* 1958;37:638–646.

70. Wightman FL, Kistler DJ, Perkins ME. A new approach to the study of human sound localization. In: Yost WA, Gourevitch G, eds. *Directional hearing*. New York: Springer-Verlag, 1987.

71. Wightman FL, Kistler DJ. Headphone simulation of free-field listening. I: Stimulus synthesis. *J Acoust Soc Am* 1989;85:858–867.

72. Wightman FL, Kistler DJ. Headphone simulation of free-field listening. II: Psychophysical validation. *J Acoust Soc Am* 1989;85:868–878.

73. Woodworth RS. *Experimental psychology*. New York: Holt, Rinehart, & Winston, 1938.

74. Yost WA. Tone-on-tone masking for three binaural listening conditions. *J Acoust Soc Am* 1972;52:1234–1237.

75. Yost WA. Discriminations of interaural phase-differences. *J Acoust Soc Am* 1974;52:1234–1237.

76. Yost WA. Lateral position of sinusoids presented with interaural intensive and temporal differences. *J Acoust Soc Am* 1981;70:397–409.

77. Yost WA. Masking level difference as a function of overall masker level internal noise hypothesis revisited. *J Acoust Soc Am* 1988;83:1522–1527.

78. Yost WA, Dye RH. Interaural intensity discrimination as a function of frequency. *J Acoust Soc Am* 1988;83:1846–1851.

79. Yost WA, Gourevitch G, eds. *Directional hearing*. New York: Springer-Verlag, 1987.

80. Yost WA, Hafter E. Lateralization of simple stimuli. In: Yost WA, Gourevitch G, eds. *Directional hearing*. New York: Springer-Verlag, 1987.

81. Yost WA, Soderquist DR. The precedence effect revisited. *J Acoust Soc Am* 1984;76:1377–1383.

82. Yost WA, Dye RH, Harder PJ. Complex spectral patterns with interaural differences dichotic pitch and the "central spectrum." In: Yost WA, Watson CS, eds. *Auditory processing of complex sounds*. Hillsdale, NJ: Erlbaum, 1987.

83. Zurek PM. Measurements of binaural echo suppression. *J Acoust Soc Am* 1979;66:1750–1757.

84. Zurek PM. The precedence effect. In: Yost WA, Gourevitch G, eds. *Directional hearing*. New York: Springer-Verlag, 1987.

*Neurobiology of Hearing: The
Central Auditory System*, edited by
R. A. Altschuler et al.
Raven Press, Ltd., New York © 1991.

16

Assessment of the Human Central Auditory Nervous System

*†Frank E. Musiek and *‡Jane A. Baran

*Section of Otolaryngology and Audiology, Department of Surgery, †Section of Neurology,
Department of Medicine, Dartmouth-Hitchcock Medical Center,
Hanover, New Hampshire 03756; ‡Department of Communication Disorders,
University of Massachusetts, Amherst, Massachusetts*

In *Neurobiology of Hearing: The Cochlea* (Volume I), Hood and Berlin reviewed the modern approaches to the assessment of the human auditory system, addressing both the peripheral and central auditory systems. This volume is directed to the central auditory system, the specific assessment of which is this chapter's focus. For the purpose of continuity there is some overlap with the assessment chapter of Hood and Berlin, but it is hoped that this is kept to a minimum.

This chapter provides a brief historical background and emphasizes the critical need for a thorough understanding of neuroanatomy, as well as the rationale for combining psychophysical and electrophysiological approaches in clinical evaluation. Test procedures in the evaluation of brainstem, hemispheric, and interhemispheric dysfunction are discussed, as well as issues pertaining to peripheral hearing loss, aging, and perceptual dysfunction in children. Extensive references are provided to direct the interested reader to additional background information on these topics.

BOCCA'S CONTRIBUTIONS

Ettore Bocca and colleagues are generally considered the first investigators to au-diologically evaluate the integrity of the central auditory nervous system (CANS). Bocca noted that patients with temporal lobe lesions complained of hearing difficulties despite normal results on basic audiometric tests (14). Due to the patients' complaints, Bocca et al. (14) decided to make their routine speech discrimination tasks more difficult, in the hope that the results would be more consistent with the patients' symptoms. The speech signals that they routinely had been using were routed through a low-pass filtering system to reduce the redundancy of the stimuli. Their findings regarding the use of filtered speech as a test for patients with cortical lesions were well documented in the 1950s and early 1960s (13). These early studies not only created the field of central auditory testing, but also served as the basis for three important concepts that are still useful: (a) pure tone threshold tests and speech discrimination tests in quiet at one intensity level are of little value in defining central auditory lesions; (b) the deficits associated with cortical lesions are often manifested in the ear contralateral to the involved hemisphere; and (c) patients with damage to the central auditory system have hearing difficulties, despite normal pure tone thresholds. This last concept continues to be very significant, but is often overlooked, especially when the patient has more acute neurological symptoms (59,112).

More than 30 years have passed since the germinal papers of Bocca and his colleagues, and although progress has definitely been made, it has been difficult and slower than many of us had hoped. One of many reasons why progress for central auditory assessment has not been rapid is that the complex manner in which the brain handles acoustic signals is not well understood. Also, the extent and true effect of a given lesion in the brain cannot always be well defined. After the brain is damaged, it changes and often continues to change with time, making test inconsistencies difficult to interpret. There are many other difficulties that affect the progress of central auditory assessment (132), but perhaps one of the main problems is the overall lack of clinical and basic research on the CANS (compared with what is known about the auditory periphery), despite the fact that it constitutes the majority of the auditory system. This trend in research is changing, however, as evidenced by what is presented in this book, and it appears that there is much more to be learned by clinical and basic scientists interested in the CANS.

ANATOMICALLY DEFINING THE CENTRAL AUDITORY NERVOUS SYSTEM

In this chapter we refer to the human CANS, since most of the clinical research data have been obtained using this model. The starting point of the ascending CANS is the cochlear nucleus complex, located at the posterior-lateral aspect of the ponto-medullary junction. Other structures in the auditory pathway of the brainstem include the superior olivary complex (caudal-most pons), the nuclei of the lateral lemniscus (mid-pons), the inferior colliculus (mid-brain), and the medial geniculate complex (caudal-posterior thalamus) (97) (see previous chapters). The projections from the

medial geniculate probably take several subcortical routes to the cortex, but the details of these are not well known (95). There are at least two main fiber groups of the medial geniculate that project to Heschl's gyrus and the insula (163,164). In addition to the superior temporal lobe, the posterior-inferior frontal lobe, the inferior parietal lobe, and the insula all have areas responsive to acoustic stimulation (22,40) (see Chapter 7).

The corpus callosum also appears to have an auditory area. The primate work by Pandya and colleagues (125), as well as studies on partial split-brain patients (5), indicates that the posterior half of the corpus callosum contains auditory fibers. The final segment of the auditory system, the descending auditory pathway, takes an anatomical course similar to that of the ascending tracts, but functions (as best we know) very differently (see elsewhere in this volume). Since the central auditory system encompasses much of the brain, it can provide the clinician with valuable data about overall CANS function. However, to use the data effectively, the clinician must use assessment tools skillfully and possess an in-depth knowledge of the structure and function of the brain.

PSYCHOPHYSICAL AND ELECTROPHYSIOLOGICAL APPROACHES

Both electrophysiological and behavioral approaches should be used in audiological testing of the CANS, with the appropriate test considered for a given situation. For example, the auditory brainstem response (ABR) is better than most behavioral tests for evaluation of brainstem lesions involving the pons but is of no value in assessing cortical lesions. On the other hand, many of the behavioral tests are more sensitive to cortical lesions than are any of the electrophysiological procedures currently in use. If the clinician is unsure if the cortex or brainstem is involved, then some combination of electrophysiological and behavioral central tests should be used. We attempt to place in perspective the use of behavioral and electrophysiological tests in assessing the brainstem, cerebrum, and interhemispheric connections.

AUDITORY EVALUATION OF THE BRAINSTEM

There are two general categories of audiological tests that can be used in evaluating brainstem integrity. The first includes those tests that are brainstem specific, that is, tests that, for the most part, are not affected by lesions rostral to the brainstem, such as the ABR (24), acoustic reflex (AR) (46), masking level differences (MLD) (27), and, to a slightly lesser degree, synthetic sentence identification with ipsilateral competing message (SSI-ICM) (56). The second group of brainstem tests are those that can be affected by either brainstem or cerebral lesions but are not specific to either. Examples of these tests would be dichotic speech tasks, filtered speech tests, speech with competing stimuli tests, and various localization tests (98,114). Both categories of tests can be influenced by peripheral hearing loss. There are other auditory tests purported to measure brainstem integrity that we cannot discuss here because of space limitations. Several references provide information about these (31,94,159). Our aim here is to discuss tests currently in use, as well as those procedures that hold promise for future use.

The Auditory Brainstem Response

Briefly, the ABR is the recording of synchronous neural discharges from the auditory nerve and brainstem in response to short acoustic stimuli, such as a series of clicks. Usually 1,000 to 2,000 responses are picked up by scalp electrodes, and filtered and averaged by a computer to yield a highly repeatable series of waves, as seen on an oscilloscope (49,52) (see Hood and Berlin, Volume I). These waves are probably generated from the auditory nerve (waves I and II) and the auditory tracts in the pons (III, IV, and V) (91). It is highly probable that there are multiple generator sites for the later waves, although specifics surrounding this issue are still unclear (24). ABR waves I, III, and V, commonly used in clinical assessment, are most likely generated caudal to the midbrain (91,173). This can be interpreted to mean that lesions involving and limited to the inferior colliculus and/or medial geniculate (as well as the cortex) may not affect the ABR (61,96).

Despite its limitations for defining rostrally positioned brainstem lesions, the ABR is probably the most sensitive audiological test for detecting brainstem pathology (3,24,101,159). The ABR can be abnormal when there is brainstem involvement, and there is considerable variability among investigators in the determination of criteria for abnormality (24,103). The most valid and reliable measure for predicting brainstem abnormality may be the degree of extension of the interwave intervals (IWI), that is, the latencies between the I–III, III–V, and I–V waves. If the lesion is in the low brainstem, the I–III interval may be extended; if the high pons is involved, the III–V interval could be extended (87,103, 158). This specific anatomical correlation is not a strong one, but usually at least one of these intervals is affected in brainstem pathology (3).

One drawback of the IWI measure is that all the waves needed for interpretation are not always obtainable, due to hearing loss, or to eighth nerve or brainstem pathology (108). If waves IV and V are absent, with waves I and III present, there is a high probability that the brainstem is involved (3,157,162). If wave III or V is present and wave I is absent, the comparison of absolute latencies with the other ear is often useful but not as predictive as the IWI (24). When early waves or all waves are absent, it is necessary to obtain an audiogram to quantify hearing loss and to help interpretation. If there is no recordable ABR and the hearing is good, the probability of a neural lesion is high; if there is considerable hearing loss, peripheral or neural involvement is possible.

When the early waves are absent, there are other latency measures (such as the absolute latency and interaural latency difference [ILD] of wave V) that can be used. The absolute latency of wave V can be affected by the degree of hearing loss—hence the diagnostic value of wave V will be compromised. However, if a delayed wave V cannot be reasonably explained by the hearing loss, there is a good possibility that a neural lesion is present. The ILD is the comparison of wave V latency between right and left ears. This measure can be difficult to interpret if hearing sensitivity is asymmetric (7). Also, it has been shown that brainstem lesions often affect ABRs from both sides. Therefore, there may be a latency abnormality bilaterally, but the ILD may be normal because both sides of the brainstem auditory tracts are involved (107).

Additional ABR measurements used in detecting brainstem dysfunction include the V-I amplitude ratio and high repetition rate effects. Neither of these is as robust or reliable as the IWI, but they can be useful in some situations. In the normal population, wave V is of greater amplitude than wave I, but this ratio can be affected by a number of nonpathological variables (24,25,113, 142) and should be used cautiously. When wave V is significantly smaller in amplitude than wave I, eighth nerve or brainstem involvement may be indicated (113,140,161).

Presenting the click stimulus at a high repetition rate (usually greater than 50/sec) may help in the detection of a brainstem lesion (139,161,174). The assumption is that at high repetition rates the system is stressed, and if a disorder exists, the latency of wave V will be shifted more than in normal subjects. Occasionally, at a high rate, wave V may even disappear in a patient with an eighth nerve or brainstem disorder (2). It is presently difficult to evaluate the high repetition rate in terms of its overall clinical value, due to the lack of comprehensive studies that have addressed this issue.

Despite some interpretive constraints, the ABR is valuable in evaluating brainstem lesions. However, its sensitivity is affected by the lesion type (Fig. 1). Intra-axial tu-

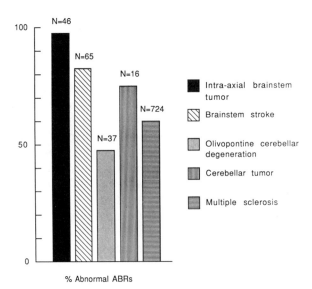

FIG. 1. The percentage of abnormal ABRs for various brainstem lesions. These percentages were computed based on a number of reports (3,24, 62,87,140).

mors, especially those originating in the pons, yield a high incidence of ABR abnormality, probably because there is a high concentration of crossing and noncrossing auditory fibers in the pons that are directly affected by this type of lesion (see elsewhere in this volume). In some common degenerative disorders, such as multiple sclerosis (MS), the auditory tracts of the brainstem may not be affected, which results in reduced overall ABR sensitivity.

The acoustic tumor (schwannoma) is a peripheral nerve lesion that usually originates in the internal auditory meatus. ABR sensitivity to the detection of acoustic tumors is generally greater than 90% (103). If this mass lesion becomes large, it often will affect the brainstem. The ABR reveals some unique findings from the ear opposite the one with a large acoustic neuroma. In these cases, the ABR's early waves (I, II, and III) are usually normal and the later waves (IV and V) are abnormal (110). This ABR finding, as mentioned earlier, is an accurate indicator of brainstem involvement.

The laterality effect of brainstem lesions on ABR is a topic of great interest. The ABR is most often abnormal from the ear ipsilateral to the side of the brainstem that has the lesion (24,101,122). It is also common to observe bilaterally abnormal ABRs in brainstem involvement. When bilateral ABR deficits occur and the lesion is limited to one side, it is the ear ipsilateral to the side that has the lesion that yields the greater deficit (24,122). When both sides of the brainstem are involved, bilateral ABR deficits are often observed (158). True midline brainstem lesions are seldom reported but probably yield bilateral ABR abnormalities, especially if they are in the low pons (96) (Fig. 2).

A contralateral (ear) ABR deficit alone is seldom reported in brainstem pathology (24,101,122), yet it is well known that the majority of auditory fibers cross at the superior olivary complex in the caudal pons, and at this level and higher the ear tested should then be influenced more by the contralateral rather than the ipsilateral fiber

tracts. This is not the case with the ABR, and this inconsistency has provoked much discussion about general brainstem neuroanatomy and the anatomical characteristics of the fiber tracts that are responsible for generating the ABR (24,96).

The Acoustic Reflex

The AR is another valuable audiological procedure for assessing brainstem integrity. (This test was discussed by Hood and Berlin in Volume I). The AR occurs when the stapedius muscle contracts when a relatively intense sound is presented. This consensual reflex is dependent on a normal middle ear system, cochlea, eighth nerve, and caudal brainstem (see Volume I). Since the brainstem is an important link in the acoustic reflex, pathology that involves the brainstem can affect the AR (16). The threshold measurement of the AR can be readily accomplished by a variety of commercial instruments that measure the acoustic immittance at the eardrum, which changes when the stapedius muscle contracts, stiffening the ossicular chain (46, 156,175). This change in immittance, measured at the eardrum, is a reliable indicator of the stapedius reflex. There are a number of characteristics of the AR besides its presence, absence, or threshold, that may be helpful in defining brainstem lesions.

An important observation in AR research was made by Greisen and Rasmussen (45) in their comparative study of ipsilateral or uncrossed AR (i.e., the reflex recorded from the same ear that is acoustically stimulated) with the contralateral or crossed AR (i.e., the reflex recorded from the ear opposite the acoustic stimulation). In two patients with brainstem lesions, these investigators noted that the ipsilateral AR was present, but the contralateral AR was absent. This concept of comparing crossed and uncrossed ARs was expanded by subsequent studies by Jerger and Jerger (58), who reported findings similar to those of Greisen and Rasmussen.

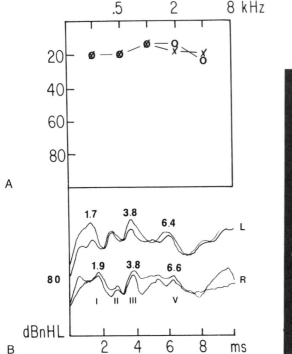

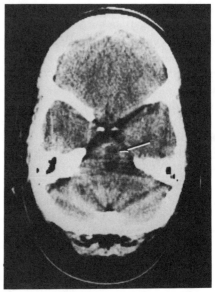

FIG. 2. Pure tone audiogram (**A**), auditory brainstem response (ABR) (**B**), and CT scan (**C**) from a 57-year-old woman who suffered a brainstem infarct at the level of the pontomedullary junction. The CT scan shows that the lesion is essentially midline and does not involve the cochlear nuclei on either side. The ABR shows normal waves I, II, and III, but wave V is abnormally delayed and reduced in amplitude bilaterally. Since the eighth nerve and cochlear nucleus are not affected, but the crossing fibers (ventral, dorsal, intermediate stria) from the cochlear nucleus and superior olivary complex should be, it could be interpreted that the first three ABR waves are generated by the eighth nerve and cochlear nucleus. This case also shows a bilateral effect of a midline brainstem lesion.

It has also been shown that the sensitivity of the AR can be enhanced by measuring the amplitude and certain morphological characteristics of the AR (17,46,63,156). The latency of the AR may be useful in detecting brainstem involvement (17,156); however, instrumentation problems can be a factor in this measurement, and considerable caution in clinical use is suggested (26,46,116).

Although there are many interesting anecdotal reports demonstrating the value of the AR in brainstem lesions, there are few reports with even a moderate number of cases. Antonelli et al. (3) showed that the AR was only moderately sensitive to intra-axial brainstem tumors. Stephens and

Thornton (159) reported that 8 of 18 patients with brainstem lesions had abnormal ARs. In a number of studies of patients with MS reviewed by Jerger and colleagues (62), about one-half of the patients demonstrated abnormal ARs. However, in the same report, using temporal measures of onset and offset, amplitude, and traditional AR indices, Jerger showed that 71% of the patients with MS had AR abnormalities. Abnormal ARs have been reported in other central nervous system disorders that compromise the brainstem, such as chronic alcoholism (154) and severe head injury (47).

The more carefully the dynamics of the AR can be defined and measured, as advocated by Jerger and colleagues (63), the more sensitive the procedure will become. In assessing CANS integrity, the AR is essentially limited to the caudal pons and must be used accordingly.

Masking Level Differences

The bilateral MLD is a behavioral test that requires the presentation of pulsed tones (usually 500 Hz) or speech (spondees or consonant-vowel nonsense syllables) stimuli to both ears diotically while a masking noise (usually broad band) is delivered bilaterally. Thresholds for the tonal or speech stimuli are established for two listening conditions termed "homophasic" (SoNo) and "antiphasic" (SπNo) (50). In the homophasic condition, both the tonal or speech stimuli and the masking noise are presented to both ears in-phase. In the antiphasic condition, one of the signals is presented 180° out-of-phase between the two ears, while the other signal is kept in-phase (50,83). The comparison of thresholds for these two conditions generally yields a difference measured in decibels, which is termed the MLD (119,170).

It has been well documented that patients with brainstem lesions often have significantly smaller MLDs than normal subjects (86,119,123,136). The incidence of MLD abnormality for patients with brainstem lesions, as reviewed by Noffsinger et al. (119), ranges from 50% to 100%. Abnormal MLDs were reported in approximately 50% of a large population of patients ($N=114$) with various types of brainstem disorders (121). The average incidence of abnormality was also about 50% in a number of studies using MLDs in MS populations (48, 62,106,120,123).

Of special interest is the study by Lynn et al. (86), which showed that patients with cerebral or rostral brainstem lesions had normal MLDs, and patients with lesions confined to the pontomedullary area of the brainstem had markedly reduced MLDs. This concept of the MLD being related specifically to the function of the caudal brainstem is also supported by correlative studies with the ABR (48,118).

Synthetic Sentence Identification with Ipsilateral Competing Message

The tests for brainstem dysfunction mentioned to this point are sensitive to lesions of the low to mid brainstem (below the midbrain) but are likely to miss isolated lesions in the rostral-most brainstem. The SSI-ICM, and other behavioral tests, help to offset this problem. Although the SSI-ICM is sensitive to both rostral and caudal brainstem lesions, it can still be affected (to a lesser degree) by cerebral involvement (53).

The SSI-ICM is composed of 10 third-order approximations of English sentences that are presented with a competing message (continuous discourse) to one ear (153). When a closed message set is used, the patient is asked to point to the sentence that is heard. The test can be presented in two ways: (a) by varying the signal-to-competition ratio or (b) by keeping the signal-to-competition ratio constant (usually 0 dB) and presenting the sentences at several intensity levels from low to high. This latter approach can also be used with monosyllabic word lists without a competing message (performance-intensity function), with results similar to those from the SSI-ICM (53,55). If this procedure is used with patients with brainstem involvement, word recognition performance decreases as intensity is increased; the term "roll-over" has been introduced to describe this phenomenon (55).

The incidence of SSI-ICM abnormality in populations with brainstem involvement is relatively impressive. Jerger and Jerger (56) reported that 11 of 11 patients with intra-axial brainstem lesions had scores in one or both ears that were below the normal criteria. In another study the patients with brainstem involvement, an average deficit of 40% was noted for the ear contralateral to the lesioned side of the brainstem (57). Reports using a modification of the SSI-ICM showed that 7 of 13 (159) and 8 of 12 (3) patients with brainstem lesions had abnormal results.

Other Behavioral Tests

There are a number of other tests that have been used to define brainstem involvement: rapidly alternating speech perception (85), binaural fusion (151), filtered speech (85), compressed speech (20), and a variety of dichotic listening tasks (114). Although some of these tests are sensitive to brainstem lesions, they are affected equally or more by cerebral lesions; hence, brainstem involvement cannot be discriminated from higher level involvement. These tests become valuable in brainstem evaluation when a lesion exists in the rostral brainstem—an area that is often beyond the anatomical range of tests such as the ABR, AR, and MLD.

The laterality effects of brainstem lesions with behavioral tests are different from those with the ABR. Although there are exceptions, lesions at or above the mid-pons (especially intra-axial lesions) often result in contralateral or bilateral ear deficits on behavioral tests (56,57). Further investigation of this issue is warranted and could prove valuable in increasing our knowledge of the structure and function of the auditory tracts of the brainstem.

AUDITORY EVALUATION OF THE CEREBRUM

As was the case with the assessment of brainstem pathology, there are two general categories of audiological tests that can be used in the assessment of cerebral integrity. The first category includes the electrophysiological test procedures that have been used to assess cerebral integrity. These include the later evoked potentials, specifically the middle late and late auditory potentials. The second group of tests includes various psychophysical or behavioral tests, such as dichotic speech tests, monaural low redundancy speech tests, temporal ordering tasks, and various localization tests (98). Although these tests are not specific to the site of lesion, they tend to be somewhat more sensitive to cerebral and/or interhemispheric lesions than to brainstem lesions, especially if a test battery approach to assessment is used. Both categories of tests can be influenced by peripheral hearing loss, and this will be addressed in greater detail subsequently.

The Middle Latency Response

The middle latency response (MLR) is one of the electrophysiological procedures that is beginning to be used to assess hemispheric integrity. First reported by Geisler, Frishkopf, and Rosenblith in 1958 (41), this auditory evoked response consists of a series of waves occurring after the ABR and before the N1 component of the late auditory evoked response. There are several negative and positive waves (Fig. 3); the most robust and consistent are the Na and Pa waves (41,168).

The MLR can be elicited by using clicks or tone pips (168), with the subject either awake or asleep; however, the amplitude of the waveform is decreased by the deeper stages of sleep (124). The MLR has an extended maturational course. In normal infants and young children, it is often absent, delayed in latency, and with less distinct waveforms than those observed in adults (77).

Filtering of the MLR is an important factor in assessing CANS integrity. The filters used should have a gradual rejection rate (e.g., 6–12 dB per octave) and relatively broad band pass characteristics (e.g., 20–500 Hz or greater). Narrow EEG filter bands with sharp roll-offs have been shown to distort the MLR, in a manner that may

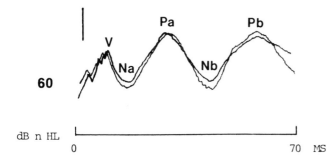

60

dB n HL

0   70 MS

FIG. 3. A middle latency response (MLR) waveform obtained from a normal hearing young adult. Wave V of the auditory brainstem response is shown preceding the MLR. The calibration marker at the left is equal to 0.4 µV.

give a false impression that a wave is present (69).

Although there is some disagreement, the majority of evidence suggests that the main component of the MLR (the Pa wave) originates in the vicinity of the primary auditory cortex. This concept is supported by mapping studies in animals (65,76,78), and by strong correlations between recordings from exposed human cortex and scalp-recorded potentials (23,144). In addition, abnormal MLRs from patients with temporal lobe lesions highlight the possibility that this potential's origin is in that area (178).

If the generation of the MLR is associated with the primary auditory cortex and surrounding areas, as the preponderance of data indicates, then abnormality in this area should compromise the MLR. A number of reports support this notion (65,76,78), but there are also some that do not (178). Multiple electrode sites can be helpful in comparing hemispheric MLR differences in amplitude, which seems to be an excellent index for detecting abnormality. Kraus et al. (75) showed that MLRs were reduced in amplitude over the damaged hemisphere when using T-3 and T-4 electrode sites. Similar results were noted in the study by Kileny et al. (71) on patients with unilateral cerebral lesions. This latter study also showed significantly reduced Na-Pa amplitudes for patients with temporal lobe involvement compared with patients with brain lesions outside the temporal lobe.

Bilateral temporal lobe damage can result

in central deafness and in most cases in absent or abnormal MLRs (44,51). These findings have implications for our understanding of the MLR's generator sites and support its clinical use. However, some patients with bitemporal lesions have had normal MLRs (178). This inconsistency in MLR results is difficult to explain and warrants further research.

The Late Auditory Evoked Responses

There are three evoked potentials that are discussed in assessing cerebral integrity. The N1 response occurs at about 100 msec, the P2 at about 200 msec, and the P3 (or P300) at about 300 msec poststimulus. The P3 is often and more appropriately referred to as an event related potential (ERP). These late auditory evoked responses (LAERs) range in amplitude from about 3 to 20 µV in normals, with the P3 generally providing the largest response (128) (Fig. 4). LAERs can be elicited using a wide variety of acoustic stimuli such as clicks, tones, or short speech segments (135). The latencies of the N1 and P2 are a function of stimulus intensity (128), while all the LAER waves are affected by a variety of drugs (42), the patient's psychological state (135), and age (104,135). The interstimulus interval can also affect the amplitudes of the LAERs. Therefore, in most studies the rate of presentation seldom exceeds one per second (128).

The N1 and P2 responses are generally

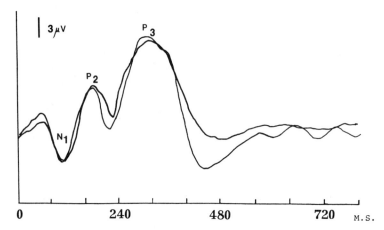

FIG. 4. Normal late auditory evoked response including the N1, P2, and P3 waves. These responses were obtained from a young adult using the odd-ball paradigm with 70 dB HL, 1,000 Hz (frequent) and 2,000 Hz (rare) tones as the stimuli.

considered exogenous potentials, and the P3 is endogenous. The exogenous potentials can be obtained with the subject in a passive listening condition (i.e., he/she does not have to manipulate the stimuli actively in some prescribed manner). The endogenous responses require that the subject processes the stimuli in some set manner as indicated by the paradigm used (155). The most common paradigm for obtaining a P3 is termed the "odd-ball" paradigm. In this procedure the subject usually is presented two stimuli, one of which occurs only 15% to 20% of the time, and the other occurring 80% to 85% of the time; these are termed the "rare" and "frequent" stimuli, respectively. The subject is asked to attend (usually by counting) to the rare stimuli and to ignore the frequent stimuli. The cognitive processes associated with attending to the stimuli result in a large potential: the P3 (135,165). Therefore, it is the "internal" or "cognitive" processes operating on the stimuli that cause the response.

The LAERs are widely distributed over the scalp, but the greatest amplitudes are recorded from the vertex, frontal, and central parietal areas (135). However, there is disagreement about the location of the generators of the LAERs. The N1 and P2 are generated, at least in part, by the primary auditory cortex with additional input from frontal and parietal areas (128,172). These cerebral areas may also be involved in the P3 response, but other areas, probably deeper in the brain, may also be involved (179).

Because the LAERs seem to involve the auditory areas of the cerebrum, it is possible that these potentials can be used to assess central auditory integrity. The N1 and P2 responses were originally used for assessing hearing sensitivity in infants (29). Only recently have the LAERs been investigated for use in testing CANS function in disease or disorder states. Peronnet and Michel (126) showed reduced or absent N1, P2 complexes recorded from electrodes placed over the hemisphere with the lesion, while responses from the normal hemisphere were larger in amplitude or were of better morphology (126). Subsequent reports have revealed similar findings and emphasize two factors: (a) as with the MLR, the electrode over or nearest the lesion site has the highest probability of demonstrating abnormality and (b) LAERs may be clinically useful in defining cerebral lesions affecting the auditory areas (95,145). This latter concept has support from several additional studies. It has been shown that N1 amplitudes are reduced for patients with lesions in the temporal-parietal region of the brain, when compared with normals, as well as for patients with lesions of the frontal lobe (73) (Fig. 5).

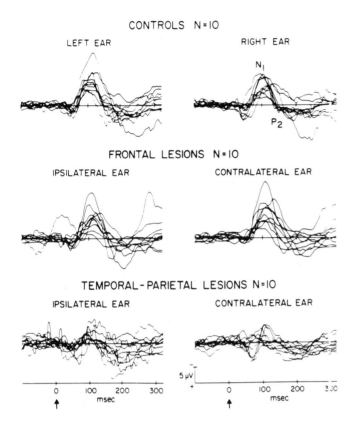

CONTROLS N=10

LEFT EAR RIGHT EAR

FRONTAL LESIONS N=10

IPSILATERAL EAR CONTRALATERAL EAR

TEMPORAL-PARIETAL LESIONS N=10

IPSILATERAL EAR CONTRALATERAL EAR

FIG. 5. The N1 to P2 complex for three groups of subjects. These are overlayed traces of these late auditory evoked responses. Ipsilateral and contralateral ears are shown with respect to the lesioned hemisphere. In this case, negative is up (N1) and positive (P2) is down. (From ref. 73, with permission.)

Recently, hemispheric asymmetries in P2 have been shown for verbal stimuli in aphasic patients, with the right hemisphere yielding larger responses than the left (147). In bilateral temporal lobe lesions it is difficult to make hemispheric comparisons with regard to the evoked response characteristics, but the LAERs appear to provide results consistent with the neurologic and radiologic findings. Totally absent LAERs have been reported in a number of cases of bitemporal lesions. These patients were centrally deaf or demonstrated severe auditory difficulties (44,64,89,90,178). Although they have not demonstrated absent LAER components, other studies on patients with bitemporal lesions have revealed decreased amplitudes and/or increased latencies for the LAER waveforms (1,88). Interestingly, there is at least one study reporting normal LAERs in patients with bilateral temporal lobe involvement (178).

The P3 has been used with a greater number of clinical populations than have the N1 and P2 responses. Since the task associated with the P3 requires the focusing of attention and other subtle cognitive processes, it has been used with disorders that may affect these functions (e.g., aging, various dementias, and psychological abnormalities). There are several studies that have shown increased latencies as a function of increasing age for the P3 (43,134,135). It appears that dementia affects the P3 latency even more than aging, as patients with dementia have significantly greater latency delays than age-matched controls (21,43). There also have been correlations of certain P3 abnormalities with psychological disorders, such as depression and schizophrenia (127). The P3 has also been used with other clinical populations, including patients with head injury (82), focal brain lesions (107), language disorders associated with stroke

(155), and Down's syndrome (84). It has been shown that patients with focal lesions that involve areas of the auditory cerebrum have P3s with significantly increased latencies and decreased amplitudes compared with an age- and audiometrically matched control group (99).

The use of LAERs in evaluating disorders that may affect the CANS is gaining attention. However, before clinical or research use of the LAERs is undertaken, several factors need consideration. In defining or detecting dysfunction of the CANS, the LAERs do not presently have the capability of some of the more sensitive behavioral tests mentioned. Combining MLRs and LAERs with certain behavioral tests could prove to be most helpful in defining higher order auditory problems. It also may be beneficial to examine the correlation between various behavioral and electrophysiological test procedures (145).

Consideration must also be given to some of the intrinsic limitations of the LAER and, to some degree, the MLR. These potentials require considerable time to administer, produce responses that can be variable within and across subjects, and, as mentioned earlier, the specific generators of these potentials are not known (70). Much more research must be done on the pathological correlates to these responses to accurately assess their diagnostic value.

Monaural Low Redundancy Speech Tests

These behavioral tests detect central auditory dysfunction by reducing the redundancy of the test stimuli by distorting the acoustic properties of the speech test materials. Bocca et al. (14,15) were the first to use a monaural low redundancy speech test (low-pass filtered phonetically balanced words) to assess CANS function in a group of patients with verified lesions of the auditory cortex. Word recognition performance in this group of subjects was reduced substantially in the contralateral compared with the ipsilateral ear. Since the time of

these pioneering investigations, there have been several other attempts to reduce the extrinsic redundancy of the typical undistorted speech stimuli by manipulating the temporal, intensity, and/or frequency patterns of the speech signal (137).

Low-Pass Filtered Speech

One of the more commonly used forms of monaural degrading of the speech signal has been the use of low-pass filtered speech (LPFS). There have been several variations of this test procedure since it was first introduced into the assessment field in the mid-1950s. Test stimuli have included different speech materials (e.g., monosyllabic words, spondees, and sentences) and a variety of different cut-off frequencies and roll-off characteristics. (The reader is directed to Rintelmann [137] and to Musiek and Baran [98] for a comprehensive discussion of these tests.) Today, one of the more commonly used and commercially available versions of the LPFS test is that developed by Willeford (176). In this version, monosyllabic phonetically balanced words are low-pass filtered using a 500-Hz cut-off frequency and a roll-off of 18 dB per octave. Results of several investigations have shown that the LPFS test is moderately sensitive to cerebral lesions (98) (Fig. 6). Typically, one notes contralateral ear deficits on this type of test in subjects with temporal lobe lesions and essentially no ear differences in subjects with interhemispheric auditory pathway involvement. In subjects with brainstem involvement, no specific pattern of performance has been identified.

Compressed Speech

A second common method of degrading or reducing the redundancy of the speech signal has involved the use of time compressed speech stimuli. Historically, this type of method of distortion has involved one of three methods: (a) having the speaker accelerate his/her speech rate, (b)

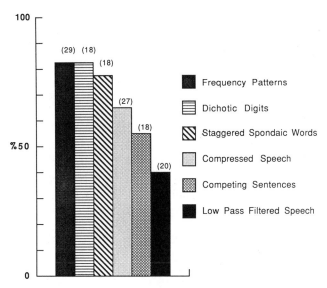

FIG. 6. The sensitivity of a variety of central auditory tests. All patients represented in this graph had normal peripheral hearing with the exception of three patients who were administered the compressed speech test. (The numbers in parentheses indicate the number of patients in the study.) The data reflect the authors' experiences with these procedures in patients who had documented cerebral lesions affecting the auditory areas. The results shown depict the percentages of patients with abnormal results in at least one ear and are derived from the following studies: frequency patterns (115), dichotic digits, staggered spondaic words, and competing sentences (93), compressed speech (6), and low-pass filtered speech (*unpublished data*).

accelerating the recorded signal by using a faster playback rate, and (c) removing segments of the signal electromechanically and then joining together the remaining segments. With the advent of sophisticated computer instrumentation, a fourth method of time compression is possible. This includes computer manipulation and/or generation of time compressed speech materials. Results of some early, but limited, investigations indicated that patients with localized lesions in the auditory cortex demonstrated reduced speech recognition scores in the ear contralateral to the affected hemisphere (80), while patients with more diffuse lesions were more likely to demonstrate reduced performance in both ears (80,138). In a study of 27 subjects with intracranial lesions involving the temporal lobe, approximately 60% of the subjects showed reduced performance in one or both ears (6) (Fig. 6). The more common

finding was for depressed performance in the contralateral ear. We are not aware of any specific investigations that have studied the effects of brainstem lesions on compressed speech test performance. However, we anticipate that, as is the case with the other monaural low redundancy speech tests used in the assessment of the CANS in subjects with brainstem pathology, the results would be mixed. Contralateral, ipsilateral, and bilateral deficits may be encountered in this population. In addition, the hit rate is likely to be low.

Dichotic Speech Tests

Kimura (72) has been credited with introducing dichotic speech tests into the CANS assessment field. In the early 1960s she administered a dichotic digits (DD) test in which digit triads were presented to a group of patients with unilateral temporal lobe involvement. Kimura found impaired digit recognition in the ear contralateral to the lesion if the stimuli were presented in a competing dichotic paradigm, while no deficits were noted if the digits were presented in a noncompeting condition, i.e., unless the left or dominant hemisphere for speech and language was affected. In that case, bilaterally depressed scores were noted most frequently.

Based on these findings and some earlier physiological evidence (141), Kimura developed a model that could be used to explain the function of the CANS in the perception of auditorily presented stimuli. The model was based on the premise that the contralateral pathways in humans are more numerous and/or stronger than the ipsilateral pathways. In cases in which there is only monaural input to the auditory system, either pathway is capable of initiating the appropriate neural response to allow accurate perception of the speech signal. In dichotic competing situations, however, the stronger contralateral pathways take precedence over the weaker ipsilateral ones, and there may even be a suppression of the ipsilateral pathways. Therefore, if one hemisphere is damaged, reduced performance in the contralateral ear is expected, as long as the test stimuli are presented in a competing dichotic paradigm. In addition, ipsilateral ear deficits are expected if the left, or dominant, hemisphere for speech and language is affected.

Although there have been several different dichotic tests used in the assessment of CANS lesions, we review three of the more popular and/or more sensitive of these tests. (For information regarding several of the other tests, the reader is referred to Musiek and Pinheiro [114] and to Musiek and Baran [98]).

Dichotic Digits

As mentioned above, a DD test presumably was the first dichotic test used to assess the integrity of the CANS (72). Since that time there have been many variations of this basic test procedure. These have included differences in the number of digits presented to each ear and in the manner of responding. For example, in some investigations, the subjects were asked to repeat the items perceived in one ear first, followed by the other ear, while in others, the subjects were asked to add together the numbers perceived in each ear and report a single number for each ear (114).

We have used a version of the DD test in which 20 pairs of digits are presented dichotically to the two ears (92). Our subjects are asked to repeat the words perceived in both ears, and the percentage of correctly identified digits is calculated. The advantage of this test over many of the other dichotic speech tests currently used in CANS assessments is that it takes less than 4 min to administer and is easily scored. Our test results, along with those of several other investigators (see ref. 98) have shown that the test is fairly sensitive to both brainstem and cortical lesions. Results of a study of 21 subjects with either brainstem or cortical lesions revealed that 18 showed abnormal performance in one or both ears (92). A comparative study that investigated the relative sensitivity of the DD, staggered spondaic words (SSW), and competing sentences (CS) tests in the assessment of CANS dysfunction in 12 subjects with brainstem lesions and 18 subjects with cortical lesions showed that the DD test yielded slightly more abnormal findings for both groups than did either of the other two tests (93) (Fig. 6).

Staggered Spondaic Words

Approximately 1 year after Kimura introduced the dichotic test paradigm into the field of central auditory assessment, Katz (66) introduced a unique modification of this psychophysical test procedure. In this test, two spondee words were presented with a staggered onset. The first half of one test item was presented in a noncompeting condition, followed by a competing condition in which the second half of the first spondee and the first half of the second spondee were presented to the two ears in a dichotic manner. Finally, the second half of the second spondee was presented in a noncompeting manner. The SSW is among the best-known and most frequently used dichotic speech tests in clinics today. (The scoring of this test is complex. The reader is referred to Brunt [18] for details regarding scoring as well as test administration procedures.) Subsequent studies by Katz and associates (67,68) have shown a close correspondence between SSW test results and site of CANS damage.

Dichotic Consonant-Vowels

In the early 1970s, Berlin et al. (10) introduced yet another dichotic speech test, dichotic consonant-vowels (CVs), into the CANS assessment area. For this test, synthetic CV stimuli are presented to the two ears dichotically, while the onsets of the two stimuli are varied. On one part of the test the alignments of the two stimuli are almost simultaneous, while in another segment of this test the onsets differ. Onset delays of 15, 30, 60, and 90 msec are used. Berlin et al. (10) found that normal subjects obtained better scores if the onsets of the lagging CVs were delayed by 30 to 90 msec; however, similar improvements were not noted for patients who had undergone temporal lobectomies.

In a subsequent study, Berlin et al. (9) administered the dichotic CV test to three lobectomy and four hemispherectomy patients. In all patients performance in the ear contralateral to the lesion declined to near chance levels after surgery, while performance in the ipsilateral ear improved. However, a significant difference was noted between the two groups in the amount of improvement for the ipsilateral ear. In the lobectomy group there was a small improvement, but the scores did not approach

100%; in the hemispherectomy group performance rose to nearly 100%. These differences could be created by a competition for neural substrate, which was effectively eliminated in the hemispherectomy group.

We are aware of only one report on the use of dichotic CVs in the evaluation of brainstem pathology (9). These authors discovered almost complete suppression of the CVs presented to the left ear of a patient with a lesion of the right medial geniculate. The ipsilateral ear score was grossly normal.

TEMPORAL ORDERING TASKS

In the early 1970s, researchers began to introduce test paradigms in which subjects were asked to differentiate two different tones or clicks of different pitches and/or different onset times (81,166). The tones were presented to either the same ear or to opposite ears, and the subjects were asked to indicate the order of the two tones. Swisher and Hirsh (166) studied performance in young adults, older adults, and brain-damaged adults (including left brain-damaged subjects with fluent aphasia, left brain-damaged subjects with nonfluent aphasia, and right brain-damaged subjects without aphasia). Their results indicated that subjects with fluent aphasia required the longest intervals to order stimuli, particularly if the two stimuli were presented to the same ear. In subjects with right hemisphere damage, the differences to make temporal order judgments between two stimuli presented to the same ear were smaller and approximated those demonstrated by the control subjects. However, greater deficits were discovered when the tonal stimuli were presented to opposite ears.

Lackner and Teuber (81) presented dichotic clicks with various onset times to both ears in 24 subjects with left hemisphere damage and 19 with right hemisphere damage. They found that subjects with left hemisphere damage required longer silent intervals between stimuli to perceive separation.

More recently, a dichotic pattern discrimination has been introduced that has shown good sensitivity to cortical and subcortical lesions (11). This test requires the dichotic presentation of patterns of click trains. The pattern or intensity of the stimuli is changed for one ear, and the patient reports when this monaural change is noted.

Efron and associates (32–35) conducted a series of experiments using nonspeech auditory signals and demonstrated contralateral ear deficits in individuals with temporal lobe lesions for a variety of auditory tasks (gap detection, sound lateralization, and temporal ordering tasks). These authors found consistent contralateral ear effects not only in subjects with posterior temporal lobe involvement, but also in those with anterior lobe resections that involved portions of the temporal lobe previously believed to have no role in auditory processing. Based on these findings, Efron and Crandall (33) postulated the existence of a contralaterally organized efferent pathway located within each temporal lobe that, when activated, significantly enhances the ability to perceive auditory stimuli on the contralateral side. This efferent multisynaptic auditory pathway has been discovered in the rhesus monkey (149).

Frequency (Pitch) Pattern Sequences

One of the more popular temporal ordering tasks used today is the frequency (pitch) pattern sequence (PATT) test developed by Pinheiro and Ptacek (133). It consists of test sequences containing three tone bursts. In each sequence, only two of the three tone bursts are of the same frequency, creating six different possible sequences. The subject is asked to verbally describe each sequence heard, and a percent correct score is derived for each ear. Patients with lesions of either hemisphere or of the interhemispheric pathways have difficulty describing

the monaurally presented test stimuli (109, 111,115,129). Results have demonstrated that this test is fairly sensitive to cerebral lesions (Figs. 6). Findings also suggest that some processing of the stimuli occurs in both hemispheres and that the auditory interhemispheric pathway must be intact for a normal verbal response on this test (111,115).

Although some patients with brainstem lesions perform poorly on the frequency pattern test (101,131), the majority of patients with this kind of lesion perform normally (115).

Auditory Duration Patterns (100)

Recently, we have begun to experiment with a test that is similar to the PATT, with the exception that rather than requiring frequency discrimination this test requires that the subject discriminate differences between tones on the basis of their durational characteristics. This auditory duration patterns (ADP) test includes 60 items with each containing three tone bursts. In each of the sequences, two of the tones are of the same duration. Like the PATT, six different sequences are possible. The test stimuli are presented monaurally, and the subject is asked to verbally describe the sequences. To date, we have reported on the performance of 18 individuals with confirmed lesions of the CANS (4). Our preliminary results have shown that this test is sensitive to CANS lesions and is relatively resistant to the effects of peripheral hearing loss.

AUDITORY EVALUATION OF THE INTERHEMISPHERIC PATHWAYS

In the late 1960s, several investigators reported reduced left ear scores on dichotic speech tests in patients who had undergone complete surgical section of the corpus callosum (90,152). Similar left ear deficits have since been reported by other investigators (98). We have been able to assess the performance of patients who have had complete surgical sections of the corpus callosum (111), as well as individuals with anterior sections of the corpus callosum (5). Unlike many earlier investigations, we tested our patients not only postoperatively, but also preoperatively. In this way we were able to determine if the deficits noted postoperatively were related to the surgical sectioning of the corpus callosum or to some pre-existing hemispheric in-

volvement. Our results showed that subjects with complete surgical sections (a) performed normally on a monaural low redundancy speech test (LPFS); (b) showed left ear deficits on dichotic speech tests (SSW and DD); and (c) demonstrated bilateral deficits on a temporal ordering task (PATT) (111) (Fig. 7).

Interestingly, we did not find similar deficits in a group of eight subjects with ante-

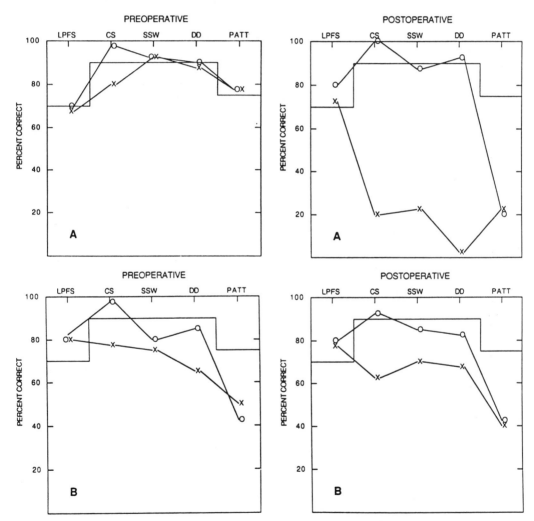

FIG. 7. A: Mean preoperative and postoperative scores on five central auditory tests for four patients with complete sections of the corpus callosum. The lower limit of normal performance is indicated by the *solid line*. Data are presented for the right (O) and left (X) ears (adapted from ref. 111, with permission.) **B:** Mean preoperative and postoperative scores for eight patients with anterior sections of the corpus callosum. Other specifications are the same as for A. (Adapted from ref. 5, with permission.)

rior sections of the corpus callosum (5), in whom preoperative and postoperative results were very similar (Fig. 6). Only on the CS and PATT tests did postoperative results differ substantially from the preoperative results. These differences, however, were due in large part to a rather dramatic postoperative effect in one subject on both tests. In this subject left ear scores dropped from 95% preoperatively to 0% postoperatively on the CS test and from 80% preoperatively to 47% postoperatively on the PATT test. It is likely that these differences were related to individual differences in the structure of the corpus callosum and/or possible variations in the surgical reference points. In addition, the limited attention and motivation of this subject at the time of postoperative testing may have affected test results.

The differences between patients with a complete versus an anterior section of the corpus callosum are presumed to have an anatomical basis. If one assumes that the auditory portion of the corpus callosum in humans is located in its posterior half (consistent with the evidence provided by Pandya et al. [125], which placed the location of auditory interhemispheric fibers in primates in the posterior portion of the corpus callosum), then sectioning of this part of the corpus callosum would result in the deficits noted in our first group of subjects since the interhemispheric transfer of auditory information would be prevented. The left ear deficits on the dichotic speech tests presumably occurred since the stronger contralateral auditory pathways from the left ear to the right hemisphere to the left hemisphere were rendered ineffective by sectioning. At the same time, the ipsilateral pathways were suppressed because of the dichotic nature of the task. No deficits were noted on the monaural low redundancy speech test, since the ipsilateral left ear to the left hemisphere pathway was not being suppressed. The bilateral deficits noted on the PATT test were expected, since both hemispheres are involved in the processing

of acoustic contours of temporal sequences (right hemisphere) that require verbal labeling (left hemisphere). Sectioning of the corpus callosum prohibited the necessary interaction of the two hemispheres, and thus performance was affected bilaterally. When we asked two of our split-brain subjects with complete surgical sections to "hum" the test stimuli on the PATT test, both were able to do this with a fairly high degree of accuracy. This is because humming is essentially a mimicking response, apparently triggered by the right hemisphere (5).

Similar test results in patients with a variety of hemispheric lesions suggest that other lesions may also affect the interhemispheric pathways. Severe left ear deficits have been reported for patients with lesions near the lateral wall of the lateral ventricle at the level of the trigone (28), for patients with MS (98,143), and for a patient with a right hemisphere stroke (95).

Almost any type of cerebral lesion can affect the interhemispheric pathways. If only the white matter is involved, the neuroaudiological profile should mimic that of the split-brain patient; however, when the lesion affects both the gray (cortex) and white matter in the left hemisphere, a slightly different neuroaudiological pattern emerges. In the latter case, dichotic speech scores should be abnormal bilaterally. This bilateral deficit results from the combination of the left auditory cortex involvement, which causes the classic contralateral ear deficit (right ear), together with the corpus callosum pathology, which disrupts the transfer of neural information from the right to the left hemisphere, causing a left ear deficit. Monaural low redundancy tasks, such as LPFS, demonstrate only a contralateral (right ear) ear deficit. This is because the task does not require interhemispheric transfer for verbal report of left ear stimuli, since the ipsilateral pathways are not suppressed. Frequency pattern results would indicate bilateral abnormalities since the necessary interhemispheric processing is disrupted (98).

EVALUATION OF THE LEARNING DISABLED CHILD

During the past decade there has been considerable interest in the central auditory evaluation of learning disabled (LD) children. Although there are great variability and much that is unknown about this population, it appears that many of these children have central auditory dysfunction (37). The underlying mechanisms are not clearly understood, but improper brain development (39) and lagging maturation (105) are theories gaining support from an audiological viewpoint. Many of the psychophysical procedures mentioned in this chapter have been used in the assessment of LD children. Investigators have reported abnormal test results for several of these tests, especially for those requiring temporal ordering and binaural listening; tests for brainstem function (such as the ABR) are rarely abnormal in this population (177). This topic cannot be discussed in detail here, but it represents a challenging and much needed area of study.

EVALUATION OF THE ELDERLY

The influence of age on the results of CANS assessment is not well documented, primarily because there are various sites of aging effects. In a 1964 publication, Schuknecht (146) identified four distinct types of presbycusis: (a) sensory presbycusis related to atrophy of the organ of Corti and degeneration of the hair cells, beginning at the basal end of the cochlea and moving toward the apex; (b) neural presbycusis related to the loss of neurons in the auditory pathways and eighth nerve; (c) stria vascularis atrophy, or metabolic presbycusis, related to the degeneration of the stria vascularis in the apical turn of the cochlea; and (d) inner ear conductive-type presbycusis, which is probably related to an increase in the stiffness of the supporting structures of the cochlear duct. These various pathologies manifest themselves in different audiometric configurations, and often more than one may coexist at the same time. In many presbycusic losses, the peripheral hearing mechanisms, as well as the central auditory structures, are involved. Therefore, the audiologist must be aware of the potential confounding effects of peripheral hearing loss on the central auditory tests being used.

Although the binaural hearing thresholds may appear to be similar, one cannot assume that both ears have the same hearing capacity at suprathreshold levels. Recruitment and problems related to temporal factors may be present. In testing the patient with presbycusis, the audiologist must consider the presence of not only a cochlear hearing loss, but also a central disability that is not related to a brain lesion. In the older patient, central auditory function may be depressed by a general loss of neurons throughout the CANS. Blood flow may be reduced by fatty deposits in the arteries supplying the brain. There may also be age-related changes in the cerebral energy metabolism that do not affect peripheral hearing. Glucose metabolism and oxygen consumption in the brain decrease with aging (150). The problem with CANS assessments is how to account for these differences and their effects on CANS function, which appear to be primarily physiological and not chronological. Therefore, establishing norms by chronological age will not necessarily solve the problem.

There have been some attempts to study CANS function in the geriatric population. Investigations of elderly patients with normal hearing sensitivity for their age and no known central lesions demonstrated higher percentages of abnormal findings on LPFS (12), time compressed speech (74,160), synthetic sentence identification (54), binaural tonal and speech procedures (such as MLDs) (38,169), and on dichotic speech measures (such as dichotic nonsense syllables) (30,79). (Additional information on this topic can be found in Bergman [8] and

Rintelmann [137].) Such findings implicate a reduction in the efficiency with which the aging CANS handles difficult auditory stimuli. In addition, these studies suggest that the reduced capacity noted in elderly patients is likely to be present throughout the CANS, i.e., from the low brainstem through to the cortex and the interhemispheric pathways. The results obtained to date have shown that age-related deficits are typically manifested bilaterally on tests in which individual ear scores are obtained, and if ear differences do appear, the size of the interaural differences are typically small.

The ability to differentiate age effects from pathological effects is of considerable importance when one is evaluating elderly patients. The differentiation is relatively easy when age-independent lesions dramatically manifest themselves in only one ear. As mentioned above, senile changes due to aging alone tend to manifest themselves bilaterally. Unfortunately, widespread CANS disease, some cortical lesions, and some brainstem lesions may also manifest themselves bilaterally. In these cases, a clear differentiation of the effects due to age and those due to a lesion is difficult if not impossible.

EFFECTS OF PERIPHERAL HEARING LOSS

As alluded to throughout this chapter, the presence of a peripheral hearing impairment may compromise the use of most, if not all, tests of central auditory function. Fortunately, many patients with CANS disorders have normal hearing. In those cases in which hearing is not normal, one must be alert to the potential confounding effects of a peripheral impairment when attempting to interpret test results.

The effect of peripheral hearing loss on electrophysiological and behavioral central tests depends on the degree and type of loss, as well as the audiometric configuration and the intensity level at which the

stimuli are presented. It is beyond the scope of this chapter to discuss in detail how these factors influence central test data, but some general principles are mentioned. Since there is a paucity of information on the effects of hearing loss on middle and late auditory responses as it relates to central auditory assessment, the main focus here is on the ABR and behavioral tests.

The ABR is generally evoked by a brief click that, when passed through TDH-39 earphones, results in spectral energy peaking at 3,000 to 4,000 Hz, making hearing status at the high frequencies a major consideration. High-frequency hearing losses tend to delay and/or distort the ABR waveform, while low-frequency deficits may have little or no effect on the ABR (see Volume I). If the peripheral hearing loss is such that the ABR waves can be obtained but they are delayed, one cannot be sure if the peripheral or central mechanism is responsible for this delay. This diagnostic dilemma remains a clinical challenge. Although formulas for offsetting the effects of cochlear hearing loss on the absolute latency of wave V or the ILD have been proposed, these have many shortcomings (60,148). Transtympanic electrocochleography can provide one way of consistently obtaining the early ABR wave (wave I), but it is an invasive procedure (36). Extratympanic electrocochleography is noninvasive, but to date it has not been thoroughly assessed with regard to providing wave I responses in clinically difficult ABR cases.

For individuals with peripheral hearing losses, it also may be difficult to ascertain whether deficits on a behavioral test battery are related to central auditory dysfunction or to the effects of a peripheral hearing impairment. This determination, however, may be possible in some instances. For example, in an individual with a symmetric hearing loss, a large interaural ear difference in the central auditory test results may be related to CANS involvement rather than to the effects of a peripheral hearing impairment. Also, in the patient with a unilateral hearing loss, a central loss in the ear with good peripheral hearing (or in both ears) implicates CANS involvement.

Because of the complications introduced into the assessment of CANS function in individuals with peripheral hearing losses, many investigators avoid central auditory testing in individuals with any degree of hearing loss. However, we believe that such testing may provide invaluable information in some cases (e.g., in those described above) in which the deficits are due to involvement of the CANS. Testing should not necessarily be precluded by the presence of a peripheral hearing loss. Furthermore, a finding of normal central auditory test results in the presence of a peripheral impairment could be used to rule out CANS pathology. The degree of central involvement is also important in the evaluation of hearing aids and the subsequent management of the patients who use them.

The specificity of a test battery can be increased by carefully selecting those central tests that are less likely to be affected by a peripheral hearing loss. Performance on tests such as the PATT and the ADP is less likely to be affected by peripheral involvement than is performance on tests that use speech stimuli. In a recent investigation, we found that the ADP test may be particularly suited for use in the assessment of individuals with cochlear hearing losses (4). It therefore appears that neuroaudiological assessment of the CANS is possible in many patients with hearing loss and is not likely to result in inaccurate interpretation as long as the audiologist selects appropriate tests to be administered and is cautious in the interpretation of the test results.

TEST BATTERY CONSIDERATIONS

Presently, no single test can yield optimal sensitivity or specificity in the evaluation of central auditory disorders. Most investigators agree that the test battery approach is needed in assessing the integrity of the CANS (61,101,117). The rationale is that the complexity of the CANS in normal and pathological states is so great that no current single test can consistently detect abnormal function. In addition, the variability and range of various pathological conditions are difficult for a single test to accommodate (132).

If a test battery is used, the examiner must determine which tests to use. (Surprisingly, this important question has seldom been addressed. Therefore, we offer our own impressions and considerations with, we hope, some solid rationales for test battery composition.) A test battery cannot require an extensive amount of time, as patients and clinicians often cannot tolerate long testing procedures. It generally is considered that the greater the number of tests used, the better the sensitivity of the battery; however, this appears to be true only to a limited extent (171). Much depends on the tests in the battery, as well as the various characteristics of the lesion (e.g., its type, size, and location). Generally, the greater the number of tests administered, the greater the number of false positives.

In selecting tests for a battery, it is prudent to use tests that evaluate different processes. Two similar dichotic speech tests, although sensitive, may not be as useful as one dichotic speech test used with a temporal ordering task, because the latter combination tests a greater variety of processes. This in turn should increase the probability of detecting abnormal function. The nature of the tests in a battery should vary depending on patient characteristics, and the clinical question that is being asked. If the goal is to evaluate auditory perception in an LD child, the test battery would be different than if the objective was to evaluate brainstem integrity in an adult. We believe that the tests used for brainstem evaluation should be different from those used for assessing the cortex because the brainstem and the cortex have different auditory functions. It can be of great value if, prior to test selection, some insight can be gained as to whether the brainstem or the cortex may be involved, allowing the clinician to better tailor the test battery to be used.

If one wishes to evaluate brainstem function, tests such as the ABR, AR procedures, and perhaps a dichotic speech task or the SSI-ICM should be strongly considered (101). If one suspects a cerebral lesion, then dichotic speech, pattern perception, and either middle or late evoked response tests should be favored. If preliminary information does not point to a specific lesion site (brainstem versus cerebrum), but a lesion somewhere in the CANS is still suspected, then some combination of tests from the two categories could be tried (e.g., ABR, dichotic speech, and pattern perception).

The evaluation of LD children for auditory perceptual difficulties requires a different approach than that for adults with definable lesions. In reviewing several studies in which test batteries were conducted with this difficult population, some trends emerge in regard to individual test comparisons. It appears that the CS test, dichotic speech procedure (102,130), and the DD test (19,102) are consistently among the more sensitive tests in the assessment of perceptual difficulties in children. The frequency pattern sequences test also seems to be one of the better tests to be used with this population (19,102,130). Tallal's temporal ordering task, although not used in a test battery paradigm, is a test that we think should be considered in developing a test battery because of its high sensitivity (167). Other tests, including electrophysiological procedures such as the late and/or middle latency potentials, may be of value in evaluating LD children, but these test data are too few or unimpressive to recommend them strongly at this time.

CONCLUSION

The clinical evaluation of the human CANS is a relatively new and challenging area. There is much that remains unknown, yet the advances being made have profound implications for clinical and basic research. The use of, and correlations between, behavioral and electrophysiological assessment procedures of the CANS in normal and diseased states will eventually yield much new information. In addition, new technology, such as magnetic resonance imaging, positron emission tomography, and cerebral blood flow analysis will enhance our ability to identify the relationships between human anatomy, physiology, and psychoacoustics. This in turn will lead to a better standard against which we can measure new tests of central auditory function.

REFERENCES

1. Albert M, Sparks R, Stockert T, Sax D. A case study of auditory agnosia, linguistic, and nonlinguistic processing. *Cortex* 1972;8:427–443.
2. Antonelli A, Bellotto R, Bertazzoli M, Busnelli G, Nunez-Castro M, Romagnoli M. Auditory brainstem response test battery for multiple sclerosis patients: evaluation of test findings and assessment of diagnostic criteria. *Audiology* 1986;25:227–238.
3. Antonelli A, Bellotto R, Grandori F. Audiologic diagnosis of central versus VIII nerve and cochlear auditory impairment. *Audiology* 1987; 26:209–226.
4. Baran JA, Musiek FE, Gollegly KM, Verkest SB, Kibbe-Michal KS. Auditory duration pattern sequences in the assessment of CANS pathology. *ASHA* 1987;29:125.
5. Baran J, Musiek F, Reeves A. Central auditory function following anterior sectioning of the corpus callosum. *Ear Hear* 1986;7:359–362.
6. Baran JA, Verkest S, Gollegly K, Kibbe-Michal K, Rintelmann WF, Musiek FE. Use of time-compressed speech in the assessment of central auditory nervous system disorders. *J Acoust Soc Am* 1985;78(suppl 1):541.
7. Bauch C, Olsen W. Interaural latency differences for cochlear and retrocochlear lesions. *ASHA* 1986;28:76.
8. Bergman M. *Aging and the perception of speech.* Baltimore: University Park Press, 1980.
9. Berlin CI, Cullen JK, Hughes LF, Berlin JL, Lowe-Bell SS, Thompson CL. Dichotic processing of speech: acoustic and phonetic variables. In: Sullivan MD, ed. *Central auditory processing disorders* (Proceedings of a Conference at the University of Nebraska Medical Center). Omaha: University of Nebraska, 1975; 36–46.

10. Berlin CI, Lowe-Bell SS, Jannetta PJ, Kline DG. Central auditory deficits after temporal lobectomy. *Arch Otolaryngol* 1972;96:4–10.

11. Blaettner V, Scherg M, Von Cramon D. Diagnosis of unilateral telencephalic hearing disorders: evaluation of a simple psychoacoustic pattern discrimination test. *Brain* 1989;112:177–195.

12. Bocca E. Clinical aspects of cortical deafness. *Laryngoscope* 1958;68:301–309.

13. Bocca E, Calearo C. Central hearing processes. In: Jerger J, ed. *Modern developments in clinical audiology*. New York: Academic Press, 1963;337–370.

14. Bocca E, Calearo C, Cassinari V. A new method for testing hearing in temporal lobe tumors. *Acta Otolaryngol* 1954;44:219–221.

15. Bocca E, Calearo C, Cassinari V, Migliavacca F. Testing "cortical" hearing in temporal lobe tumors. *Acta Otolaryngol* 1955;45:289–304.

16. Borg E. On the organization of the acoustic middle ear reflex: a physiologic and anatomic study. *Brain Res* 1973;49:101–123.

17. Bosatra A, Russolo M, Puli P. Oscilloscopic analysis of the stapedius muscle reflex in brainstem lesions. *Arch Otolaryngol* 1976;102:284–290.

18. Brunt MA. The staggered spondaic word test. In: Katz J, ed. *Handbook of clinical audiology*. Baltimore: Williams and Wilkins, 1978;334–356.

19. Brunt M. Central auditory processing problems: a selective test battery for children. Presented to the *American Speech-Language-Hearing Association*, New Orleans, November 18, 1987.

20. Calearo C, Antonelli A. Audiometric findings in brainstem lesions. *Acta Otolaryngol* 1968;66:305–319.

21. Canter N, Hallett M, Growdon J. Lecithin does not affect EEG spectroanalysis or P-300 in Alzheimer's disease. *Neurology* 1982;32:1262–1266.

22. Celesia G. Organization of auditory cortical areas in man. *Brain* 1976;99:403–414.

23. Celesia G, Pauletti F. Auditory input to the human cortex during states of drowsiness and surgical anesthesia. *Electroencephalogr Clin Neurophysiol* 1971;31:603–609.

24. Chiappa K. *Evoked potentials in clinical medicine*. New York: Raven Press, 1983.

25. Chiappa K, Gladstone K, Young R. Brainstem auditory evoked responses: studies of waveform variations in 50 normal human subjects. *Arch Neurol* 1979;36:81–87.

26. Clemis J, Sarno C. The acoustic reflex latency test: clinical application. *Laryngoscope* 1980;90:601–611.

27. Cullen J, Thompson C. Masking release for speech in subjects with temporal lobe resections. *Arch Otolaryngol* 1974;100:113–116.

28. Damasio H, Damasio A. Paradoxic ear extinction in dichotic listening: possible anatomic significance. *Neurology* 1979;19:644–653.

29. Davis H. Principles of electric response audiometry. *Ann Otol Rhinol Laryngol* 1976;85 (suppl 28):82–92.

30. Dermody P. Auditory processing factors in dichotic listening. Presented at the 91st Meeting of the Acoustical Society of America, Washington, DC.

31. Durlach N, Thompson C, Colburn H. Binaural interaction in impaired listeners. *Audiology* 1981;20:181–211.

32. Efron R. The central auditory system and issues related to hemispheric specialization. In: Pinheiro ML, Musiek FE, eds. *Assessment of central auditory dysfunction: foundations and clinical correlates*. Baltimore: Williams and Wilkins, 1985;143–154.

33. Efron R, Crandall PH. Central auditory processing: effects of anterior temporal lobectomy. *Brain Lang* 1983;19:237–253.

34. Efron R, Crandall PH, Koss D, Divenyi PL, Yund EW. Central auditory processing. III. The "cocktail party" effect and anterior temporal lobectomy. *Brain Lang* 1983;19:254–263.

35. Efron R, Yund EW, Nichols D, Crandall PH. An ear asymmetry for gap detection following anterior temporal lobectomy. *Neuropsychologia* 1985;23:43–50.

36. Eggermont J, Don M, Brackmann D. Electrocochleography and auditory brainstem electric responses in patients with pontine angle tumors. *Ann Otol Rhinol Laryngol* 1980;89:1–19.

37. Ferre J, Wilber L. Normal and learning disabled children's central auditory processing skills. *Ear Hear* 1986;7:336–343.

38. Findlay RC, Schuchman GI. Masking level differences for speech: effects of ear dominance and age. *Audiology* 1975;15:232–241.

39. Galaburda N, Kemper T. Cytoarchitectonic abnormalities in developmental dyslexia: a case study. *Ann Neurol* 1979;42:428–459.

40. Galaburda A, Sanides F. Cytoarchitectonic organization of the human auditory cortex. *J Comp Neurol* 1980;190:597–610.

41. Geisler C, Frishkopf L, Rosenblith W. Extracranial responses to acoustic clicks in man. *Science* 1958;128:1210–1211.

42. Goldstein R. Electroencephalic audiometry. In: Jerger J, ed. *Modern developments in audiology*. New York: Academic Press, 1973;407–433.

43. Goodin D, Squires K, Starr A. Long latency event-related components of the auditory evoked potential. *Brain* 1978;101:635–648.

44. Graham J, Greenwood R, Lecky B. Cortical deafness. *J Neuro Sci* 1980;48:35–49.

45. Greisen O, Rasmussen P. Stapedius muscle reflexes and otoneurological examinations in brainstem tumors. *Acta Otolaryngol* 1970;70:366–370.

46. Hall J. The acoustic reflex in central auditory dysfunction. In: Pinheiro M, Musiek F, eds. *Assessment of central auditory dysfunction: foundations and clinical correlates*. Baltimore: Williams and Wilkins, 1985;103–130.

47. Hall J, Huangfu M, Gennarelli T. Auditory

function in acute head injury. *Laryngoscope* 1982;93:383–390.

48. Hannley M, Jerger J, Rivera V. Relationships among auditory brainstem responses, masking level differences, and the acoustic reflex in multiple sclerosis. *Audiology* 1983;22:20–33.

49. Hecox K, Galambos R. Brainstem auditory evoked responses in human infants and adults. *Arch Otolaryngol* 1974;99:30–33.

50. Hirsh I. The influence of interaural phase on interaural summation and inhibition. *J Acoust Soc Am* 1948;20:536–544.

51. Ho K, Kileny P, Paccioretti D, McLean D. Neurologic, audiologic, and electrophysiologic sequelae of bilateral temporal lobe lesions. *Arch Neurol* 1987;44:982–987.

52. Jacobson J. *The auditory brainstem response.* San Diego: College Hill Press, 1985.

53. Jerger J. Diagnostic audiometry. In: Jerger J, ed. *Modern developments in audiology.* New York: Academic Press, 1973;75–115.

54. Jerger J, Hayes D. Diagnostic speech audiometry. *Arch Otolaryngol* 1977;103:216–222.

55. Jerger J, Jerger S. Diagnostic significance of PB word functions. *Arch Otolaryngol* 1971; 93:573–580.

56. Jerger J, Jerger S. Auditory findings in brainstem disorders. *Arch Otolaryngol* 1974;99:342–350.

57. Jerger J, Jerger S. Clinical validity of central auditory tests. *Scand Audiol* 1975;4:147–163.

58. Jerger S, Jerger J. Diagnostic value of crossed versus uncrossed acoustic reflexes: VIII nerve and brainstem disorders. *Arch Otolaryngol* 1977;103:445–453.

59. Jerger J, Jordan C. Normal audiometric findings. *Am J Otol* 1980;1:157–159.

60. Jerger J, Mauldin L. Prediction of sensorineural hearing level from the brainstem evoked response. *Arch Otolaryngol* 1978;103:181–187.

61. Jerger J, Neely J, Jerger S. Speech, impedance, and auditory brainstem response audiometry in brainstem tumors. *Arch Otolaryngol* 1980;106:218–223.

62. Jerger J, Oliver T, Chmiel R, Rivera V. Patterns of auditory abnormality in multiple sclerosis. *Audiology* 1986;25:193–209.

63. Jerger J, Oliver T, Rivera V, Stach B. Abnormalities of the acoustic reflex in multiple sclerosis. *Am J Otolaryngol* 1986;7:163–176.

64. Jerger J, Weikers F, Sharbrough W, Jerger S. Bilateral lesions of the temporal lobe. *Acta Otolaryngol Scand [Suppl]* 1969;258:1–151.

65. Kaga K, Hink R, Shinoda Y, Suzuki J. Evidence for primary cortical origin of middle latency auditory evoked potentials in cats. *Electroencephalogr Clin Neurophysiol* 1980;50:254–266.

66. Katz J. The use of staggered spondaic words for assessing the integrity of the central auditory system. *J Aud Res* 1962;2:327–337.

67. Katz J, Basil RA, Smith JM. A staggered spondaic word test for detecting central auditory lesions. *Ann Otol Rhinol Laryngol* 1963;72:906–917.

68. Katz J, Pack G. New developments in differential diagnosis using the SSW test. In: Sullivan MD, ed. *Central auditory processing disorders. Proceedings of a conference at the University of Nebraska Medical Center.* Omaha: University of Nebraska, 1975;84–107.

69. Kileny P. Auditory evoked middle latency responses: current issues. *Semin Hear* 1983; 4:403–413.

70. Kileny P, Kripal J. Test-retest variability of auditory event-related potentials. *Ear Hear* 1987; 8:110–114.

71. Kileny P, Paccioretti D, Wilson A. Effect of cortical lesions on middle latency auditory evoked responses (MLR). *Electroencephalogr Clin Neurophysiol* 1987;66:108–120.

72. Kimura D. Some effects of temporal lobe damage on auditory perception. *Can J Psychol* 1961;15:157–165.

73. Knight R, Hillyard S, Woods D, Neville H. Effects of frontal and temporal-parietal lesions on the auditory evoked potential in man. *Electroencephalogr Clin Neurophysiol* 1980;50:112–124.

74. Konkle DF, Beasley DS, Bess F. Intelligibility of time-compressed speech in relation to chronological aging. *J Speech Hear Res* 1977;20:108–115.

75. Kraus M, Ozdamar O, Heir D, Stein L. Auditory middle late responses (MLR) in patients with cortical lesions. *Electroencephalogr Clin Neurophysiol* 1982;54:275–287.

76. Kraus N, Smith D, Grossmann J. Cortical mapping of the auditory middle latency response in the unanesthetized guinea pig. *Electroencephalogr Clin Neurophysiol* 1985;62:219–226.

77. Kraus N, Smith D, Reed N, Stein L, Cartee C. Auditory middle latency responses in children: effects of age and diagnostic category. *Electroencephalogr Clin Neurophysiol* 1985;62:343–351.

78. Kraus N, Smith D, Reed N, Willott J, Erwin J. Auditory brainstem and middle latency responses in non-human primates. *Hear Res* 1985;17:219–226.

79. Kurdziel SA, Noffsinger D. Unusual time-staggering effects via dichotic listening with aged subjects. Paper presented to the American Speech-Language-Hearing Association, Chicago, IL, 1977.

80. Kurdziel S, Noffsinger D, Olsen W. Performance by cortical lesion patients on 40% and 60% time-compressed materials. *J Am Audiol Soc* 1976;2:3–7.

81. Lackner J, Teuber H-L. Alterations in auditory fusion thresholds after cerebral injury in man. *Neuropsychologia* 1973;11:409–415.

82. Levin H. Neurobehavioral recovery. In: Becker D, Pavlishock J, eds. *Central nervous system trauma status report.* Bethesda, MD: National Institutes of Health, 1985;281–302.

83. Licklider J. The influence of interaural phase relations upon masking of speech by white noise. *J Acoust Soc Am* 1948;20:150–159.

84. Lincoln A, Courchesne E, Kilman B, Galam-

bos R. Neuropsychological correlates of information processing by children with Down's syndrome. *Am J Ment Defic* 1985;89:403–414.

85. Lynn G, Gilroy J. Evaluation of central auditory dysfunction in patients with neurological disorders. In: Keith R, ed. *Central auditory dysfunction.* New York: Grune and Stratton, 1977;177–222.

86. Lynn G, Gilroy J, Taylor P, Leiser R. Binaural masking level differences in neurological disorders. *Arch Otolaryngol* 1981;107:357–362.

87. Lynn G, Cullis P, Gilroy J. Olivopontocerebellar degeneration: effects on auditory brainstem responses. *Semin Hear* 1983;4:375–384.

88. Miceli G. The processing of speech sounds in a patient with cortical auditory disorder. *Neuropsychologia* 1982;20:5–20.

89. Michel F, Peronnet F, Schott B. A case of cortical deafness: clinical and electrophysiological data. *Brain Lang* 1980;10:367–377.

90. Milner B, Taylor L, Sperry RW. Lateralized suppression of dichotically presented digits after commissural section in man. *Science* 1968;161:184–185.

91. Moller A. Physiology of the ascending auditory pathway with special reference to the auditory brainstem response (ABR). In: Pinheiro M, Musiek F, eds. *Assessment of central auditory dysfunction: foundations and clinical correlates.* Baltimore: Williams and Wilkins, 1985; 43–66.

92. Musiek FE. Assessment of central auditory dysfunction: the dichotic digit test revisited. *Ear Hear* 1983;4:79–83.

93. Musiek FE. Assessment of three dichotic speech tests on subjects with intracranial lesions. *Ear Hear* 1983;4:318–323.

94. Musiek F. The evaluation of brainstem disorders using ABR and central auditory tests. *Monogr Contemp Audiol* 1983;4:1–24.

95. Musiek F. Neuroanatomy, neurophysiology, and central auditory assessment. Part II: The cerebrum. *Ear Hear* 1986;7:283–294.

96. Musiek F. Selected aspects of ABR and auditory psychophysical tests in brainstem lesions. Presented at the International Congress on Brainstem Auditory Evoked Potentials, Oct. 21, 1986, New York.

97. Musiek F, Baran J. Neuroanatomy, neurophysiology, and central auditory assessment. Part I: Brainstem. *Ear Hear* 1986;7:207–219.

98. Musiek F, Baran J. Central auditory assessment: 30 years of challenge and change. *Ear Hear* 1987;8:22S–35S.

99. Musiek F, Baran J, Pinheiro M. P-300 results in patients with lesions of the auditory areas of the cerebrum *(submitted).*

100. Musiek F, Baran J, Pinheiro M. Duration pattern recognition in normal subjects and patients with cerebral and cochlear lesions. *Audiology (in press).*

101. Musiek FE, Geurkink N. Auditory brainstem response (ABR) and central auditory tests (CAT) findings for patients with brainstem le-

sions: a preliminary report. *Laryngoscope* 1982;92:891–900.

102. Musiek F, Geurkink N, Keitel S. Test battery assessment of auditory perceptual dysfunction in children. *Laryngoscope* 1982;92:251–257.

103. Musiek F, Gollegly K. ABR and VIII nerve and low brainstem lesions. In: Jacobsen J, ed. *The auditory brainstem response.* San Diego: College Hill Press, 1985;181–202.

104. Musiek F, Gollegly K. Maturational considerations in the neuroauditory evaluation of children. In: Bess F, ed. *Hearing impairment in children.* Parkton, MD: York Press, 1988;231–252.

105. Musiek F, Gollegly K, Baran J. Myelination of the corpus callosum and auditory processing problems in children: theoretical and clinical correlates. *Semin Hear* 1984;5:231–242.

106. Musiek F, Gollegly K, Kibbe-Michal K, Reeves A. Electrophysiological and behavioral auditory findings in multiple sclerosis *(submitted).*

107. Musiek FE, Gollegly K, Kibbe-Michal K, Verkest S. The ABR interaural latency difference (ILD) in brainstem lesions. *ASHA* 1987;29:189.

108. Musiek F, Josey A, Glasscock M. Auditory brainstem response in patients with acoustic neuroma: wave presence and absence. *Arch Otolaryngol Head Neck Surg* 1986;112:186–189.

109. Musiek FE, Kibbe K. An overview of audiological results in patients with commissurotomy. In: Reeves AG, eds. *Epilepsy and the corpus callosum.* New York: Plenum Press, 1985;393–399.

110. Musiek FE, Kibbe K. Auditory brainstem response wave IV-V abnormalities for the ear opposite large cerebellopontine lesions. *Am J Otol* 1986;7:253–257.

111. Musiek FE, Kibbe K, Baran JA. Neuroaudiological results from split-brain patients. *Semin Hear* 1984;5:219–229.

112. Musiek F, Kibbe-Michal K, Geurkink N, Josey A, Glasscock M. ABR results in patients with posterior fossa tumors and normal pure tone hearing. *Otolaryngol Head Neck Surg* 1986;94:568–573.

113. Musiek F, Kibbe K, Rackliffe L, Weider D. The ABR I-V amplitude ratio in normal, cochlear, and retrocochlear ears. *Ear Hear* 1984;5:52–55.

114. Musiek F, Pinheiro M. Dichotic speech tests in the detection of central auditory dysfunction. In: Pinheiro M, Musiek F, ed. *Assessment of central auditory dysfunction: foundations and clinical correlates.* Baltimore: Williams and Wilkins, 1985;201–218.

115. Musiek FE, Pinheiro ML. Frequency patterns in cochlear, brainstem, and cerebral lesions. *Audiology* 1987;26:79–88.

116. Niswander P, Ruth R. A discussion of some temporal characteristics of electroacoustic impedance bridges. *J Am Aud Soc* 1979;5:151–155.

117. Noffsinger D, Kurdziel S. Assessment of central auditory lesions. In: Rintelmann M, ed.

Hearing assessment. Baltimore: University Park Press, 1979;351–378.

118. Noffsinger D, Martinez C, Schaefer A. Auditory brainstem responses and masking level differences from persons with brainstem lesions. *Scand Audiol [Suppl]* 1982;15:81–93.

119. Noffsinger D, Martinez C, Schaefer A. Pure tone techniques in evaluation of central auditory function. In: Katz J, ed. *Handbook of audiology,* 3rd ed. Baltimore: Williams and Wilkins, 1985;337–354.

120. Noffsinger D, Olsen W, Carhart R, Hart C, Sahgal V. Auditory and vestibular aberrations in multiple sclerosis. *Acta Otolaryngol Scand [Suppl]* 1972;303:4–63.

121. Noffsinger D, Schaefer A, Martinez C. Behavioral objective estimates of auditory brainstem integrity. *Semin Hear* 1984;5:337–349.

122. Oh S, Kuba T, Soyer A, Choi I, Bonikowski F, Vitek J. Lateralization of brainstem lesions by brainstem auditory evoked potentials. *Neurology* 1981;31:14–18.

123. Olsen W, Noffsinger D, Carhart R. Masking level differences encountered in clinical populations. *Audiology* 1976;15:287–301.

124. Osterhammel P, Shallop J, Terkildsen K. The effect of sleep on the auditory brainstem response (ABR) and the middle latency response (MLR). *Scand Audiol* 1985;14:47–50.

125. Pandya D, Karol E, Heilbronn D. The topographical distribution of interhemispheric projections in the corpus callosum of the rhesus monkey. *Brain Res* 1971;32:31–43.

126. Peronnet F, Michel F. The asymmetry of auditory evoked potentials in normal man and patients with brain lesions. In: Desmedt J, ed. *Auditory evoked potentials in man: psychopharmacology correlates of EPs.* Basel: Karger, 1977;130–141.

127. Pfefferbaum A, Wenegrat B, Ford J, Roth J, Roth W, Kopell B. Clinical applications of the P-3 component of event-related potentials: II. Dementing, depression, and schizophrenia. *Electroencephalogr Clin Neurophysiol* 1984; 59:104–124.

128. Picton T, Woods D, Baribeau-Braun J, Healey T. Evoked potential audiometry. *J Otolaryngol* 1977;6:90–119.

129. Pinheiro ML. Auditory pattern perception in patients with left and right hemisphere lesions. *Ohio J Speech Hear* 1976;12:9–20.

130. Pinheiro M. Tests of central auditory function in children with learning disabilities. In: Keith R, ed. *Central auditory dysfunction.* New York: Grune and Stratton, 1977;223–256.

131. Pinheiro ML, Jacobson G, Boller F. Auditory dysfunction following a gunshot wound of the pons. *J Speech Hear Disord* 1982;47:296–300.

132. Pinheiro M, Musiek F. Special considerations in central auditory evaluation. In: Pinheiro M, Musiek F, eds. *Assessment of central auditory dysfunction: foundations and clinical correlates.* Baltimore: Williams and Wilkins, 1985; 257–266.

133. Pinheiro ML, Ptacek PH. Reversals in the perception of noise and tone patterns. *J Acoust Soc Am* 1971;49:1778–1782.

134. Polich J, Howard L, Starr A. Effects of age on the P-300 component of the event-related potential from auditory stimuli: peak definition, variation, and measurement. *J Gerontol* 1985; 40:721–726.

135. Polich J, Starr A. Middle, late, and long latency auditory evoked potentials. In: Moore E, ed. *Bases of auditory brainstem evoked responses.* New York: Grune and Stratton, 1983;345–361.

136. Quaranta A, Cervellera G. Masking level differences in central nervous system diseases. *Arch Otolaryngol* 1977;103:42–44.

137. Rintelmann WF. Monaural speech tests in the detection of central auditory disorders. In: Pinheiro M, Musiek F, eds. *Assessment of central auditory dysfunction: theoretical and clinical foundations.* Baltimore: Williams and Wilkins, 1985;173–200.

138. Rintelmann WF, Beasely D, Lynn G. Time-compressed CNC monosyllables: case findings in central auditory disorders. Paper presented to the Michigan Speech and Hearing Association, Detroit, 1974.

139. Robinson K, Rudge P. Abnormalities of the auditory evoked potentials in patients with multiple sclerosis. *Brain* 1977;100:19–40.

140. Rosenhall U, Hedner M, Bjorkman G. ABR and brainstem lesions. *Scand Audiol [Suppl],* 1981;13:117–123.

141. Rosenzweig M. Representation of the two ears at the auditory cortex. *Am J Physiol* 1951; 167:147–158.

142. Rowe M. Normal variability of the brainstem auditory evoked responses in young and old adult subjects. *Electroencephalogr Clin Neurophysiol* 1978;44:459–470.

143. Ruebens A, Froehling B, Slater G, Anderson D. Left ear suppression on verbal dichotic tests in patients with multiple sclerosis. *Ann Neurol* 1985;18:459–463.

144. Ruhm H, Walker E, Flanigan H. Acoustically evoked potentials in man: mediation of early components. *Laryngoscope* 1967;77:806–822.

145. Scherg M, von Cramon D. Psychoacoustic and electrophysiologic correlates of central hearing disorders in man. *Eur Arch Psychiatry Neurol Sci* 1986;236:56–60.

146. Schuknecht H. Further observations on the pathology of presbycusis. *Arch Otolaryngol* 1964; 80:369–382.

147. Selinger M, Prescott TE, Shucard DW. Auditory event-related potential probes and behavioral measures of aphasia. *Brain Lang* 1989; 36:377–390.

148. Selters W, Brackmann D. Acoustic tumor detection with brainstem electric response audiometry. *Arch Otolaryngol* 1977;103:181–187.

149. Seltzer B, Pandya DN. Afferent cortical connections and architectonics of the superior temporal sulcus and surrounding cortex in the rhesus monkey. *Brain Res* 1978;149:1–24.

150. Smith CB. Aging and changes in cerebral energy metabolism. *Trends Neurosci* 1984;7:203–208.

151. Smith B, Resnick S. An auditory test for assessing brainstem integrity: a preliminary report. *Laryngoscope* 1972;32:414–424.

152. Sparks R, Geschwind N. Dichotic listening in man after section of the neocortical commissures. *Cortex* 1968;4:3–16.

153. Speaks C, Jerger J. Method for measurement of speech identification. *J Speech Hear Res* 1965;8:185–194.

154. Spitzer J, Ventry I. Central auditory dysfunction in chronic alcoholics. *Arch Otolaryngol* 1980;106:224–229.

155. Squires K, Hecox K. Electrophysiological evaluation of higher level auditory processing. *Semin Hear* 1983;4:415–433.

156. Stach B, Jerger J. Acoustic reflex patterns in peripheral and central auditory system disease. *Semin Hear* 1987;8:369–378.

157. Starr A, Achor J. Auditory brainstem responses in neurological disease. *Arch Neurol* 1975;32:761–768.

158. Starr A, Hamilton A. Correlation between confirmed sites of neurological lesions and abnormalities of far-field auditory brainstem responses. *Electroencephalogr Clin Neurophysiol* 1976;41:595–608.

159. Stephens S, Thornton RA. Subjective and electrophysiological tests in brainstem lesions. *Arch Otolaryngol* 1976;102:608–613.

160. Sticht T, Gray B. The intelligibility of time compressed words as a function of age and hearing loss. *J Speech Hear Res* 1968;12:443–448.

161. Stockard J, Rossiter V. Clinical and pathologic correlates of brainstem auditory response abnormalities. *Neurology* 1977;27:316–325.

162. Stockard J, Stockard JE, Sharbrough F. Detection and localization of occult lesions with brainstem auditory responses. *Mayo Clin Proc* 1977;52:761–769.

163. Streitfeld B. The fiber connections of the temporal lobe with emphasis on rhesus monkey. *J Neurol Sci* 1980;11:51–71.

164. Sudakov K, MacLean P, Reeves A, Marino R. Unit study of exteroceptive inputs to the claustrocortex in the awake, sitting squirrel monkey. *Brain Res* 1971;28:19–34.

165. Sutton S, Tueting P, Zubin J, John E. Information delivery and the sensory evoked potentials. *Science* 1967;155:1436–1439.

166. Swisher L, Hirsch IJ. Brain damage and the ordering of two temporally successive stimuli. *Neuropsychologia* 1972;10:137–152.

167. Tallal P, Stark R, Kallman C, Mellits D. Developmental dysphasia: relation between acoustic processing deficits and verbal processing. *Neuropsychologia* 1980;18:273–284.

168. Thornton A, Mendel M, Anderson C. Effects of stimulus frequency and intensity on the middle components of the averaged auditory electrocephalic response. *J Speech Hear Res* 1977;20:81–94.

169. Tillman TN, Carhart R, Nicholls S. Release from multiple maskers in elderly persons. *J Speech Hear Res* 1973;16:152–160.

170. Tobin H. Binaural interaction tasks. In: Pinheiro M, Musiek F, eds. *Assessment of central auditory dysfunction: foundations and clinical correlates.* Baltimore: Williams and Wilkins, 1985;155–172.

171. Turner R, Nielsen D. Application of clinical decision analysis to audiological tests. *Ear Hear* 1984;5:125–133.

172. Vaughan H, Ritter W. The sources of auditory evoked responses recorded from the human scalp. *Electroencephalogr Clin Neurophysiol* 1970;28:360–367.

173. Wada S, Starr A. Generation of auditory brainstem responses: III. Effects of lesions of the superior olive, lateral lemniscus, and inferior colliculus on the ABR in guinea pig. *Electroencephalogr Clin Neurophysiol* 1983;56:352–366.

174. Weber B, Fujikawa S. Brainstem evoked response (BER) audiometry at various stimulus presentation rates. *J Am Aud Soc* 1977;3:59–62.

175. Wiley T, Block M. Overview and basic principles of acoustic immittance measurements. In: Katz J, ed. *Handbook of clinical audiology,* 3rd ed. Baltimore: Williams and Wilkins, 1985;423–437.

176. Willeford J. Assessing central auditory behavior in children: a test battery approach. In: Keith RW, ed. *Central auditory dysfunction.* New York: Grune and Stratton, 1977;43–72.

177. Willeford J. Assessment of central auditory disorders in children. In: Pinheiro M, Musiek F, eds. *Assessment of central auditory dysfunction: foundations and clinical correlates.* Baltimore: Williams and Wilkins, 1985;239–256.

178. Woods D, Clayworth C, Knight R, Simpson G, Naeser M. Generators of middle and long latency auditory evoked potentials: implications from studies of patients with bitemporal lesions. *Electroencephalogr Clin Neurophysiol* 1987;68:132–141.

179. Wood C, Ellison T, Goff W, Williamson P, Spencer D. On the neural origin of P-300 in man. *Progr Brain Res* 1980;54:51–56.

*Neurobiology of Hearing: The
Central Auditory System*, edited by
R. A. Altschuler et al.
Raven Press, Ltd., New York © 1991.

17

Prosthetic Stimulation of the Central Auditory System

J. M. Miller, J. K. Niparko, and Xiaolin Xue

Kresge Hearing Research Institute, University of Michigan, Ann Arbor, Michigan 41809-0506

The cochlear prosthesis (CP) has provided contact with the auditory environment and an aid to lipreading to more than 2,000 deaf people in the United States. Some of these individuals have achieved a significant degree of nonvisually aided open-set speech discrimination. The success of this device, particularly with recent data on multichannel devices (47,67), and the lack of obvious morbidity, are encouraging the application of the CP to expanded populations. Depending on the author, of the two million profoundly deaf citizens of the United States, CP implant candidate estimates range from 200,000 upward (61). If current investigations on the application of multichannel prostheses in the severely, but not profoundly impaired deaf populations prove successful (U.S. Food and Drug Administration, Investigational Device Exemption, Cochlear Corp., Melbourne, Australia), the candidate populations of the CP will increase dramatically.

For one small subpopulation of the profoundly deaf, the CP is not a potential therapy. These include several thousand profoundly deaf persons in the United States who have no auditory nerve that can be electrically stimulated.[1] Patients in this category include those with bilateral surgically removed acoustic neuromas (von Recklinghausen's disease). However, they also include those with total calcification of the inner ear as a result of severe meningitis, congenital inner ear agenesis (Michel's deformity), and some cases of temporal bone fracture. By far, the vast majority are those patients with bilateral acoustic neuromas. These patients may be candidates for a central nervous system (CNS) prosthesis, one that could provide auditory sensations as a result of direct stimulation of second order neurons of the auditory system—cells of the cochlear nucleus (CN). If benefit from central auditory tract stimulation is dependent on factors similar to those associated with cochlear stimulation, such patients would appear in many cases to be ideal. In many cases residual hearing is present until the time of surgery and implantation. It would be expected that in the majority of these cases, a full or near normal neuronal population of excitable elements exists at the level of the CN. Obviously, for some patients, such as those with Michel's deformity, this may not be the case. Moreover, in many cases acoustic neuroma removal is required in young adults, at a most productive time in their life. Thus, while the patient population is not large, the potential benefit for these individuals is indeed great.

In addition to compelling clinical justifi-

---

[1] The numbers quoted for patients in this category are derived from estimates of patients with acoustic neuromas taken from ref. 79.

cation to objectively assess the feasibility of developing a CNS prosthesis, there is a clear basic science rationale. The implementation of the CP has clearly served as an impetus for basic science research, including technical and theoretical issues related to electrodes and processor development, thereby providing information on a variety of basic issues concerning the auditory periphery. Thus, work on the prosthesis has motivated basic biophysical studies of electrical impedance characteristics of inner ear structures and is leading to finite and field models of current paths in the inner ear of importance both for the CP and our understanding of normal transduction processes. CP-related research has also led to the development of deaf animal models for experimental studies of cochlear function, has encouraged correlations of various causes of deafness with histopathology, including the study of the sequence of degeneration of sensory and neural elements of the inner ear, and is providing a strong impetus for studies of the encoding of sensory information and its plasticity. In the case of the CN, detailed information on the anatomy, physiology, and histochemistry of this structure continues to grow. Animal studies demonstrate that electrical excitation of functional subunits within the CN can provide meaningful cues for behavior. The prospect of gaining information on the perceptual significance of excitation of discrete clusters of cells and the way in which they may vary with parametric manipulation of stimulation may provide a strategy to address fundamental issues of neurophysiology and sensory behavior. The implication of such studies for the representation and processing of complex signals and issues of signal detectability is most intriguing. Thus, it may be possible to activate small clusters of cells that form functionally distinct categories organized along more complex (or at least different) perceptual dimensions than exist at the level of the eighth nerve. Certainly, as research continues in areas of artificial intelligence, neural

nets and connectivity, and the signal processing fields of bioengineering, there is good reason to expect that innovative means of activating the CN can be developed. Of course, primary questions in this area concern the risks involved with chronic implantation of a tethered foreign body and direct stimulation of the CNS. It is clear from the work to date that these are significant issues that must place constraints on the application of such a therapy in humans. However, these concerns do not provide a justification for inhibiting scientific study and efforts to develop this technology.

HISTORICAL PERSPECTIVE

Biological Observation

The application of electrical stimuli to the CNS has a long and rather illustrious history. Its original application in 1870 by Fritsch and Hitzig to elicit specific motor responses in humans provided the first convincing evidence for the concept of "localization of function" in the nervous system. In the 1930s, it was first used chronically in animal investigations to study the role of cortex in learning (76,77). Since then it has been used in studies to elucidate the wiring diagrams underlying certain learned behaviors as well as for clinical purposes. Clinically it is most known for its use in the treatment of epilepsy, chronic pain, and spastic motor disorders (54). Direct neurostimulation of the CNS has contributed to the study of sensory function by delineating functional neuronal circuits involved with or underlying perception (89). This early work primarily involved the visual nervous system, in part because of the accessibility of the visual cortex. These studies demonstrated that animals could readily learn to perform detection and discrimination tasks signaled by electrical stimulation (33–36) and that many features of performance were similar to those expected in response to external visual signals processed by the retina. Differences in performance were explicable on the basis of a "short circuiting" of the pathway inherent in tapping into the circuit at a point that bypassed peripheral portions of the system (88,89). These studies also demonstrated that such behaviors could be stable over long periods. However, under some conditions of stimulation, permanent elevation in the threshold current necessary for detection, temporary threshold shifts (11), and local damage to neural tissue in the vicinity of the electrode (86) have been reported.

The first attempt to stimulate the central auditory system in humans as a potential therapy for deafness was performed at the level of auditory cortex by Dobelle and colleagues (31). This approach was taken on the basis of observations by Brindley and colleagues (18–20) who demonstrated that with surface stimulation of sites on visual cortex, the perception of a punctuate light localized in the visual field (a phosphene) was elicited. The position in the visual field varied with site of cortical stimulation. Size, brightness, and color varied to some extent with parameters of stimulation, although significant variability was seen across subjects. Many of these findings have been corroborated in studies of CNS auditory centers by Dobelle et al. (31). (Additional findings from these studies are discussed later in this chapter.) Unlike observations by Brindley for the visual system, no simple auditory percept comparable to a phosphene (i.e., "audene") was elicited. Stimulation elicited auditory memories, e.g., the memory of a portion of a song or a conversation or a phrase, rather than simple auditory percepts. It has been suggested that these findings indicate a fundamental difference in the processing of information along the central auditory versus visual pathways, as well as a difference in the representation of information at the level of auditory cortex versus visual cortex. However, given that the electrodes in these

human auditory experiments were placed in the lateral surface of the temporal gyrus rather than on primary auditory cortex, that the electrodes were large, and that a large current was required to elicit these perceptions (6 mA), a more accurate explanation may be that there was relatively poor stimulus control in these studies and that they tell us little about the effects of discrete excitation of primary auditory structures.

Bioelectric Considerations

Clearly the future development and application of this technology to humans should incorporate considerations of local passive characteristics of neural tissue, as well as the active properties of the system, in designing electrodes and specifying stimulus parameters for activation of central auditory units. Discrete stimulation of neural elements with injected current depends on resistance and capacitance of adjacent tissues; the pattern of current flow as determined by the configuration of the electrodes; the shape, duration and magnitude of the current pulses; and the distance and orientation of the neural elements relative to an electrode. With monopolar cathodal stimulation, only axons lying in a "shell" around the electrode are stimulated. Elements immediately adjacent to an electrode may not be stimulated because suprathreshold monopolar cathodal current (8 times threshold) may block action potential propagation. These factors have been well described in an excellent review by Ranck (101). Interestingly, considerations enumerated in Ranck's review suggest that with proper control, discrete activation of a spherical shell of neural tissue restricted to a 250 μm diameter is possible. Recently it has been demonstrated that with bipolar stimulation the current is localized within a flat profile and that the current profile can be optimized by varying the electrode geometry (118).

Stimulus polarity and current-distance relationship determine which element of a neuron is stimulated with electrical current. When current is passed from a monopolar electrode to a nearby axon, it takes less cathodal current than anodal current to stimulate the fiber. This phenomenon occurs because a fiber is depolarized when there is current flow from the cell membrane of a fiber in an outward direction toward the cathode. When a monopolar electrode is placed near a cell body, as occurs with stimulation of the pial surface of the cortex, the opposite is true. Anodal current enters and hyperpolarizes apical dendrites, then leaves and depolarizes the cell body and/or axon. This model of electrical fields complement the observations of van den Honert and Stypulkowski (113), in that reversing polarity produces differences in threshold and profiles of excitation in auditory neurons with scala tympani stimulation.

CURRENT HUMAN INVESTIGATIONS

In setting expectations for a CN implant to habilitate the deaf patient who is not a candidate for a CP, it is reasonable to look to findings of the effects and effectiveness of the CP. For the single-channel, monopolar CP, the effect of stimulation is to excite a rather large percentage of all remaining afferent nerve fibers quite synchronously. With variation in intensity, the population excited may vary over a limited range. With variation of frequency of stimulation, the neural discharge rate is modified. Even presently used multichannel systems are limited in their control over the percentage and location of fibers activated because of the shunting effects of perilymph. Moreover, in the extreme case of the patient who has only five auditory nerve fibers left (63), CNS activation must be considered to be severely restricted, and yet this patient received benefit from the CP. These observations suggest that even a

rudimentary activation of the CN may be useful therapeutically, provided it can be accomplished within acceptable levels of risks.

It may be argued that if we can excite primarily that population of CN cells receiving afferent eighth nerve fibers with surface electrodes, we may provide benefit comparable to that observed with single-channel CPs (38,39). Or, if on the basis of biophysical properties of the tissue or of physiological characteristics of the wiring of the CN, the response of those cells that would normally receive the eighth nerve input will dominate the population response to electrical stimulation, we may provide meaningful perceptions at least comparable to those obtained with simple CPs.

Support of this notion may be found in the intraoperative stimulus trials by Simmons et al. (107), in which stimulation of the auditory nerve trunk as it entered the brainstem produced sound sensations. This was done under local anesthesia using behavioral responses, and given the nature of the stimulus, it is likely that direct excitation of CN cells was a contributing factor in the perception elicited. From the chronic human work performed to date (39,40), it appears that perceptions evoked by CN stimulation are similar to those observed with cochlear stimulation. Such observations lead to at least one speculation (64), that with monopolar CP stimulation, in some patients, the site of effective excitation of the auditory system may be cells of the CN.

In 1979, House and colleagues (38) placed the first chronic electrodes into the CN for purposes of auditory habilitation. The bipolar pair of penetrating electrodes, with tip separation 1.5 mm, was positioned to stimulate "deep cells" of the ventral cochlear nucleus (VCN). The 0.5-mm ball, platinum-iridium (Pt-Ir) electrodes terminated in a percutaneous connector anchored to the skull and permitted direct access to the electrodes. Acoustic sensations could be elicited with currents as low as 4 μA and demonstrated a dynamic range of 6 to 10 dB. As expected, thresholds tended to be lower and dynamic ranges larger for lower frequency stimulation as compared to high-frequency stimulation. Frequency difference limens were large (about 250 Hz at 500 Hz) and intensity limens of 5% to 15% were observed. Variation in intensity of stimulation produced qualitative changes in perception. Thus, at 90 Hz the subject reported the perception of a "stretching rubber band" at low intensity, which changed to the perception of a drum, and finally to the sound of a fog horn as intensity was increased. Characteristics of the perception varied with frequency of stimulation. The intensity-dependent changes might be expected with changes in excitation of functionally distinct subpopulations of cells in the CN. Because the VCN implant bypasses the frequency analyzer function of the cochlea, high intensities of stimulation may produce widespread activation of functioning cells and result in the perception that is the same for all frequencies. For this patient, all high-intensity stimuli, regardless of frequency, yielded the perception of a fog horn.

Of significance, the perceptions changed in time until the device failed at 2 months, at which time it was explanted. Changing perceptions included the development of dysesthesia in the ipsilateral hip, suggesting a migration of the electrode tip, which was confirmed at explantation. This implant was replaced with a surface electrode.

Since this case study, four reports have appeared on the effects of chronic CN stimulation for habilitation of the deaf by House and colleagues (39,40,60,84). As of mid-1987, seven patients have been studied in this program, four female and three male, ranging in age from 19 to 57 years. Each has received a bipolar surface CN implant in association with removal of bilateral acoustic tumors. The electrode surface area is approximately 1.9 mm². Some consistent observations of the effect and benefit of CN stimulation have been made in these pa-

tients. Following implantation, electrode impedance appears to increase over the first 2 weeks in association with, but not strictly dependent on, stimulation and then stabilizes at a value ranging from 4 to 10 Kohm. Current thresholds increase somewhat with time, stabilizing at values ranging from 10 to 180 μA at 1 kHz across patients. Thresholds varied directly with frequency, in general, similar to that observed in CP patients. Dynamic ranges were 4 to 10 dB, with a mean of 6 dB. In only one patient was some indication found for discrimination of site of stimulation with these large surface electrodes. An interesting, but unexplained, observation was that during daily testing sessions the impedance of the electrodes decreased.

Like many CP patients, the primary benefit of CN implants appears to be environmental contact and enhanced lipreading. Suprasegmental information was transmitted by the device. Performance was comparable to that achieved by single-channel House/3M CP patients on consonant, voicing, speech pattern, and contrast tests. Little evidence for open-set discrimination was observed. Overall, these patients performed similarly but slightly below single-channel (House/3M) CP patients. Major quantitative variations in perceptions were observed across these subjects, which led us to suggest that it will be necessary to develop flexible signal processors for this patient population.

There have been few complications associated with implantation of the CN surface reported. The patient first implanted with a penetrating electrode experienced tingling sensations in the hip, apparently secondary to electrode migration. A second patient experienced vertigo and nystagmus during the first week following surgery. Except for these instances, nonauditory sensations have not been observed. Another device failed after 3 days and the implant was removed; apparently it was not replaced. It appears that the most frequent complication they encountered was topical infection about the percutaneous connectors, which occurred in four of the seven patients. In addition, House and colleagues suggest that setting realistic expectations for this patient population is difficult. Unlike the typical CP patient with profound deafness for some time, many of these patients experience significant hearing abilities immediately before implantation. Thus, the transition is not from profound deafness to rudimentary hearing, but from hearing to a crude contact with the world of sound. Appropriate rehabilitation will include much more than just learning to distinguish and identify sound signals.

While the limited medical complications reported in these recent studies should encourage continued work, it is necessary to note that across studies of CNS prostheses, substantial complications have been observed occasionally in the past. In the visual system, the last of Brindley's three patients required explanation due to severe infection; although the first two showed no infection. While in the case of other prostheses, a large number of patients have been implanted and treated with no complications (112); in other cases cerebral spinal fluid leaks have been reported. Also, in two unfortunate cases, a cerebral infarct resulted in a hemiparesis and one postoperative death occurred due to brain hemorrhage (27,29).

ANIMAL INVESTIGATIONS

The first studies demonstrating selective activation of the auditory system with behaviorally meaningful cues were work performed by Miller et al. (90) and Gerken and colleagues (45,49–51). These authors found that in animals trained to detect and respond to acoustic stimulation, the substitution of electrical stimulation at sites along the central auditory pathway from the CN through the auditory cortex led to immediate transfer of the behavioral response to the electrical stimulus. Such immediate generalizations were modality specific, i.e., an animal trained in a visual detection task would not respond to stimulation to auditory structures and vice versa; and in the brainstem Gerken demonstrated that behavioral responses were only elicited when stimulation was carefully restricted to auditory structures. Findings of Miller et al. (90) demonstrated that the latency of behavior response to electrical stimulation, compared to that observed with acoustic stimulation, was shortened by an amount equal to the latency of the auditory evoked responses recorded via the stimulation electrodes. Thus, they were equivalent to that expected, if the normal auditory pathway involved in the behavior was "short-circuited" (Fig. 1).

Frederickson and Gerken (45) investigated the interaction of central and acoustic stimulation. Their observations indicate that the electrically elicited cues are specific auditory percepts. Acoustic stimulation selectively elevated behavioral threshold for electrical stimulation of both the CN and acoustic nerve but did not affect responses elicited with stimulation to the adjacent nonauditory neural structures. Figure 2 illustrates the primary observations of this excellent study, demonstrating a threshold shift to electrical stimulation at various sites in the brainstem when the stimulus was masked by wideband noise. These authors also demonstrated that the amount of threshold shift was directly proportional to the intensity of the stimulus masker. Maximum masking occurred when the interval between masker and electrical stimulus was equal to the latency of acoustically elicited activity in brainstem cells at the implant site. Tonal masking was differentially effective for different stimulation sites within the auditory system (Fig. 3), with variation consistent with the cochleotopic organization of the central auditory pathways. The characteristics of these interactions led Frederickson and Gerken to conclude that the masking is based on a di-

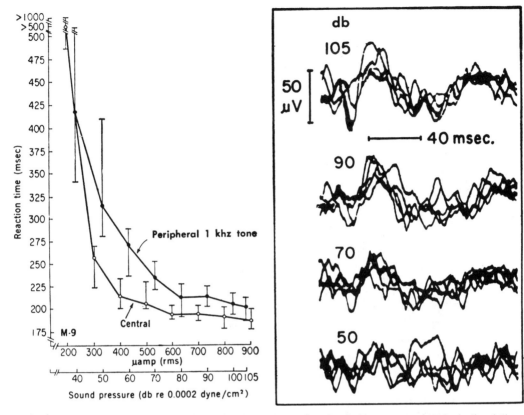

FIG. 1. Reaction times observed in a monkey to acoustic stimulation versus electrical stimulation of the auditory cortex. At high intensity levels, a constant latency shift of 15 μsec is observed, which is equivalent to the latency of the evoked response recorded for auditory cortex from the stimulation electrodes to acoustic stimulation (see inset). This is consistent with the view that with electrical stimulation we have tapped into the neural circuit involved in the acoustical elicitation of this behavioral response and, thus, have short-circuited the peripheral processing and conduction time to auditory cortex. (From ref. 90, with permission.)

rect interaction of the two stimuli on a common selective population of auditory cells. Moreover, Gerken (50) demonstrated cochlear lesions decreased the threshold for a behavioral response elicited by electrical stimulation at sites from the CN to the medial geniculate. He interpreted these findings as indicating a denervation hypersensitivity.

Clark et al. (26) demonstrated similar characteristics of behavioral responses elicited to acoustic and electrical stimulation of the central auditory pathways sites. Response characteristics elicited by electrical stimulation of the cochlea also were similar

to those derived from stimulation of the lateral lemniscus and auditory cortex. These authors found different limens for rate of stimulation ranging from 50% to 100% for test signals at 200 and 400 Hz.

The studies by Berard et al. (13) of behavior and evoked responses to superior olivary complex (SOC) electrical stimulation in the rat demonstrated stable performance and evoked response characteristics across subjects with thresholds of detection at 15 to 25 μA (peak) and thresholds for aversive reactions at approximately 40 μA (peak). Electrodes were described as bipolar semimicroelectrodes. Figure 4 demon-

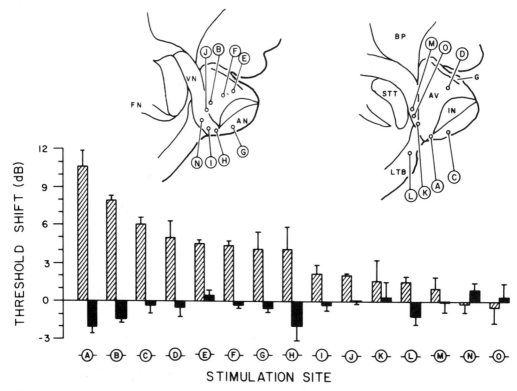

FIG. 2. Shift in electrical detect threshold caused by acoustic masking. Sites of stimulation are indicated with letters in the diagrammatic drawings of the cross section of the auditory nuclei of the cat above and correspond to the letters listed below the bars in the graph of threshold shifts. (From ref. 45, with permission.)

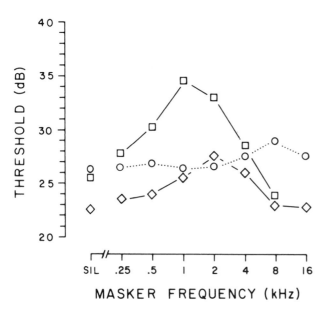

FIG. 3. Effects of change in frequency of acoustic masker stimulus on the threshold shift observed with electrical stimulation for three different sites of stimulation: Site A (*square*) was most sensitive to 1-kHz masker, site B (*diamond*) was most sensitive to a 2-kHz masker, and site D (*circle*) was most sensitive to an 8-kHz masker. These stimulation sites correspond to those indicated in Fig. 2. The differential frequency sensitivity may reflect a tonotopic organization of the central auditory pathways. (From ref. 45, with permission.)

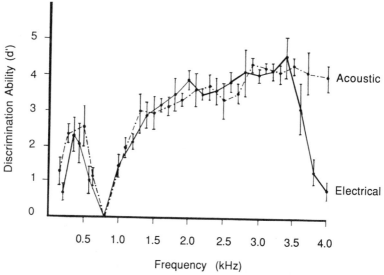

FIG. 4. Frequency discrimination ability to acoustic and electrical stimulation. In all cases discrimination performance at each frequency indicated was compared to the discrimination of an 800-Hz standard. (Redrawn from ref. 13, with permission.)

strates the mean discrimination ability of three subjects for various frequencies of acoustic and electrical stimulation compared to an 800-Hz standard. Biphasic square pulses of 100-μsec duration were used for the electrically stimuli. These data suggest that acoustic and electrical stimulation of the SOC may yield similar perceptions along at least some dimensions.

CLINICAL RISKS AND TECHNICAL CHALLENGES

The surgical exposure and implantation of a CN electrode, excluding stimulation, involves clear risks. For patients undergoing a translabyrinth approach for removal of an acoustic neuroma, the additional exposure required for electrode placement may be small (84,85). Obviously, this will vary with the site and size of the tumor. Even with those requiring little additional exposure and the use of surface electrodes, the manipulation of electrodes into position and their accurate fixation and stabilization present added risks. Anatomical work by

Terr and Edgerton (110) and McElveen et al. (84) has provided detailed descriptions of the surface characteristics of brainstem structures in the vicinity of the CN in humans and are appropriate first steps in developing the information base needed to minimize these risks. These studies make it clear that only limited portions of the CN have surface exposure available to the surgeon and that access is restricted by intricate vascular beds and other neural structures. However, Terr and Edgerton (110) provided a number of fairly distinct anatomical features that can provide landmarks for the surgeon. The study by McElveen et al. (84) of autopsy material concludes that sufficient exposure of this surface of the CN can be obtained for safe and accurate placement of surface stimulation electrodes. From the description in both papers it appears, however, that such placement is not trivial and is, even under the best conditions, not without significant risks.

Large surface electrodes thus far employed clinically and the higher currents required for surface stimulation compared to depth stimulation (55) may predictably result in substantial current spread. In the vicinity of these electrodes are the flocculus cerebellar peduncles, glossopharyngeal nerve, vestibular nuclei, and pontobulbar nuclei. However, clinical experience, as reported in studies by House and colleagues in humans suggests, little apparent adventitious excitation. CN electrode stimuli do not appear to excite regional structures, due perhaps to the orientation of fiber tracts, the low level of stimulation required for excitation of CN cells, and the accuracy of electrode placement (85).

If the results of stimulation of the cochlea are used as a model for development of CN stimulation devices, it is reasonable to assume that small multichannel penetrating electrodes may offer significant benefits over those that can be provided with large surface electrodes (57). However, penetrating electrodes provide a host of technical as well as conceptual problems. Most clear is the difficulty of fabrication and fixation after placement. Over the past three decades, multichannel microelectrode probes have been developed for neuronal recording and stimulation. In the past, techniques to fabricate such electrodes required bundling together microelectrodes using adhesives or magnetic changes (68,108). Advances in thin-film technology now enable dimensional control on planar probes to microscopic levels using photolithographic techniques. A polysilicon layer embedded in dielectric layers is deposited on a silicon wafer as interconductors between stimulating sites and bonding pads (9). The stimulating sites are deposited with iridium or iridium-oxide materials that are capable of large charge transfer (112). In conjunction with efforts to fabricate silicon substrate microelectrodes, polyimide and silicon ribbon cable technology may provide the critical interconnect between the percutaneous plug and the stimulating microelectrode (59). In fact, thin-film electrodes integrated with silicon cable have recently been fabricated by Anderson and colleagues at the University of Michigan. These investiga-

tors have shown that multichannel electrodes may be capable of exciting differentially subpopulations of cells within the CN complex as reflected in evoked gross potentials and that stable excitation is possible at stimulation levels well below the threshold for tissue damage (43,94).

Fixation and the prevention of migration, on the other hand, may present a more significant problem. Hitselberger et al. (60) described a case study strongly suggestive of migration of a penetrating electrode. Observations with Pt-Ir penetrating electrodes in animals confirm this (96). Given that the brainstem moves relative to surrounding cranial bone, it appears that the tethering cable cannot be relied on to fix the electrode position and that fixation must be obtained at the brain/electrode interface. In addition, we speculate that it may be possible to construct electrodes with physical features, e.g., phlanges at the electrode hub that will provide stabilization with respect to neural tissue that will allow them to float with the neural structures. Clearly, the construction and placement of an electrode that will induce little trauma with insertion, remain anchored, and function for many years present a significant challenge.

The potentially damaging effects of chronic electrical stimulation have been a major concern in the development of the CP as well as various CNS sensory and motor prostheses (37,69,72,80). Preliminary data suggest that in the short-term stimulation currents required for physiological activation of the auditory pathway are below the level for producing damage (94). This agrees with observations on stimulation at other nervous system sites (see below). However, in all cases observations have been of relatively short duration, typically days to a few weeks. Hence, generalization of these data to the human, with a much longer expected time of application, must be done with caution. Certainly the work of Gerken demonstrating stable behavioral responsiveness in cats, studied over months with typically minimal and restricted neural damage, is supportive of this approach. More detailed consideration of the safe levels of electrical stimulation of the CNS should be done within the context of an understanding of the mechanisms of damage.

MECHANISMS OF ELECTRICALLY INDUCED TISSUE DAMAGE[2]

The mechanisms of damage resulting from the injection of current into biological tissue have been well reviewed (32,56). Charge transfer from an electrode to biological tissue is dependent on two electrochemical mechanisms. One is a capacitive mechanism, which results when a relatively high dielectric boundary exists between electrode and tissue. When an alternate voltage is imposed across the boundary, charges are accumulated differentially on each side of the dielectric, which alternate in polarity with the characteristics of the stimulus. This charging and discharging of material on each side of the dielectric result in current flow in the biological medium without the direct transfer of charge carriers between electrode and tissue. This charge transfer will depend on the characteristics of the electrode and the dielectric boundary. In all cases, it is limited to a charge density above which the dielectric boundary may break down. The direct transfer of charge takes place as a result of reversible and nonreversible reduction-oxidation reactions at the electrode-tissue interface. The second mechanism is one in which no dielectric boundary exists, and charge carriers transfer between electrode and tissue as a result of reduction-oxidation reactions. Reversible reactions are confined to the electrode-tissue interface. Irreversible reactions generate new chemical species that migrate into the tissue and may cause damage.

Most investigations in this area aim to define carefully the level at which irreversible reactions take place and are predicted on the assertion that current injected at levels below this limit are safe. Thus, one definition of safe limits of stimulation is the "electrochemical safe" limit, i.e., the level below which no products of electrolysis are generated in the tissue (23,24). These products, including water electrolysis products (e.g., O_2 and H_2), are uniformly toxic. Brummer studied the nongassing limits of platinum, the level at which O_2 and H_2 evolution occurred, using both microscopic determination of gas bubble formation and electrical measurement. For platinum, the level at which H_2 and O_2 formed was 400 μC/real-cm^2/ϕ and Cl-oxidation products were not found until higher levels were reached. Their studies led them to conclude that the safe stimulation charge should be restructured to ≤ 400 μC/real-cm^2/ϕ for platinized electrodes and 9 μC/geom-cm^2/ϕ for smooth electrodes.[3] The recommended limits represent an outside safety limit.

Limits recommended by Brummer are above the threshold for platinum dissolution but at a level that restricts dissolution to equal to or less than one part in a 10^5 injected charge for both gas evolution and platinum dissolution. The estimated safe limits for Pt-Ir were below those specified for platinum (22). At this time, the data do not clearly show the effect of platinum deposition in biological tissue or its threshold for damage. In the cochlea, as well as the brain, platinum salts are believed to be toxic (6,14,62,104). Agnew et al. (8) and others have established limits for the dissolution of platinum in neural tissue at less than 40 μC/geom-cm^2/ϕ, a somewhat higher value than that estimated by Brummer at

---

[2]Since completion of this chapter, an excellent book has been published (1), including review papers and recent data relevant to these issues. In particular, we commend papers by Ronner (105), Agnew et al. (3), Leake et al. (71), and McCreery and Agnew (82).

---

[3]It is important to note that most authors quote the higher figure and apply it equally to all electrodes, whether platinized or smooth.

approximately 20 μC/real-cm^2/ϕ. (The fact that one is specified in terms of real and the other in terms of geometrically calculated measured electrode surface area does not account for these substantially different findings.) Forty μC/cm^2/ϕ approximates the upper threshold estimate for histopathology using similar electrode material with similar stimulation protocols reported by Babb et al. (10), Brown et al. (21), Gilman et al. (52), and Agnew et al. (5). While it was observed that pathology increases with increasing corrosion of the electrode (21), we cannot evaluate if this represents a causative relationship using currently available data. The observations that cathodal-first pulses are more damaging than anodal-first pulses and that the thresholds for damage and for platinum deposition are both lower with cathodal-first pulses than anodal-first pulses (7,14), indicate that electrochemical factors may contribute in a causative manner to both platinum deposition and damage. However, the observation that the threshold for neural excitation is lower for cathodal pulses indicates that such pulses may lead to greater metabolic activity and stress than anodal-first pulses. The observation that cathodal-first pulses are more damaging is consistent with a role for both electrochemical factors and metabolic factors in stimulation-induced damage to the nervous system.

Agnew et al. (8) also examined the histopathology induced by the injection of platinum salts in neural tissue. The amount injected (approximately 20 μg) equaled that lost with 3 μA, driven at 50 PPS ϕ.25 msec/ϕ, through a 1.4-mm diameter platinum disk electrode (0.012 μC/cm^2/ϕ) for 36 hr. This amount produced extensive neural damage that, in many ways, was similar to that seen with electrical stimulation; however, some significant pathologic differences were observed (e.g., presence of Zebra bodies). At this time, the literature does not permit us to conclude what harmful effects occur when minute quantities of platinum are driven into the cochlea or brain by

electrical stimulation. We do know that platinum dissolution can occur at stimulation levels achievable by some CP (15). The exact form platinum may take in tissues, its concentration, distribution, and rate of elimination or accumulation are unknown. It is clear that given the long-term expectations we have for Pt-Ir CP electrodes implanted in children, these questions should not be ignored, and we will need these data for the development of a safe CNS prosthesis.

Finally, from work by Brummer and Turner (23,24), Bernstein et al. (14), and Shepherd et al. (106) it is clear that it is not always possible to generalize results from testing electrodes *in vitro* to observations made *in vivo*. For instance, rhodium appears from *in vitro* studies to be an excellent choice of material for electrodes, because of its high resistance to corrosion and dissolution. However, when driven *in vivo* it was found to be much more susceptible to dissolution than Pt-Ir. The only explanation offered was that with stimulation, even at relatively low levels, the pH of the medium in the immediate vicinity of the electrode was decreased from 7.4 to 7.3 or less, and this change was sufficient to dramatically affect the dissolution properties of rhodium. On the other hand, the work of these authors indicated that small amounts of protein added to *in vitro* studies may raise the threshold for gas formation for platinum and that the threshold pitting of electrodes is significantly higher *in vivo* than in saline *in vitro* tests. Such observations should increase our caution in generalizing results from one set of investigation conditions to another, whether it be *in vitro* to *in vivo*, from animal preparation to human, or perhaps even from adult humans to children.

The definition of safe limits of stimulation in terms of "electrochemical safety" is based on the assumption that damage is caused by the deposition of new harmful products into the tissue as a result of chemical reactions and that these reactions can be localized and minimized if only reversible reduction-oxidation reactions associated with charge transfer at low levels occur. This theory also holds that such harmful reactions can be completely avoided through the use of capacitive electrodes, such as tantalum electrodes with a totally insulated boundary (e.g., tantalum pentoxide), in which all currents reflect the movement of ions that are normal to the tissue environment and are attracted or repelled by the charge of the electrode.

These assertions, as well as the notion that capacitive mechanisms for charge transfer are ideal from a safety point of view, have been questioned as a result of recent investigations, principally by Agnew and colleagues at the Huntington Medical Research Institute. Agnew et al. (2) observed that capacitive and noble metal (Pt-Ir) electrodes did not differ in their damage threshold. For a given set of stimulus parameters, the characteristics of damage were identical for both types of electrodes. This suggests that electrical stimulation of neural tissue induces damage primarily from processes associated with the passage of current through tissue, rather than from electrochemical reactions at the electrode-tissue interface. This observation makes it clear that defining the safe limits of electrical stimulation in terms of levels at which irreversible oxidation reactions occur is inadequate. These findings are consistent with other observations in this growing literature indicating varying degrees of damage at low levels of stimulation. Clearly, levels at which obvious irreversible chemical reactions occur, such as the theoretical nongassing limit of given electrode material (23,24), are an inadequate measure of safety. Damage of cochlear tissue occurs at levels well below these values (114).

In the absence of stimulation, pathology associated with biocompatible electrodes is restricted. On the basis of observations made in implanted but unstimulated cortex using pure platinum, Pt-Ir (90%/10%), and iridium electrodes, Agnew et al. (5) report

local widening of extracellular space, extravasated red blood cells, as well as other intravascular elements, macrophages, and some cellular debris. Occasional neutrophils were observed along the electrode tract. With longer term implantation (6), a thin gliosis about the electrode tract, lipid-filled macrophages, some mononuclear cells, and connective tissue cells have been observed. These reactions were directly adjacent to the electrode tract. While it can be assumed that some neural membranes were directly torn during implantation, no obvious neural changes were observed as a result of the presence of passive electrodes that were composed of appropriate nonreactive material (2). Implantation in the CN (94–96) revealed excellent tissue tolerance to both silicon substrate and Pt-Ir electrodes with only thin gliosis about the electrode tract observed. Cell counts within the CN were not significantly different between stimulated and unstimulated conditions. Moreover, tethering the electrode did not affect the degree of neuronal tolerance.

With low local electrical stimulation a variety of changes have been reported. These include changes in the concentration and distribution of K^+ and Ca^+ in tissues immediately surrounding the stimulating electrodes and changes in vascular permeability and pH (4,28,53,81,83,100,109). With moderately long-term stimulation (more than 36 hr), intraneural sequestration of Ca^+ as calcium hydroxyapatite crystals has been reported (4). Gilman and colleagues (53) report swollen mitochondria under similar conditions, and these findings are corroborated by Agnew and colleagues (2). Agnew et al. (5) reported that under acute stimulation conditions, widespread extracellular edema, swollen axons and dendrites with mild to moderate neuronal damage. With small electrodes, 20 hr of stimulation in the CN at and above an evoked potential threshold of 150 μA (approximately 600 μC/cm^2/ϕ) produced increased gliosis along the electrode tract, reactive cell infiltrates, and neuronal loss, typically in the region corresponding to the electrode terminus (94). With longer term stimulation, Agnew et al. (6) found increased glial thickness with an accumulation of giant cells and fibrocyst, swollen and atrophied neurons, areas of necrosis extending well beyond the electrode, and platinum deposition with the stimulation site representing the center of these changes. These changes varied directly with stimulus parameters. The volume of affected tissue appeared to be directly dependent on the charge density in these investigations (6).

Most recently, Agnew et al. (2) reported that the pattern of affected cells may be represented as a cone of tissue changes with the base more superficial and centered at the pulsed surface electrode. Immediately following stimulation, as quickly as 7 hr, primary changes included mild intracellular edema, marked vacuolation, and shrunken, hyperchromic neurons. These changes were associated with a presence of macrophages and neutrophils indicating phagocytic activity. Glial cells immediately associated with damaged neurons consistently appeared quite normal. After 1 week of recovery time from such stimulation, all signs of changes seen immediately following stimulation were reduced and still observable only at the electron microscopic level. There was clear evidence that the reduction reflected the phagocytic scavenging of damaged cells and their remnants. All of these latter changes observed with short-term electrical stimulation were found to be identical, both with capacitive (tantalum electrodes) as well as pulsed platinum electrodes, and the amount of damage was essentially identical for equicoulombic pulses.

Interestingly, the threshold for damage appears to depend on the size of the electrodes used. In recent physiological and histological studies (6,83), reversible changes in excitability with no evidence of structural damage were seen following 24 to 161 hr of 24 PPS, 200 μsec charge-balanced pulses, up to 800 $\mu C/cm^2/\phi$. These observations were made with 20 μm Pt-Ir and Ir microelectrodes implanted in cerebral cortex. These safe limits were five to 10 times threshold for activation of neurons in this area, although at highest levels, changes in excitability requiring 1 week for recovery were observed. Clear structural damage was observed at values four times (3,200 $\mu C/cm^2/\phi$) the defined safe limit.

It appears that there are two principal factors that underlie electrically induced damage. One is based on the development of new chemical products and reactions that are harmful to biologic tissue. These reactions depend on charge density, that is, they are electrochemically driven. The second set of factors are related to activation of the tissue and the metabolic environment surrounding the tissue and are more dependent on effectiveness of the stimulation across a volume of tissues; they may be more dependent on total injected charge over time. Thus, a number of factors affect the type of electrochemical reactions that occur at the electrode-tissue interface and the response of the tissue. Most important are the chemical characteristics of the electrode and the medium, the current and charge densities, and the parameters of the stimulation waveforms. However, recent work also suggests that the electrode surface area may play a significant role not only in determining total charge and charge density in tissue, but also in determining the rate of change of current density through a volume of tissue that subsequently determines the total population of activated neural elements. It appears that harmful local metabolic environmental changes induced by activation occur at lower levels of stimulation than previously suspected, and our notion of safe limits of electrical stimulation must be adjusted accordingly.

It is consistent with this view that the upper limit of safety for prosthesis stimulation must be defined by two criteria: one that will limit forces that define electrochemical safety and one that will limit those factors that determine metabolic safety. Charge density may be the determining limit of electrochemical safety, while total charge per time, or average current level, may more closely reflect metabolic safety. As pointed out by Agnew et al. (2,6), (a) charge per phase is correlated with the volume of neurons activated, (b) the mechanism underlying damage observed with lower levels of stimulation may be dependent on the volume of neurons activated in a specific area and the level of neuronal driving (i.e., "some type of mass action phenomena"), and (c) charge density may specifically determine the level of driven activity by setting the magnitude of depolarization and hyperpolarization of neural membranes in the vicinity of the stimulating electrode and charge per phase will determine "the volume of tissue through which the stimulus current will depolarize neuronal processes having particular thresholds and chronaxies."

Obviously, metabolic damage is based on active processes. We may expect that the system will sustain high levels of stimulation and neural driving of short duration, and occasional pauses in stimulation may significantly increase the threshold for metabolically induced damage. Studies are needed to answer these important questions. These considerations follow well from the studies of the Huntington Laboratory, which suggest a relationship of damage to charge density and total charge. From their data, we suggest that a trading relationship may exist between these two measures, that with a decrease in one, the other may be allowed to increase to some limit. For cortical brain tissue, the safety limit suggested by their data is 20 $\mu C/cm^2/\phi$ and 0.15 $\mu C/cm^2/\phi$. These figures are conservative, in that they reflect those levels of stimulation at which little or no damage was observed, with the next levels demonstrating clear damage. However, on the other hand, the data on which they are based are derived from relatively short-term chronic investigations. In no cases were observations based on stimulation paradigms of 16 to 18 hr per day, 7 days a week, for many years, as defined by expected human use.

BASIC CONSIDERATIONS

In considering the design of electrodes and the development of processor strategies for activation of the CN, the extensive and detailed data base of the physiology and anatomy of the CN that has been acquired during the past decade must not be ignored. These data can provide the base for rationally defining research strategies to implant and stimulate this complex structure. These data can set the boundaries for appropriate expectations from such stimulation and most surely will help to define the important features of electrode construction and placement, signal processor design, and appropriate characteristics of drivers to activate these electrode surfaces to yield biologically meaningful neural activation. Moreover, these data can provide the basis for specifying meaningful hypotheses to guide research in this area.

From Lorente de Nó (74,75) through the careful work of Osen (97,98), Cant and Morest (25), Moore (91) and others, extensive information is now available on the afferent innervation of the CN complex and its subdivisions, the morphological characteristics of the different cell types, and specific intrinsic and extrinsic projections (see Chapters 1–3 and 5, *this volume*). Histochemical studies have provided information on the distribution of excitatory and inhibitory transmitters and their receptors in the CN (see Chapter 3). These data have yielded a picture of a complex system of well-defined cell types with specific internal and external connections, which allow the interplay of excitatory and inhibitory influences that can affect the spatial and temporal encoding of auditory information. Indeed, electrophysiological studies from Kiang et al. (65,66), Evans and Nelson (41,42), Palmer and Evans (99), Rhode and Smith (102,103),

Young (117) have demonstrated functional subclassifications of cells that, at least in general, appear to relate well to the structural information available on this nuclear complex (25a; and Chapters 3 and 4 for review). The overall structure is that proposed by Lorente de Nó (73–75) of cell subpopulations with distinct features that should be capable of transmitting with fidelity information of the eighth nerve, but also capable of extraction, analysis, and re-encoding auditory information before transmission to higher stations of the system.

In light of the number of factors to be considered, the design and development of a CN prosthesis represent a formidable task. If the specific interplay of activity of each functional unit of cells is essential for the ascending output from the CN to have physiological meaning, the task of stimulation may be impossible, or if the processing of auditory information at this level results in the representation of qualitatively complex acoustic features in the discharge of specific cells or clusters of cells, the development of a usable prosthesis may be impossible. However, to the extent that the system is plastic, to the extent that stimulation in some areas may be dominated by a cell type that yields a predictable and relatively simple percept, and to the extent that we might activate selectively a portion of the system that serves largely a relay purpose or that we can affect predominantly those second order cells that are driven selectively by eighth nerve fibers, it may be possible to develop a CN prosthesis.

Rhode and Smith (102,103; and Chapter 3, *this volume*) have carefully described the electrophysiological classes of cells and their distribution in the CN of the cat. One subclass includes those with a primary-like discharge, so called because of their similarity of the discharge pattern of eighth nerve fibers to a tone burst. These response types have been associated with bushy and spheroid cells, which have been described well for the cat by Osen (97,98) and Cant

and Morest (25), and by Moore and Osen (92,93) for humans. These cells are restricted to the VCN and predominantly to the anterior ventral cochlear nucleus. The output projection of these cells is to the contralateral SOC and directly into the lateral lemniscus. This system has been described as a comparatively simple first order relay station of the auditory pathway. One consideration then for the stimulation of the CN would be to attempt to selectively, or at least predominantly, activate primary-like cells with the expectation that this might provide perceptions analogous to those observed with cochlear stimulation (38). Indeed, Anderson and colleagues (58) have speculated that with appropriately designed penetrating electrodes in the CN it might be possible to provide more discrete activation of cochleotopically organized elements than that possible with electrodes surrounded by the shunting perilymph of the scala tympani.

At the level of visual cortex, there is extensive electrophysiological evidence for an organization of cells based on multidimensional perceptual factors. One set of factors is spatially restricted features of the stimulus, which leads to the representation of specifically oriented lines and bars in visual cortex. This, in turn, leads to the suggestions that direct electrical stimulation of sites of visual cortex may produce relatively complex percepts involving lines and bars with particular angles. Moreover, evidence from physiological recordings indicate that percepts might vary qualitatively, taking on new dimensions in the visual field depending on the stimulation in areas 17, 18, or 19. However, observations reported by Brindley and colleagues (18–20) and by Dobelle et al. (30) on the percepts of four patients stimulated with electrodes on visual cortex indicate that relatively simple percepts are elicited. Largely, these were steady phosphenes (some flickered) that varied in size from a "rice grain" to a "coin held at arms length." Their location within the visual field varied in a predictable manner with stimulation site. Interestingly, the basic characteristics of these percepts were similar, whether they were elicited by stimulation of striate cortex or association visual cortices. These observations suggest that, in spite of the apparent complexity of organization of the CN complex, electrical stimulation may yield relatively simple percepts, which may support the clinical utility of a CN implant to provide relatively basic information and acoustic contact with the world. It may also be that the simplicity of percepts elicited with visual cortex stimulation reflects the rather gross nature of the stimulus generated with surface electrodes. The challenge of this CN prosthesis may be to provide sufficiently discrete patterns of activation at sites within the complex to take advantage of the subpopulations of different cell types that process auditory information.

With multiple site stimulation, changes in visual percepts were observed by Brindley and colleagues, indicating an interaction of electrical fields. The stability of the image varied at times and discrete patterns "filled in." Little success was found in providing discrete patterned percepts with such stimulation. With gross stimulation of the CN, comparable to that previously used in the visual cortex, we may be able to elicit simple and predictable percepts that can provide environmental contact and perhaps an aid to lipreading for the profoundly deaf. By analogy to the CP, it may be that unless discretely patterned percepts can be provided by discrete stimulation of subpopulations of CN cells, it will probably be impossible to provide speech recognition capabilities solely by a CN prosthesis. It is also possible that the representation of discrete *temporal* patterns required for complex acoustic perceptions may be more readily achieved with current technology than the discrete *spatial* patterns required by the visual system. This consideration leads to a set of interesting questions to be answered as work progresses on testing and developing a CN prosthesis.

As previously noted, the major candidate population for a CN implant would be those with bilateral acoustic neuromas, and these patients in most cases would be recently deafened with a relatively normal CN, provided brainstem compression by the tumor was not extensive. A small candidate group would include patients with long-standing profound deafness, with no cochlea or eighth nerve, e.g., Michel's deformity. In these patients, the effect of long-term deafness on morphological characteristics of the CN and associated changes in physiological properties of the tissue is a concern. From experimental animal preparations, we know changes in these structures occur (111,115,116), and recently this has been documented in humans by Miller et al. (87). Specific information on changes in cellular response properties with prolonged deafness is not yet available. However, previous work (16,17,44) indicates a hypersensitivity in the responsiveness of the central auditory pathways to cochlear electrical stimulation in congenitally deaf animals. Initial results with CN-implanted animals in our laboratory indicate that electrically evoked middle latency response thresholds remain stable 1 year after ototoxic deafening. Moreover, our current views of the effects of deprivation and deafness on auditory nerve and central auditory structures may undergo significant change with the recent findings of the "sustaining" effects of electrical stimulation on the auditory system of the deafened animal (70,78,87).

In this regard, in the visual system at the level of cortex, Brindley (18) reported fading and size changes in phosphenes elicited by electrical stimulation in a long-term blind subject. These did not occur in a patient with short-term blindness. Whether early stimulation may counter such changes in the CNS and whether these findings may apply to percepts elicited with brainstem stimulation is a matter of speculation. From behavioral work in animal preparation (50), it would appear that deafness in the relatively short run leads to a hypersensitivity

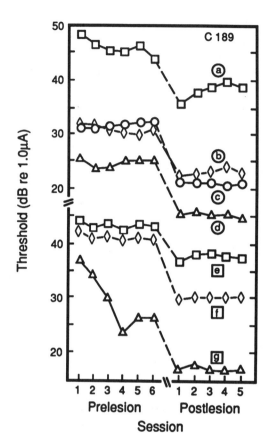

FIG. 5. Electrical stimulation thresholds prior to and following bilateral cochlear destruction. Each function demonstrates the results from a different stimulation site along the central auditory structures (e and g, medial geniculate nucleus; b and f, inferior colliculus; g and d, cochlear nucleus; c, superior olivary complex). (From ref. 50, with permission.)

consistent with the physiological observations of Bock and colleagues.

Figure 5 is a summary of Gerken's findings (50) showing pre- and postlesion thresholds for stimulation in sites from the CN (g) through the medial geniculate nucleus (a). Overall, a mean threshold shift of approximately 8 dB was observed. Depending on the course of such excitability changes, hyperexcitability could be either an advantage for the development of CN implant, by lowering the threshold for activation, or it could inhibit development of a multichannel CN implant by limiting the extent to which discrete populations of cells may be selectively excited. Information is not yet available as to the extent to which the observed hyperexcitability reflects excitation of a larger cell population.

CONCLUSIONS

Clearly, there are a number of problems and challenges that face this field. To some extent, the fundamental questions are similar to those facing development of other neural prostheses, particularly CP. They involve questions of safety and processing schemes for discrete excitation of selective neural elements to provide biologically meaningful signals in a stable and safe manner. For the central auditory system, these challenges are magnified by increased problems of stability, the small volume of functionally distinct units requiring selective excitation, and the potentially increased risk of current spread to adjacent structures. However, these are challenges to the imagination and experimentation, not barriers to research. The clinical needs are clear, and the fundamental knowledge that may be accrued from work in this area can have significant benefits for our understanding of sensory processes, auditory perception, and nervous system function.

ACKNOWLEDGMENTS

This work was supported in part by NIH grant P01-DC00274-06S1, NIH contract NS52387, FDA contract #223-87-6028, the Deafness Research Foundation, and the Office of the Vice President for Research at the University of Michigan. We gratefully acknowledge the invaluable suggestions of Dr. Sandy Spelman, University of Washington, on the section "Mechanisms of Electrically Induced Tissue Damage," the very helpful corrections and additions provided by Dr. F. Terry Hambrecht of the NIH Neural Prosthesis Program, and the assistance of Yvonne Beerens and Denise Dyson in the preparation of this manuscript.

REFERENCES

1. Agnew WF, McCreery DB. *Neural prostheses: fundamental studies.* Englewood Cliffs, NJ: Prentice Hall, 1990.
2. Agnew WF, McCreery DB, Bullara LE, Yuen TGH. Development of safe techniques for selected activation in neurones. Neural Prosthesis Project NINCDS Contract No. N01-NS-62397, Quarterly Progress Report, April 1, 1987.
3. Agnew WF, McCreery DB, Yuen TGH, Bullara LE. Effects of prolonged electrical stimulation of the central nervous system. In: Agnew WF, McCreery DB, eds, *Neural prostheses: fundamental studies.* Englewood Cliffs, NJ: Prentice Hall, 1990;225–252.
4. Agnew WF, Yuen TGH, Bullara LA, et al. Intracellular calcium deposition in brain following electrical stimulation. *Neurol Res* 1979; 1:187–202.
5. Agnew WF, Yuen TGH, McCreery DB. Morphologic changes following prolonged electrical stimulation of the cat's cortex at defined charge densities. *Exp Neurol* 1983;79:397–411.
6. Agnew WF, Yuen TGH, McCreery DB, Bullara LA. Histopathologic evaluation of prolonged intracortical electrical stimulation. *Exp Neurol* 1986;92:162–185.
7. Agnew WF, Yuen TGH, Pudenz RH, Bullara LA. Electrical stimulation of the brain. IV. Ultrastructural studies. *Surg Neurol* 1975;4:438–448.
8. Agnew WF, Yuen TGH, Pudenz RH, Bullara LA. Neuropathology effects of intracerebral platinum salt injections. *J Pathol Exp Neuropathol* 1977;36:533–546.
9. Anderson DJ, Najafi K, Tanghe K, et al. Batch-fabricated thin-film electrodes for stimulation of the central auditory system. *IEEE* (special edition on electrical stimulation) *(in press).*
10. Babb TL, Soper HV, Lieb JP, et al. Electrophysiological studies of long-term electrical stimulation of the cerebellum in monkeys. *J Neurosurg* 1977;47:353–365.
11. Bartlett JR, Doty RW, Lee BB, et al. Deleterious effects of prolonged electrical excitation of striate cortex in macaques. *Brain Behav Evol* 1977;14:44–66.
12. Beebe X, Rose TL. Charge injection limits of activated iridium oxide electrodes with 0.2 μsec pulse in bicarbonate buffered saline. *IEEE Trans Biomed Eng* 1988;35:494–495.
13. Berard DR, Coleman WR, Berger LH. Electrical stimulation of the superior olivary complex can produce cortical evoked potential and behavioral discrimination correlates of pitch perception in the rat. *Int J Neurosci* 1983;18:87–96.
14. Bernstein JJ, Johnson PF, Hench LL, et al. Cortical histopathology following stimulation with metallic and carbon electrodes. *Brain Behav Evol* 1977;14:126–157.
15. Black RC, Hannacker P. Dissolution of smooth platinum electrodes in biological fluids. *Appl Neurophysiol* 1979;42:366–374.
16. Bock GR, Frank MP, Steel KP. Preservation of central auditory function in the *deafness* mouse. *Brain Res* 1982;239:608–612.
17. Bock GR, Horner K, Steel KP. Electrical stimulation of the auditory system in animals profoundly deaf from birth. *Acta Otolaryngol (Stockh)* 1985;421:108–113.
18. Brindley GS. Sensory effects of electrical stimulation of the visual and paravisual cortex in man. In: Jung R, ed. *Handbook of sensory physiology.* New York: Springer-Verlag, 1973; 583–594.
19. Brindley G, Donaldson P, Falconer D, Rushton J. The extent of the region of occipital cortex that when stimulated gives phosphenes fixed in the visual field. *J Physiol (Lond)* 1972;225:57–58.
20. Brindley G, Lewin W. The sensations produced by electrical stimulation of the visual cortex. *J Physiol (Lond)* 1968;196:479–493.
21. Brown WJ, Babb TL, Soper HV, et al. Tissue reactions to long-term electrical stimulation of the nervous system with platinum electrodes. *IEEE Trans Biomed Eng* 1977;24:59–63.
22. Brummer SB, McHardy J, Turner MJ. Implantable electrodes. Visual Prostheses Contract

#NO1-NS-3-23313, Ninth Quarterly Progress Report, April 1, 1975.

23. Brummer SB, Turner MJ. Electrical stimulation with pt. electrodes: I-A method for determination of "real" electrode areas. *IEEE Trans Biomed Eng* 1977;BME-24:436–439.

24. Brummer SB, Turner MJ. Electrochemical considerations for safe electrical stimulation of the nervous system with platinum electrodes. *IEEE Trans Biomed Eng* 1977;BME-24:59–60.

25. Cant NB, Morest DK. The structural basis for stimulus coding in the cochlear nucleus of the cat. In: Berlin C, ed. *Hearing science*. San Diego: College Hill Press, 1984;371–422.

25a. Caspary D. Cochlear nuclei: functional neuropharmacology of the principal cell types. In: Altschuler R, et al., eds. *Neurobiology of hearing: the cochlea*. New York: Raven Press, 1986;303–332.

26. Clark GM, Nathar JM, Kranz HG, Maritz JS. A behavioral study on electrical stimulation of the cochlea and central auditory pathways of the cat. *Exp Neurol* 1972;36:350–361.

27. Cooper IS, Amin I, Riklan M, Waltz JM, Poon TP. Chronic cerebellar stimulation in epilepsy. *Arch Neurol* 1976;33:559–570.

28. Dauth GW, Defendini R, Gilman S, et al. Long-term surface stimulation of the cerebellum in the monkey. *Surg Neurol* 1977;7:377.

29. Davis RM, Cullen RF, Flitter MA, et al. Control of spasticity and involuntary movements. *Neurosurgery* 1977;1:205–207.

30. Dobelle WH, Mladejovsky MG, Girvin JP. Artificial vision for the blind: electrical stimulation of visual cortex offers hope for a functional prosthesis. *Science* 1974;183:440–444.

31. Dobelle WH, Stensaas SS, Mladejovsky MG, Smith JB. A prosthesis for the deaf based on cortical stimulation. *Ann Otol Rhinol Laryngol* 1973;82:445–463.

32. Donaldson N de N, Donaldson PEK. When are actively balance biphasic ("Lilly") stimulating pulses necessary in a neurological prosthesis? I. Historical background; Pt perting potential; Q studies. *Med Biol Eng Comput* 1986;24:41–49.

33. Doty RW. Conditioned reflexes formed and evoked by brain stimulation. In: Sheer DE, ed. *Electrical stimulation of the brain*. Dallas: University of Texas Press, 1961;397–412.

34. Doty RW, Kimura DS, Mogenson GJ. Photically and electrically elicited responses in the central visual system of the squirrel monkey. *Exp Neurol* 1964;10:19–51.

35. Doty RW, Rutledge LT. Surgical interference with pathways mediating responses conditioned to cortical stimulation. *Exp Neurol* 1962;6:478–491.

36. Doty RW, Rutledge LT, Larsen RM. Conditioned reflexes established to electrical stimulation of cat cerebral cortex. *J Neurophysiol* 1956;19:401–415.

37. Duckert LG, Miller JM. Morphological changes following cochlear implantation in the animal model. *Acta Otolaryngol [Suppl] (Stockh)* 1984;411:28–37.

38. Edgerton BJ, House WF, Hitselberger W. Hearing by cochlear nucleus stimulation in humans. *Ann Otol Rhinol Laryngol* 1982;91:117–124.

39. Eisenberg LS, House WF, Mobley JP, et al. The central electro-auditory prosthesis: clinical results. In: Andrade J, ed. *Artificial organs: The WJ Kolff Festschrift*. New York: VCH Publishers, 1987;91–101.

40. Eisenberg LS, Maltan AA, Portillo F, et al. Electrical stimulation of the auditory brain stem structure in deafened adults. *J Rehabil Res Dev* 1987;24:9–22.

41. Evans EF, Nelson PG. The responses of single neurones in the cochlear nucleus of the cat as a function of their location and the anesthetic state. *Exp Brain Res* 1973;17:402–427.

42. Evans EF, Nelson PG. On the functional relationship between the dorsal and ventral divisions of the cochlear nucleus of the cat. *Exp Brain Res* 1973;17:428–442.

43. Evans DA, Niparko JK, Miller JM, et al. Multiple-channel stimulation of the cochlear nucleus. *Otolaryngol Head Neck Surg* 1989;101:651–657.

44. Frank MP, Steel KP, Bock GR. Electrical stimulation of the cochlear nerve in *deafness* mice. *Arch Otolaryngol* 1983;109:526–529.

45. Frederickson CJ, Gerken GM. Functional characteristics of cochlear nucleus in behaving cat examined by acoustic masking of electrical stimuli. *J Neurophysiol* 1978;41:1535–1545.

46. Fritsch GT, Hitzig E. Über die elektrische erregbarkeit des grosshirns. *Arch Anat Physiol Wiss Med Leipzig* 1870;37:300.

47. Gantz BJ, Tyler RS, Knutson JF, et al. Evaluation of five different cochlear implant designs: audiologic assessment and predictors of performance. *Laryngoscope* 1988;98:1100–1106.

48. Gerken GM. Electrical stimulation of the subcortical auditory system in behaving cat. *Brain Res* 1970;17:483–497.

49. Gerken GM. Behavioral measurement of electrical stimulation thresholds for medial geniculate nucleus. *Exp Neurol* 1971;31:60–74.

50. Gerken GM. Central denervation hypersensitivity in the auditory system of the cat. *J Acoust Soc Am* 1979;66:721–727.

51. Gerken GM, Sandlin D. Auditory reaction time and absolute threshold in cat. *J Acoust Soc Am* 1977;61:602–607.

52. Gilman S, Dauth GW, Tennyson VM, et al. Chronic cerebellar stimulation in the monkey. Preliminary observations. *Arch Neurol* 1975;32:474–477.

53. Gilman S, Dauth G, Tennyson V, et al. Clinical morphological biochemical and physiological effects of cerebellar stimulation. In: Hambrecht F, Reswick JB, eds. *Functional electrical stimulation: applications in neural prostheses*, vol 3. New York and Basel: Marcel Dekker, 1977;191–223.

54. Groth K. Deep brain stimulation. In: Byklebust J, Cusich J, Sances A, Larson S, eds. *Neural stimulation*, vol II. Boca Raton, FL: CRC Press, 1985;11–22.

55. Hambrecht FT. Neural prosthesis. *Annu Rev Biophys Bioeng* 1979;8:239–267.

56. Hambrecht FT, Reswick JB. *Functional electrical stimulation: applications in neural prosthesis* (Biomedical Engineering and Instrumentation Series, vol 3). New York and Basel: Marcel Dekker, 1977;435–482.

57. Heederks W, Hambrecht FT. Applications in neural control in 1990's. *Proc IEEE* 1988;56:1115–1121.

58. Hetke JT, Anderson DJ, Evans DA, et al. Tissue volume selectivity in the cochlear nucleus to electrical stimulation with multichannel silicon substrate arrays. Abstracts of the 12th Midwinter Meeting, Association for Research in Otolaryngology, St. Petersburg Beach, FL, 1989;146–147.

59. Hetke J, Najafi K, Wise K. Flexible miniature ribbon cables for long-term connection to implantable sensors. Fifth International Conference Solid-State Sensors and Actuators, Montreux, Switzerland, June 25–30, 1989.

60. Hitselberger WR, House WF, Edgerton BJ. Cochlear nucleus implant. *Otolaryngol Head Neck Surg* 1984;92:52–54.

61. Hopkinson NT, et al. Cochlear implants: report of the Ad Hoc Committee. *ASHA* 1986;28:29–52.

62. Johnson PF, Hench LL. An in vitro analysis of metal electrodes for use in the neural environment. *Brain Behav Evol* 1977;14:23–45.

63. Johnsson L, House W, Lithicum F. Otopathological findings in a patient with bilateral cochlear implants. *Ann Otol Rhinol Laryngol* 1982;91:78–84.

64. Kiang NYS. Suggestion made during discussion. Cochlear prosthesis. An International Symposium by the New York Academy of Sciences. *Ann NY Acad Sci* 1983;405.

65. Kiang NYS, Morest DK, Godfrey DA, Guinan JJ, Kane EC. Stimulus coding at caudal levels of the cat's auditory nervous system. I. Response characteristics of single units. In: Møller AR, ed. *Basic mechanisms in hearing*. New York: Academic Press, 1973;485–488.

66. Kiang NYS, Pfeiffer RR, Warr WB, Backus ASN. Stimulus coding in the cochlear nucleus. *Ann Otol Rhinol Laryngol* 1965;74:463–485.

67. Kohut RI, Carney AE, Eviatar L, et al. Cochlear implants: National Institutes of Health Consensus Development Conference Statement, 1988;7:1–25.

68. Kruger J, Bach M. Simultaneous recording with 30 microelectrodes in monkey visual cortex. *Exp Brain Res* 1981;41:191–194.

69. Larson SA, Asher DL, Balkany TJ, Rucker NC. Histopathology of the auditory nerve and cochlear nucleus following intracochlear electrical stimulation. *Otolaryngol Clin North Am* 1983;16:233–248.

70. Leake PA, Snyder RL, Chambers PL, et al. Consequences of chronic electrical stimulation in an animal model of congenital profound hearing loss. Abstracts of the Twelfth Association for Research in Otolaryngology, 1989;268.

71. Leake PA, Kessler DK, Merzenich MM. Application and safety of cochlear prostheses. In: Agnew WF, McCreery DB, eds. *Neural prostheses: fundamental studies*. Englewood Cliffs, NJ: Prentice Hall, 1990;253–296.

72. Leake-Jones PA, Walsh SM, Merzenich MM. Cochlear pathology following chronic intracochlear electrical stimulation. *Ann Otol Rhinol Laryngol* 1981;90:6–8.

73. Lorente de Nó R. *The primary acoustic nuclei*. New York: Raven Press, 1981.

74. Lorente de Nó R. Anatomy of the eighth nerve: the central projections of the nerve endings of the inner ear. *Laryngoscope* 1933;43:1–38.

75. Lorente de Nó R. Anatomy of the eighth nerve. III. General plans of the structure of the primary cochlear nuclei. *Laryngoscope* 1933;43:327–351.

76. Loucks RB. Preliminary report of a technique for stimulation or destruction of tissues beneath the integument and the establishing of conditioned reactions with faradization of the cerebral cortex. *J Comp Psychol* 1933;16:439–444.

77. Loucks RB. The experimental delimitation of neural structures essential for learning; the attempt to condition striped muscle responses with faradization of the sigmoid gyri. *J Psychol* 1935–1936;1:5–44.

78. Lousteau RJ. Increased spiral ganglion cell survival in electrically stimulated, deafened guinea pig cochleae. *Laryngoscope* 1987;97:836–842.

79. Martuza RL, Eldridge R. Neurofibromatosis 2. *N Engl J Med* 1988;318:684–688.

80. Maslan M, Miller JM. Electrical stimulation of the guinea pig cochlea. *J Otolaryngol Head Neck Surg* 1987;96:349–361.

81. McCreery DB, Agnew WF. Changes in extracellular potassium and calcium concentration and neural activity during prolonged electrical stimulation of the cat cerebral cortex at defined charge densities. *Exp Neurol* 1983;79:371–396.

82. McCreery DB, Agnew WF. Mechanisms of stimulation-induced neural damage and their relation to guidelines for safe stimulation. In: Agnew WF, McCreery DB, eds. *Neural prostheses: fundamental studies*. Englewood Cliffs, NJ: Prentice Hall, 1990;297–317.

83. McCreery DB, Bullara LA, Agnew WF. Neuronal activity evoked by chronically implanted intracortical microelectrodes. *Exp Neurol* 1986;92:147–161.

84. McElveen JT, Hitselberger WE, House WF. Surgical accessibility of the cochlear nuclear complex in man: surgical landmarks. *Otolaryngol Head Neck Surg* 1987;96:135–140.

85. McElveen JT, Hitselberger WE, House WF, et

al. Electrical stimulation of cochlear nucleus in man. *Am J Otol* 1985;6:88–91.

86. Miller JM. Neural circuits and reaction time performance in monkeys. Doctoral degree of philosophy thesis. Department of Physiology, University of Washington, 1965.

87. Miller JM, Altschuler RA, Niparko JK, et al. Deafness-induced changes in the central nervous system and their reversibility and prevention. In: Salvi R, Henderson D, eds. *Effects of noise on the auditory system.* Toronto and Philadelphia: BC Decker (*submitted*).

88. Miller JM, Glickstein M. Reaction time to cortical stimulation. *Science* 1964;146:1594–1596.

89. Miller JM, Glickstein M. Neural circuits involved in visuomotor reaction time in monkeys. *J Neurophysiol* 1967;30:399–414.

90. Miller JM, Moody DB, Stebbins WC. Evoked potentials and auditory reaction time in monkeys. *Science* 1969;163:592–594.

91. Moore JK. Cochlear nuclei: relationship to the auditory nerve. In: Altschuler RA, Bobbin RP, Hoffman DW, eds. *Neurobiology of hearing: the cochlea.* New York: Raven Press, 1986; 283–302.

92. Moore JK, Osen KK. The cochlear nuclei in man. *Am J Anat* 1979;154:393–418.

93. Moore JK, Osen KK. The human cochlear nuclei. *Exp Brain Res* 1979(suppl II);36–44.

94. Niparko JK, Altschuler RA, Evans DA, et al. Auditory brain stem prosthesis: biocompatibility of stimulation. *Otolaryngol Head Neck Surg* 1989;101:344–352.

95. Niparko JK, Altschuler RA, Xue X, et al. Surgical implantation and biocompatibility of CNS auditory prosthesis. 17th Annual Meeting, Abst. Soc. Neurosci., New Orleans, LA, 1987; 543.

96. Niparko JK, Altschuler R, Xue X, et al. Surgical implantation and biocompatibility of CNS auditory prostheses. *Ann Otol Rhinol Laryngol* 1989;98:965–970.

97. Osen KK. Cytoarchitecture of the cochlear nuclei in the cat. *J Comp Neurol* 1969;136:453–484.

98. Osen KK. The intrinsic organization of the cochlear nuclei in the cat. *Acta Otolaryngol* 1969;67:352–359.

99. Palmer AR, Evans EF. Intensity coding in the auditory periphery of the cat: responses of cochlear nerve and cochlear nucleus neurones to signals in the presence of bandstop masking noise. *Hearing Res* 1982;7:305–323.

100. Pudenz RH, Agnew WF, Yuen TGH, Bullara LA. Electrical stimulation of brain. In: Hambrecht FT, Reswick JB, eds. *Functional electrical stimulation applications in neural prostheses.* New York: Marcel Dekker, 1977;437–458.

101. Ranck JB. Which elements are excited in electrical stimulation of mammalian central nervous system: a review. *Brain Res* 1975;98:417–440.

102. Rhode WS, Smith PH. Encoding timing and intensity in the ventral cochlear nucleus of the cat. *J Neurophysiol* 1986;56:261–286.

103. Rhode WS, Smith PH. Physiological studies on neurons in the dorsal cochlear nucleus of cat. *J Neurophysiol* 1986;56:287–307.

104. Robblee LS, McHardy J, Agnew WF, Bullara LA. Electrical stimulation with PT electrodes. VII. Dissolution of PT electrodes during electrical stimulation of the cat's cerebral cortex. *J Neurosci Methods* 1983;9:301–308.

105. Ronner SF. Electrical excitation of CNS neurons. In: Agnew WF, McCreery DB, eds. *Neural prostheses: fundamental studies.* Englewood Cliffs, NJ: Prentice Hall, 1990;169–196.

106. Shepherd RK, Murray MT, Houghten ME, Clark GM. Scanning electron microscopy of chronically stimulated platinum intracochlear electrodes. *Biomaterials* 1985;6:237–242.

107. Simmons FB, Mongeon CJ, Huntington DA. Electrical stimulation of acoustical nerve and inferior colliculus. *Arch Otolaryngol* 1964;79: 559–567.

108. Saburi M, Niki K, Kobayashi S, Aikawa S. A magnetically coupled multi-microelectrode system. *IEEE Trans Biomed Eng* 1983;BME-30:6.

109. Tennyson VM, Kremzner LT, Dauth GW, et al. Long-term surface stimulation of the cerebellum in the monkey. II. Electron microscopic and biochemical observations. *Surg Neurol* 1977;8:17–29.

110. Terr LI, Edgerton BJ. Surface topography of the cochlear nuclei in humans: two- and three-dimensional analysis. *Hearing Res* 1985;17:51–59.

111. Trune DR. Influence of neonatal cochlear removal on the development of mouse cochlear nucleus: I. Number, size and density of its neurons. *J Comp Neurol* 1982;209:409–424.

112. Van Buren JS, Wood JH, Oakley J, Hambrecht FT. Preliminary evaluation of cerebellar stimulation by double-blind stimulation and biological criteria in the treatment of epilepsy. *J Neurosurg* 1978;46:407–416.

113. van den Honert C, Stypulkowski PH. Physiological properties of the electrically stimulated auditory nerve. II. Single fiber recordings. *Hearing Res* 1984;14:225–243.

114. Walsh SM, Leake-Jones PA. Chronic electrical stimulation of auditory nerve in cat: physiological and histological results. *Hearing Res* 1982;7:281–304.

115. Webster DB. Auditory neuronal sizes after a unilateral conductive hearing loss. *Exp Neurol* 1983;79:130–140.

116. Webster M, Webster DB. Spiral ganglion neuron loss following organ of corti loss: a quantitative study. *Brain Res* 1981;212:17–20.

117. Young ED. Response characteristics of neurons of the cochlear nuclei. In: Berlin CI, ed. *Hearing science.* San Diego: College Hill Press, 1984;423–460.

118. Xue X. Acute and chronic behavior of stimulating electrodes. Ph.D. thesis, University of Michigan, 1990.

Neurobiology of Hearing: The
Central Auditory System, edited by
R. A. Altschuler et al.
Raven Press, Ltd., New York © 1991.

18

Development and Plasticity of the Ferret Auditory System

David R. Moore

University Laboratory of Physiology, Oxford OX1 3PT, United Kingdom

The selection of species for experimental studies of the neurobiology of hearing is based on many, often conflicting considerations. In addition to purely biological considerations, economic and clinical factors must be taken into account. In this chapter I discuss some of the experiences of our laboratory in the use of mature and perinatal ferrets for hearing research over the past 8 years. I then present a review of the recent experiments we have performed on the development and plasticity of the ferret auditory system. Our experiments have shown that the functional onset of hearing in the ferret begins at a very late age, around the end of the first postnatal month. Structural and functional susceptibility to manipulations of the ear and to environmental influences is, by measures of degeneration in at least some nuclei, lost at a very early stage of development, well before the onset of hearing. For other pathways, subserving binaural interaction, there is a longer lasting susceptibility to manipulations of the ear and the acoustic environment.

THE FERRET AS A MODEL FOR STUDIES OF HEARING

The Adult Ferret

The ferret (*Mustela putorius furo*) is a mustelid carnivore that has probably been domesticated for more than 2,000 years (15). Commercial ferret stocks are predominantly fitch (yellow-buff fur with black guard hair and patches of black or dark brown on the tail, limbs, and torso) or albino (nonpigmented iris, white hair). Although the albino is recessive to the pigmented wild phenotype (16), albinos are prevalent and these and other hypopigmented animals (e.g., "red-eyed" ferrets [49]) are often indiscriminantly interbred by commercial suppliers.

By superficial, morphologic criteria the auditory system of the ferret resembles that of the cat (43,51). However, the external ears are relatively small and immobile (51). As in other species, the ears contain a complex series of convolutions that impart a characteristic spectral transform to incident sound (6,7). The external auditory meatus is small in diameter and passes through a near right-angle bend about two-thirds of the distance from the tragus to the tympanic membrane. The middle ear is enclosed within an extremely hard and highly trabeculated temporal bone, through which the lateral half of each of the 3.5 turns of the cochlea is also accessible from a surgical window cut in the dorsocaudal aspect the bulla.

Hearing in ferrets has been tested by training them to make behavioral responses to remotely presented sounds (free-field

stimulation) within sound- and echo-atten-
uated rooms. The audiogram of the ferret
(Fig. 1) (25) is similar to that of other carnivores, with a frequency range (at 70 dB
SPL) of 0.02 to 45 kHz. Ferrets localize
transient sounds with considerable precision (around 10° for midline stimulus positions [22]). As in other species, sound localization in the lateral field is destroyed by
lesioning the contralateral auditory cortex
(AC) (22), although absolute sensitivity is
largely unaffected by the same lesion (23).
Physiological studies of the inferior colliculus (IC) (1,51), superior colliculus (SC)
(26,27), and AC (24) have demonstrated
that ferret auditory neurons have basically
the same response properties as those in
other, more extensively studied animals. In
the IC and AC neurons have secure,
sharply tuned responses to pure-tone stimulation, and each of these nuclei contains a
tonotopic representation. SC neurons are
less securely driven by acoustic stimuli, but
they do have spatially selective responses
and there is a topographic representation of

auditory space along both the rostrocaudal
(azimuth) and mediolateral (elevation) dimensions of the nucleus.

These observations have several implications for the use of adult ferrets in hearing research. Commercially, ferrets are
readily available and relatively inexpen-
sive. It is, however, highly desirable either
to establish a breeding colony or to obtain
animals from commercial suppliers who
maintain careful genetic records. Two studies have shown quantitative differences between hypopigmented and fitch ferrets in
auditory system morphology (2) and connectivity (49), and several lines of evidence
from the auditory (e.g., refs. 11,13) and visual (e.g., ref. 38) systems of cats carrying
albino genes emphasize the need for caution in interpreting sensory data from any
hypopigmented animals.

Anatomically, the ferret presents two major difficulties for hearing research. Because the ear canal contains a bend, it is not
possible to see the eardrum using conventional otoscopy. We use tympanometry as a

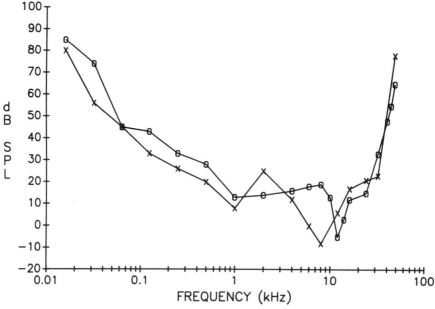

FIG. 1. Audiograms for two ferrets trained to make a behavioral response to presentation of pure-
tone stimuli in the free field. (From ref. 25, with permission.)

routine screening procedure for the outer and middle ear (18), and it may be possible to adopt surgical endoscopic techniques to redress this problem. The second difficulty is the extreme hardness of the ferret skull and, consequently, of the temporal bone. Rapid surgical exposure of the middle ear is difficult without the use of noisy drills. Thus, cochlear physiology becomes a major procedure requiring considerable patience and, in our laboratory, the use of small, hand-operated drills. The anatomy of the ferret central auditory system is much like that of the cat (23,43) and is a satisfactory model for cytological, immunohistochemical, and tracer studies.

Physiologically, ferrets have retained normal threshold levels and other response indices during long periods (up to 72 hr in our laboratory) of deep barbiturate anesthesia. One characteristic that distinguishes ferrets from cats is that in animals anesthetized to areflexia, the level of spontaneous activity in IC neurons and the proportion of neurons possessing spontaneous activity is higher in ferrets (51). This may be a reflection of the higher basal metabolic level of ferrets, since it is now well established that, at least in auditory brainstem neurons, depth of anesthesia is inversely related to the level of spontaneous activity (3,34). If this finding is confirmed at other levels of the brain, the ferret may become a preferred species for studies of the central auditory system because of the importance of inhibitory processes in auditory neural coding.

Behaviorally, the ferret appears to be an excellent species for hearing research. As might be expected from an animal with a highly gyrencephalic forebrain (37), it is easily trained and possesses certain attributes of hearing (e.g., in lateral field sound localization; [23]) that have more in common with humans and other primates than with rodents. Because of its relative cost-efficiency, the ferret may therefore be useful for studies of hearing disorders requiring a large number of animals possessing an auditory sense that is as close as possible to that of the human.

The Perinatal Ferret

The primary interest of the ferret to neurobiologists has been its immaturity at the time of birth. Ferrets are born following a 42 day gestation. They begin to "hear" some time between postnatal day (P) 27 and P32, the exact age being dependent on the response measure examined. I showed some years ago that the age at which startle responses to loud sounds could first be observed (P32) coincided well with the time of opening of the external auditory meatuses and the first evoked responses to intense tones by single neurons in the IC (42). Recently, a detailed, quantitative study of the development of the auditory brainstem response (ABR) in the ferret has been completed in our laboratory (52). Half of the ferrets examined produced an ABR to high-intensity, transient stimuli at P27, and all animals responded by P31. ABR thresholds decreased quickly from these ages, achieving adult levels by P40 (Fig. 2A). Response latency, measured at a constant suprathreshold level, matured by P35, for wave I of the response, and by around P40 for wave IV (Fig. 2B). Thus, by each of these measures, auditory function in the ferret begins late in life then matures rapidly.

Obvious advantages of the late onset of hearing in the ferret are the ability to observe relatively early events of normal development and to perform experimental manipulations of the ear without the need for difficult and inefficient *in utero* studies. For example, the cochlear nucleus (CN) of the neonatal ferret, although recognizable, differs qualitatively from that of the adult (Fig. 3). The major subdivisions of the CN are indistinct; the granule cell layer is contiguous with that of the cerebellum and the neurons are poorly differentiated. In contrast, the newborn cat CN, while differing quantitatively from that of the adult, is

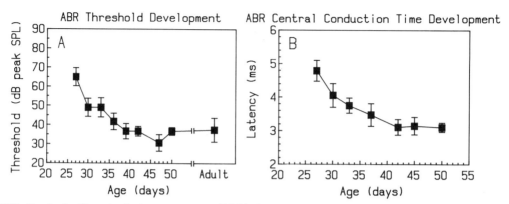

FIG. 2. A: Auditory brainstem response (ABR) threshold development. Each point is the mean (±s.d.) of at least six readings. **B:** ABR latency development for the same ferrets.

nevertheless relatively mature; CN subdivisions and individual neuron types are readily distinguishable by P2 (36).

Despite the immaturity of the ferret at the time of birth, relative to most other mammals, many significant developmental events have already taken place. We have recorded the spontaneous activity of IC neurons as early as P4 (42), suggesting that several aspects of cellular function are operative from soon after the time of birth, when the auditory system is still cytologically very immature (Fig. 3). Anterograde tracers horseradish peroxidase (HRP) and wheat germ agglutinin-HRP (WGA-HRP) injected into the cochlea on the day of birth label auditory nerve fibers that arborize throughout the rostrocaudal extent of the CN, including the dorsal CN (DCN) (*unpublished observations*). In this respect the newborn ferret may be more mature than some rodents (60). To study the early events in auditory system development, it may therefore still be necessary to perform *in utero* experiments. Alternatively, one can choose a species that permits greater freedom of access to the embryo (e.g., chicken [58]). The main advantage of the ferret from a developmental perspective is that it has a broader window for observation than most other animals, particularly those commonly used as models for the human auditory systems (cats, nonhuman primates).

PLASTICITY OF THE FERRET AUDITORY SYSTEM

Unilateral Cochlear Removal

It is now more than 40 years since Levi-Montalcini (39) published her classic paper describing the effects of early extirpation of the otocyst on the development of neurons in the chicken CN. That research has led to a number of important findings in the chicken (58), but studies of the effects of primary deafferentation on the mammalian auditory system had been rather uncommon until the 1980s. Powell and Erulkar (56) showed neuron shrinkage in the CN and superior olivary complex (SOC) following cochlear removal in adult cats. However, it was not until Trune's study (62) that the developmental aspects of this issue were first addressed. His results were dramatic; cochlear removal in P6 mice reduced neuron numbers throughout the CN by 66%. In the gerbil, cochlear ablation at P0–P1 also produced changes in the laterality of connections between the CN and the IC (29,47,53) and an increased excitatory influence of stimulation of the intact ear on neurons in the IC on that side (Fig. 4) (28,30). Cochlear removal in adult animals did not produce these changes.

The first indication of dissension in the apparently simple age-relationship between cochlear removal and CN degeneration was

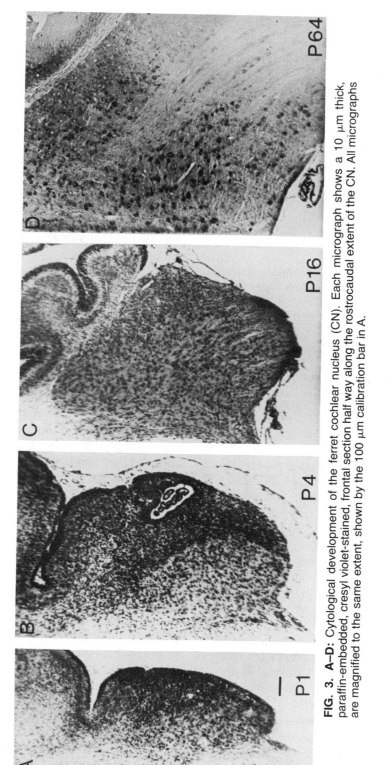

FIG. 3. A–D: Cytological development of the ferret cochlear nucleus (CN). Each micrograph shows a 10 µm thick, paraffin-embedded, cresyl violet-stained, frontal section half way along the rostrocaudal extent of the CN. All micrographs are magnified to the same extent, shown by the 100 µm calibration bar in A.

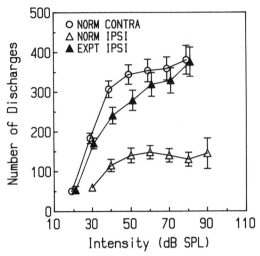

FIG. 4. Physiological effect of neonatal removal of one cochlea on the response of gerbil inferior colliculus (IC) neurons to stimulation of the intact ear. Each point is the mean (±s.d.) discharge level of 10 to 102 single neurons stimulated with best frequency pure tones. NORM CONTRA and NORM IPSI refer to control data from normal, adult animals. EXPT IPSI are data from the neonatally operated animals. (From ref. 30, with permission.)

reported by Reale et al. (57). They presented anecdotal evidence that neonatal cochlear removal in the cat did not lead to any dramatic cell loss in the deafferented CN. This result was confusing. All the previous work on rodents had documented substantial or total CN cell loss. One possible reason for the different result was that the cat is more mature at the time of birth than are most rodent species; auditory function in the cat begins in the first postnatal week (14). However, cochlear removal in the chicken, a relatively precocial animal, produced the same result at 6 weeks post-hatch (i.e., more than 7 weeks after the onset of auditory function) as at any earlier age (4). So if the relationship was with relative age, it was not a simple one.

We believe that we have provided a partial resolution to this issue through studies of cochlear removal in the ferret (Fig. 5) (44). Removal at P5 produced a massive (>50%) loss of neurons in the CN. Delaying

the removal by less than 3 weeks, to P24, completely abolished this degenerative response. Since P24 is still almost a week before the onset of hearing in the ferret, it might not seem surprising that Reale et al. (57) failed to find CN cell loss in their cats. This still leaves the problem of explaining the difference between mammals and birds. Although this may be related to different innervation patterns in the CN, it may also be related to other developmental regulatory processes (e.g., hormones). It is possible that a solution to this problem will also address the fundamental question of which mechanisms underlie developmental sensitive periods.

An important consequence of neonatal cochlear removal in gerbils is the rewiring that takes place in the auditory brainstem (29), resulting in changes in the physiology of the IC (Fig. 4). What is not known from the gerbil work is the time course over which this rewiring can take place. To address this and other issues, we developed the CN-IC pathway (Fig. 6A) as a model system for studies of peripherally induced changes of binaural connections in the brain. Through a series of experiments on normal, adult ferrets it was shown that the symmetry of the number of neurons in each CN that were retrogradely labeled following an injection of WGA-HRP into one IC could, under appropriately controlled conditions, be reliably reproduced from one animal to the next (43). The resulting "laterality index" (Fig. 6B) was then compared in groups of ferrets that had received unilateral cochlear removals at various postnatal ages. Laterality indices following removals at P14, P24, or P40 all differed significantly from those following removals at P90 and from normal animals (Fig. 6B) (50). These results confirmed and extended the earlier gerbil work of Nordeen et al. (53) by showing that neonatal removals also produced changes in the CN-IC pathway of ferrets and that the changes were limited to a developmental sensitive period that finished between P40 and P90. It should be noted

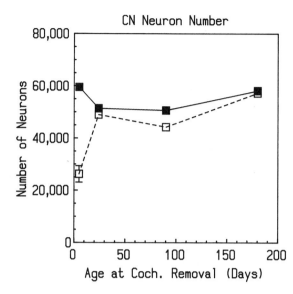

FIG. 5. Effect of right cochlear removal in the ferret on cochlear nucleus (CN) neuron number. Each point is the count for a single animal, except for the right side (*unfilled squares*) of the P5 group, which is the mean (±2 s.d.) of three animals. All animals survived for at least three months following the cochlear removal. (From ref. 44, with permission.)

that, in contrast to the work previously described on CN neuron loss, the sensitive period for the CN-IC pathway extended well beyond the time of the onset of hearing. This misalignment of the two sensitive periods shows that the degeneration of the CN is not a necessary condition for the formation of the altered CN-IC connections. The results also suggest that auditory experience may be important for the formation or consolidation of the CN-IC pathway.

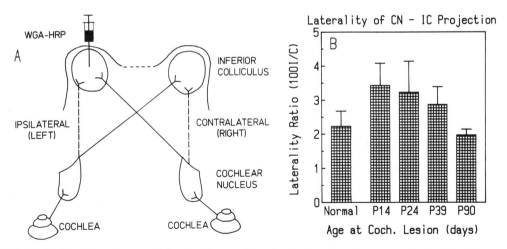

FIG. 6. A: Model system used for studying auditory brainstem development and plasticity. The retrograde tracer wheat germ agglutinin-horseradish peroxidase (WGA-HRP) was injected into the left inferior colliculus (IC). Labeled neurons were counted in each cochlear nucleus (CN). Note that the right side was used for cochlear removals and earplugs. **B:** Effect of right cochlear removal in the ferret on the laterality ratio of the number of neurons labeled in the left (ipsilateral) and right (contralateral) CN following injections of HRP in the left IC (see inset). Each histogram bar is the mean (+ s.d.) of at least four animals. All animals survived for three months following the cochlear removal.

Auditory Experience

A large body of literature now suggests that experience plays an important role in the formation of auditory system cytology (40,63,65), neuron morphology (9,10,17), physiology (8,27,31,32,46,59,61), and in sound localization (33). Unfortunately, much of this literature is of questionable validity, since in many cases it was not clear that the means used to alter auditory experience, typically some form of unilateral occlusion of the ear canal, did not also damage the cochlea. Indeed, some studies have suggested that unilateral attenuation of acoustic input may not alter central auditory system cytology (64) or physiology (5), at least by the indices examined.

To investigate the role of auditory experience in the development of the ferret brainstem, we have reared animals with a unilateral earplug producing a hearing loss of up to 60 dB. These animals were studied both anatomically and physiologically (27, 45). For several, admittedly indirect, reasons we believe that the earplugs in these

ferrets produced only a conductive hearing loss. First, in some cases, the physiological thresholds of neurons in the IC contralateral to the ear that was plugged during rearing achieved normal levels following removal of the plug and stimulation of that ear. The other results obtained from these animals did not differ from those animals in which a residual threshold elevation was observed. Second, most SC neurons had, at all stimulus levels, normal directional tuning when the earplug was in place (27), (Fig. 8A), indicating that the plugged ear was physiological to the extent that it was capable of contributing to the formation of spatial receptive fields. Third, there was no evidence of cochlear pathology in the plugged ears and, in 10 of 12 cases, there was no sign of middle ear pathology.

We found that a reduction in the level of airborne sound reaching the ear during rearing does not lead to reductions in the volume of the CN on the side of the plug (Fig. 7A) or to reductions in either the size or number of individual neurons in the CN (45). These results support the finding of

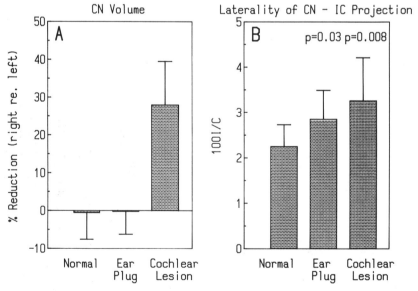

FIG. 7. Effect of rearing (from P24) ferrets with a unilateral plug of the right ear on: **A,** the reduction in volume of the right relative to the left cochlear nucleus (CN) and **B,** the laterality ratio of ferret CN neurons (see inset and legend to Fig. 6). All bars show the mean (+s.d.) of at least nine ferrets. In both A and B the lesion group shows the results of a unilateral cochlear lesion at the same age. (From ref. 45, with permission.)

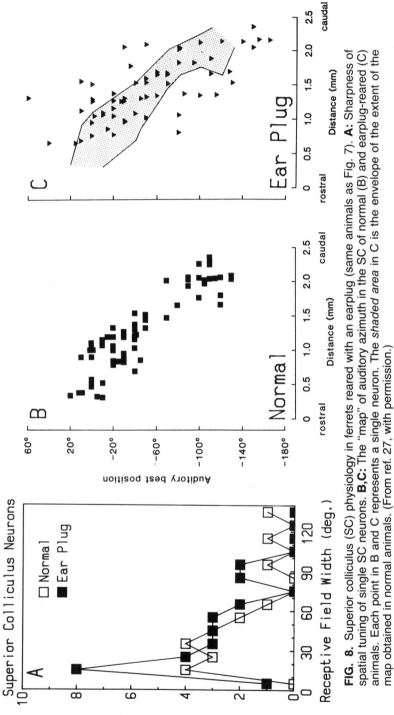

FIG. 8. Superior colliculus (SC) physiology in ferrets reared with an earplug (same animals as Fig. 7). **A:** Sharpness of spatial tuning of single SC neurons. **B,C:** The "map" of auditory azimuth in the SC of normal (B) and earplug-reared (C) animals. Each point in B and C represents a single neuron. The shaded area in C is the envelope of the extent of the map obtained in normal animals. (From ref. 27, with permission.)

Tucci and Rubel (64) that a conductive hearing loss in the hatchling chicken does not result in obvious degenerative changes in the CN. On the other hand, we did find that ear plugging in the ferret led to a change in the symmetry of the CN-IC pathway (Fig. 7B). Thus, acoustic experience can influence the formation or consolidation of connections in the auditory brainstem.

In the SC, ferrets reared and tested with a unilateral earplug showed two major differences from what would be expected to result from the placement of a plug in one ear of a normal adult ferret at the time of testing. First, as outlined above, individual neurons maintained a sharpness of spatial tuning that was in the normal range (Fig. 8A). Plugging one ear at the time of testing in normal animals profoundly disrupts spatial tuning of SC neurons (41,54). So the auditory system of the plug-reared ferrets had adjusted to compensate for the altered binaural cues experienced during the first few months of life. Second, the "map" of auditory space in the SC (26) (Fig. 8B) was preserved in these animals (Fig. 8C). With the plug inserted, the relation between recording position of a neuron in the SC and the location of that neuron's receptive field best position was also roughly normal. With the plug removed, and binaural cues shifted back toward normal values, the neuron best positions moved away from the previously plugged ear by up to 30°. The compensation to altered binaural cues that had occurred during development was thus a systematic one. As in the barn owl optic tectum (31), the representation of auditory space in the ferret SC adjusted to distorted cues to maintain a correct topographic relation both to the surface of the nucleus and to the well-known representation of visual space across that surface.

Relation to Normal Development

One of our goals in recent work has been to establish how the effects of auditory deafferentation and deprivation are related to the normal, postnatal development of the auditory brainstem in the ferret. Clearly, since experience is influential, developmental changes that extend beyond the age at which auditory function begins need to be identified. Since the anatomy of the CN-IC pathway was used to study many of the effects of manipulations of the auditory periphery, we began to address the normal developmental issue by retrograde labeling of CN neurons from injections of WGA-HRP in the IC (48). One of the general difficulties of performing quantitative anatomical studies across animals of different ages is that biological changes may be confounded by changes in the efficacy of the technique. In an attempt to overcome this problem, we again chose the symmetry of the number of CN neurons labeled on each side rather than the absolute number as our primary measure. The variability of the laterality indices obtained for animals of P26 or older was comparable with the adult level (Fig. 9A), suggesting that the index was a robust measure with which different age groups could be compared. In a younger group of ferrets (P18) the variability was much larger, excluding those animals from statistical comparison. Nevertheless, the mean laterality index was consistent with the pattern that emerged when older ferrets were examined.

The mean laterality index obtained for P26 ferrets was significantly larger than that obtained for P39 or adult animals, whereas the latter groups did not differ from one another (Fig. 9A). These results have two points in common with the effects of ear manipulations. First, the extent by which the laterality index in the P26 animals exceeded the adult index was around 50%; about the same increase as that obtained following cochlear removal at P24. Second, the increase in the laterality index was, in both cases, entirely attributable to an increase in the number of neurons retrogradely labeled in the CN on the same side as the tracer injection. These similarities suggest that, as in other neural systems

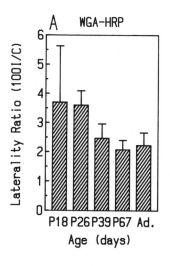

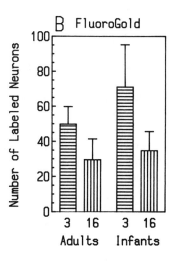

FIG. 9. Normal development of projections from the cochlear nucleus (CN) to the inferior colliculus (IC) in the ferret. **A:** Laterality ratios (see Fig. 6) derived from injections of HRP at the ages indicated. Ad, adult. **B:** Number of left CN neurons retrogradely labeled following an injection of FluoroGold in the left IC at the age and for the survival times indicated.

(12,35), the plasticity observed in the ferret auditory brainstem may be the result of a failure of regressive events that occur in normal development. However, the data obtained from normal P39 animals were adult-like (Fig. 9A), whereas cochlear removals performed at P39 still resulted in a significant increase in the CN-IC laterality index (Fig. 6). Moreover, for animals in which the cochlear removal was performed at a younger age (P24), changes in the laterality of the CN-IC projection did not begin to take place until over 11 days after the removal and continued to occur for more than 30 days (50). Thus, for this pathway, the sensitive period for the effect of cochlear removal exceeded the time course over which developmental changes normally occurred.

Despite the failure of the developmental change in the CN-IC pathway to explain the effects of cochlear removal, it is interesting to pursue the mechanisms by which the normal decrease in the ipsilateral CN-IC projection does take place. In other systems, neuron death and process (axon, synapse) elimination are two mechanisms that have been widely identified and studied (12). We have performed an experiment, based on similar studies of the rodent retinotectal system (20,21), to determine whether neuron death is involved. Fluoro-Gold (FG), a cytologically persistent retro-

grade fluorescent tracer, was injected into the IC of P26 and adult ferrets. Half of the animals in each group were perfused 3 days and half 16 days after the injection. For the short survival cases, the results were consistent with those obtained with WGA-HRP (Fig. 9B); significantly more neurons were labeled in the CN ipsilateral to the injected IC in the P26 than in the adult group. For the long survival cases, P26 and adult injected animals had the same number of labeled CN neurons. Thus, for the group injected at P26, survival through the period P26 to P39, during which the number of labeled neurons in the ipsilateral CN-IC pathway was shown above to decrease, revealed that the decrease was due to a loss of neurons.

The interpretation of this result is that CN neuron death during the period between P26 and P39 can account for all of the previously observed decrease of labeled neurons over the same period. If axon retraction had occurred, the number of labeled neurons observed in the CN following injection of FG at P26 and survival for 16 days would still have exceeded that seen in the equivalent adult group, since the larger number of neurons that had incorporated the FG at P26 would still be present to be counted following the long survival; in the event they were not, having died during the long survival time. The long survival, adult group formed an essential control to check the possibility that the labeled neurons did not die because of the presence of the label, or that the label did not leach out of the CN neuron bodies. In fact, the number of labeled neurons following long survival in the adult group was somewhat lower than following short survival, suggesting that one or both of these processes did occur. However, the finding that the P26 long survival group reduced to the same level as the adult long survival group shows that developmentally associated neuron death also occurred.

The suggestion that neuron death may be the process underlying the reduction in the size of the developing ferret ipsilateral CN-IC pathway is not novel, since "naturally occurring neuronal death" may be a ubiquitous feature of brain development (12). There is, however, another aspect of these results that is surprising. Over the period during which the ipsilaterally projecting CN neurons were dying, there was no decrease in the number of contralaterally projecting neurons (48). It would therefore appear that neuron death in this nucleus does not occur *en masse* but at different rates or times depending on the destination of the axons. To establish how the neurons that project to the IC relate to neuron death in the whole CN, we performed a final experiment in which we counted neurons in Nissl-stained sections through the normal, neonatal ferret CN. In the normal, adult ferret the CN contains about 50,000 large (i.e., nongranular) neurons (44). Of these, about 20% project to the contralateral IC and about 0.4% to the ipsilateral IC (49). Preliminary results from two ferrets examined at P26 and from one ferret examined at P32 suggest that the total CN neuron population does not decrease between these ages and that by P26 the number of neurons is roughly adult-like. It would therefore seem that the very small proportion of CN neurons that project to the ipsilateral IC are exceptional in dying as late during development as they do.

CONCLUDING REMARKS

The evidence that sensorineural or conductive hearing loss in early infancy can produce permanent changes in the structure and function of the brain is now overwhelming. In this chapter I have shown that, in the ferret, some of these changes are dependent on or show increased sensitivity to hearing loss that is started only at a very early stage of development. Other changes may occur following later onset hearing loss. Most but not all of the changes are occurring at a time when the brain is normally undergoing developmental alterations of neuron number and size.

Although the mechanisms underlying these changes are presently unknown, evidence from the chicken (19) and gerbil (55) auditory systems suggests that presynaptic activity in the cochlear nerve is necessary for the maintenance of at least CN neurons in the early neonatal period. In the ferret, we have hypothesized that a competition between the ears takes place for synaptic space on binaurally innervated neurons in the auditory brainstem (45). This competition may be sensitive to the level as well as the presence of activity in the cochlear nerves. Through a combination of these processes the brain is adapted to the input provided by the ear and by the acoustic environment in which the animal lives.

I hope that the experiments described in this chapter have also shown the usefulness of the ferret for studies of development and plasticity of the auditory system. Although the adult animal does present some problems, particularly for cochlear physiology, we have now obtained several results that would not have been possible without *in utero* surgery in other carnivores or in primates. We have shown that in certain fundamental respects the ferret auditory system and, in particular, its response to cochlear removal differ at least quantitatively from that of the chicken. Our intention over the next few years is to concentrate on the development and plasticity of auditory function, using longitudinal studies of the ABR and behavioral testing following various forms of hearing loss in infancy. For these purposes the ferret would seem to combine several desirable characteristics.

ACKNOWLEDGMENTS

The research described in this chapter is the result of contributions from many individuals. I especially wish to thank, in alphabetical order, Simon Carlile, Pat Cordery, Mary Hutchings, Andy King, Nancy Kowalchuk, Kathy Laman, and Adrienne Morey. Gunther Rose, in a seminar in this laboratory in 1980, originally drew my attention to the potential of the ferret for developmental auditory research. The work described here has been funded by grants from the Medical Research Council, The Lister Institute, The Royal Society, the University of Oxford Research and Equipment Committee, and the E. P. Abraham Research Fund.

REFERENCES

1. Addison PD. Coding for auditory localization in the midbrain of the ferret. Ph.D. thesis, University of Oxford, 1984.
2. Baker GE, Guillery RW. Evidence for the delayed expression of a brainstem abnormality in albino ferrets. *Exp Brain Res* 1989;74:658–662.
3. Bock GR, Webster WR, Aitkin LM. Discharge patterns in single units in inferior colliculus of alert cats. *J Neurophysiol* 1972;35:265–277.
4. Born DE, Rubel EW. Afferent influences on brain stem auditory nuclei of the chicken: neuron number and size following cochlea removal. *J Comp Neurol* 1985;231:435–445.
5. Brugge JF, Orman SS, Coleman JR, Chan JCK, Phillips DP. Binaural interactions in cortical area AI of cats reared with unilateral atresia of the external ear canal. *Hear Res* 1985;20:275–287.
6. Carlile S. The auditory periphery of the ferret. I. Directional response properties and the pattern of interaural level differences. *J Acoust Soc Am* 1990;88:2196–2204.
7. Carlile S. The auditory periphery of the ferret. II. The spectral transformations of the external ear and their implications for sound localization. *J Acoust Soc Am* 1990;88;2180–2195.
8. Clopton BM, Silverman MS. Plasticity of binaural interaction. II. Critical period and changes in midline response. *J Neurophysiol* 1977; 40:1275–1280.
9. Conlee JW, Parks TN. Age- and position-dependent effects of monaural acoustic deprivation in nucleus magnocellularis of the chicken. *J Comp Neurol* 1981;202:373–384.
10. Conlee JW, Parks TN. Late appearance and deprivation-sensitive growth of permanent dendrites in the avian cochlear nucleus (Nuc. magnocellularis). *J Comp Neurol* 1983;217:216–226.
11. Conlee JW, Parks TN, Romero C, Creel DJ. Auditory brainstem anomalies in albino cats. II. Neuronal atrophy in the superior olive. *J Comp Neurol* 1984;225:141–148.
12. Cowan WM, Fawcett JW, O'Leary DDM, Stanfield BB. Regressive events in neurogenesis. *Science* 1984;225:1258–1265.
13. Creel DJ, Conlee JW, Parks TN. Auditory brainstem anomalies in albino cats. I. Evoked potential studies. *Brain Res* 1983;260:1–9.
14. Foss I, Flottorp G. A comparative study of the development of hearing and vision in various species commonly used in experiments. *Acta Otolaryngol (Stockh)* 1974;77:202–214.
15. Fox JG. Taxonomy, history, and use. In: Fox JG, ed. *Biology and diseases of the ferret.* Philadelphia: Lea and Febiger, 1988;3–13.
16. Fox JG. Reproduction, breeding and growth. In: Fox JG, ed. *Biology and diseases of the ferret.* Philadelphia: Lea and Febiger, 1988;174–183.
17. Gray L, Smith Z, Rubel EW. Developmental and experiential changes in dendritic symmetry in n. laminaris of the chick. *Brain Res* 1982;244:360–364.
18. Hutchings ME. The gerbil as an animal model of otitis media with effusion. *J. Physiol (Lond)* 1987;396:175P.
19. Hyson RL, Rubel EW. Transneuronal regulation of protein synthesis in the brain stem auditory system of the chick requires synaptic activation. *J Neurosci* 1989;9:2835–2845.
20. Insausti R, Blakemore C, Cowan WM. Ganglion cell death during development of ipsilateral retino-collicular projection in golden hamster. *Nature* 1984;308:362–365.
21. Jeffery G, Perry VH. Evidence for ganglion cell death during development of the ipsilateral retinal projection in the rat. *Dev Brain Res* 1982; 2:176–180.
22. Kavanagh GL, Kelly JB. Contribution of auditory cortex to sound localization by the ferret *(Mustela putorius). J Neurophysiol.* 1987;57: 1746–1766.
23. Kavanagh GL, Kelly JB. Hearing in the ferret *(Mustela putorius):* effects of primary auditory cortical lesions on thresholds for pure tone detection. *J Neurophysiol* 1988;60:879–888.
24. Kelly JB, Judge PW, Phillips DP. Representation of the cochlea in primary auditory cortex of the ferret *(Mustela putorius). Hear Res* 1986;24: 111–115.

25. Kelly JB, Kavanagh GL, Dalton JCH. Hearing in the ferret *(Mustela putorius):* thresholds for pure tone detection. *Hear Res* 1986;24:269–275.

26. King AJ, Hutchings ME. Spatial response properties of acoustically responsive neurons in the superior colliculus of the ferret: a map of auditory space. *J Neurophysiol* 1987;57:596–624.

27. King AJ, Hutchings ME, Moore DR, Blakemore C. Developmental plasticity in the visual and auditory representations in the mammalian superior colliculus. *Nature* 1988;332:73–76.

28. Kitzes LM. Some physiological consequences of neonatal cochlear destruction in the inferior colliculus of the gerbil. *Brain Res* 1984;306:171–178.

29. Kitzes LM. The role of binaural innervation in the development of the auditory brainstem. In: Ruben RJ, Van De Water TN, Rubel EW, eds. *Biology of change in otolaryngology.* Amsterdam: Elsevier, 1986.

30. Kitzes LM, Semple MN. Single unit responses in the inferior colliculus: effects of neonatal unilateral cochlear ablation. *J Neurophysiol* 1985; 53:1483–1500.

31. Knudsen EI. Experience alters the spatial tuning of auditory units in the optic tectum during a sensitive period in the barn owl. *J Neurosci* 1985;5:3094–3109.

32. Knudsen EI. Early blindness results in a degraded auditory map of space in the optic tectum of the barn owl. *Proc Natl Acad Sci USA* 1988;85:6211–6214.

33. Knudsen EI, Esterly SD, Knudsen PF. Monaural occlusion alters sound localization during a sensitive period in the barn owl. *J Neurosci* 1984;4:1001–1011.

34. Kuwada S, Batra R, Stanford TR. Monaural and binaural response properties of neurons in the inferior colliculus of the rabbit: effects of sodium pentobarbital. *J Neurophysiol* 1989;61: 269–282.

35. Land PW, Lund RD. Development of the rats uncrossed retinotectal pathway and its relation to plasticity studies. *Science* 1979;205:698–700.

36. Larsen SA. Postnatal maturation of the cochlear nucleus complex. *Acta Otolaryngol Suppl (Stockh)* 1984;417.

37. Lawes INC, Andrews PLR. The neuroanatomy of the ferret brain. In: Fox JG, ed. *Biology and diseases of the ferret.* Philadelphia: Lea and Febiger, 1988;66–99.

38. Leventhal AG, Vitek DJ, Creel DJ. Abnormal visual pathways in normally pigmented cats that are heterozygous for albinism. *Science* 1985; 229:1395–1397.

39. Levi-Montalcini R. Development of the acoustico-vestibular centers in the chick embryo in the absence of the afferent root fibers and of descending fiber tracts. *J Comp Neurol* 1949; 91:209–242.

40. McGinn MD, Faddis BT. Auditory experience affects degeneration of the ventral cochlear nucleus in mongolian gerbils. *Hear Res* 1987; 31:235–244.

41. Middlebrooks JC. Binaural mechanisms of spatial tuning in the cat's superior colliculus distinguished using monaural occlusion. *J Neurophysiol* 1987;57:688–701.

42. Moore DR. Late onset of hearing in the ferret. *Brain Res* 1982;253:309–311.

43. Moore DR. Auditory brainstem of the ferret: sources of projections to the inferior colliculus. *J Comp Neurol* 1988;269:342–354.

44. Moore DR. Auditory brainstem of the ferret: early cessation of developmental sensitivity to cochlear removal in the cochlear nucleus. *J Comp Neurol* 1990;302:810–823.

45. Moore DR, Hutchings ME, King AJ, Kowalchuk NE. Auditory brainstem of the ferret: some effects of rearing with a unilateral ear plug on the cochlea, cochlear nucleus, and projections to the inferior colliculus. *J Neurosci* 1989;9:1213–1222.

46. Moore DR, Irvine DRF. Plasticity of binaural interaction in the cat inferior colliculus. *Brain Res* 1981;208:198–202.

47. Moore DR, Kitzes LM. Projections from the cochlear nucleus to the inferior colliculus in normal and neonatally cochlea-ablated gerbils. *J Comp Neurol* 1985;240:180–195.

48. Moore DR, Kowalchuk NE. Development of crossed and uncrossed projections from the cochlear nucleus to the inferior colliculus in the ferret. *Soc Neurosci Abstr* 1987;13:80.

49. Moore DR, Kowalchuk NE. An anomaly in the auditory brain stem projections of hypopigmented ferrets. *Hear Res* 1988;35:275–278.

50. Moore DR, Kowalchuk NE. Auditory brainstem of the ferret: effects of unilateral cochlear lesions on cochlear nucleus volume and projections to the inferior colliculus. *J Comp Neurol* 1988;272:503–515.

51. Moore DR, Semple MN, Addison PD. Some acoustic properties of neurons in the ferret inferior colliculus. *Brain Res* 1983;269:69–82.

52. Morey AL, Carlile S. Auditory brainstem of the ferret: maturation of the brainstem auditory evoked response. *Dev Brain Res* 1990;52:279–288.

53. Nordeen KW, Killackey HP, Kitzes LM. Ascending projections to the inferior colliculus following unilateral cochlear ablation in the neonatal gerbil, Meriones unguiculatus. *J Comp Neurol* 1983;214:144–153.

54. Palmer AR, King AJ. A monaural space map in the guinea-pig superior colliculus. *Hear Res* 1985;17:267–280.

55. Pasic TR, Rubel EW. Rapid changes in cochlear nucleus cell size following blockade of auditory nerve electrical activity in gerbils. *J Comp Neurol* 1989;283:474–480.

56. Powell TPS, Erulkar SD. Transneuronal cell degeneration in the auditory relay nuclei of the cat. *J Anat* 1962;96:249–268.

57. Reale RA, Brugge JF, Chan JCK. Maps of auditory cortex in cats after unilateral cochlear ablation in the neonatal period. *Dev Brain Res* 1987;34:281–290.

58. Rubel EW, Parks TN. Organization and development of the avian brain-stem auditory system.

In: Edelman GM, Gall WE, Cowan WM, eds. *Auditory function.* New York: Wiley, 1988;3–92.

59. Sanes DH, Constantine-Paton M. The sharpening of frequency tuning curves requires patterned activity during development in the mouse, *Mus musculus. J Neurosci* 1985;5:1152–1166.

60. Schweitzer L, Cant NB. Development of the cochlear innervation of the dorsal cochlear nucleus of the hamster. *J Comp Neurol* 1984;225:228–243.

61. Silverman MS, Clopton BM. Plasticity of binaural interaction. I. Effect of early auditory deprivation. *J Neurophysiol* 1977;40:1266–1274.

62. Trune DR. Influence of neonatal cochlear removal on the development of the mouse cochlear nucleus. I. Number, size and density of its neurons. *J Comp Neurol* 1982;209:409–424.

63. Trune DR, Morgan CR. Stimulation-dependent development of neuronal cytoplasm in mouse cochlear nucleus. *Hear Res* 1988;33:141–150.

64. Tucci DL, Rubel EW. Afferent influences on brain stem auditory nuclei of the chicken: effects of conductive and sensorineural hearing loss on n. magnocellularis. *J Comp Neurol* 1985;238:371–381.

65. Webster DB. Conductive hearing loss affects the growth of the cochlear nuclei over an extended period of time. *Hear Res* 1988;32:185–192.

Subject Index